DATE DUE

OCT 1 2 1994	APR 2 9 1999
NOV - 2 1994	NOV - 4 1999
NOV 2 4 1994	DEC 1 5 1999
	MAR 1 7 2000
MAR 2 1 1995	
Apr. 03/95	DEC 1 2
APR 2 0 1995	
NOV - 6 1995	
FEB 2 2 1996	
SEP 3 0 1996	
OCT - 9 1996 OCT 2 4 1996	
NOV 1 2 19	
FEB 2 7 1997	
NOV 1 2 1997	
Nov 26	
NOV 2 4 1998	

BRODART   Cat. No. 23-221

EXPERIENCES OF SCHIZOPHRENIA

EXPERIENCES OF SCHIZOPHRENIA

An Integration of the Personal,
Scientific, and Therapeutic

Michael Robbins, M.D.

THE GUILFORD PRESS
New York   London

Last digit is print number: 9 8 7 6 5 4 3 2 1

Library of Congress Cataloging-in-Publication Data

Robbins, Michael, M.D.
    Experiences of schizophrenia : an interpretation of the personal,
scientific, and therapeutic / by Michael Robbins.
        p.   cm.
    Includes bibliographical references and index.
    ISBN 0-89862-997-7
    1. Schizophrenia.   2. Schizophrenia—Treatment—Case studies.
I. Title.
    [DNLM: 1. Schizophrenia—therapy.   WM 203 R635e]
RC514.R55   1993
616.89'8206—dc20
DNLM/DLC
for Library of Congress   92-48311
                                                              CIP

*In memory of Elvin Semrad, who taught me
how to sit with schizophrenic patients and bear
the thoughts and feelings their predicament
evokes in me, so that I in turn might be able to
help them learn how to bear the unbearable.*

*To my patients, who taught me much of what I
know about schizophrenia.*

*And to the McLean Hospital of yesteryear,
which sometimes supported treatments such as
those I describe in this book, particularly to
those staff who helped to create the holding
environment without which the crucial early
stages of these treatments could not have taken
place, often resisting destructive pressure and
hostility from my patients, members of their
families, hospital administration, and other
staff—and in some instances, I regret to say,
from myself as well—in order to do so.*

Acknowledgments

I gratefully acknowledge the critical readings of earlier drafts of the manuscript and valuable suggestions made by Sheldon Roth, MD, and Paul E. Stepansky, PhD. John E. Gedo, MD, has not read the manuscript and therefore is in no way accountable for any flaws it may contain, but his concept of multiple hierarchical models of the mind and his openness to the possibility of an expanded yet intellectually rigorous psychoanalytic theory has served as an intellectual inspiration in my efforts to go beyond my clinical work and speculate about meanings, causes and theories. I would like to express my appreciation to the staff of the McLean Hospital library, particularly Deborah Pennino and Lyn Dietrich, for their patient and cheerful assistance in locating reference material, and my thanks to my editor, Kitty Moore, for her valuable suggestions and encouragement.

Preface

These brief remarks are intended for the prospective reader who would like a taste of what the book is about and why I undertook to write it.

My career as a psychoanalyst has been somewhat atypical insofar as I have spent a substantial portion of it in hospital psychiatry: in administrative, therapeutic, and teaching capacities. This was not so curious a choice when I embarked upon my career some three decades ago—at what turned out to be the end of the era in which schizophrenia was considered to be a psychological illness, and romanticized and inflated claims were made that psychoanalysis could cure it—as it is now, at a time when schizophrenia is generally considered to be an organic illness, and is treated with brief hospitalization, psychotropic medication, and supportive and rehabilitative measures. Nowadays dynamic psychotherapy is not taught or practiced at all in many reputable mental hospitals and medical schools. Surprising as it may seem to some who are steeped in the lore of the current moment, I have been fortunate enough to experience some success in treating selected schizophrenic patients utilizing a primary psychological focus. While I understand that all human thought and behavior, normal and pathological, has an organic substrate which it is necessary to comprehend as thoroughly as possible, I have come to view schizophrenic thinking, feeling, and behavior not as a meaningless epiphenomenon entirely reducible to organic pathology, but as a meaningful expression of the human personality.

Some years ago I became aware that scientific and popular comprehension of schizophrenia was changing so radically that what I was doing and what I had learned had become a kind of endangered species. Few people in positions of authority any longer know that such an approach is even possible to say nothing of whether it might be preferable in some instances. Many have come to look upon psychological forms of treatment as poor medical practice if not a form of witchcraft, and few if any hospital facilities still exist where such work might be done. So I decided to attempt to codify my experience, utilizing extensive case material. In so doing I embarked on a path which led to some unexpected changes in my own attitudes and beliefs, and to a book which is very different from the one I initially envisioned.

As the book unfolded I realized that the social-scientific trend in post–World War II psychiatry that had motivated me to write it, away from an exclusively psychological approach and toward an equally exclusive organic one, was part of a greater cyclical fluctuation of viewpoints which have historical antecedents. I came to believe that this cyclical fluctuation is the product of a flawed kind of scientific thinking which philosophers call monism. I became aware that, while in some respects I had been caught up in monistic thinking, in others I had not. For example, though a substantial portion of my career has involved efforts to ascertain which schizophrenic persons might benefit from psychologically focused treatment and to provide it, I have always believed that such treatment is not the only valid way to approach schizophrenia, and that the success of my own efforts was critically linked to the contributions of neuroscience, interpersonal and social psychology, sociology, and cultural anthropology. From such thinking it was but a small step to realize that it is both possible to account for the phenomenology of schizophrenia within the language and operations of each of the human sciences, and essential if one is to have anything approaching a comprehensive view of the illness. An exclusive and myopic preoccupation with any single human science leaves the clinican and the theoretician in the position of learning more and more about less and less. Moreover, such typical controversies which arise from monistic ways of thinking as whether schizophrenia is an organic or a psychological condition are not only misguided and wasteful of resources, but obscure a far more important issue, namely, how the activities and contributions of the various human sciences relate to one another, and what forms of interdisciplinary collaboration are possible.

I have attempted a selective summary of current knowledge about schizophrenia from the vantage points of each of the various human sciences, viewed through the lens afforded by my particular psychological and psychoanalytic perspective. It is sometimes easy to overlook the fact that, after thousands of years in which our understanding of human beings was confined to the fields of mythology and philosophy, in a single century we have experienced the explosive birth of the human sciences. Simply providing an encyclopedic compendium of knowledge about a subject such as schizophrenia leaves one in danger of drowning in a sea of unintegrated information. So I have also proposed an overarching model derived from systems theory to synthesize the contributions of the various human sciences, and I explore some of the ways this model might enrich our understanding of schizophrenia and might offer theorists and clinicians from each of the human sciences new possibilities for intrascientific expansion and interscientific or interdisciplinary collaboration. For those who, like myself, are interested in a particular psychological focus on the schizophrenic person, I have made some original contributions to theory and treatment, as well.

As my own ideas evolved during the writing of the book, one thing that did not change was my clinical case orientation. I have interwoven and illustrated my arguments not only with a multitude of specific clinical illustrations, but with a casebook, including five of the most detailed reports of treatment of schizophrenic persons from inception to termination that are to be found in the literature on psychopathology. I have included two cases which I consider to be failures along with the three successes, as failure is a reality of work with persons with illnesses as serious as schizophrenia, and as I believe failures constitute unique opportunities for learning.

The book is written for everyone in the human sciences who is interested in the study and treatment of mental illness, for those who are interested in philosophical and practical questions about the relationships among the scientific disciplines, and for persons curious about the relationship between the individual, the family, and the structure of society. In addition, the detailed case accounts should appeal to anyone with a lively interest in human beings—in understanding how and why we think, feel, and relate to one another as we do.

Contents

Part III: Viewpoints on Schizophrenia: A Pluralistic Model

Part IV: The Treatment of Schizophrenia

Part V: Cases: The Middle Range of Outcome

Part VI: Conclusion

Introduction

Originally, I set out to pen a study of schizophrenia using extensive material from my personal clinical experience and my particular perspective as a psychoanalyst who values the contributions of the other human sciences. In the course of setting down my ideas I reached some unsettling conclusions: One is that the human sciences have yet to devise a respectful and orderly way to coexist and collaborate. Another is that, at least with regard to a mental illness such as schizophrenia, the human sciences and their interactions, far from being sources of objective knowledge and truly mutative treatment, naturally tend to be reflections of the very elements of primitive mentation that characterize the disease process itself. As a consequence, while this book remains a study of schizophrenia and its treatment, it has also evolved into a larger study of the very organization and operation of the human sciences.

The history of our understanding and treatment of schizophrenia, the quintessential madness, reflects problems that are inherent in the cultural process of acquisition and accretion of knowledge. These include the very human tendencies to overvalue the particular perspective and belief system around which we currently organize ourselves, to rationalize its superiority to what appears to be the errors of the past, and to defend it against contemporary competing points of view. Much as we may wishfully perceive ourselves to be objective and even scientific evaluators of our situation, history teaches us that it is impossible to escape the perceptual and conceptual bonds of the culture and society in which we live. The philosophical position that corresponds to this primitive, extremist, either-or way of thinking is known as monism, and while it may be compatible with the acquisition of knowledge in depth, with knowing more and more about less and less, it is antithetical to the acquisition of knowledge in breadth. In these pages I intend to elucidate a multiplicity of ways in which monistic thinking has determined our understanding of schizophrenia, and to propose more useful and comprehensive ways to view the illness.

1

The approximately two-centuries-old process of social enlightenment and activism in Western culture with regard to the plight of the mentally ill has tended in two diverse directions: one medical-scientific and the other moral-psychological. In the present century these two models have oscillated in dominance and the proponents and adherents of whichever model is currently in favor have, for the most part, tended to ignore or dismiss those of the other. Kraepelin (1896/1919), whose conception of schizophrenia as a disease of the frontal lobes characterized in all instances by a deteriorating course and unfavorable outcome was probably determined by contemporary discoveries concerning the nature and treatment of neurosyphilitic dementia, is largely responsible for the modern belief that schizophrenia is a brain disease. As no specific lesion or toxic agent has been definitively identified, the influence of the neuropathological school that Kraepelin personified gradually waned by midcentury. By the time of the post–World War II romance between psychoanalysis and schizophrenia, popularized in Joanne Greenberg's pseudonymous account (Green, 1964) of her treatment by Frieda Fromm-Reichmann (*I Never Promised You a Rose Garden*), and movies like *Spellbound*, made with the consultation of the director's own analyst, it was widely held that schizophrenia is a psychological process related to pathogenic child-rearing practices and entirely amenable to psychoanalytic intervention.

Disappointment in these equally one-sided psychoanalytic beliefs and the grandiose therapeutic expectations that accompanied them, along with the proliferation of drugs that appear to ameliorate at least some psychotic symptomatology and the publication of exciting data that suggest that schizophrenia is an inherited disorder and even point toward specific areas of brain abnormality, has led most people back to the ideas of Kraepelin and to the reductionistic hypothesis that schizophrenia is an organic illness, albeit not necessarily one whose prognosis is quite so hopeless as he believed, whose characteristic mentation is merely an epiphenomenon, a kind of toxic delirium lacking intrinsic meaningfulness. From this neo-Kraepelinian perspective the disturbances of thought that characterize schizophrenia, such as hallucinations and delusions, are believed to have no intrinsic meaning, and to be useful only insofar as they, like smoke that leads to the fire, may point us to the affected areas of the brain, for example, the temporal-limbic system. This concrete medical disease model is predicated on a clear distinction between the host personality and the organic illness that afflicts it, and it renders more or less irrelevant the contributions of the humanistic disciplines including psychoanalysis and social psychology, except as they may inform us about such factors as the causes and control of stress. Although some who embrace such a model are reluctant to abandon a humanistic approach entirely, and so use such terminology in their approach as "stress diathesis" or "biopsychosocial,"* they nonetheless characterize stress as though it were a physical, rather than

---

*Engel (1977, 1980), who originated the term *biopsychosocial* did not intend it to be used in the manner I am describing, as we shall see in Chapter 2).

a psychological, entity, and concern themselves not with the dynamics of personality structures and human interactions but with such variables as personal compliance or lack thereof with the treatment regimen, or family or host attitudes that may appear to ameliorate or exacerbate the symptoms and course of the illness. Armed with this medical-scientific model it is deemed unnecessary for the clinician to make more of an acquaintance with the person of the patient than is necessary to make the diagnosis and ascertain how he is coping with his illness and complying with prescribed treatments.

The medical viewpoint just summarized is more than the prevailing conception of schizophrenia; it has become the direction of psychiatry itself. In his introduction to the most recent volume of an important monograph series, Van Praag (1992) writes the following:

> Psychiatry is moving, still relatively slowly, but irresistibly, from a more philosophical, contemplative orientation to that of an empirical science. . . . Biological psychiatry provided psychiatry not only with a basic new science and new treatment modalities, but also with the tools, the methodology, and the mentality to operate within the confines of an empirical science, the only framework in which a medical discipline can survive. (p. v)

Psychiatry is becoming indistinguishable from neuroscience and is gravitating toward a monistic and reductionistic position not unlike that occupied by psychoanalysis 30 years ago.

An ever-diminishing minority continue to approach schizophrenia with psychological models, which are looked upon as relics of antiquity, even of the age of magic and witchcraft. From the psychological perspective the illness is considered inseparable from the psychological structure and function of the personality; therefore, it is believed essential to look beyond behavioral symptoms and signs, and beyond neurobiological lesions and disorders, into complex mental processes and into the interpersonal relationships of the patient with important others in order to discover the dynamic meanings and connections that determine and structure the pathological process. Such a model also implies that effective treatment will necessitate some alteration of the basic structure of the personality and perhaps of the social network of personal relationships that sustain it. Unfortunately, "beyond" has too often meant that the findings of neuroscience are forgotten or ignored; perhaps the fact that the contemporary psychological viewpoint is not generally taken seriously is a consequence of this.

It is widely believed that these two viewpoints, organic and psychological, are incompatible and that only one of them can be correct; in other words, there is a common assumption that our approach to the understanding and treatment of mental illness must be monistic. When the limitations of one approach become apparent, the pendulum of opinion seems to swing toward the other in an equally extreme manner. Of course, not everyone is beguiled by either-or thinking. Even back in Kraepelin's time Elmer Southard (1912), who pioneered some of the studies of cerebral pathology, condemned one-sided theories that ascribed mental disorders either to "blots and spots in the brain" or to "tangles and twists in the mind." More recently, Eisenberg (1986) referred to such cyclical fluctuations of belief within psychiatry as shifts back and forth between a position of "mindlessness," by which he refers to the radical reductionist orientation of neuroscience, and a position of "brainlessness," by which he refers to psychological theories that deny the importance of organic process. From a philosophical perspective the oscillation of belief systems about schizophrenia is but an instance of the ages-old debate about the relationship between body and mind (or, as the ancients conceived it, body and soul). Another way to think about the problem is that we, lacking an integrated view of schizophrenia, tend to perceive it in a fragmented, extreme, *pars pro toto* manner, which bears some resemblance to the pathology of the illness itself.

The specific problem of elucidating the nature of schizophrenia and the related but more general problem of extreme and single-minded fluctuations in belief systems are questions of great social and scientific import. The latter issue has far-reaching implications for the form and function of the human sciences, individually and collectively. As for the former problem, there are about 1.5 million diagnosed schizophrenics in the United States, about 14% of whom are currently in hospitals (Torrey, 1988). U.S. Public Health Service statistics suggest that schizophrenia is at least 15 times more prevalent than AIDS. Sartorius et al. (1986) claim there are 20 million schizophrenics in the world. while Strauss and Carpenter (1981) believe the illness afflicts 0.5–3% of the population. In addition to the ruination of their individual lives, the problem they represent for society—whether measured in terms of economics, social responsibility, violence and destructiveness—or in other ways, is almost beyond comprehension.

My credentials for undertaking to elucidate these subjects include my professional background as a psychoanalyst and approximately 30 years of work as therapist, consultant, teacher, and ward administrator in and around mental hospitals with schizophrenic patients. The case histories in this book include the total treatment, start to finish, of five DSM-III-R schizophrenic patients. The primary lens through which I view schizophrenia was forged for me by my original mentor in the field, Elvin Semrad, who taught me to sit with patients, literally and figuratively, and to listen and try to bear and understand the nature of the distress they were presenting to me so that eventually, hopefully I might help them put it in some more constructive perspective. I was taught to attend to my own impulses to prematurely (before achieving understanding) mitigate the unbearable pain of being there (both the patient's and my own), to resist temptations to yield to the precipitous use of medication, advice, and behavior modification, and even to efforts at quantification and theorization. In retrospect, I would be hard pressed to say how much of this posture is an enlightened form of masochism originating in an era before significant drug treatment became available and how much is a kind of Buddhistic acceptance of the remarkably helpless position in which this awesome condition places both patient and those who aspire to be helpers. What I think is indisputable, as I trust the case reports that constitute my unique contribution of data to the book will illustrate, is that this is a remarkably useful and virtually forgotten way to learn, one now all but foreclosed to the present generation of clinicians who do not become intimate with their patients but get to know them only enough to observe their symptoms, correlate them with a DSM III diagnosis and prognosis, and then prescribe medications, programs, and behaviors designed to control and if possible obliterate the symptomatology.

Beyond the utility of the posture I was taught for learning about schizophrenia was its aid in enabling me to help some patients to understand themselves and their world better, to work to correct what they came to perceive as areas of difficulty and immaturity within themselves, and as a result to become more autonomous, effective and satisfied human beings. I do not mean to imply that such an approach is helpful in all instances of schizophrenia; even in some instances when it was, I would have to admit—when I view them in retrospect from the contemporary platform of knowledge afforded by such fields as psychopharmacology—that the suffering of some individuals was unduly prolonged. Among the five detailed case presentations in this book are two instructive failures, which constitute my acknowledgment that no treatment is always successful. During the course of my efforts I have learned something about the other human sciences that hold schizophrenia in their view, and about their approaches to treatment. I have relied heavily on the holding environment of a hospital and the social-cultural attitudes and issues it represents, on family therapy based on an understanding of family dynamics, and on psychotropic medication based on current knowledge of organic processes.

This book represents my effort to (a) demonstrate that an approach to selected cases of schizophrenia based on the etiologic and therapeutic assumptions of postclassical psychoanalysis, combined with judicious use of other treatment modalities and their associated theories, is not only efficacious but, when feasible perhaps even the treatment of choice, and (b) argue that failure to recognize this fact is an implicit negation of the humanity of schizophrenic persons. But the book is not simply a re-presentation of old psychoanalytic wine in new bottles. While my approach to schizophrenic patients is humanistic, predicated on the belief that the mental phenomena characteristic of the illness are historically and adaptively meaningful aspects of the personality or psychology of the sufferer, and on its corollary that looking upon the mentation of a schizophrenic as nothing more than a toxic by-product amounts to a rejection of him or her as a person, psychology is by no means sufficient to understand and to treat schizophrenia. It is necessary to have a pluralistic, relativistic view and to appreciate the contributions of the various sciences and disciplines that study it. In particular, some of the most exciting and promising contemporary developments in our understanding of schizophrenia come from the neurosciences. I believe that these have the potential to enrich psychoanalytic theory and reciprocally, that the generation of sophisticated neuroscientific hypotheses requires a detailed understanding of the psychology—not just the symptoms and signs—of schizophrenia.

But this book is not simply an argument for the necessity of theoretical and clinical pluralism, or an echo of the common practice in case discussions of using the slogan "multidisciplinary approach" to rationalize the addition of ideas from many fields as though theories could be admixed like the dishes at a buffet. Little in the way of overarching theory has been developed to systematize the organization of and relationships among the human sciences. I have modified what is sometimes referred to as General Systems Theory, which was developed in post–World War I Germany by a group of scientist-philosophers, including Ludwig von Bertalanffy, Paul Weiss, and Werner Heisenberg, in order to describe a formal structural relationship not only between neuroscience and clinical psychology or psychoanalysis but involving other sciences critical to an understanding of schizophrenia, such as cultural anthropology, social psychology, family systems theory, and behavioral and cognitive psychology. The result, which I call the hierarchical systems model, is predicated on the fact that we tend to perceive and intuit the world as a phenomenological hierarchy of structural systems, assemblages, or gestalts, ranging from microscopic to macroscopic, from concrete and specific to abstract and general, and from lesser to greater evolution, development, or complexity. The relationships among the various human science systems in such an array are ones of creative transformation rather than simple linear causality. The implications of such a schema are manifold. Like the blind men describing the elephant, we cannot assume that the particular scientific stance or perspective we take as observers represents all that is to be seen of a phenomenal array such as schizophrenia, and while it may be necessary to comprehend that phenomenal array, it may not be sufficient to interpret all its meanings. Using hierarchical systems theory, I have tried to describe the multiple facets of schizophrenia and to explore the ways in which the various scientific viewpoints interdigitate with one another, and the potential of each to enhance the explanatory capability of the others.

The same hierarchical systems schema that is so useful interscientifically in delineating a complementary place for each of the human sciences proves to be equally useful intrascientifically in expanding the scope of psychoanalysis to accommodate qualitatively different but interconnected models of the mind, and thereby to encompass the primitive mental phenomena characteristic of schizophrenia as well as those of the psychoneuroses.

In its relativity and uncertainty of perspective the view of the human sciences and of schizophrenia that I propose parallels the way in which modern physics has come to view the natural universe. And it raises new and troublesome but, hopefully, productive questions. For example, we can no longer content ourselves with asking whether an illness such as schizophrenia is either organic or psychological. And it will be necessary to question whether there is a clear distinction between the so-called illness on the one hand and society's higher or more abstract level of comprehension, objectification, and treatment of it on the other. As we attempt to conceive of schizophrenia and its treatment from progressively more macroscopic perspectives we shall identify a core gestalt of problems or issues that emerge and reemerge successively transformed and reorganized. We may reach the disquieting conclusion that what passes for scientific comprehension and treatment of schizophrenia may be little more than reflection, transformation, and enactment at a higher system level of the illness process itself.

Each of us has a unique perspective, and for better and for worse mine is that of a psychoanalyst; thus, in developing a pluralistic hierarchical systems model for the human sciences and for schizophrenia, I can no more avoid speaking as one than a leopard can change its spots. I believe that it is possible to write a number of books similar to this one insofar as they begin with the same hierarchical systems perspective, but different from it insofar as they reflect a perspective and expertise unique to the scientific discipline of the author. Others may justifiably question my emphasis or perhaps bias, but not, I hope, the pluralistic schema I have constructed to embrace all the human sciences that bear on schizophrenia and their contributions. Indeed, I hope that this may be one outgrowth of my effort, for I think it will only be after a number of such books have been written that the full scope or story of schizophrenia and the interactive potential of the disciplines that contribute to its understanding and treatment will have unfolded for our appreciation.

The book is organized as follows: Part I presents a critical review of the nature of schizophrenia and the ways in which it has been conceptualized. In particular, I take note of the flaws of monistic, reductionistic models and of the naive interactionist thinking that is commonly resorted to as an alternative. In their stead I elaborate a hierarchical systems theory and demonstrate its special value in accommodating shifts of perspective among a variety of equally valid scientific models of explication and treatment, and enabling mutually enriching collaborations among the various sciences and their related treatment philosophies. Part I concludes with a discussion of the methodology and data on which this book is based, and a critical evaluation of the value and the limitations of the two most common sources of data: (a) the scientific experiment, with its deconstruction of complex phenomena into parts involving discrete variables and linear, cause–effect hypotheses that can be measured in large groups of subjects and results that may be statistically tabulated, and (b) complex and extensive reports of a relatively few psychological and interpersonal systems that cannot be described by any mathematical model currently available to us.

Part II consists of a detailed presentation of two cases, chosen to illustrate the extremes of treatment outcome: extraordinary success and abysmal failure.

Parts III and IV, on the nature of schizophrenia and its treatment, respectively, constitute the substance of the theoretical presentation. Each part is organized along hierarchical systems lines, viewing schizophrenia variously from the microscopic level of neuroscience; from the personal-psychological level, including the dyadic relationship and the family system; and, finally, from the perspective of sociology and culture. Three more detailed case reports, illustrating the middle range of outcomes in cases where a central psychological focus was utilized, conclude the book.

Placement of the case reports in the book is somewhat arbitrary. Clinical material is not confined to these but interspersed throughout the book for illustrative purposes. Because of their complexity the case reports are not intended to illustrate particular points in the text but to illustrate the synthesis of thinking that characterizes use of hierarchical systems theory with a central psychological focus. Therefore, it should not interfere with obtaining a grasp of the general exposition of the book if the reader chooses to peruse the case reports in some other sequence according to his or her personal inclination.

Part I

The Groundwork

Chapter 1

What Is Schizophrenia?

History of the Concept

Those in search of the mysteries of schizophrenia need look no further than the vexing questions of how to define and detect the condition and how to comprehend its natural course. Despite exhaustive, expensive, and time-consuming research for definitive concrete and "objective" markers of the disease, including such current candidates for a so-called biological marker as particular evoked EEG potentials, eye movement disturbances, or curiosities such as visible capillaries at the base of the fingernail bed, schizophrenia remains as Kraepelin originally described it in 1896 (1919): a syndrome, or symptom and sign cluster, without associated organic lesion, defined by its clinical phenomenology and detected by mental status examination and anamnesis.

Kraepelin believed what he called dementia praecox (prior to his contribution madness went by a variety of names) to be an organic disease of the frontal lobes—an endogenous psychosis, that is, one without gross anatomic lesion or toxic factor. His use of the term *dementia*, which, according to Ellenberger (1967), was coined by Morel in 1856, indicates his belief that, invariably, the illness has a deteriorating course and a poor prognosis. Since Kraepelin's contribution the diagnosis, like that of cancer, has, for better or worse, been inextricably intertwined with pessimism, and cases that present like dementia praecox but seem to recover are often retrospectively rediagnosed. Bleuler (1911), however, was not convinced that schizophrenia, as he named it, invariably had a deteriorating course, and his view that it is a group of conditions with a variety of courses and outcomes is more consistent with our current belief that the schizophrenic syndrome is an end point for disease processes whose etiology runs the gamut from organic, to psychological, with multiple permutations and combinations of the two. When there is concurrent evidence of a neurological lesion, regardless of how "schizophrenic" the clinical picture looks, the diagnosis of organic brain syndrome is usually made.

Disquieting as all this may be for those devoted to objective scientific (read "quantifiable") thinking, matters would be even worse were it not for the fact that the syndrome has been detected in virtually all countries and cultures with approximately equal incidence (Sartorius et al., 1986), and its descriptive parameters have not changed substantially in the hundred or so years since it was clearly differentiated from neurosyphilitic dementia. To be sure, the modal content of delusions seems to shift in parallel with cultural preoccupations, and extremes of hebephrenia and catatonia are encountered less frequently, but the former relates to content rather than to the structural core of the disease process and the latter is probably a consequence of alterations in treatment philosophy, including the introduction of neuroleptic medication and the gradual replacement of back wards with more vigorous behavioral rehabilitative programs, both of which tend to forestall deterioration.

Schizophrenia as a Social Construct

The definition and diagnosis of schizophrenia is undeniably unusual, compared to other illnesses. Historically, schizophrenics have come to the attention of society as infrahuman objects of fear and loathing because of their alien and disturbing demeanor and thinking, and they have tended to arouse social pressure to quarantine and even eradicate them. Until the advent of moral treatment in the 19th century, incarceration and various forms of punishment were used to combat what was largely perceived as a form of degeneracy. Even now, in contemporary times, schizophrenia remains first and foremost a social construct, a statement of social deviance and unacceptable conduct. This means that in almost every instance the condition is initially brought to attention, though perhaps not diagnosed, by an agency that is representative of society (the family, school, social welfare agency, workplace, or legal system) and that has been perturbed by an individual's social disturbance. In most instances the initial designation of derangement is made without the concurrence of the person destined to be the patient. Treatment measures are initiated involuntarily or, at best, with passive compliance on his part. Moreover, probably in no other instance of disease has the search for an organic correlate proven so lengthy and inconclusive. These facts differentiate schizophrenia from most of the typical "medical" illnesses, in which the initial designation of illness is made by the patient, treatment is initiated by patient complaint, and unequivocal correlative organic lesions are eventually discovered. Notable exceptions include some of the organic brain syndromes, but even in those instances (for example, in Alzheimer's disease) organic corroboration is usually possible. The same holds for the traditional psychiatric illnesses, at least with regard to the paradigm of complaining patient. This means that we cannot deny the element of truth in the radical social critique of the notion of schizophrenia as a disease, namely, that it is society's effort to control deviance.

Nonetheless, I do not think this requires us to reach the same conclusion as that of the radical social critics, namely, that schizophrenia is not an illness, or that it is society, rather than the individual, that is ill. Only among those who have not had intimate contact with individual schizophrenics and who tend to rationalize the content of their thinking along lines of artistic expression or social protest can there exist serious doubt as to the existence of a syndrome or disease beyond the normal range of personality deviance. Such critics of the schizophrenia concept lack the experience to place content—socially deviant ideas—in the context of structure; that is, they ignore the extreme social withdrawal, the overall mentation so bizarre that the person is virtually impossible to empathize with, and the basic failure of the self-regulatory and adaptive functions of mind, which result in failure of all but rudimentary self-care. The total picture is every bit as inimical to life as some of the most severe forms of "medical" illness, and it compellingly demands intervention in any society sufficiently civilized that its members are unwilling to allow their fellows to perish.

All the patients I shall present came to recognize that they were quite ill and in need of help and that they would have died or been chronically disabled without it. They were able to specify in some detail what the illness meant in terms of psychological and interpersonal limitations. While some critics may suggest that such patients were "brainwashed" into such an admission, evidence of their greatly enhanced capacity for self-assertion, conflict, and even constructive deviance with elements of society at the time they reached their recognition of illness would seem to belie such an explanation. In fact, the recovered schizophrenic usually presents more of a "problem" to his family and is a more formidable assertive force in society than he ever was in the untreated state.

There is no way that a sincere, intelligent observer can confuse the solipsistic, nonadaptive posture of the schizophrenic, which I will try to describe, with adaptive if disturbing social deviance, as is sometimes possible in instances of hypomania. The social or political deviant, in contrast, actively enlists the sympathies of, or already belongs to, a passionate, minority group. As it is not nearly so easy as the fears of the layman might suggest to confuse schizophrenia with social deviance, it is my opinion that social misuse of the power to diagnose schizophrenia is in most instances a conscious and willful occurrence rather than a frightening mistake perpetrated by a conscienceless society.*

Nonetheless, the radical social critique of the schizophrenia concept as a guise for scapegoating and for authoritarian political suppression of deviance should not be dismissed lightly. It is a theme to which I return throughout the

---

*I am aware of the various studies in which normal subjects have posed as patients on hospital wards or in clinics, without actually simulating illness, and been mistaken for schizophrenics. But I believe these tell us more about the training and competence of the mental health personnel involved than they do about the validity of the diagnosis of schizophrenia.

book in order to demonstrate that the romantic mythology that has arisen around schizophrenia conceals some surprising truths.

Schizophrenia as a Relativistic Construct

The definition and diagnosis of schizophrenia is dependent on the vantage point of the observer in yet another way; that is, there is a certain circularity between our theoretical perspective and what it is we believe we perceive. To give an example, depending on whether one's theoretical orientation is that of psychoanalysis, family systems theory, or neuroscience, one may define schizophrenia as a disease of childhood onset or one of adult onset. With the ascendancy of the neuroscientific perspective, adult onset is commonly accepted as fact, but, as we shall see, there is much room for doubt. These aspects of definition, in turn, bias both the nature, methodology, and conclusions of research into schizophrenia. For example, Beiser (1992) recently presented a follow-up study of the occupational adjustment of schizophrenics. Although his own data reveal that their occupational adjustment was significantly worse than that of affective psychotics before their acute episode, and that the schizophrenics end up much lower on the occupational ladder, because he defines the illness as commencing with the acute episode and the subsequent slope of decline in work adjustment is similar to that of affective psychotics, he concludes the deterioration in job functioning of schizophrenics is no worse than that of persons with affective psychosis.

Early Attempts at Definition

Bleuler (1911) said "I have chosen the name schizophrenia because the 'splitting' of the different psychic functions is one of its most important characteristics" (p. 1). As we shall see, his observation remains valid today. He also proposed that there are fundamental, or primary, symptoms and accessory, or secondary, symptoms. The primary group includes dissociation of affect from thought; disruption or disorganization of the train of association; ambivalence, defined as the simultaneous presence of contradictory affects and ideas rather than the common usage that defines it as ordinary "mixed feelings"; autism (a term Bleuler coined that has found its way into ordinary vocabulary); and disturbance of activity and volition. Bleuler listed delusions and hallucinations as "accessory" symptoms. His division among primary and secondary symptoms very roughly approximates the contemporary distinction between "negative" and "positive" symptoms.

Schneider (1959) proposed a definition in some respects quite opposite to Bleuler's, based on a similar dichotomy between what he calls first- and second-order symptoms. Some of Schneider's first-order symptoms (hallucinations, delusions, ideas of reference, and thought control) are what Bleuler would term accessory manifestions. Langfeldt, in 1939, returned to the vexing debate between Kraepelin and Bleuler about outcome and proposed that there are two classes of schizophrenia: process and reactive. The former resembles Kraepelin's dementia praecox, and has a deteriorating course and poor outcome, whereas the latter is clearly a response to stress or trauma, and has a better prognosis.

The distinction between so-called positive symptom schizophrenia, characterized by a continuing behavioral and affective aliveness and symptomatology (however bizarre), as well as by disruptive behavior, and negative symptom schizophrenia, characterized by such things as apathy, passivity, withdrawal, and flattened affect—a distinction we tend to attribute to Strauss and Carpenter (1972) and Strauss, Carpenter, and Bartko (1974)—was in fact first proposed in the 19th century by Hughlings Jackson (1931–1932). He divided schizophrenic symptomatology into two groups: positive, presumably related to the intact but disinhibited functioning of lower centers of the brain, and negative, a product of destruction of the higher centers, presumably a reversal of the evolutionary process. In 1980 Crow took this distinction a step further and proposed that these might in fact be two separate disease entities.

Contemporary Diagnostic Criteria

More recently, systematic diagnostic criteria have been proposed in the various versions of the official *Diagnostic and Statistical Manual of the American Psychiatric Association* (DSM) and by Feighner and associates (Robins & Guze, 1970; Feighner, Robins, & Guze, 1972). Feighner lists three sets of criteria: The first, involving the present illness, consists of at least six consecutive symptomatic months prior to the evaluation and an absence of significant affective illness symptomatology. The second involves at least one of the following mental status findings: delusions or hallucinations without perplexity, and illogical or disorganized verbalization. The third relates to the presence in the personal and family history of at least three of the following five: unmarried, poor premorbid adjustment, onset prior to age 40, family history of schizophrenia, and no significant substance abuse history.

The cases in this book meet not only the Feighner criteria but also the DSM-III-R criteria for diagnosis of schizophrenia, which are rather similar with the exception of the past history items. Each comprises three broad categories: characteristic mental status symptoms and signs, chronicity and deterioration of function, and differential diagnosis exclusion of other conditions. For a diagnosis of schizophrenia at least two of the following mental status features must be present: delusions, hallucinations, disorganized and peculiar speech, catatonic behavior, and flat or inappropriate affect. Symptoms, both prodromal and florid, must have been present for at least 6 months and there must be proof of poor self-care, deterioration of function, and social

withdrawal. It is necessary also to rule out organic factors, including substance abuse and affective disorder.

Thought Disorder and Affect Disorder

One consequence of the newer classificatory systems is to encourage more
discrimination between affective and thought disorders. Conditions characterized by affective excess—once called schizophrenia, affective type—are nowadays classified as manic disorders. The diagnosis of schizophrenia tends to
be reserved for conditions where manifest affect is blunted or diminished and
the cognitive disturbance is more prominent. However valuable this shift has
been in assisting clinicians to identify patients who might benefit from lithium
or antidepressant medication, a classificatory schema based on descriptive
psychiatry alone has limitations. In Chapter 6 we shall see that one of the most
productive current neuroscience hypotheses involves the dominant temporal
lobe and limbic system, particularly structures involved with affect production
and regulation. And we shall see as we review cases in depth, that from a
psychological perspective schizophrenia is characterized by inappropriate affect, the absence of expectable affect, and hypersensitivity to emotional stimulation, as well as by a destructiveness seemingly related to poorly represented
and controlled rage. From a developmental perspective, as well, the traditional
diagnostic dichotomy between affect and cognition makes little sense, for
affect and thought emerge from an undifferentiated self–object matrix (Loewald, 1971). In other words, schizophrenia may profitably be considered an
affective disorder. A similar assertion has been made by McGlashan and Keats
(1989, p. 101). Or to put it differently, efforts to distinguish between schizophrenia and manic–depressive psychosis on the basis of the presence or absence of manifest affect may represent a false dichotomy, for problems representing, structuring, and controlling affect pervade both these conditions
and manifest themselves at times in excessive or inappropriate emoting and at
other times in a seeming absence of affect. We shall return to this differential
diagnosis problem in a moment.

The Kraepelinian Diagnostic Legacy

Despite the fact that the five cases in this book meet DSM-III-R criteria, some
readers will not be convinced these individuals were in fact schizophrenic.
Hearing recurrent efforts to rediagnose Joanne Greenberg (Green, 1964),
Fromm-Reichmann's famous "rose garden" patient (a current one is to label
her a multiple personality), and repeatedly encountering among members of
audiences to whom I present the case of Emily the rejoinder that she could not
have been schizophrenic because she did so well, has made me realize that
most of us have difficulty accepting the retrospective diagnosis of schizo-

phrenia for any patient who has been so successfully treated that he or she seems more or less normal. Most of us, however sophisticated, tend to the Kraepelinian equation of schizophrenia with an alien state of bizarreness, chronicity, and a prognosis of, at best, better adaptation but without alteration in the fundamental condition. While in principle, at least, Bleuler's belief that it is incorrect to define schizophrenia in terms of deterioration and poor outcome is widely accepted, and while the circular reasoning and therapeutic nihilism involved in defining a disease by its outcome is antithetical to the processes of both scientific inquiry and therapeutic endeavor, Kraepelin's beliefs still have a powerful hold on most of us. I think one reason is that our shocked sense of incomprehensibility and alienation upon encountering schizophrenic persons is such that, no matter how "scientifically" and open-mindedly we may attempt to approach them, we unconsciously tend to conceive of them as qualitatively different from ourselves, as nonhuman. It is also true that many schizophrenics do not think of themselves as human, like other people. When meanings and comprehensibility unfold in the course of treatment and the patient "joins the human race," we tend to think of him disjunctively, as very different from before. Even if we have experienced the process from the start it is sometimes difficult to realize that the recovered patient is in fact the same person; thus, it is hardly surprising that it requires a great leap of faith on hearing or reading a retrospective account to believe that the person who has ended up so well was in fact schizophrenic to begin with.

A Clinical Description

I would like to supplement the necessarily dry and sparse description from DSM-III-R with a brief account of some of what I consider the salient descriptive features of the illness. I shall return to many of these in greater detail throughout the book. For more detail about the thought disorder itself the reader is especially referred to Kasanin's (1944) edited volume, to Werner (1940), and Hanfmann and Kasanin (1942). Schizophrenia is characterized by the persistence of the following clinical picture in the absence of evidence of significant neuropathology, including toxicity or trauma: There is an overall bizarreness of behavior and thinking. Self-care is grossly impaired and often utterly ineffectual, even self-destructive. Body movement and gesture, as well as behavior and ideation, have a stereotypic, repetitive mechanical or robotic quality. Manifest affect is grossly incongruous with ideation and objective reality and may be seriously blunted and flattened. Because thought association is fragmented, incoherent, or "loosened," it makes little "sense," even to one trained psychoanalytically to attend to the associative stream and its unconsciously motivated determinants; that is, there are no apparent unconscious linkages or integrating elements. "Ambivalence," the manifestation of the virtually simultaneous existence of utterly contradictory, polarized ideas, affects, and volition, may be so severe as to lead to virtual paralysis of expression and action, a paralysis to which such terms as blocking and catatonia have been applied. Schizophrenic thinking proceeds according to idiosyncratic rules of "logic" and principles of cognition that are not readily inferred or empathized with by the normal observer as is the case with the neurotic, hence the at times frightening sense of being in the presence of a bizarre or alien being. There are hallucinations, usually auditory, and delusions. The content of the delusions most often indicates an absence of boundaries between self and world; that is, one senses that the "things" referred to are not the things themselves but unwitting representatives of parts of the patient's mind. In other words, what ought to be the contents of thought tend to contaminate and at times almost obliterate perception so that they are taken by the patient for external reality. Overall, the schizophrenic appears to be living in a world other than that of ordinary cultural consensus, however vehemently he may insist it is more real than that which the observer perceives. This last conclusion is, of course, one of the most potentially dangerous aspects of subjective diagnosis, as is illustrated by the use in Soviet Russia of the ideologically inspired concept of "sluggish schizophrenia" as a rationalization for incarceration of political dissidents. The concept of consensual reality to which I refer is quite different and is in no way culturally or politically expedient. It includes recognizing the normalcy in some instances of minority, nonconforming, socially rebellious, and even revolutionary attitudes, even the "bizarreness" of behavior associated with them, and recognizing the contextual bizarreness in some instances (for example, the case of Celia in Chapter 21) of superficially normal behavior that makes no trouble for anyone.

By asserting that the clinical picture must be persistent, I mean there must have been at least several episodes, each lasting at least a few days. If and when episodes of gross bizarreness subside, careful acquaintance with the subject should elicit for a long period thereafter, albeit in muted form, many of the aforementioned features. Not all of these features—and I have made no effort to exhaustively mine the wealth of clinical description of schizophrenia—need to be present to make the diagnosis. And more than a few may dominate a clinical picture that is most probably not schizophrenic. The diagnosis of schizophrenia is an overall impression or gestalt of bizarre other-worldliness that is not difficult for experienced clinicians to agree upon, and is clearly more than the sum of the parts into which it can be dissected.

Differentiation from Manic–Depressive Psychosis

In the foregoing discussion of changes in diagnostic fashion related to the separation of so-called disorders of cognition from those of affect, I suggested that, contrary to predominant current opinion, both may be affective disorders. Now I should like briefly to contrast features I find characteristic of manic–depressive psychosis with those more typical of schizophrenia. The former is characterized by major mood swings of prolonged amplitude: many months of deep depression followed cyclically by many months of increasingly expansive grandiose thinking, paranoid attitudes and controlling behavior, which are associated with flight of ideas, diminished need for sleep, sprees of constant activity, and voracious consumption. The hypomanic patient is often extremely creative and productive, and even in the manic phase, in contrast with the disorganized inept schizophrenic, he tends to dominate and control social settings and to be perceived by many as plausible, normal, and even exceptional. Many socially productive and even creative individuals have been afflicted with this condition, which has been inextricably intertwined with both their productivity and social charisma. This form of illness is infrequently encountered. It is similar to the borderline personality insofar as there are cyclic alternations of behavior (depressed and manic phases, respectively) but different insofar as these cycles are prolonged in duration rather than rapidly alternating or even simultaneously enacted, such as one encounters in the primitive personality disorders.

Natural Course

If the definition and diagnosis of schizophrenia remain ambiguous and controversial, the natural course of the illness is not much better known, which is remarkable considering the fact that we are approaching the hundredth anniversary of the formal diagnosis, and the vicissitudes of madness have been well known since ancient times. Only in the last 15 years or so have the results of systematic follow-up studies begun to appear in the literature. As it is next to impossible to find an untreated population, these studies for the most part involve patients treated with a potpourri of methods, including hospitalization, somatic therapies, neuroleptic medication, rehabilitation programs, and various forms of psychotherapy.

Our confusion about the natural course of schizophrenia also relates to the likelihood that, as Bleuler (1911) first suggested, it really comprises a group of conditions with different etiologies and therefore different outcomes. The controversy between the neo-Kraepelinians (for whom schizophrenia is synonymous with deterioration, so that if there is "cure" or at least achievement of high function the original diagnosis of schizophrenia is subject to doubt) and those who subscribe to Bleuler's doctrine of variability of outcome has not been settled by the studies of the last 15 years, some of which appear to support the Kraepelinian position and others the Bleulerian.

Some of the earlier studies suggest that a substantial number of schizophrenics may actually improve over time and achieve a modest functional capability, with no specific or intensive treatment save general rehabilitation programs and psychotropic medications (Bleuler, 1968; Strauss & Carpenter, 1977; Tsuang, Woolson, & Fleming, 1979; Huber, Gross, Schuttler, & Linz, 1980). Two of these studies (Bleuler's and Huber's) have been subject to criticism on methodologic and diagnostic grounds (Harding, Brooks, Ashikaga,

Strauss, & Breier, 1987). But the Vermont longitudinal study, conducted in the mid-1950s by Harding et al. (1987), which was more rigorous in design, reached similar conclusions. In that study 118 chronically hospitalized patients were selected for placement in a rehabilitation-deinstitutionalization program. These lower-class middle-aged patients had averaged 6 consecutive years of hospitalization, 10 years of total disability, and 16 years of illness at the time of original placement, and they had been refractory to treatment with what phenothiazines were then available. By the time of the retrospective assessment of these patients 25 years later, 25% of the original group had died (of causes not indicated) and another 6% could not be located or refused to participate. Of the 70% who were reviewed, 60% scored in the healthy range on the Global Assessment Scale, 68% manifested no schizophrenic symptomatology, and a remarkable 45% showed no psychiatric symptoms whatsoever. The functioning of the asymptomatic group is not described in detail, however, and there are some disturbing notes. Eighty-four percent remained on antipsychotic medication, and 18% had been hospitalized for their illness within the past year. The majority were unemployed, and only 40% of those of working age had held a job at some time during the preceding year. And among patients in what is described as the "middle range of outcome" a number still reported delusions and hallucinations—although they had learned not to talk about them. The results of the study are reported in such a distant statistical manner that it is difficult to get a picture of the subjects as human beings, but my impression is that "good outcome" is measured not in relation to normal functioning but in relation to the Kraepelinian belief that deterioration is normal and expectable. Moreover, McGlashan (1988) has recently pointed out that the somewhat favorable outcomes reported in the good outcome group might in part be an artifact of the original selection criteria for the rehabilitation program. Candidates were picked because they were already improving in their current situation; moreover, because of their extreme poverty they were highly motivated to learn job skills and to work.

One of the earliest studies, the Iowa 500 (Morrison, Winokur, & Crowe, 1973; Tsuang, Woolson, & Fleming, 1979), which is unique insofar as modern treatment techniques were unavailable to this state hospital population, comes closest to being a true study of the natural course of illness. The investigators concluded that schizophrenia is a chronic, serious, often disabling disease. Several more recent follow-up studies, based on a population of schizophrenics very different from the Iowa 500, arrive at a similar conclusion.

McGlashan (1984) followed 163 chronic schizophrenics most of whom were upper-middle-class patients admitted to Chestnut Lodge in their late twenties, often after multiple hospitalizations. These stayed at the Lodge an average of 3 to 4 years and usually had considerable psychotherapy. McGlashan reviewed their course 15 years later. His findings are not so sanguine as those of the Vermont study, but it is not clear whether he observed different outcomes or used a different lens to view them and different criteria to assess them. Thirteen percent of his cohort had committed suicide, two-thirds remained chronically ill, and the other third had improved. Since McGlashan's study provides examples of his outcome categories, it is possible to picture the people he refers to. One good outcome case is a man (with obviously superior abilities to begin with) who had done excellent college work and had nearly earned a degree prior to his hospitalization, after which his condition gradually deteriorated. He was admitted to Chestnut Lodge and stayed there for almost 6 years, until age 35. At age 41, when he was recontacted, he was married and held a good job but was still on haloperidol. He reported problems in his marriage, anxiety, and depression, and he was noted to have inappropriate affect and tangential thinking. In this "good outcome" case use of a higher magnification lens than that in the Vermont study reveals that the psychotic illness is still very visible, though social deterioration has been arrested.

Two recent studies lack the human richness of McGlashan's report but are similarly rather negative in their conclusions. Breier et al. (1991) found that the condition of a group of 58 young chronic schizophrenics from the NIMH program followed up at 2 to 12 years after hospitalization was generally worse; over 75% had had serious relapses and rehospitalizations, and 38% had made at least one suicide attempt. Carone, Harrow, and Westermeyer (1991) followed for a period of 5 years what would seem to be a more hopeful population—79 young acute schizophrenics without a long history of illness—and reached a similarly unfavorable conclusion. Only 15% of the outcomes were positive, and 10% of the group had committed suicide. It appears that no form of treatment made a significant difference. In a 1992 survey of studies of the fate of first admission schizophrenics, a group with a relatively favorable prognosis, Ram et al. note a relapse rate of 60% within the first 2 years.

McGlashan (1988) presents an excellent summary, from which I borrow, in part, of what we may tentatively conclude about the natural history of schizophrenia based on these cases: First, the onset of manifest clinical illness is usually in late adolescence or young adulthood, whether or not problems were visible on close inspection earlier in life. I should like to add to this the caveat that it is important to try to distinguish between the first acute outbreak of illness and the actual commencement of the illness, which may be much earlier (a topic I discuss beginning in Chapter 7).

Second, a number of researchers—Gittelman-Klein (1969), Flor-Henry (1978, 1990), Lewine (1980, 1988), Seeman (1982, 1985, 1986), Gur et al. (1985), Nasrallah et al. (1986), Haas (1987), Goldstein and Link (1988), Haas, Glick, Clarkin, Spencer, and Lewis (1990), and DeLisi, Dauphinius, and Hauser (1989)—have noted that the onset of schizophrenia is earlier and its course, with regard to cognitive impairment, predominance of negative symptomatology, and response to neuroleptic medication, tends to be worse in male than in female patients. Goldstein and Tsuang (1990) and Josiassen, Roemer, Johnson, and Shagass (1990) report that male schizophrenics are more withdrawn than females, and McGlashan and Bardenstein (1990) report that female schizophrenics have more affective symptomatology. Haas et al. (1990) write that schizophrenic females respond more favorably to family treatment intervention than do males, and Angermeyer, Kuhn, and Goldstein (1990) report that their own findings and their review of other studies suggest better outcomes in the treatment of female schizophrenics.

Third, schizophrenia is often a chronic, disabling illness.

Fourth, the average outcome is worse than that of any other mental illness.

Fifth, the mortality rate of schizophrenics from other conditions is significantly higher than that of the general population. In particular, there is a very significant risk of suicide: 13% over a 15-year period in McGlashan's 1984 study, 10% in the more recent (1991) review by Carone and associates, and somewhere between these two figures in a survey of studies undertaken by Caldwell and Gottesman (1990). McGlashan found the suicide rate among schizophrenics to be higher than that among those with bipolar affective disorder (0%) and those with unipolar disorder (8%).

Sixth, the condition of schizophrenics typically deteriorates during the first 10 to 15 years following clinical onset, and subsequently reaches a stable state or plateau.

When all is said and done, however, statistical reports cannot entirely convey the richness of informed subjective impressions. I conclude this chapter with a statement that vividly reflects some of my own experience:

> The following scenario takes place too often. A young adult develops symptoms of schizophrenia and is hospitalized in a private psychiatric setting for symptom stabilization and diagnosis. Several additional short-term hospitalizations take place in the first couple of years of unfolding illness until the insurance resources are exhausted (typically a lifetime limit of $30,000 to $50,000). The patient is then at risk for homelessness or custodial hospitalization in a state facility. Premature death by suicide or other concurrent illness is a definite danger. (Sharfstein, 1991, p. 396)

Chapter 2

A Hierarchical Systems Model for Mental Illness

Monism

The new consideration of the problem of schizophrenia and its treatment which I shall propose requires first that we be aware of the problem posed by monistic thinking, the conceptual filter to which I referred in the Introduction, which has determined the shape of most existing schemata for understanding mental illness. Monism in the human sciences is the belief that the phenomena under scrutiny may be exhaustively accounted for by a single science, or, to say it differently, that they may be reduced to the concepts of that science. When considering schizophrenia, for example, monists explicitly assert or implicitly function as though the particular science to which they adhere, be it neuroscience, psychoanalysis, family systems theory, sociology, or cultural anthropology, is sufficient to account for all of the characteristic mental processes. The effect of monistic thinking on the relationships among the human sciences is most starkly represented in the ages-old struggle of philosophy and science to resolve the mind–body problem, currently embodied in the controversy about whether and how material scientific ways of thinking about mind may be reconciled with psychological ones.

Contemporary expressions of monism such as logical positivism and its specific derivative scientific materialism (Huxley, 1898) hold that thoughts and feelings are epiphenomena without intrinsic meaning; by-products of an organic essence, the smoke produced by the fire. Positivists hold that those who regard mind and meaning as existential entities with causal substance are engaging in an illusion, like a primitive tribesman who attributes corporeal essence to the images he sees on a movie screen. They believe that psychoanalytic efforts to comprehend these things are primitive efforts at knowing that will be rendered superfluous and whose prescientific nature will be clearly

revealed once neuroscience has succeeded in identifying the intrinsic underlying organic elements and their scientific relationships. When this reduction
is achieved such disciplines as psychoanalysis will presumably be consumed
and digested, so that their metabolic end-products will be recognizable only to
those with training in the neurosciences. Such reasoning is most commonly
applied to pathological conditions of mind known or suspected to have an
organic substrate, such as schizophrenia, in the course of discussions that
dismiss the importance of psychological theories of etiology and modes of
treatment. But because all mental activity, both the normal variations and the
pathological manifestations, has an organic substrate, and genetic variations
in the nervous system are increasingly suspected in a variety of pathological
conditions hitherto deemed psychological, such as anxiety and obsessive compulsive neurosis (Pardes et al., 1989), and, as twin adoption studies are beginning to suggest, may characterize many normal personality variants, as well,
we may expect to encounter the reductionist position with increasing frequency and stridency in the years to come.

Contemporary pressures to replace psychological models of mind with
organic ones are quite direct in some instances, and subtly disguised in others.
Some neuroscientists are quite blunt about their monistic bias. For instance,
here is how one prominent schizophrenia researcher looks upon psychological
accounts of that illness: "all areas of science have dusty shelves full of discarded theories and schizophrenia research is no exception. They include
psychoanalytic theories. . ." (Torrey, 1988, p. 161). He adds that psychoanalytic ideas about schizophrenia are like "old books on phrenology" (p. 378).
Other neuroscientists are more subtle and sophisticated, and in other contexts
would doubtless defend the intrinsic significance of things such as meaning,
emotion, and relationship. Nonetheless, in their activities as scientists they
perceive such things as insubstantial. For example, the general editor of a
psychiatric monograph series states in the introduction of the most recent
volume that "psychiatry is moving, still relatively slowly, but irresistibly, from
a more philosophical, contemplative orientation to that of an empirical science
. . . *the only framework in which a medical discipline can survive*" (Van Praag,
1992, p. v, italics mine).

The stress model of illness, generally attributed to Cannon (1935) and
Selye (1950), is an example of monistic and reductionistic thinking which is
particularly insidious insofar as it is disguised as an appreciation of psychological forces. It is gaining increasing prominence in general psychiatry, where its
best-known application—the stress-diathesis model—has been to schizophrenia (Zubin & Spring, 1977; Marsella & Snyder, 1981; Gottesman & Shields,
1982; Kringlen, 1987). The stress-diathesis model holds that the biological
diathesis produces enduring traits or vulnerabilities that become activated if
and when predisposing factors in the environment reach a critical threshold.
On close inspection, however, it becomes apparent that stress is defined as a
physical and not a psychological event (Selye, 1956); a state of the organism
secondary to the physical impact of forces which are conceived of as being

qualitatively no different than bacteria, viruses, toxins, injury, and the like. The independent reality and causal significance of psychic factors of meaning and feeling which make events or even thoughts stressful for one individual and not for another is not appreciated. The patient is conceived of as a psychologically unremarkable host who is responding to the physical stress of a generic environmental event such as death of a relative, job loss, a move; that is, an event that would be stressful for all human beings and therefore requires no intervening uniqueness of mind. My point is not to criticize stress models per se, so long as they are accurately represented as neuroscientific. They provide a theoretical rationale for the somatic therapies, as we shall see in Chapter 18. However, I do object to their mis-use to give token service to the importance of mind and the psychological disciplines which attempt to comprehend its workings while in fact dismissing them.

Nor do I mean to imply in the foregoing discussion that monism and reductionistic thinking is a condition which afflicts only and all neuroscientists, to which psychoanalysts (and other human scientists) are immune. Some of the most respected biologists and physicists have been pluralists, for example, MacLean (1985). And conversely and paradoxically Freud appears to have espoused a materialistic monist position early in his career (Jones, 1953), though it is perhaps not quite so surprising if one considers his training as a neuroscientist. For example, in his *Project for a Scientific Psychology*, Freud (1895) wrote, "The intention is to furnish a psychology that shall be a natural science: that is, to represent psychical processes as quantitatively determinate states of specifiable material particles" (p. 295). While Freud eventually came to hold different views he never abandoned this one. In 1914 he suggested that "it is special substances and chemical processes which perform the operations of . . . special psychical forces" (p. 78). Again, in his discussion of the life and death instincts, he states: "The deficiencies in our description would probably vanish if we were already in a position to replace the psychological terms by physiological or chemical ones. . .we may expect it [biology] to give us the most surprising information and we cannot guess what answers it will return in a few dozen years to the questions we have put to it. They may be of a kind which will blow away the whole of our artificial structure of hypothesis" (Freud, 1920, p. 60, parenthetic word mine).

It may come as a further surprise to note that even among contemporary psychoanalysts one may encounter internal inconsistency in the form of paradoxical materialistic, reductionistic beliefs. For example, in Schwartz' 1988 argument in favor of reification he states ". . . that feelings too *are* ultimately neurobiological 'things' " (p. 366, italics mine) and proposes that neuroscience and psychoanalysis should share a common conceptual language. Other expressions of materialistic monism penned by psychoanalysts may be found in contemporary writings about schizophrenia. Grotstein (1990) has proposed a "dual track" hypothesis with which he views schizophrenia simultaneously as a state of organic pathology and a meaningful psychological disturbance. However, his position appears to be organic reductionistic in that he believes the core mental experience in schizophrenia, which he depicts as a sense of nothingness, a nameless dread, a sense of chaos, and calls a "black hole" experience, is actually an absence of mentation or a psychological vacuum corresponding to the organic level deficit. Willick (1990) goes further, and seems convinced that schizophrenia is an organic illness whose mental manifestations are meaningless. He claims that negative symptoms "are most likely caused by a primary biological disturbance. . . . Other symptoms do appear to be a consequence of regression brought about by the illness disrupting the mental organization . . . reactions to or attempts to deal with the trauma of the dimly perceived but poorly understood organic deficiencies" (pp. 1067–1068).

Moreover, by denying the immediate relevance of the impressive array of neuroscientific findings about the origin and nature of mental activity, normal and pathological, to their theoretical beliefs and clinical practice, many psychoanalysts (who, if directly asked, would certainly affirm the importance of the neurosciences) are thinking monistically. In this context Grotstein's work, just alluded to, stands out as a conscious effort to reject monism, albeit in my estimation an unsuccessful one. The findings of neuroscience have yet to make any significant impact on psychoanalytic theory, which continues to rest more or less uneasily on the postulate of a common biological and psychological beginning for everyone—*the* psychic apparatus—and of a single developmental line stemming therefrom, punctuated by an idiosyncratic profile of arrest, fixation, and regression.

Furthermore, when we turn to psychoanalysis' relationship with such higher order disciplines (in the sense of levels of organization) as the social psychologies (interpersonal and family systems), sociology, and cultural anthropology, we discover that psychoanalysts often tend to be monists, at times blithely utilizing intrapsychic psychoanalytic theory to analyze interpersonal and social phenomena and at other times implying that these phenomena are reducible to intrapsychic representations of relations among objects. This is a subtle assertion that the phenomenal world is nothing but a figment of the mind, a state of affairs that would render these other disciplines superfluous.

The Fallacy of Monism

Monistic and reductionistic thinking in the human sciences is now generally discredited (see, for example, the Koestler & Smythies, 1969, summary of the 1968 Alpbach symposium; Sperry, 1969; Popper & Eccles, 1981). Earlier in the century the natural sciences discarded it as inadequate to the complexity of their task. The achievement of the simplest reduction—of chemistry to physics—is now more or less conceded to be impossible. Physics developed principles of relativity and uncertainty instead, and biologists turned to General Systems Theory. Belief in the sufficiency of a single conceptual system is based on linear causal thinking and the fallacious equation of analysis with synthesis, that is, the belief that the process of analysis or deconstruction of a complex phenomenon into component parts is reversible. It does not take into account that nature consists of complex dynamic systems that are related not by simple reduction but by a process of hierarchical transformation or reorganization or emergence along dimensions of evolution, development, or magnification. Laplace contended that it should be possible to predict the entire future of the universe from a thorough analytic knowledge of all of its parts. However, higher levels of system organization cannot be constructed or predicted from the array of their discretely analyzable constituents; in the process of analysis something essential is lost. The biologist-philosopher Paul Weiss (1977) has put it succinctly and elegantly: "The study of parts—analytical information about parts—paid off magnificently as long as we indulged primarily in learning more and more about less and less, relying on the ingrained conviction that from the parts of that diminutival knowledge we would be able to reconstruct, 'synthesize' (at least in our mind) the typically patterned order of the phenomenon that we had deliberately disordered in our analytical procedure as if we could resurrect the phoenix from its ashes" (p. 24). More concretely, the physicist Neils Bohr (1937) notes that the linear reductionistic study of life, taken to its extreme, literally destroys its subject.

Nozick (1981) points out that logical positivist and scientific materialist or reductionist accounts of the human being are not only philosophically and scientifically unsound, but also morally bankrupt. "In devaluing people, the reductionist violates the principle that everything is to be treated as having the value it has. Reductionism is not simply a theoretical mistake, it is a moral failing (p. 631)." By reducing the diversity, complexity, and richness of the phenomenal world, reductionists devalue human life and experience.

Naive Interactionism

If we reject monoscientistic and monotheoristic solutions to the problems I have outlined then we are confronted with a whole new set of problems: Intersystemically, when we appreciate the validity and importance of viewpoints and data from various scientific disciplines we implicitly assume the task of integrating very different theoretical languages, methodologies, and forms of data. Intrasystemically (within the theoretical system of a given science) we are confronted with the problem of determining which areas require new models or theories, and constructing ones that can systematically co-exist. The intrasystemic problem of constructing new but compatible models (as physics has done) within psychoanalytic theory for phenomena, such as schizophrenia, that have been refractory to adequate explanation by the classical model is examined in Chapter 8.

Wittingly or otherwise, most of us confront this problem daily in our work, during clinical case discussions or difficult points in an individual treatment. Reluctant to abandon the insights and techniques of any field that seems of pragmatic value in a given case, but unable to resolve more fundamental issues about how different scientific theories and technologies relate to one another, we engage in naive interactionism, additive thinking, or conceptual grafting, mixing neuroscientific, psychoanalytic, family systems, and social psychological terminology as though these share a common theoretical base. It is like knowing that the combustion of gasoline in an automobile engine activates the pistons which turn the crankshaft. This is important practical information for the auto mechanic, but as applied science or technology it overlooks the fact that the languages of two distinctive disciplines—physical chemistry and physics—are being treated as undifferentiated and miscible. Pragmatically useful as this may sometimes be, such hybridized reasoning is no more theoretically sound than monism. It is really a form of applied science or technology, and it overlooks crucial distinctions between hierarchical levels of organization and the theoretical or scientific systems which account for them.

The common clinical and sometimes scientific practice of speaking as though the forces conceptualized at one system level, usually a lower one such as neuroscience, may act in a linear causal fashion within a system conceptualized at a different level, usually higher, such as behavior and thinking, represents such a fallacy. It is called upward and downward causation (Sperry, 1969; Campbell, 1974). While the fallacy of upward causation is now better appreciated than it once was, similarly fallacious reasoning is currently embodied in the concepts of downward causation and transduction (Delbruck, 1970; Weiner, 1970, 1972) to account for the observed fact of neural plasticity; namely, that experience, including pathogenic environmental "stress" and psychological therapies, appears to structurally modify the central nervous system.

Hierarchical Systems Theory

I should like to propose an alternative to monistic forms of thinking and to the naive interactionistic perspective most of us resort to daily in order to free ourselves from its constraints: a supraordinate or metatheoretical structure or viewpoint that respects pluralism in the human sciences. In the pages that follow I shall address the question of how this hierarchical systems model provides for systematic relations among the human sciences, and in Chapter 8 I examine how it also creates space for internal expansion of psychoanalytic theory to encompass multiple and interdigitating theoretical models of the mind such as are necessary to embrace such extremes of pathology as the neuroses and schizophrenia.

The concepts I shall describe represent the confluence of historical roots from several disciplines. To my knowledge they are first encountered within the field of medicine and the organic approach to pathology in the 19th century work of Hughlings Jackson (1931–1932), who suggested that organisms are integrated in a hierarchical series of increasingly complex neural levels, and that in the course of development the expression of lower levels is progressively inhibited by the functioning of higher ones. Jackson utilized this ontogenetic hierarchical model to construct an hypothesis about schizophrenia which has resurfaced in the last decade or so as the distinction between so-called positive and negative symptoms (Crow, 1980).

In the early part of the 20th century, Adolph Meyer (1957) took the next step and introduced the concept of "psychobiology" to denote that human beings are meaningfully integrated at a mental level as well as a neurobiological one. He believed that phenomena characteristic of one level, such as the organic, may affect events and processes at other levels, such as the mental.

Although I have suggested that Freud was in some respects a monistic thinker, as with so many things in the complexity of his mind he also anticipated developments in systems theory. He was aware of Jackson's work and he conceived of a transformational hierarchy of systems both neurological and psychological with recurring analogous structures.

> The physiological events do not cease as soon as the psychological ones begin; on the contrary, the physiological chain continues. What happens is simply that, after a certain point in time, each (or some) of its links has a psychical phenomenon corresponding to it. Accordingly, the psychical is a process parallel to the physiological—a "dependent concomitant." (Freud, 1915a, p. 207)

Toward the end of his life Freud (1940) restated this position:

> We know two kinds of things about what we call our psyche (or mental life): firstly, its bodily organ and scene of action, the brain (or nervous system), and, on the other hand, our acts of consciousness, which are immediate data and cannot be further explained by any sort of description. Everything that lies between is unknown to us, and the data do not include any direct relation between these two terminal points of our knowledge. If it existed, it would at the most afford an exact localization of the processes of consciousness and would give us no help towards understanding them. (p. 144)

Freud's concept of metapsychology may also be seen as an acknowledgment of the importance of a variety of systems or perspectives within psychoanalysis.

The approach I propose is most closely related to what is popularly known as General Systems Theory and attributed to the biologist-philosopher Ludwig von Bertalanffy (1952, 1967a, b, 1968). More accurately, systems philosophy is the creation during the 1920s and 1930s of a group comprising prominent German biologists and including persons from disciplines as disparate as fiction writing (Arthur Koestler), psychology (Heinz Werner, 1940), particularly the Gestalt school (Perls, Hefferline, & Goodman, 1951), and physics (Heisenberg, 1958). The biologist Paul Weiss, whose earliest published writing on the subject, a paper first published in 1925 and translated into English and republished in 1959, slightly antedates the work of von Bertalanffy, is for me the most articulate spokesperson of this group.

Systems theory begins with recognition of the insufficiency of the linear summation of parts model of the human sciences, which is at the root of monistic thinking, with its implicitly mechanistic and reductionistic description of life. Von Bertalanffy (1967b) asserts that "compared to the analytical procedure of classical science, with 'linear' causality connecting two variables as basic category, the investigation of organized wholes of many variables requires new categories of interaction. . . . This leads to a 'perspective philosophy' . . . reality is a hierarchy of organized wholes" (p. 14). As Weiss (1977) puts it, "the ordered state (organization) of a living entity can, therefore, not be conceived of as the blind outcome of microprecisely defined serial cause–effect chain reactions, as in an assembly plant" (p. 29). The physicist Neils Bohr (1937) introduced what he called the principle of complementarity in an attempt to apply Heisenberg's uncertainty principle to the human sciences, and argues for the separate study of the human as a system. Von Bertalanffy (1968) proposes that living systems ". . . maintain themselves in a state of high order and improbability, or may even evolve toward increasing differentiation and organization as is the case in organismic development and evolution" (pp. 143–144). He uses the concept "anamorphosis" to describe the progressive differentiation and reorganization of biological systems at hierarchically higher levels into wholes that cannot be accounted for by summing their parts. He emphasizes that his use of terms such as higher and lower orders or levels simply denotes differences in perspective, not in importance or validity. This observation is most germane to the current reductionist dispute between neuroscientists and psychologists. Paul Weiss writes that nature is ordered as a hierarchical continuum in which more complex, larger units are supraordinate to less complex, smaller ones. He uses the terms larger and smaller in the same way von Bertalanffy used higher and lower. His comment that "it is one thing not to see the forest for the trees, but then to go on to deny the reality of the forest is a more serious matter, for it is not just a case of myopia, but one of self-inflicted blindness" (1969, p. 11), could serve as a cautionary note for contemporary reductionists.

In other words, we may view the human sciences on a hierarchical systems continuum from molecular biology (a term Weiss introduced) to, let us say, cultural anthropology. Weiss (1969) points out that "all living phenomena consists of group behavior" (p. 8), hence, all theories deal with the integration and interrelationships among differentiated phenomenal aspects or elements. The physicist Werner Heisenberg (1958) sums up the matter succinctly and reiterates that the primary focus in any human systems analysis involving mental phenomena (not epiphenomena!) must be at that level:

> The degree of complication in biology is so discouraging that one can at present not
> imagine any set of concepts in which the connections could be so sharply defined

that a mathematical presentation could become possible. If we go beyond biology and include psychology in the discussion, then there can scarcely be any doubt but that the concepts of physics, chemistry, and evolution together will not be sufficient to describe the facts. On this point the existence of quantum theory has changed our attitude from what was believed in the nineteenth century. . . . We would, in spite of the fact that the physical events in the brain belong to the psychic phenomena, not expect that these could be sufficient to explain them. We would never doubt that the brain acts as a physical-chemical mechanism if treated as such; but for an understanding of psychic phenomena we would start from the fact that the human mind enters as object and subject into the scientific process of psychology. (pp. 105–106)

More recently the concept of systems as dynamic groups in transformation has been given new life in the form of what was first called Chaos theory (Gleick, 1987) and more recently is being renamed as "complexity" theory (Spruiell, 1993). In the process, and with the advent of computers and the discovery by Mandelbrot (1977) of fractal geometry, Heisenberg's pessimism that complex systems are susceptible to mathematical analysis is also being called into question.

Ramifications of General Systems Theory, Meyerian psychobiology, and even complexity theory, have begun to penetrate psychiatry, in its interface with general medicine (Engel, 1977, 1980), and psychoanalysis (Gedo & Goldberg, 1973; Moran, 1991; Spruiell, 1993). I shall discuss its intrasystemic impact on psychoanalysis in Chapter 8. George Engel (1977, 1980) focused on the interscientific problem in his role as a medical-psychiatric liaison physician and proposed a hierarchical schema known as the biopsychosocial model. However, Engel was primarily interested in teaching the relevance of psychoanalytic ideas to physicians working with organically ill patients, and although his biopsychosocial model possesses some of the formal characteristics of a hierarchical systems theory, for the most part it has been used simply to affirm the importance of a psychological level of understanding in persons with a coexisting but distinctive organic illness rather than to suggest that the very same disease process may be simultaneously conceptualized at different hierarchical levels. What I mean is well illustrated in the instance of schizophrenia, a condition which Engel did not study with his model. His thinking has become the basis for what is nowadays popularly known as the biopsychosocial approach to schizophrenia, which is based on what I consider to be a crucial misunderstanding both of Engel's apparent intent and of the nature of schizophrenia, involving the monistic belief that it is a purely organic disease, albeit one with psychological ramifications to the personality. Biopsychosocialists remain convinced that the understanding and treatment of schizophrenia is based on an organic model, but affirm the importance of comprehending its psychological effects on the coping mechanisms of an otherwise relatively normal host, and treating these with a kind of supportive, cognitive, behavior modification psychotherapy. In this sense the schizophrenic is treated no differently than the presumably normal person afflicted with a heart condition. The model I shall propose, by contrast, asserts that psychopathology does not *exist* concretely at any single level, therefore that no single science has a monopoly on its comprehension and treatment, but it may be viewed with equal validity from a hierarchy of systems and the sciences which conceptualize them, and the different viewpoints may be mutually enriching. For example, the growing body of neuroscience knowledge about constitutional vulnerability may help the psychoanalyst to construct a different model of the schizophrenic psyche, at the same time that psychological observations of basic schizophrenic weakness of affinity both for integrating his own thoughts and for relating to others may assist the neuroscientist in the search for particular uniquely organized aspects of the central nervous system (Robbins, 1992).

Hierarchical systems theory deals with the organization of the human world, including the individual and his society and culture, into discontinuous but sequentially related dynamic entities or systems. Hierarchical systems are characterized by the qualities of transformation and emergence. The elements of a lower level system are essential to the emergence and continuity of a higher level one, but are not sufficient to account for it. In general, new and unique principles of structure, organization, meaning, and function characterize each level of a system hierarchy. Integration and differentiation seem to be processes crucial to such transformations and assemblages. As Weiss (1969) describes it, "hierarchical concepts of organization . . . imply some sort of discontinuity encountered as one crosses interfaces between lower and higher orders of magnitude (p. 8)." Each level of organization, from the microscopic to the macroscopic, depends on its predecessor but is theoretically autonomous and free-standing, based on new principles of structure, function, and meaning that can be neither predicted from that predecessor nor entirely reduced to it. Systems may be arranged in hierarchies according to successive transformations or reorganizations along the continua or dimensions of time (growth, development, evolution), magnitude (based on observational perspective, vantage point), and complexity, or level of concreteness-abstraction. Human systems tend to resist entropy and maintain themselves in a state of equilibrium or homeostasis or cohesion, solving routine problems and self-adjusting in the process; in addition, they may creatively evolve or transform themselves into other systems of higher order. This implies the presence of an energic factor.

Let us turn from some characteristics of systems themselves to issues that arise in the study and theory of systems. Hierarchical systems theory defines the sciences and their associated methodologies which are applicable to any given entity or whole, in this instance the human being, and studies the structure and function of each system or level, the principles and processes of transformation and reorganization at successive levels, and the nature of the interdependency of one level with another. One may observe a given system from a given perspective over time, whether one is a neurobiologist observing the function of an organ system, a psychologist observing human development, a therapist observing the evolution of a family system, a biologist observing evolution, or a cultural anthropologist observing social change. Or one may study a human being, normal or pathological, holding the element of time constant, and may observe the hierarchical layering of systems on such dimensions as field size (magnification) or concreteness-abstraction. This is accomplished by successively using the different conceptual lenses peculiar to different sciences such as molecular biology, neurobiology, neurochemistry, psychoanalysis (intrapsychic psychology), interpersonal psychology, family systems, sociology, and cultural anthropology. In each instance the observations yield a hierarchy of systems with unique structure and organization that are neither reducible to lower levels nor predictable from them. Knowledge of one systems level yields indispensable information about the parameters, possibilities, and limitations of the next, much as the foundation of a building establishes certain parameters for the superstructure, but there are no simple predictive or reconstructive-reductive rules of transition, transduction, or translation, and the very definition of the transition as novel seems to preclude any traditional understanding of the transition by principles of linear casuality or assembly, directing us instead to the realm of creativity, which still remains the basic reasoning process of all sciences.

The person, comprehended by psychoanalytic theory but also by the lower level neurosciences and higher level interpersonal, group dynamic, and sociological theories simultaneously represents a holistic reintegration of elements from the organismic hierarchy and a differentiated element in still higher order social entities. Weiss (1969) says, "what the 'level' we are speaking of signifies is really the level of attention of an observer whose interest has been attracted by certain regularities of pattern prevailing at that level, as he scans across the range of orders of magnitude ... as he would turn a microscope from lower to higher" (p. 16).

A condition such as schizophrenia can be conceptualized using such a metatheory from multiple frames of reference, ranging from particle physics to biology, psychological theory, interpersonal and family dynamic theories, sociology, or cultural anthropology, depending on one's purpose at the moment. While such a pluralistic viewpoint is heuristically and pragmatically useful, as I shall demonstrate in Parts II and III; conceptualization of schizophrenia as a hierarchical series of transformations and reorganizations of fundamental phenomena at various levels is also a very different way to think of the illness. When we myopically immerse ourselves in but a single one of these levels, our knowledge of schizophrenia is bound to be limited in critically important ways, like the blind man's concept of the elephant. When we utilize a hierarchical systems model schizophrenia appears not so much to be a one dimensional, concrete process as a multidimensional and relativistic one which may be viewed from many windows.

Parameters and Constraints of Hierarchical Systems

From the perspective of systems theory, monistic and reductionistic thinking may be thought of as an aberration of systemic energy and cognition. In the intersystemic realm this means that the curiosity of investigators operating within a given scientific discipline does not remain confined to the particular system under consideration, where it might exhaustively express itself studying all human phenomena from the perspective of that system, but instead degenerates into a combination of greed and sloppy thinking about the boundaries between systems and their concepts, leading to misinformed and disrespectful efforts to consume and destroy adjacent higher order systems.

In the intrasystemic realm monistic thinking tends to express itself in a similar manner, but whereas in the intersystemic realm one encounters a variety of sciences to begin with so that the only recourse of a monist is to deny the existence of the others or to claim they are unnecessary and insubstantial because they deal with epiphenomena, an individual science is more likely to begin modestly, with a single theory, as did physics and indeed psychoanalysis as well, and manifest an inflexible resistant attitude toward the development of multiple models even when the classical model seems inadequate to the task of accounting for all observable phenomena.

The theories of contiguous hierarchical systems, such as neuroscience and psychoanalysis in the intersystemic hierarchy, must conform to certain parameters and respect certain constraints. While there is no a priori limit to the phenomena for which a given system can account, each system must respect the autonomy of its hierarchical neighbor and be compatible with it. The concepts and principles of organization that characterize each level are unique, meaning that lower levels cannot predict or consume higher ones and knowledge of higher ones is insufficient to reconstruct lower ones, but at the same time the principles of a higher level must be comprehensible in terms of those of the lower level.

Psychology in a System Hierarchy: Psychoanalysis' Intersystemic Relations

The presence of a neurobiological substrate to all behavior and thought, both that which characterizes the spectrum of so-called normal variability and that which we think of as psychopathological, and the necessity of encouraging vigorous neuroscientific theory making and data gathering even in sometimes mistakenly hallowed areas such as emotion, aesthetics, soul, theology, and even psychotherapy should be beyond dispute. But no matter how exhaustive and successful such investigations may ultimately be, they can never be sufficient to comprehend the unique psychological level of organization which depends on but cannot be reduced to a more atomistic neurobiological substrate. We must beware the misconception that neuroscience explanations are causally sufficient, for it leads to devaluation of the separate and autonomous realms of psychology and meaning. Conversely, providing an adequate psychological explanation of a person's character and problems in no way precludes that there is an equally valid and useful explanation of these things at the neuroscientific level.

What are the parameters of psychoanalysis within a hierarchical systems schema and what constraints are placed upon it? First and foremost, the theories of psychoanalysis must be compatible with (or, at minimum, not incompatible with) lower level neuroscientific systems and their findings. Psychoanalysis must take into account that all individuals are not created equal or endowed by their creators with a uniform or in the case of some forms of psychopathology even similiar psychological constitution. Classical psychoanalytic theory assumes constitutional and environmental configurations more or less common to all human beings: the instinctual drive derivatives, possibly varying in intensity, a psychic apparatus, perhaps with variations in ego "strength," and certain paradigmatic infantile experiences. The assumption of uniformity may not be a problem so long as psychoanalysis confines itself more or less to neurotic patients, whose similarities far outweigh their differences, and whose differences may satisfactorily be accounted for by postulating relatively minor (but to the individual significant) differences in early experience, or in drive strength, ego strength, and wish or fantasy configuration. Such assumptions, however, are not adequate to the challenge posed by more disturbed persons, for example, schizophrenics. I suspect in the long run they may not prove so satisfactory even for our understanding of neurotic patients.

Earlier I noted how Freud anticipated the importance of a hierarchical systems perspective for psychoanalysis. More specifically, he also wondered about the reasons for choice of one type of neurosis rather than another, and he proposed, but did not develop, the concept of a complemental series, in which the interaction of a hereditary predisposition with early infantile experience produces a fixation point and a susceptibility to later adult experience (1916, p. 362). In 1905 he wrote, "The constitutional factor must await experiences before it can make itself felt; the accidental factor must have a constitutional basis in order to come into operation" (p. 239). In 1913 he said that factors determining the specific choice of a neurosis "are in the nature of (hereditary) dispositions and are independent of experiences which operate pathogenically" (p. 317).

From a hierarchical systems perspective the contribution of neurobiology that is of significance for psychoanalytic theory, elaborated in Chapter 6, is that there are one or more genotypes that predispose toward schizophrenia. From a psychoanalytic vantage point the schizophrenic must attempt to negotiate the same developmental tasks and milestones, and respond to the same social and interpersonal stresses as do others, but their *meaning* to him and his *mode of resolution* of them may differ as the constitutional differences in his psychic makeup interact with his experiences with primary caretakers (who are themselves, in varying degrees and styles, normal and pathological). Parents of constitutionally vulnerable children face an extraordinary challenge, which we might expect them to cope with in ways consistent with their unique configurations of capability and limitation. Phenotypic (characterological) vulnerability emerges in the context of primary parenting that is not good enough, and that exploits rather than repairs the emerging mental manifestations of specific genetic weakness. In other instances, since studies summarized in Chapter 6 indicate that genetic predisposition alone is by no means sufficient to produce clinical schizophrenia, and since the brain is a plastic organ which may be structurally modified, for good or for ill, by life experience, constitutionally vulnerable children probably grow up to be relatively normal, perhaps in some instances even exceptional, because of the healing influence of unusually devoted and creative parents.

Neuroscience has commanded so much attention of late that it is easy to overlook the fact that psychoanalysis also has systems relationships with social psychology, including interpersonal psychology and family systems; as well as with sociology and cultural anthropology. In each of these, in contrast to its position with regard to the neurosciences, psychoanalysis is the lower level discipline in the hierarchy. Important as it is to comprehend individual human personalities, it cannot be expected that such knowledge will suffice to explain higher level social and cultural phenomena. Just as neuroscientists are increasingly becoming aware that a sophisticated knowledge of mental functioning may be required to generate useful neuroscientific hypotheses, for example, about conditions such as schizophrenia (MacLean, 1985), so it is more than likely that observations from these higher order disciplines may ultimately enrich psychoanalysis. I have alluded to two such areas: the effects of various forms of psychopathological parenting both singly (the dyad) and multiply (the family system) on the psychic apparatus and developmental pathway, and the effects of major cultural variants on individual development and normative pathology. If it appears that I am suggesting a form of downward causality which I just denounced as a fallacy, I reiterate that the effects of culture, for example, must simultaneously be conceptualized within their own system (cultural anthropology) and as forces acting within the conceptual confines of other systems, for example, individual psychology, and even neural organization (perhaps through the mediation of the limbic system; see MacLean, 1990, and Weiger & Bear, 1988).

The remainder of the book may be viewed as a detailed application of hierarchical systems theory to the comprehension and treatment of schizophrenia. We shall see the remarkable ways in which the core illness process is creatively transformed and reorganized at multiple systems levels, and how one level both reverberates with, reorganizes, and compensates for disturbances of organization at the preceding one. Before embarking on this journey, I should like to note one fundamental consequence of having to abandon the single-window view of schizophrenia to which we have become accustomed—in this age most likely that of neuroscience—for a multiple systems perspective: it may surprise us to find that some of the basic questions we have about the illness—its essence, when does it begin, what are the variables which exacerbate or ameliorate it—may yield very different answers depending upon the discipline or perspective in the scientific hierarchy from which we choose to address them, and that these answers may become yet more complex if we attempt to correlate the findings of one level with those of another.

Chapter 3

Data and Methodology

The data for this book come from existing research and theory from the various human sciences and from my personal clinical experience with schizophrenics, which ranges from administrating mental hospital wards, evaluating countless patients, and, especially, treating patients with a multimodal approach in which psychoanalytic psychotherapy, hospital treatment, family therapy and neuroleptic medication are central ingredients. This experience is summarized in Chapter 13 and illustrated in the five detailed case reports that constitute the clinical substance of this book.

The psychological self, or person, is the central focus of inquiry in this book. From it other inquiries commence, both macroscopic (interpersonal, social, cultural) and microscopic (neuroscientific), and to it they ultimately return. Hence, the psychological case report is the central datum, not replacing the quantitative, statistically enumerable data of the experimental scientist but helping to order it at its most meaningful level. Much as most of us like to read case reports, and may lament their absence from books and papers on theory and treatment, there is widespread skepticism with regard to their objectivity and validity, to say nothing of their scientific value. So before proceeding to the substance of the book it is necessary to review thorny questions concerning whether a focus on the whole person is scientifically meaningful, whether case reports constitute suitable data, and how they might best be presented and interpreted.

The Whole Person or Individual Case and the Two-Variable Cause–Effect Experiment Using a Large Statistical Sample

Making the study of the whole person, conceived of as a complex dynamic system, the central focus of inquiry is consistent with the hierarchical systems model proposed in Chapter 2, and with the modern science and mathematics of systems known as Complexity theory. I hope to recast the controversy between the clinician and the statistical scientist from a heated polemic between right and wrong to a more reflective question of intention and focus, just as we would not assert that the electronic microscopic view of a phenomenon is right and the wide angle photographic view wrong, but would ask about the purpose for which each was to be used.

In few areas is it more apparent than in schizophrenia research that there is an intimate relationship between the hypotheses generated by the dominant theoretical model, the research strategy employed, the selection of data to investigate the hypotheses, and the conclusions derived therefrom that seem to corroborate the model. While this phenomenon may be more evident in the case of the psychoanalytic theorist who simultaneously conducts a clinical treatment and attempts to utilize it as an example of his theory, it is at least equally true of statistical research. The researcher who gathers data from a model which holds that schizophrenia is not distinguishable from the personality of the sufferer reaches entirely different conclusions about the nature of relevant data (intimate knowledge of the personality of the patient) and methodology (participant observation) than does the researcher who believes that disease and personality are distinctive and unrelated entities. Statistical studies generated by a traditional medical model generally seek to quantify signs and symptoms of illness as dependent variables. Attention to personality, feelings, and complex mental processes, except with regard to such gross variables as stress or compliance, is deemed unnecessary. The data from which conclusions are drawn consist of fragments or bits of information with a concrete, measurable quality. This entire process and way of thinking not only reflects and reifies the theoretical preconception of the illness as a physical process, but strikingly parallels the Bleulerian conception of schizophrenia as a disease characterized by mental fragmentation, thought concreteness, an autistic or unrelated world, and absent affect. In other words, there is a circular, closed, internally reinforcing relationship between the hypotheses and methods of medical-statistical research and the conclusions it reaches about the nature of schizophrenia, which are presented as being objective. (Later, particularly in Chapter 11, I speculate on the basis of this observation that the hypotheses and methods employed in much of the currently fashionable medical-statistical research into schizophrenia may be sociocultural reflections of the disease process itself disguised as its objectification and treatment.)

The clinical data from a single analyst's sample are considered by the statistical scientist, who accumulates numerically large samples in the course of testing a hypothesis, neither sufficiently objective to be valid nor sufficiently numerous as to constitute an adequate sample. From the vantage point of the analyst, however, the statistical scientist operating within the medical research model and its linear causal framework sacrifices the experience of the richness, abstraction, affectivity, and interwoven complexity of human life in order to achieve what may be the illusion of certitude. Most of the specimens or samples collected by the clinical, descriptive or anecdotal researcher are so conceptually complex that they defy quantitative enumeration, at least with currently available methods.

While there are significant differences between the hard "scientific" and the more subjective, impressionistic clinical psychological approaches, in some respects distinctions commonly made between the two may be more apparent than real. The belief that the data of the statistical researcher is more valid and reliable because it represents a large sample of schizophrenics whereas the descriptive researcher is reporting on one, or at best, a few cases may not bear close scrutiny. The statistical researcher sacrifices depth of experience with patients and with the illness in question for what, in return, may be a very superficial (and hence quite possibly distorted) knowledge of his "statistically significant sample." This may be even more true of research on psychotic patients than with statistical research using other subjects, for the researcher often relies on subjective reporting of data and the schizophrenic subject tends to be mistrustful or suspicious of others, including the experimenter, not to mention being a notoriously unreliable observer and reporter of self and external world. Moreover, data for quantitative studies are usually obtained from patients who have been treated and "normalized" into at least the semblance of a cooperative state with neuroleptic medication, raising further questions about the validity of the data and suggesting the possibility that the research conclusions are artifactual to the treatment process. The empirical researcher may have gathered through superficial and casual contact a very little bit of data about a large number of cases, and his findings should be viewed with at least the degree of healthy skepticism he himself directs toward the psychological clinician. One might make the case that the clinical investigator who has studied a relatively few cases in great depth has at least as much accurate information about schizophrenia as does the empirical researcher, though, like the blind man and the elephant, his perspective is unique. Knowledge acquired primarily from in-depth psychological studies of schizophrenics is different from that of the medical-statistical researcher, not necessarily better or worse, but definitely richer and more complex, and for that reason if for no other is worthy of presentation.

But it is also inaccurate to infer that the breadth of the clinical research experience from which I have drawn the sample of five cases presented in this book is limited to and identical with those cases. These cases were selected because they are typical examples of a much larger clinical experience with schizophrenics—an experience spanning 30 years of running wards and doing consultations, evaluations, and supervision, as well as treatment—not because they seem unique or even atypical. They are, in their own way, a meaningful, if not statistically legitimatized, sample.

Enumerative and Eliminative Inductivism

Adducing multiple instances of a phenomenon in a single case (and, better still, in multiple cases) to support a hypothesis is the process of enumerative inductivism, or what Grunbaum (1984) refers to as the "tally argument" of psychoanalysis. Many, including Grunbaum, Popper (1962), and Edelson (1984, 1988), have raised doubts that simply tallying positive instances is sufficient to confirm a hypotheses, but there is no doubt it can make it more or less probable. Reviewing several cases in depth brings with it the opportunity to discover inconsistent or disconfirming ideas and phenomena, particularly when, as in this book, some of the cases are deliberately chosen to illustrate failure of a particular approach to treatment. This is the closest we can come to eliminating alternative explanations and the effect of spurious variables. This process is referred to as eliminative inductivism. To some extent the actual operation of these processes in my thinking must be inferred by the reader since I present the cases and the theory and technique separately, although reference is made throughout the book to case material as illustration and support for some hypotheses and in refutation of others. For example, I use enumerative inductivism to refute the hypothesis that schizophrenia is an adult illness that arises in a previously normal individual and his family.

How the Data Were Gathered

If the data-gathering process is seriously flawed, then it hardly matters how rigorously canons of scientific reasoning are applied to analyze the results. Typically, the author of hypotheses illustrated with clinical material is suspected of having confounded and confused his beliefs and inferences with his so-called data. So the reader will doubtless want to know more about how I acquired the data that make up the substance of the book, how valid it might be, and how I went about preparing the case reports. In the 10-minute break between the end of one therapeutic hour and the commencement of the next, I type a summary of the session just completed, which is a few sentences to half a page or more in length. I attempt to capture the themes and sequences of the material, and as much of the specifics as I can recall to illustrate them. These include the state of the patient's relatedness to me and to his inner life, unusual comments and gestures, dream and fantasy content, and thematic sequences. No doubt the material is colored by my memory distortions, as well as by my theoretical biases and interests of the moment. However, I have been training myself to do this for about 30 years, and I sometimes check the accuracy of my memory against the content of tape recordings, to say nothing of the feedback provided by my patients in subsequent sessions. To supplement my own material and check some of its accuracy of detail and sequence I have carefully reviewed the extensive hospital records of each of the five patients whose cases I present, including notes by nursing staff, social worker, and psychiatric administrator, as well as summaries of review conferences in which input from consultants was obtained.

How the Reports Were Written

In preparing the cases for this book, I made successive condensations from the large books of notes I accumulated on each patient and from hospital records. I was surprised at the richness of detail of the raw data. The new connections and meanings I discovered in the course of reviewing material gathered as much as 20 or more years ago impressed me, at least, that in taking the notes I had been doing much more than codifying my own biases and theories.

Problems Inherent in Condensing and Reporting Clinical Data

The problems in the study of schizophrenia that confront both the quantitative scientist and the psychological investigator are related to the failure of integration and differentiation that are characteristic of this illness and we will return to them again and again throughout the book. The statistical scientist elects to view the phenomenology of schizophrenia as a collection of linear, causally related pieces or elements, whereas the humanistic scientist, whose primary focus is on the psychology of the schizophrenic self attempts to map interrelationships among elements constituting a large and complex entity that can be viewed in multiple dimensions, through multiple sensory-perceptual modalities, and at many levels of magnification. Each method has advantages and problems. However reassuring we may find its concrete data, arranged in linear causal patterns, the quantitative approach enhances discontinuity or fragmentation of a complex phenomenon and is ill equipped to perceive and comprehend its patterning and organization. In the case of schizophrenia, such an approach is consonant with the failure of integration that is characteristic of the illness to begin with. And it reflects the assumption, which I have already questioned, that the disease is indeed separate from meaningful organization of the personalty of the host.

In the process of attending to the larger picture of personality organization the psychologically focused scientist who compiles intensive case studies encounters a very different manifestation of the problem of integration and differentiation, namely, the tendency to impose on the material a false sense of coherence and meaning. In the condensation process there is a certain inevitable imposition of sense, which may not be inherent in the raw material. Both the author and the readers of case reports think of them as stories or narratives, and, in doing so, assume the existence of whole or integrated "characters," psychologically differentiated from one another, as well as thematic coherence (a plot) and a course of events (or a sequence of scenes and acts). In schizophrenia, where the self is fragmented and incoherent and not well differentiated from the selves of others, such assumptions may be unwarranted, especially in the early stages of treatment. Does the narrative that emerges after smoothing infinite jagged edges and discontinuities of schizophrenic unintegration and undifferentiation—the countless changes during each treatment hour in words, actions, gestures, facial expressions, and affects—have a misleading coherence and meaningfulness that reflects the organizing theoretical beliefs of the storyteller-clinician more than the uniqueness of the patient?

Some of these problems of condensing and presenting a lengthy treatment case may be illuminated by the new mathematics of fractal geometry (Mandelbrot, 1977). In a paper entitled "How Long Is the Coast of Britain?" Mandelbrot's answer is either that it is infinite in length or that its length is dependent on the measuring scale utilized. The closer one looks at the coastline, or the finer one's measuring device, adjusting from the macroscopic aerial view to the microscopic or submicroscopic level, the more the result approaches infinity. This phenomenon of infinite length imbedded within a finite area is known as a Koch curve. In one sense the notion of mapping a coastline is a technological-scientific fiction, albeit in another it remains not only useful but even essential to comprehending reality and making order out of chaos. If we accept the necessity and the scientific validity of the mapping enterprise, whether it be of a coastline or of a psychological therapy, even as we recognize that the result is inevitably in some sense a fiction, it is important that we ask ourselves questions about the purpose of the map (in the case of the coastline it may relate to topics as diverse as auto travel, fishing, or the construction of harbors) and that we be aware of the scale employed to actualize that purpose.

In my construction of the reports that constitute the clinical data of this book, I set out to condense 1,000 to 1,200 therapy hours. It seemed necessary, for reasons of economy of space and adherence to the generally accepted conventions of comprehensibility and story telling, to eliminate redundancy and repetition, chaotic or stray thoughts, and meanderings, distractions, and disruptions that did not seem of significance to me. But perhaps what seemed irrelevant or chaotic to me might have contained the essence of the matter for you. As I condensed the clinical data, reports took shape that convey more of a sense of flow, thematic continuity, meaning, purpose and progress than I experienced at any moment in these lengthy treatments.

I would like to illustrate with the cases of Emily and Celia, which represent the extremes of length in this book. I have had occasion to present the case of Emily orally to many different audiences. As it is difficult to find a forum for an oral presentation that is much longer than an hour, I was constrained to streamline the presentation. As a result, the report of Emily's treatment underwent the greatest number of successive condensations and is the briefest of my reports. To my surprise, a characteristic audience response is one of disbelief that Emily was schizophrenic. While there are other reasons for this (one of which was elaborated in Chapter 1, namely, the tendency to equate "schizophrenic" with "unredeemably alien"), the point I wish to make here is that because I had sacrificed so much of her incoherence, randomness, disintegration and internal contradiction, so much of her bizarreness, silences, repetitiveness, unrelatedness, and absence of movement, in favor of a story of change and recovery, it seemed I had made the schizophrenic aspect—and the description of Emily does satisfy DSM-III-R criteria—barely credible. The report of Celia, by contrast, is the longest in the book. It was the last I wrote, and the more I thought about the issues involved, the more difficult it became to justify both major omissions of information and the use of any particular criterion for deciding what they ought to be.

But no one could write a book with five cases like the one of Celia, to say nothing of including an effort to make theoretical coherence of them. There is no way a publisher could reproduce an actual case and no way a reader could be expected to have funds to buy such a book, much less the time and interest to immerse himself in it in the requisite depth and complexity. The essential distinction here is between living one's experience and finding some viable way to communicate it to another. Editorial reaction to the initial draft of the case of Celia was that it had to be condensed because no reader would be willing and able to follow the repetitiveness and disorganization. But that is like saying, "Make the schizophrenic coherent so the reader may be spared contact with him."

One final observation about the process of condensing. It involves selecting and writing down "representative episodes." But there are two ways to do this, each with advantages and disadvantages. The first is to select a "real" episode that stands for many roughly similar ones. The advantage is a closer adherence to reality, but the disadvantage is that this involves sacrificing numerous individual and potentially enriching variations. The second method is to create a fictional representative episode that contains both the general theme and many of the individual variations, as though these had all occurred at once. In this instance enrichment is provided at the cost of reality. For the most part I have done the former. When episodes have been condensed and are presented as a single vignette, I have made it clear that I am generalizing.

To summarize, I have attempted to establish the validity, under well-defined circumstances, of developing, illustrating, and (at least to some degree) validating hypotheses from the intensive study of clinical case material. In so doing I do not imply that case studies are the only valid source of data and information about schizophrenia; that would be contrary to the basic assumptions of a hierarchical systems theory.

Confidentiality

Aside from disquieting the statistical scientist, the use of extensive clinical data raises questions about patient–therapist confidentiality. The public need for accumulation and dissemination of scientific knowledge in formats such as this book must be balanced against the right of the patient/subject to privacy and confidentiality of communication.

This means that data and information from and about the patient and the treatment must be confined to the immediate participants. That is, data that allow more or less unequivocal and specific identification of the subject by another person must not be printed. There are a number of methods for avoiding breaches of confidentiality, which I have judiciously resorted to, except as noted.* These include:

1. Fabrication of misleading data. This was not done for the obvious reason that the case reports are not fiction.

2. Distortion of data where the altered fact is so similar to the original that the reader is not substantively misled. For example, if the patient went to Harvard, in the report it is written that he attended Yale. I have disguised obvious identifying information. This was done with caution because it is not always possible to know, even when one has studied someone else in the depth required to conduct treatments such as those I will describe, all the various symbolic guises in which basic information has become encoded; that is, in altering a seemingly innocuous fact one can never be certain that one is not also rendering some of the patient's intrapsychic life correspondingly incomprehensible to the reader.

3. Generalization of data. For example, if the patient went to Harvard, the report states that he had "some higher education."

4. Omission of data. The patient went to Harvard, but nothing about his higher education is mentioned.

5. Using selected cases and arranging time and place of publication so as to sequester the data from an audience of persons capable of making a specific identification. To continue the Harvard example, the report would be published in a place where it would be unlikely to be encountered by Harvard people.

This last method, above all, is what has enabled me to publish such detailed material with reasonable confidence that I have protected my former patients' confidences. With regard to the particular cases in this book, none is recent with the exception of the case of Celia, whose treatment terminated within the last several years. The patients, along with the hospital staff who

---

*I used techniques 2, 3, and 4 whenever material about the patient seemed sufficiently remarkable or unusual as to hint at specific identification.

worked with them and others who knew them at the time, went their various ways 15 to 25 years ago. Moreover, there is significantly less likelihood of breaching confidentiality by writing about hospitalized schizophrenics than there is by writing about patients from a more traditional psychoanalytic practice, who are likely to be psychiatrists, psychoanalysts, and assorted other mental health personnel, or at least persons from the analyst's social milieu. None of the patients whose cases are presented here were or are, to my knowledge, related in any way to the mental health community. They are from different parts of society and are therefore unlikely to come in contact with this book or its readers. Moreover, by virtue of their problems, they were peripherally, if at all, involved in the world before they entered the hospital and treatment, so they are not likely to be identified by readers who knew them as sick persons. In the course of their treatment my patients were removed from their environments not only by virtue of hospitalization but because in most instances it occurred at a significant distance from their homes. In the process most lost contact with whatever acquaintances they did have. The successfully treated patients eventually left the hospital and made new lives for themselves—or perhaps it would be more accurate to say that they made lives for themselves for the first time—lives involving others from whom their illness histories were often withheld or by whom such histories, when presented, were greeted with disbelief since they were so discrepant with the person's current relatively healthy state. (During the termination phase of her treatment Emily put it succinctly when she remarked that she had stopped trying to tell her new friends about her illness and treatment not because she was reluctant for them to know but because of their incredulity: "No one believes me when I tell them how crazy I was!") As for the patients whose treatment failed and who went on to be chronically hospitalized, only their families, who are unlikely to read this book, would ever recognize them. What I am trying to say is that the subjects of the case histories in this book are people who lacked significant social identities to begin with. In those instances where treatment succeeded they developed new and healthy identities so utterly different from and, on the surface, unrelated to the old, and new relationships with persons outside the mental health field, that it would take a detective to trace them from this book.

Part II

Cases:
The Extremes of Outcome

Chapter 4

Emily:
An Unusually Successful
Treatment

History

Emily was raised in a depressed, nonverbal family. Her mother, who was from a rural background, had wanted to become a doctor but became a nurse instead. She met Emily's father while he was in medical school. She worked throughout most of Emily's childhood, and shortly after she divorced Emily's father, when Emily was around puberty, she changed careers and gained considerable success as an executive in the entertainment industry. She was a chronically depressed person, and her masochistic life was testimonial to her articulated belief that life was painful. Emily's father came from a socially prominent family. His own father was a very successful physician. By contrast, Emily's father's accomplishments as a physician were marginal, and he suffered from chronic feelings of inadequacy. By the time Emily was born, he was a depressed, suspicious, isolated general practitioner who had come to specialize in performing vasectomies in his office.

Mother wanted a boy for her third child. The delivery was difficult. Emily was said to be unhappy from the very start of life. She was breast-fed for 3 months and switched to the bottle because of colic. Emily was separated from mother for a time toward the end of her first year because mother became ill and required hospitalization and surgery.

By all accounts Emily was an irritable and isolated child. She was acutely sensitive to loud noises and would cringe and hide when airplanes passed overhead. She had nocturnal phobias and eventually a school phobia. She had temper tantrums that escalated in intensity. At such times her parents would ignore her or put her in her room. As a small child Emily began a pattern of scratching her abdomen until it bled, which got her much attention from mother. Father took her on some hiking and canoeing expeditions with him, but for the most part ignored her except when she hurt herself and required medical attention. He sutured several of her wounds, and gave her physical examinations until the time of the divorce. Attention from mother consisted of being dressed in outfits that were frilly but rather inappropriate in relation to her peers, and being forced to participate in mother's causes as a civil rights crusader. When mother was not pushing Emily into difficult situations she tended to leave her alone a great deal. When mother would return home from an absence she would ask Emily if she had missed her, and would be delighted if the answer was no. Like many things mother did, this response reflected her philosophy of life, namely, that children had to learn to accept reality (that is, suffering) and learn to be strong.

But Emily became quite fearful of separating from mother. This was most pronounced when she began school; mother had to take her there and remain with her. Because of mother's crusade against the required pledge of allegiance in school, Emily was required, as early as kindergarten, to walk out of the classroom when the other children saluted the flag. Mother's philosophy about this was that the needs of the individual (in this case, Emily) had to be balanced against the needs of society. As one might expect, Emily was soon perceived as strange and tended to be scapegoated by her peers. When she was 8, other children referred to her as "piggie girl" and ostracized her. When she was beaten up by some boys on her way home from school, mother's response was, "Don't worry about it; they did it because they love you."

Emily's parents' marriage, which was never happy, deteriorated gradually. When Emily was 9 or 10 her parents separated, and as she entered adolescence they divorced. A year or two later mother began an affair with a successful professional man who was also divorced. This man, unlike Emily's father, was quite extroverted and very fond of Emily; his attraction to her contained a latent sexual element, and the attention made Emily most uncomfortable. Emily's menarche, at 11 or 12, was celebrated with champagne by mother.

Though she tended to be isolated from peers, Emily was academically successful at school, and tended to be a teacher's pet. When Emily was 14, mother and her lover were married. As mother became increasingly preoccupied with her growing career and her new marriage, she tended to leave Emily alone. Emily was manifestly naive, and tended to get herself into potentially dangerous situations through such behaviors as hitchhiking, frequenting locations where there was potential for her to be assaulted, and acting passive and compliant when she was mistreated by others.

Emily was sent to boarding school, where, though she remained quietly depressed, and apparently began to hallucinate robed figures advising and admonishing her, it appears retrospectively that she radiated a kind of charisma that attracted the attention of her teachers. She obtained glowing reports for her achievements, which included painting. During her senior year her male English teacher, who seems to have been depressed, took to calling her "Virginia Woolf." Emily began secretly to think of herself as van Gogh.

After graduation Emily began college, but she was unable to concentrate and dropped out after a semester. She began to hallucinate. Her dress and hygiene deteriorated. She wandered from city to city, like a bum. Her judgment and ability to care for herself were obviously impaired, and it is a wonder she escaped serious injury. She went to live with her father, (who had also remarried), held several menial jobs briefly, and got entangled in a sexual relationship with a foreign student from a culture that tends to devalue women. Finally, even her ordinarily inattentive father was moved to express his concern about her, which led to a quarrel and caused Emily to return to her mother and stepfather. There she spent most of her time in the attic, writing in her diary and painting, but destroying anything mother seemed to like.

Emily had fits in which she smashed things, and she ingested several overdoses of pills. She began to cut and burn her body in symbolic patterns. In her diary she wrote of despair, suicide, and her belief that she was a possession of mother's; the writing, which I eventually saw, was often incoherent and even bizarre in content. Finally, mother became alarmed and arranged for her to see a psychiatrist. About a year before I met her Emily attempted to kill herself after completing a picture of a princess looking out on the world through the window of a castle battlement. She slit her wrists and overdosed while mother was away from home, but was discovered and hospitalized for almost a month. After her discharge she ran away. When she was found and rehospitalized, her psychiatrist recommended long-term treatment; Emily was transferred to the hospital, distant from her home, where I met her.

At the time of Emily's admission to the hospital psychological testing revealed a person who did not experience herself as autonomous and whose defenses were unstable. Emily was delusional and her logic was autistic. She tended to make arbitrary, grandiose, global syntheses of information and to engage in paranoid thinking.

Treatment

Year One

Emily was 19 when our therapy commenced, and 25 when it was completed. She was attractive and slightly overweight. She chain-smoked and showed not even ordinary anxiety about meeting me. She was friendly and obviously intelligent, but there was a vacant, mechanical, compliant quality about her. She spoke softly and without affect, and the content of her remarks was vague and abstract. She said she felt adrift. She did not understand her feelings or the reasons for her actions. I tried to empathize with what she must have been feeling, and restricted myself to attempts to rephrase what she was telling me and to find out whether she thought I had comprehended. She seemed to feel understood, and expressed some surprise and relief.

At our second meeting, around Easter, Emily's head was bandaged and she was much more distant and suspicious. She did not look at me as she recited an elaborate delusion about killers and victims involving herself and the ward staff, a delusion that had culminated with her carving a cross in her forehead. She fell silent, then gradually became agitated. Rather than commenting about the provocative content of the delusion I asked her about her immediate state of mind. She felt she was avoiding something that she experienced as dangerous, though she could not say what. She became quite disturbed, and I thought she was upset with me; in fact, she thought my question was important, and we concluded by deciding together that we would have a try at therapy.

Our third hour followed a similar pattern. Emily described extreme and disparate states of consciousness or mood, "good" states and rageful paranoid states, but her speech was flat, she chain-smoked, and she did not look at me as she talked. Again, rather than comment about the content of what she told me, I wondered aloud about her immediate state of mind, and again she seemed pleased. During the fourth hour she more or less enacted contrary states of mind; in one of these she claimed she wanted to relate to others and have constructive goals while in the other she was enigmatic, withdrawn, prone to tantrums, and preoccupied with her mother. When she spoke in one of these states of mind, she tended to attribute the motivation for the other to outside influences, which she then proceeded to attack and devalue. After helping her clarify what she was saying, I commented that it was hard for me to know what she wanted and that it was therefore difficult to make any kind of treatment agreement with her. In the fifth hour it became clearer that her meaningful communications were not so much verbal as behavioral; these were in the form of destructive, attention-getting enactments that were somehow related to her mother.

In my condensed presentation of Emily's treatment, you will mercifully be spared her long, tedious periods of silence and withdrawal, sometimes lasting a month or more, in which she would say but few words to me. You will have to imagine her affective cycles, including fits of rage during which I occasionally sensed—and she much later confirmed—that I was in danger of being attacked (not an inconsequential danger, as Emily was tall and solidly built). It will also be difficult to convey her disintegration. Her speech would say one thing, her behavior another, and her affect yet another, often seemingly unrelated. The repetitive back-and-forth movement between progress and self-destructive regress also can only be hinted at. This report unavoidably conveys a false sense of coherence and continuity.

Emily was verbal and compliant, but it soon became apparent that the person who spoke with me had no contact with her feelings or with the person who was episodically out of control on the ward where I met with her. She hallucinated mystical robed figures speaking to her critically or seductively. From time to time she became enraged and panicked, convinced that the ward staff were about to execute or poison her—or had already done so. At these times she smashed objects, assaulted staff, and burned and cut herself in patterns associated with a private symbolism. The staff experienced her as frighteningly out of control. These gross psychotic episodes led to her restraint and seclusion, and they were a constant counterpoint to our work for the first 14 months. I soon sensed that Emily obtained some gratification from the attention she got from staff for this behavior. After 2 weeks of therapy her ward administrative psychiatrist placed her on trifluoperazine, on which she remained for 3 years. Initially, the dose was 10 mg daily; it was raised to as much as 40 mg in the subsequent tumultuous months.

Emily found life intolerably burdensome: she had to satisfy relentless internal and hallucinated critics, she felt obligated to make mother feel good, and now I was forcing her to learn to be intimate. She had attended a rural private school, and she told me she preferred goats to people. She punished herself and her mother by being self-destructive, which also served to get her taken care of and to make mother feel needed.

Emily became more self-destructive during my first vacation, after 5 months of therapy. When I returned, her posture was robotic. She laughed hysterically and informed me that three white-robed figures were ridiculing her. She told me she had wanted to kill herself while I was gone. She expressed fear that she might become involved with me and lose her specialness, which she associated to her relationship with mother and to the belief that she was Vincent van Gogh (in fact, Emily had a considerable but undeveloped interest in art). After telling me this she doubled over, shrieked with pain, and said the three robed men were laughing at her.

After 7 months of work together I told Emily that our meetings would be interrupted while I underwent knee surgery. She was initially sad but then said she wanted to go home and be a great artist while living in mother's attic, where she envisioned mother taking care of her unconditionally. She then imagined me tearing a baby from its mother's breast. She became withdrawn and paranoid, hallucinated more, looked menacing, told me everything was connected and had special meaning, and sat on the floor of the seclusion room (where we were then meeting because of her uncontrolled destructiveness), tracing womblike patterns in the dust with her finger.

When we resumed meeting after my surgery, Emily sucked her thumb, rocked, talked baby talk, and maintained that she was 6 years old. She wanted me to take care of her and wanted mother, who was visiting, to take her home. After mother left she sadly told me that no one in her family knew how to love, and she asked for my help. The night of this striking revelation, in a state of terror because her hallucinatory men were threatening to kill me, she called me at home. I suggested that she might be angry at me; although she confused the feeling with physical ugliness, she admitted she was enraged that I had "made" her need me and then was not always there to take care of her. The following hour she denied anger at me, but after I left the ward she had a rage reaction, bloodied both hands, and had to be placed in restraints (a condition in which she now spent much of her time, including her therapy sessions). The dose of trifluoperazine was raised to 40 mg. During this period Emily told me two dreams: In the first, she was trying, unsuccessfully, to get a tiger into a car in which she was having therapy. In the second, she was trying to build a world with pipe-cleaner men but failed, and a woman came to take care of her.

At Christmas, during the ninth therapy month, she presented me with a gift: a beautiful painting. Long afterward, she informed me it represented a fetus trapped in a teardrop womb inside a tree trunk, but at the time she could tell me nothing about it. Then she decided to give up and go home; she began an active campaign to leave the hospital. I suggested that her plan to live in mother's attic and be a famous artist was a womb fantasy. I added that she was enraged that I did not treat her like an invalid. She promptly forgot what I said but decided she would remain at the hospital, adding that her mother thought she was perfect just as she was.

In the eleventh therapy month Emily took to her bed (in her single room) and refused to see me. She stared at the ceiling and was mute. After a month of being almost totally bedridden and mute and in response to pressure from the ward staff, she called and asked to see me again. She told me, without affect, that she was very angry that she had let me "get inside" and that she had been trying to get rid of the world. The month had been quite comfortable, she added, and she reported a dream of walking tirelessly and effortlessly through beautiful woods. But, she concluded, she knew no one would take care of her the way she wished.

Year Two

Though she attended her sessions, Emily remained virtually mute with me for more than a month in the early part of the second year of treatment, and she seemed quite untroubled about it. Over the first 4 months her trifluoperazine was gradually reduced from 40 mg to 10 mg as she was no longer perceived to be such a destructive menace on the ward. I cast about for ways to relate to her, and tried to enlist her in a discussion of "my problem" by asking her what one does when rejected and left alone. She suggested, without any manifest concern, that I could daydream or read a book. She remarked flatly that she wanted to stop therapy, but when I asked if she was going to do anything about it she remained rooted to her chair.

Emily began to tell me how her mother never seemed to recognize that she (Emily) had problems and how she treated her as though she were perfect. She told me how she played along, by laughing and being superficial, and how, during mother's visits, the two of them would blame the hospital and me for the fact that she was still there. Emily used these interactions as "fixes" in order to feel "high," and mother would leave perplexed about why Emily mutilated herself and required seclusion between her visits. Emily then made an unconvincing, hence unsuccessful, effort to tell mother how upset she was. I suggested that I might join the meetings that were being held between Emily, her mother, and the social worker in order to assist her to communicate with mother. Soon after, Emily came to therapy, in the heat of summer, dressed in a red ski cap and long red socks with holes. Her expression was wooden, her affect flat, and she was very agitated. She voiced fear and anger that my participation in family meetings might disrupt her relationship with mother. Suddenly, Emily removed her cap, remarking challengingly that she had made it herself and that mother would like it but she believed I did not. I responded that she thought mother would like both her creativity and her crazy behavior, whereas I distinguished the two, and that what she made was nice but wearing it here was inappropriate. In the following hour her leg shook uncontrollably, she smiled bizarrely, and described silly behavior and a conversation in which she had participated on the ward as though it were profound. I expressed my concern that her condition was worsening. She wanted me to comfort her and reassure her that everything would be all right, but I responded that I could not.

Emily told her mother and stepfather what I had said about her condition, but they responded that she seemed better to them. Regarding the question of my participation in family meetings Emily reported, "Mother thinks you are too blunt; you must not let your kids get away with anything!" After her parents left, the staff discovered that Emily had severely mutilated herself. When I came to the ward for her next appointment, I found her in the quiet room, spread-eagled on a mattress on the floor in four-point restraints, laughing and singing loudly and bizarrely. I could not hide my distress at her degradation. At the time I looked upon my show of emotion as a breach of neutrality, however unavoidable, but years later Emily informed me that my involuntary response had been a turning point in her treatment, and I have learned over the years that the success of many treatments, particularly of more disturbed persons, seems to hinge around similar therapeutic "mistakes." I think it was the unplanned, out-of-character nature of this therapeutic event, which was "beyond" technique, that contributed to its value. In any event, Emily told me that she had carved NO HOPE on one arm; I subsequently learned from a letter that her mother sent me that she told mother that she had carved HELP on the other.

Emily remained in restraints for the next 2 weeks, acting bizarre and euphoric. I decided it was time I began to attend family meetings, and the social worker reluctantly agreed, although she thought my presence would be disruptive to Emily's mother. I met with mother, stepfather, Emily, and the social worker every other week for the next 5 months, and our work was extremely productive. Around the time we commenced, Emily's behavior explosions permanently ceased, but she began a monthlong fast, accompanied by the delusional conviction that she did not require food.

My first discovery in the family meetings was that it was mother and not Emily who experienced the distress of being hospitalized. Mother felt all the physical and emotional pain that Emily seemed not to, down to the sensation of being cut and burned. Stepfather cried when I pointed this out, and said that their marriage was deteriorating, but he was quite willing to make the sacrifice "for Emily's sake." We began to uncover a multiplicity of ways in which family members conspired to deny Emily's separateness and to avoid overt expression of anger and conflict. The parents tended to soothe Emily, to cut her off when she tried to speak, and to speak for her, asserting that they knew her thoughts. This was sometimes an invitation for her to act out *their* feelings, and at other times, as Emily later put it, a way of "stealing [her] thunder." That is, if mother knew about Emily's anger and understood and accepted it before Emily expressed it, then they were one and there could be no conflict. Parents also tended not to take Emily seriously. When Emily first began to tell mother how angry she was at her, mother became confused and refused to believe it. I pointed out that it had more impact on mother when Emily mutilated herself than when she expressed her feelings verbally. Stepfather's response at this point in the meeting was to give Emily a very sensual hug because she was "bleeding." I had to point out that this was an instance where she had not cut herself!

After several family sessions Emily reported two dreams: In the first, she and mother were guarding their house against an enemy attacking from the rear. In the second, Emily was preparing for her coronation, to succeed mother as queen. The coronation turned out to be a disappointment, however, and mother got all the attention. I wondered, in response, whether she perceived me as the enemy and whether that meant that I should stop attending the meetings. Emily said she hoped not, and told me how important my participation had become to her. I suggested that, if this was true, perhaps she could begin to verbalize the negative feelings about me that her dreams suggested, and she began to do so. Gradually, the intense anger Emily and her mother felt for one another also emerged in the family meetings, despite the belief each held that the other was too depressed and fragile to deal with that anger.

All was not well, however. Emily continued to fast; she lost 25 pounds over the month and became visibly gaunt. The staff became concerned she might require forcible feeding. In response to my concern Emily insisted she did not need to eat because mother was taking care of her. I told her I did not believe this, and she cried and responded that I had helped her to understand things about herself she preferred not to know. Then she said she believed that by fasting she could shrink herself and become mother's little baby.

Eventually, Emily began to express excitement that the family meetings were providing the first new direction in her life, and she decided to resume eating. She told me she wanted my help to learn to be more grown-up. Emily's subsquent feelings of depression, loss, and helplessness suggested some separation from mother and the loss of her illusion of security, and she began for the first time to take part, with some pleasure, in hospital relationships and activities.

After 16 months of treatment trifluoperazine was reduced to 10 mg. In anticipation of interruption of treatment for my summer vacation Emily first became enraged that she did not possess me and then confused, with paranoid thoughts and self-destructive urges. On my return she was withdrawn and did not make eye contact. First, she said, she had tried to control the separation by acting like me and encouraging other withdrawn patients to relate. Then she had smeared spaghetti over her entire body and had turned to a staff member who had helped her. She told me matter-of-factly that she guessed she didn't need me anymore. She had also gotten involved with a young man who, she asserted, was brilliant; she believed this was so because she couldn't understand a thing he said. He had told her not to look at anyone else; he also told her that if she didn't look at me, then I didn't exist. We realized that she, like her mother, had trouble distinguishing genius from psychosis. I made a slip and called her by the first name of another withdrawn patient of mine. With some embarrassment I acknowledged that she had succeeded in making me feel rejected the way she must have felt while I was away. She, in turn, cried and raged at me, but she began to realize, in connection with my habit of taking vacations, that nothing is totally satisfying and everything has limits.

Emily began to express dissatisfaction with the preoccupation with suffering, depression, and unreality that characterizes hospital patients in general, and her family in particular, and to wonder if there might be a more positive world "out there." Her interests and activities blossomed, and partly in response to impending limitations in her hitherto generous insurance coverage she began to make discharge plans. She still wished for an endless womblike existence in the hospital, and she reported dreams in which she wanted to scream, masturbate, and otherwise let go but was unable to. She tearfully identified herself with a movie hero who achieved greatness through hard work.

Meanwhile, I gradually became aware that the attitude of ward staff and other patients had become rather hostile toward me as I came on the ward for Emily's appointments. My surmise that Emily was presenting distorted versions of our conversations to them in order to elicit their anger at me was subsequently confirmed by talks with her and with staff. When confronted with this, Emily began to express rage at the idea that I might be experiencing success as her therapist, wishes to mutilate me and reduce me to her "size," and doubts about my sanity. She told me, and I subsequently confirmed, that a junior staff member had said that a remark Emily told him I had made to her was crazy. Coincidentally, her administrator reduced her trifluoperazine to 5 mg. Rather frightening outbursts of rage at me from Emily alternated with maniacal laughter associated with ideas of being a fairy in flight and a prostitute whose body was literally not her own and with the belief that someone was trying to poison her.

Things seemed out of control, and I finally shared with Emily my feeling of powerlessness to reach her, and remarked that she seemed convinced that one or both of us had to be destroyed. We agreed to increase the frequency of her sessions from three to four a week, a frequency we maintained throughout the balance of the treatment process. Emily became somewhat calmer and was able to review her hospitalization and illness reasonably appropriately, say good-byes, and prepare for discharge. She decided to rent an apartment with a chronic schizophrenic male patient whose acquaintance she had made in the hospital, and with whom she had a casual relationship, despite her administrator's urging that she live in a more structured setting such as a halfway house. In retrospect, I realize that these discharge preparations were quite incomplete, and that in failing to support her administrator's suggestion I had once again colluded with Emily's grandiosity, but at the time I felt constrained by the financial pressures that her family reported.

After 23 months of hospitalization and 20 months of therapy Emily was discharged, her hair in pigtails and dressed like a little girl, in gauzy white (particularly inappropriate as it was a snowy day). I gave her a gift, a small book of walks or hikes of exploration one could take in the city area where she would be living, with an inscription saying that I believed there was a world outside the hospital and I hoped she would find it. Emily was touched and felt she should give me something in return. Perhaps I would be ill, she said, and she could take care of me, or she could give me sex, she continued, but that would be prostitution.

Emily became upset because her parents failed to respond emotionally to her discharge. She wrote them an angry letter and proceeded to gorge herself with food, to become paranoid, and to want my understanding without talking. She dreamed of being mother's sliced turkey and of messing her body but having her art work praised; then she dreamed of a phone call in which mother misidentified her and hung up, leaving a "dead line." However, she proceeded to plan a holiday trip home. Then she dreamed that since we could not find an office to meet in for therapy, we went to her parents' vacation home. We were in a car and I was trying to drive but she was blocking my view of the road and of her parents. Stepfather took over and almost hit a little car, which she associated with herself. Mother said, "Don't hit the little car," but gleefully she proceeded to smash it. The dream ended with Emily thinking that I was caressing her, but looking up to discover that it was her mother.

When she returned from her short holiday Emily had to face her roommate's regressed behavior as well as the fact that her trip home had been an effort to live out mother's fantasies and to believe that she was not only cured but perfect. Emily became disorganized and paralyzed with ambivalence and could not leave my waiting room; I arranged for a brief return to the hospital. There I discovered that Emily had secretly stopped taking trifluoperazine before her trip home, and a 10-mg dose was resumed. As we began to talk about her poorly planned discharge, Emily expressed both her expectation that I would take perfect care of her and her rage at me for failing to do so. Although Emily began to feel enthusiasm about her life again, it was now accompanied by new feelings of vulnerability and dependency. She dreamed I was a bulldozer filling in a great hole so she wouldn't disappear and also that she had purchased a defective outfit of clothing and was trying, in the face of a variety of obstacles, to return it. She realized that her mother's denial of problems, infantilization of her, and grandiose beliefs about her had kept her from learning to face and resolve problems.

Emily arranged to separate from her schizophrenic roommate and to move to more suitable living quarters, which took several weeks. She enrolled in a literature course in preparation for starting college in the fall, joined a partial-hospitalization program, and began an important friendship with a woman who was able to be remarkably realistic, persevering, and resilient despite major physical handicaps and ill fortune.

When Emily told me with dismay that she had had a horrible weekend because she had fought with her schizophrenic roommate over his inconsiderate behavior, had gone to the hospital to sleep overnight, and, as a result, had not done as much work as she would have wished on a course paper, I pointed out all the thinking, struggling, and coping that had been involved, and added that coping with problems like these was a part of everyone's life.

As my vacation approached, Emily again experienced the rageful wish to eliminate me, but after she came at the wrong time for her appointment she remarked that she was finally understanding what she called my "lectures on limits," namely, that if you love someone you allow them to be separate. She wanted to let me go, but in return she felt entitled to whatever thoughts and feelings she might have about it. These turned out to include wishes to mutilate me and cut off my legs so I could not leave. Emily feared these wishes might come true, and she recognized that this, in a sense, was what her mother had done to her.

Year Three

My return after my vacation marked the beginning of our third year. Emily burst into tears when she saw me and told me how well she had done. She was beginning to value her body. She cried over the scars from her self-mutilation and attended a weight control group. As she struggled with her familiar sense of herself as a mess needing to be fixed, she began to talk about her father, a doctor who had specialized in performing vasectomies in his office at home. She recalled how he had sutured wounds on her scalp and knee poorly, and without anesthesia, and she remembered the numerous physical examinations he had performed on her before he left the family around the time of her puberty. She began to wonder if he liked to hurt people.

Emily's hallucinations diminished, but one night while in the city she became paralyzed with terror and a sense of impending attack. Literally unable to move, she called me at home, and I drove into the city and brought her back to the hospital. In our next therapy hour she told me she was discovering sadistic wishes toward father. Emily scratched absentmindedly at her scars and appeared to be bandaging her finger with tissues as she recalled the pleasure father seemed to take in doctoring her. She laughed inappropriately as she talked about her wish to have him "fix" her, and she acted as though she were being tickled as she scratched at herself. In the days that followed she began to binge eat and talked angrily of wishes to castrate father, eat him, and excrete him. A sense of gratitude toward me alternated with hatred that I made her aware of pain; perhaps, she thought, I had even inflicted it on her. To her surprise she realized that, however perversely he had treated her, she had loved her father, and this realization provided her with an impetus to separate from her mother.

I was away for 2 weeks. Again Emily stopped trifluoperazine. On my return I found her huddled in a corner in protection against some imagined assault, sobbing convulsively; she seemed to be living out a memory or fantasy (much later she concluded that it was probably the latter) of father doing a vaginal examination on her to remove some "bumps" when she was 8 or 10 years of age. She recalled how mother had palpated Emily's breasts early in adolescence and worried that she might have cancer. As Emily became aware of her wishes to be father's neutered daughter, mother's cancerous patient (before her marriage mother had been a nurse), and my psychotic patient, she became paralyzed with rage at herself and at others, and filled with paranoid terror and self-destructive wishes. Again Emily was discharged.

I told Emily I would be taking some time off in about 2 months when my wife gave birth. Emily reported more positive feelings about her body and new insights, which she felt she had gotten from me. She had a fantasy that I had impregnated her. After a gynecologic examination she was enraged and disappointed that the doctor had not wanted to sleep with her, and she all but propositioned me. I remarked that some of her recent interest in her body was healthy, but that her notion that there were no limits or boundaries in the relationship between parents and children and between doctors and patients was a destructive one.

Emily got a job and planned to take college entrance examinations. At the same time she withdrew from me and began a pattern of nocturnal adventures; staying out late, frequenting clubs and bars, drinking heavily, and acting quite seductively, though it was my impression that she did not actually become sexually involved with anyone. During the day she did not want to wake up, missed therapy appointments, and felt much disappointment and rage. Gradually we began to reconstruct her memories of nocturnal excitement and fantasies about father, which had been stimulated by such things as his bedtime back rubs; these were often followed by sleeplessness, and fears of animals and intruders, against which she would rouse father from bed to "protect" her. In the morning father would "flash his penis" in the bathroom while he groomed himself, then leave for the day; Emily would have a tantrum and rejoin her mother.

Emily's full realization of father's hurtfulness, seductiveness, and rejection happened to coincide with the birth of my baby and a weeklong separation. She felt rage that my wife and not she had gotten the penis and the baby. She talked of her confusion between sex and hurting. Her skin itched, her knee had "arthritis," and the chant "Kill, kill" went through her head.

Gradually Emily concluded that it might be better to put her energy into new activities and relationships rather than into lost causes. She enrolled in an acting class, where she learned she had talent, got a better job, and even wrote to father to suggest he provide some money for her education (he had provided no financial support since the divorce). She dreamed she got married and father killed himself on the steps of the church. Nevertheless, there was a resurgence of diurnal acting out, and an intensification of her hallucinations. Emily called people "cunts" and "pricks," and I think that is literally how they looked to her. She recalled, with excitement, how she would sit on the hospital ward and laugh as people literally turned into monkeys in front of her eyes, and how she could hallucinate psychedelic wonders and experience great highs. She felt entitled to skip her therapy hours, but when I pointed out that she would not want me to treat her that way, she raged at me. Then she began to control her behavior again. She recalled her hospital discharge almost a year earlier, when she had dressed in white; she told me how she had believed that she was about to "marry the world" and how enraged she was that she hadn't — found the great seductive, infantilizing presence she had been seeking.

At holiday time Emily visited her brother, whom she described as much like father, and his wife. She felt imprisoned and enraged in an environment she described as angry, nonverbal, action-oriented, and infantilizing. Shortly afterward she had severe back spasms and had to be hospitalized for a week and immobilized. Before and after this hospitalization she had to lie facing me on the couch in my office because of her physical distress (the treatment was usually conducted sitting face-to-face). Feelings of not having control over her body led Emily to work on her convictions that she was omnipotent, immortal, and invulnerable. She recalled diving off a chair onto a concrete floor at age 3 (she imagined she was diving into water) and cutting her chin severely. She talked of magic rituals that, she had been convinced, warded off danger and controlled her world. A nightmare of being stalked by a figure of death led to a discussion in which she became more accepting of her mortality.

To my surprise, having to use the couch was not threatening to Emily; instead it led to moving experiences of feeling good about her body and feeling close to me. She told me of a dream in which I had come to lie on the couch with her. I began to kiss her, but, to her surprise, she pushed me away. She talked about a growing sense of propriety as well as the threatening intensity of her feelings. She dreamed she was at a beach party, and a bonfire was burning out of control. A friend was lying in a pose Emily herself sometimes assumed, smoking a cigarette. The friend told Emily she had slept with me, and Emily protested that she didn't believe I would do such a thing. Her associations were to relinquishing pleasures like sex and cigarettes for more integrated ones like the closeness she felt with me. A new and distinctive softness began to replace the familiar flatness of her voice. Her body tingled "like winter" or "like dancing," and she was afraid she might faint. She found the experience orienting but difficult to bear; I felt moved.

When Emily felt good she felt as though she were flying, a sensation she found frightening. Mother's philosophy was that life was misery, and people should be down to earth and learn to live with their feet firmly planted on the ground. I asked Emily what she thought the natural course of these flying feelings might be if they were not "grounded" by misery and suffering. She had difficulty thinking about this and turned her attention to an impending visit from mother, recalling mother feeling her breasts for cancer. She experienced burning anger, had sadistic fantasies about mother's body, and felt an urge to have a climactic, murderous confrontation. She contrasted this with the soft, warm, playful, dizzy, "feel all colors" sensation she felt for me. I remarked that she trusted me. My comment astonished her, and in a spontaneous outburst she quoted Miranda's soliloquy from *The Tempest* about her discovery of a "brave new world" of people other than her father.

In the last months of our third year, entirely on her own initiative, Emily stopped taking trifluoperazine, joined a group called Smoke Enders and, with surprising ease, relinquished her chronic two- to three-pack-a-day smoking habit; gradually terminated her partial hospital program; and decided to learn to type. She could feel the difference without the trifluoperazine and remarked how she had to talk to herself and will herself to remain in control.

Emily talked with humor about how hard it was to incorporate all the instructions about self-care she had received from her various doctors and the Smoke Enders group and concluded that she guessed we both cared about her and we both cared about me and that was "neat." But she feared she would lose her appeal to mother if she relinquished her vices and took good care of herself, and she feared setting limits regarding her physical privacy, limits based on her new sense of modesty, when mother came to visit lest mother think her crazy! She reasserted her "right" to be self-destructive and in a rage shared fantasies of incinerating me and knifing me to shreds. Finally, she concluded that she was clinging to the valuation of craziness she shared with her mother because it provided romance, privacy in the form of enigmatic withholding, and a sense of triumph and pride. I remarked that we all needed privacy, pride, and romance in our lives but perhaps there were more constructive ways to get these things.

Year Four

At the beginning of our fourth year Emily reported pleasure in her accomplishments, but she cried and said it felt like her mother was dying. She had believed that she would become the messiah of death and destruction and would preach mother's philosophy to the world—indeed, this was the symbolism of the cross carving that had marked my initial Easter meeting with her. As she talked she had to restrain powerful urges to withdraw into a rageful, annihilating hauteur rather than work to prove herself in a forthcoming college interview. She wondered if her messianic fantasies might have been a childish effort to deal with a family full of unverbalized anger and depression, where action was unrestrained and good feeling was not safe because of the absence of boundaries.

Emily began to talk about good feelings as though they were external intrusions. When I pointed this out, she recalled her hypersensitivity to sound and light, which in turn led her to deny perceptions, shut off feelings, cut off thoughts, and tense her lower back and pelvic muscles. This seemed to be a factor in her back spasms. She felt rage as she began to recall bathroom scenes with father, and her fantasies that he would use her for a toilet and kill her. She dreamed of two women, one embracing a man and the other hating men and admonishing the first to end the embrace, and recognized that both were herself. She dreamed of concealing a bandage in a tampon container but having it taken away by a man. Her association was that the penis was a vampire organ that would drain her blood and kill her and that her defense had been to imagine herself with a penis (her arms) and the ability to control the blood flow (by self-mutilation). She experienced new wishes to kiss in lieu of the old urges to smoke cigarettes.

A month before my summer vacation Emily's depressive reaction to the impending separation led her to voice the conviction that she had been breast-fed and abruptly weaned and that she had never accepted a substitute until she encountered me and the verbal presence I represented. She recalled clinging to mother, refusing to learn new things, and embracing the bad feelings that mother so readily responded to. When I reviewed her admission history, I learned that her mother had reported that Emily was weaned at 3 months because of "colic."

She became excited by her history professor and by her fantasies about his penis but experienced anxiety, gagged hysterically, and felt she didn't want to swallow. She recalled father naked in the bathroom and realized she had transferred her wish for a breast to one for a penis; she recalled imagining being a toilet for father's sperm or excrement, which would get inside and eat away at her. She began to wonder how well she had internalized the soothing functions of our relationship and whether she would need to seek a breast/penis substitute during my absence. She became transiently psychotic and fearful of loss of control, so we made an agreement that she would avoid heterosexual activity while I was gone. In response Emily felt like a ballerina who executes a complex series of steps, lands on her feet, and throws up her arms in joy, triumph, and mastery. She dreamed about kissing her history teacher and me while having a comfortable agreement not to go further. She anticipated a positive summer and interesting things to tell me in the fall.

Her prediction proved accurate. When we resumed Emily had successfully begun college. She had a brief flurry of angry oppositionalism to me, during which she recognized that during her adolescence her friends all seemed to hate their mothers, while her mother remained her "best friend." She talked of her fear to move to a place of her own and recalled that her adolescent runaways had always been to YWCAs in other cities, where she would proceed to isolate herself. She became preoccupied with somatic symptoms, imagined she had a fatal disease, and then recognized her wish to use self-destructiveness to terminate her forays into the outside world. This recognition led to a discussion of how she avoided unfamiliar sensations, particularly sensual ones. In two succeeding therapy hours Emily was first convinced that I flaunted an erection in front of her and then that a woman friend was pregnant. This led again to fantasies of being used by father as a toilet and being annihilated, and of her menses as a kind of toilet-flushing. As she recalled father's extensive caressing of her in the guise of a physical examination, she felt a back spasm, and when she moved a bit in my direction on the couch where she sat, her thigh muscles went into spasm. She laughed ruefully, took my footstool, and interposed it between us.

As Emily realized that her self-mutilation had involved efforts to control fear, rage, and sexual feelings toward the father she perceived as sadistic, she became more conscious of her own sadism. With laughter at once gleeful and uneasy she revealed fantasies of vengeful intercourse with father involving cutting a "vagina" into his chest and getting in there with her penis-arm-knife to mutilate his insides and dismember him. She wondered how dangerous she might have been to others had she not turned this rage on herself. Fantasies about her relationship with her mother—in which Emily was a princess (mother's name was Victoria) or the Messiah (her mother had used Emily to act out her own protest against prayer in the schools)—were associated with her feelings of omnipotence. She experienced wishes to have her rage contained by a man who would hold her, and she recalled how father would isolate himself elsewhere in the house when she had tantrums as a child.

Emily was behind in her first semester college work, and it was unclear whether she would complete it on time. As tension built she became increasingly rageful and launched attacks on me. She realized that she had always used tantrums to avoid confrontation between her sense of omnipotence and reality. Sexual fantasies about me turned to rageful wishes to pound me into clay. She cursed and came near to attacking me physically. She dreamed of being helpless while a madwoman attacked her. She was so angry she wanted to vomit. With just a small amount of schoolwork remaining to be done, Emily became paralyzed with ambivalence and made the case for becoming psychotic again: she would be able to feel special, and she would not have to face feelings and problems. But she realized it would also mean pushing away the friendship and love of others, and she became sad. She completed her schoolwork on time.

Emily planned a 2-week vacation to visit her parents, and then shortened the trip without telling me. When she was told that the therapy hours she had canceled might now be unavailable, she seemed unable at first to grasp the fact; when she did, she became enraged. Emily returned from the visit in a state of euphoria, bragging that she was everyone's dream girl: she had passively accepted mother's dogmatism and intrusiveness (that is, she was mother's "special shit"), stepfather's thinly veiled sexual embraces (his "playboy bunny"), and the attraction of sister's boyfriend (and victorious in competition with her sister, who experienced herself as Emily's inferior). I did not share her enthusiasm, but responded dryly that she lacked an identity or a dream of her own, and let others use her without limit. I wondered what she might be enacting for me. She angrily retorted that I was "an asshole," and then imagined becoming my perfect cure. But she realized that the price of being a dream girl—suffocation, rage, and self-destruction—was the real "pain in the ass." Emily began to experience a novel sensory-perceptual aliveness, associated with a heightened awareness of her own body and feelings and of others as separate and fascinating beings. She began to generate and act on fantasies of her own. She prepared for a physical examination, which stirred anger and fear related to her father, by planning and acting in such a way as to make the encounter satisfying, and she succeeded. By contrast, she did not anticipate a major scheduled dental procedure, and came in with an enormously swollen jaw and a sordid tale of suffering. She realized, in retrospect, that she had not voiced her doubts when the dentist reviewed the procedure with her and told her he anticipated no problems. She had tried to be his dream girl and not complain, though the procedure was excessively lengthy and painful. As she realized this she experienced biting rage.

As she became more emotional and adventurous Emily felt terrified, out of control, overstimulated, and dizzy. She recalled how hypersensitive and avoidant of stimulation she had been as a child (mother told her she would hide her head in her hands when an airplane flew overhead). After a particularly exciting experience she felt disoriented and developed a fever; she wondered if the new experience was in fact an illness. I called it "growth shock." Emily made many efforts to control these new and exciting feelings by turning them into something dangerous and bad that she could then avoid. For example, she liked ice cream but would tell herself, "It's so good it's disgusting!" Then she would literally come to believe that all food was poison. She remembered how wonderful mother said she was when she acted crippled and inept, and she recalled childhood adventures that led to accidents and to painful suturing without anesthesia by her father and without anyone holding her. She realized that making things bad and painful was a form of clinging to her parents and the security of their anhedonic attitudes, that turning unfamiliar sensations of pleasure into badness was a form of self- control and security. We realized that she had gradually worked out an elaborate set of rules and rituals based on the equation that bad equals good, and vice versa, rules and rituals that turned out to be those given her by her hallucinated robed figures.

As she felt more separate from mother, Emily planned an exciting vacation trip with a friend. She had images of flying and dancing. She felt curious about the unknown but insecure as well. Emily wanted to touch and examine my hand. When I allowed her to do this, she seemed to feel more secure about her trip and about her exploration of unfamiliar subjects. She realized in wonderment that I was alive and had feelings like she did but that I was a separate and distinct person.

Year Five

As we began the fifth year of treatment, I observed that Emily's body movements, once wooden and robotic, were becoming more fluid and graceful.

When she told me she had not allowed a man she dated to hold her hand because she knew he was involved with another woman, I reminded her that I was involved with another woman. Her requests to hold my hand ceased. Although she wanted to hold my hand again in anticipation of a trip that frightened her, because I represented security, she decided not to act on her wish when she realized that I also represented the most frightening aspect of the unknown world, the penis. This led to more work on her sexual feelings, which were unintegrated and largely experienced as external; for example, in dreams that insects were crawling in and out of her vagina. At this stage awareness of a sexual fantasy or mention of a sexual word could literally make her cringe or jump, or could trigger vaginismus. She dreamed of fleeing from an injured man with a knife and being unable to lock the door of the room she had fled to, of trying to call for help but making no sound, and, finally, of becoming a boy with a woman soothing him. She imagined she had once been a boy and that father had castrated her, but then she realized her sexual disability was an identification with him. She recalled how she had tried to suppress her feelings when father would rub her back at night. Emily dreamed that when she went to a doctor for an internal exam and was told she had an infection, she responded, indignantly, "No I don't; that's me," by which she meant that those were her feelings and they were good. She worried that her attachment to me would cause her mother pain, but at this point she was feeling more estranged from her family, and remarked that her home had been a kind of hospital, with father (a doctor) and mother (nurse by training) both invested in suffering, disability, and impotency.

When I returned from a vacation Emily reported that she had finished most of her year's schoolwork and had been able to evoke mental images of our dialogue in situations requiring judgment and self-regulation. Yet she seemed detached, guarded, and fearful. She began to protest about being separate. If she got better she would have to relinquish relationships with her parents and with me, and for what? Even so, she said, she had hung up on mother during one of her depressive litanies in order to finish a school paper and get some sleep for her early morning therapy hour. Wanting to give me the "cold shoulder," she began to act withdrawn and explosive but responded with amusement when I told her I thought she no longer had to act that way. In fact, Emily's self-image was becoming that of a serious, emotionally intense person who planned for the future and was pleased to receive compliments for her maturity. She made new friends, moved into an apartment of her own, enrolled in a painting class, and decided to transfer to a more challenging university for her junior year.

After the first painting class Emily came to me in a frenzy, which escalated until she shouted, banged her fists on the table, and sobbed. After she had calmed down we talked of her difficulty dealing with stimulation, and she likened the painting class experience to learning to dive into the water headfirst. I recalled her headfirst dive to the basement floor as a child, and the grandiose fantasies that had preceded it. Her next class seemed "dull gray."

Mother came to visit, and Emily was able to set some limits, including vetoing mother's wish to sleep in Emily's small studio apartment. She remarked, with asperity, that it was not mother she wanted sleeping next to her. She hungered for real intimacy and had some new experiences, including going to the beach (where she had hitherto feared exposing her body) and participating in a women's rights march.

It was midsummer, and as we anticipated another of my brief vacations and then the fall of Emily's sophomore year, we discovered we had each been thinking about reducing the frequency of our meetings to three times per week. Emily talked about her new hunger for relationships, which enraged the "crazy" part of her and also saddened her for she could foresee an inexorable movement away from me that, she predicted with considerable accuracy, would lead to an end to our work in 1 or 2 years.

In the fall of her sophomore year we reduced the frequency of our meetings from four to three per week. Emily's new apartment was robbed, and she felt angry and violated. She was painfully aware of longings to be hugged and loved, but not taken care of. She handled all necessary matters without turning to mother, and our discussions clarified the state of poverty and deprivation in which she had been living, one that seemed so natural to her that she had never talked about it. The apartment had been chosen for its low rent and was in fact in a dangerous neighborhood. Emily's furnishings were meagre. What little clothing she owned was mostly unsuitable. In response to a compelling but foreign inner presence she ate junk food even though she did not like it. Mother called junk food and sweets "poison" but often offered candy to Emily. Mother talked about how Emily deserved the best, but she was very stingy with money and, as I knew from her problem paying Emily's therapy bills on time, was often late or short with Emily's modest allowance. At the same time, mother never encouraged Emily to work and often reiterated her grandiose belief that Emily could do anything she wanted, whenever she made up her mind to do so. In response Emily believed that she could take advanced courses without having had the basic ones and that she could function without adequate food, clothing, or sleep. As we talked about Emily's diet of sweets and great expectations, I commented that it was as though she was expected to thrive on a sugar teat rather than the real thing.

As we talked about how Emily might have a lifestyle more compatible with feelings of self-esteem, and more in keeping with the success and affluence of her parents, she felt increasingly angry with her mother. But she feared that if she were to rise above the general level of misery and suffering in her family, she would incur the rage and envy of family members and would leave her mother with nothing. She made several efforts to talk with mother about this. The first one failed when mother "stole her thunder" by claiming she understood completely because she and Emily were just alike. Emily was in high spirits after the second try, however, reporting that mother had called her "crazy" and unable to understand or deal with reality. Mother had never spoken to her like this before, and it felt good. As she concluded her narrative she quoted a passage from A. A. Milne, in which Christopher Robin says "I think I will stay six forever and ever," thus acquainting me with one of the origins of her delusion during the first year of therapy. We shared a laugh.

Emily began to challenge what she called her "fuck up" identity in relation to the males in her family by becoming interested in science and math, hitherto the province of her brother and father. She told me she had "fucked up" a math exam by staying up the night before, but her self-destructiveness seemed to lack its former power; we had to laugh when she subsequently told me she had gotten one of the highest grades in the class. She struggled to complete her university applications in the face of a tendency to deprive herself of food and sleep; she became disorganized, whiny, and self-pitying and then thought of the currently popular song "Vincent," which proclaimed that van Gogh had been too special, brilliant, and sensitive to live in this awful world. Emily realized she had been enacting her mother's hatred. She felt an angry, tearing sensation, and she imagined a cornered rat, her psychotic part, clawing and biting her. She began to believe that she had a high potential for achievement, and her resolve to transfer to a top university intensified.

Our attention shifted to the issue of sexuality, which Emily kept avoiding by lashing out whenever she would begin to feel close to me. She realized she could not integrate her sexual and loving feelings, and the awareness that she now had a loving relationship with me encouraged her to work on this. She reviewed numerous memories of having been a passive victim of intrusion and overstimulation by men in her family, experiences that had led to difficulties accepting her sexual feelings as internal. And she realized she had developed a system of self-protection that included inhibition, rejection of her emotions, and projection of rage.

Year Six

As we commenced our sixth and final year, Emily's concerns shifted to fearfulness that mother and her women friends were hostile to her blossoming femininity and her interest in men. She worked on fears and fantasies that she would be neutered and that either she or mother would not survive the changes in her. She recalled with embarrassment and anger how she had carved a cross in her forehead at the hospital while under the delusion that she was the Messiah. She realized she had been sacrificing herself for mother. Now that she was no longer mother's "sidecar shit," to use the symbol of a dream, she imagined mother collapsed, like a broken, lifeless puppet. Emily purchased more feminine clothing, deepened some important relationships with women, and made successful friendship overtures to Mark, a classmate, despite an aversive physical response to his attractiveness—a "no" in her head and a kind of whiny negativism that sounded to me as though she were protesting, "I am only a child!" She displaced some of her competitive concerns from mother to Deborah, an accomplished and attractive woman who eventually became Emily's closest female friend.

Emily now felt that she had a personality of her own. She elaborated fantasies about intimacy, pregnancy, childbirth, graduation, career, and exhibiting her painting, which was becoming a more central pursuit in her life. Fantasy became a kind of trial thinking preceding action. Seeing me was now experienced as touching home base, as a stepping stone and no longer an end in itself. Emily felt I was now inside her as a benign and supportive presence. For the first time she began to paint on her own, and she reported a constructive inner dialogue between her self-doubts and more encouraging thoughts that incorporated the voice of her painting teacher and my voice, which was less readily identifiable.

Emily canceled a therapy hour so she could pursue an opportunity that had unexpectedly arisen to get to know Mark better. She was accepted by her first-choice university. She dreamed that she shook mother like a rag doll, heedless of cries from family members that she was heartless, and then called an ambulance to take her away. When her family visited, Emily used humor to make it clear to mother that she now had a life of her own from which mother was excluded. On the other hand, she was indignant when I expressed my doubts about the correctness of her mother's belief that maternal grandmother had Huntington's chorea and that Emily might contract it, then she realized both she and mother had wishes to reinstate the status quo.

With me Emily seemed adolescent and rebellious. She experienced me as an intrusive father in relation to her developing sexuality. The relationship with Mark was developing at a slow and satisfactory pace. Emily had some difficulty distinguishing her consuming interest in him from her relationship with her mother, and distinguishing orgastic from psychotic forms of letting go. And she imagined I would dislike her for completely excluding me from her mind at times of passion with Mark. She marveled that she had experienced orgasm just from kissing him. They had their first real fight, which served to bring them closer. But Emily wanted all this to be private. She bridled at my comments and told me, not unkindly, that she could do things herself now and that she had a man of her own.

Emily had some difficulty focusing and finishing her thoughts; she related this to fears of where she might be heading in her life and, specifically, to fears of termination. She was irritable because there was so much she wanted to do and such limited time. In contrast, there were hours when she had little she needed to talk to me about. When my summer vacation approached, Emily acted unaware of the fact and then, at the end of an hour, told me the following dream: She went to purchase an umbrella and selected a beautiful purple one. She brought it to the salesman, who said it was nice, but not waterproof, and perhaps she should not buy it. With this dream she realized she was preparing to grieve our termination.

Emily said she was planning to make love with Mark for the first time (without commenting on the fact that she had chosen a time when I would be away). The backlash occurred when she went walking with him in new shoes that were too tight, denied the pain, and got bad blisters. This reminded her of delusionally instigated self-punishments she inflicted for allowing herself to get close to me.

When we resumed her therapy in the fall, Emily felt like an aviator about to take off, not fearfully but with excitement. In contrast, she realized that our relationship had about run its course; we would no longer be struggling to be closer but to say goodbye. Emily thought about the old days at the hospital. Many of the friends she had made there had not been as fortunate as she. She remarked that hers had been a sad story but one with a happy ending. When she brought up a sleep problem, our discussion led nowhere and she realized this was her effort to present herself as crazy and hold on to me.

As Emily began her junior year at the new university, her life did seem to be taking off. She demonstrated an amazing maturity and self-sufficiency, much of it seemingly reflexive, even though we missed a number of appointments (because of difficulties coordinating her new schedule with mine). She dreamed of a disagreement with mother: mother became a monster who attacked and clawed her face, but Emily fought back.

Emily decided that 4 months would bring her to the end of her first semester and give her sufficient time to reach an equilibrium with mother and say goodbye to me. She set a termination date and then concluded a discussion of some problems with Mark by saying, quite oblivious to the significance of her remark, "I know we can work it out; after all, neither of us is insane!"

But Emily avoided the termination work. When I eventually commented on this she accused me of devaluing her, as mother did, and lacking confidence that she could meet her commitment. In a rage she began, provocatively, to imagine committing suicide in order to despoil "my" work and destroy me. My crime, she said, was to deprive her of the worry and feeling-free schizophrenic state. Soon she turned the anger on mother for not valuing her accomplishments, but it turned out that Emily had shared few of them with her. I pointed out that she was not assuming responsibility for the work she had done and the person she had chosen to become. After a dream in which she, in the driver's seat, backed up her car but failed to see an obstacle and a murderous mother then tried to take over, Emily decided she should visit her parents and tell them more about herself. In doing so she learned that what she had taken for lack of interest on their part represented mother's concept of how to let her separate and stepfather's belief that she was too fragile to tolerate a response from him. Emily received real emotional responses from both, including learning about mother's longstanding doubts that she would ever get better.

With 2 months remaining I continued to wait for Emily to begin saying good-bye, while she acted enigmatic and sulky, in a manner reminiscent of the early days of our relationship. Even after we reviewed her wish to assign me responsibility for "seducing" her into the relationship and its consequences, this behavior continued. I began to worry about whether Emily was ready to terminate, as well as to feel angry, impatient, and devalued. I did not look forward to her therapy hours, and even harbored wishes she were gone, which, I realized, reflected quite an accomplishment on Emily's part considering all we had been through together. In casting around for reasons to avoid intervening and becoming more active in the termination process, I was reassured when Emily told me about a Thanksgiving celebration at her apartment in which she shared preparations and feelings with Mark and an invited group of friends. And it sounded as though she was doing extremely well at school.

Finally, Emily clarified that she had also been waiting for me to do something. If I really believed she could take care of herself and no longer needed to see me, she reasoned, then why didn't I act that way, stop behaving like a therapist with a problem patient, and start acting like a separate person with feelings of my own? Somewhat taken aback, I said I would try, and I moved into this unfamiliar territory by telling her how turned off I had been by her recent behavior. Emily could readily understand this. After some further discussion in which she reviewed some of the changes in herself and reiterated positive feelings about me, she told me she just wanted to be quiet and look at me. But I felt distant and unmoved, like a spectator of her accomplishments and an object of her interest. In accordance with our new understanding I shared my feeling of loss of a sense of "we-ness." Once again Emily interpreted the situation. She said I was acting the way she and her mother had acted, that I was reluctant to let her go, feeling rejected and hurt by her separateness, and that I was looking for problems to keep us together. I had the disorienting sensation that our roles were reversing, but I needed to explore this new direction with her. I thought about the reasons for my reluctance to let her go, ranging from more realistic concerns to various fantasies I entertained about having a nontherapeutic relationship with her. I shared with her the uncertainty I had about terminating with someone as ill as she had been, and I told her I would miss the pleasure of relating to her now that she was her own person. Emily was moved.

The feeling of "we-ness" was briefly restored as we shared the sense of loss of a relationship no one else could possibly understand. We both felt we had made peace with her leaving. My doubts about her readiness had forced Emily to question herself, and she told me that in all respects the first semester had gone well. Emily remarked on her fearfulness about moving, changing, heading she knew not where. But then she asserted, firmly, that she didn't want to talk about it. She knew that in the future there would be many things she would never again discuss with anyone, for she could carry her own emotional baggage, an accomplishment that left her feeling at once pleased, sad, and alone. When I commented on her freedom I made a slip, and said I wondered what choices "we" would make! Emily intensified her effort to tell me how much our relationship had meant to her. She recalled my gift when she left the hospital and told me of her frustration because she could think of nothing to give me now that would adequately reflect her feelings. With a little more than a week remaining, a sense of calm descended on both of us, a feeling that our work was finished.

In our last hour Emily symbolically relinquished her precious and enigmatic insanity. She gave me journals containing a decade of her psychotic writing, along with her permission to do with them whatever I might wish. She told me how angry she felt toward people who glorify insanity. She said she had learned to lie, without qualms, to people who asked about the scars on her arms, not because she was reluctant to talk about her past, but because her experience had been that the changes in her were so profound that people did not believe her when she would tell them she was once insane. With the notebooks there was a card that read, in part:

Thank you for helping me get on the right path. I think the only way to express adequately how much you mean to me is by living my life as fully as I can.

I have had several letters from Emily in the years since termination, and it appears she is doing just that. She graduated summa cum laude, the top student in the Fine Arts Department of the university, and she won a major art prize. She played a prominent role in campus life as well. Emily went on to launch a career as artist and art teacher, a career that continues to grow. She and Mark lived together for a few years, and then she decided, as their relationship was not progressing, that it would be better for her to be on her own. Close friendships with women friends have flourished. She has little contact with her parents, but noted in one letter that mother looked better than she had in years: "Clearly, our separation has done her good." Emily concluded a recent note as follows: "So that's how things are in my life—pretty good. As far as my psychological growth and development are concerned, I don't think anyone could have hoped for any better, even you!"

Chapter 5

Edward:
A Multisystem Failure

History

The story of Edward's life, which will preface the account of my effort to treat him, is the least reliable of the histories in this book. While Edward's own unreliability as historian, due to the extent of his distortions of current events, is not uncommon, his parents' limited knowledge about him was truly remarkable. Father was largely absent during Edward's growth, and mother's perception of Edward was filtered through a haze of solipsistic self-absorption. My belief is that the patterned enactments that emerged on the ward during Edward's hospital stay and in family therapy provide a more valid window into his history and that of his family than the verbal anamnestic material.

Edward was the eldest of four children. His three sisters ranged in age from 2 to 8 years younger. There was no family history of mental illness. Father seemed consumed by his successful business enterprises and wanted the home to be a place where he could be at peace, that is, where he would not be required to relate to anyone beyond superficialities. While he was not exactly passive he left household operation to Edward's mother, and as a family member he had little to say. While his views about family members and relationships, when eventually elicited in family therapy, seemed more realistic than his wife's, they were not as realistic as those of Edward's sisters. Mother was emotional, hypersensitive, and easily aroused to intense anger, though her capacity to forget anything that disturbed her, whether it be her own outbursts or indications of her children's problems, enabled her to minimize her impact on others and theirs on her. She was convinced she understood all the other family members and their needs, even when it seemed objectively clear that she did not, and she tended to use her sharp tongue to attack and invalidate anyone who disagreed with her.

Edward learned to read by age 3 and began nursery school at 4. The family moved to another state when he was 9, and Edward was unable to make friends in the new environment. In fact, it seems that throughout his childhood he was socially isolated and unable to relate much to others. He experienced himself as alien and different, a bored, aloof observer who was contemptuous of his peers. He withdrew into reading and other isolated academic pursuits, and as an adolescent tended to stay up late at night and, when not in school, to spend much time sleeping during the day. He seemed to identify with his mother's sadistic control and his father's withdrawal and acted the role of junior dictator over his sisters during long periods of time when mother took to bed (she may have mis-used prescription drugs) or was away from home and occupied with charitable activities. Edward told me he had a girlfriend for a brief period of time toward the end of high school, although they did not have a sexual relationship; I could not be certain whether this "relationship" was anything more than a figment of his imagination. Edward's interest in science and math led him to enroll in a technical university, where his bookish iso-lation was more or less acceptable, But he was no longer the academic star he had been in high school, which proved a severe blow to his self-esteem.

Edward was a 21-year-old college senior when he was admitted to the hospital. He had gotten drunk, become confused, panicked, and tried to scale the side of his dormitory building. He was discovered by fellow students, who thought he was a burglar and then realized, because of his bizarre behavior, that he was ill. On admission he was noted to be grossly psychotic, and shortly thereafter he was found smearing and eating his feces. He was immediately placed on haloperidol, 30 mg.

It was difficult to reconstruct the events preceding Edward's psychotic break. It seems that he had always felt out of place at the university, "like a small fish in a big pond." But his social isolation and apparent scientific preoccupation had not been so out of the ordinary as to attract attention in a university that had acquired something of a reputation for harboring emo-tional eccentrics. In the fall of his sophomore year, about 2 years prior to his hospitalization, Edward had become increasingly preoccupied with efforts to formulate a cosmic theory that included everything, particularly language, science, and nuclear fission. He began to invent his own language. He con-cluded that people were plotting against him, and that the thoughts of others were being broadcast into his mind, and vice versa. Amidst this decompensa-tion he retained some awareness of feeling confused, isolated, and despairing, and some capacity to conceal the extent of his decompensation from others. At midyear vacation recess during his sophomore year his family observed that he seemed confused and irritable, and he talked with them about dropping out of school. When he returned to school it was arranged for him to see a psycho-analyst for weekly therapy. At the start of his junior year his grades began to slide, and Edward began to use marijuana, LSD, and alcohol. He became more depressed and irritable, and there was a gradual deterioration in his living habits and self-care, culminating in the events leading to his hospitalization.

A psychological test battery administered 1 ½ weeks after Edward's admission indicated bright normal intelligence, an acute psychosis, and a longstanding severe impairment of thinking—in short, a chronic schizophrenic in a state of acute decompensation. His thinking was concrete and autistic, and his judgment very poor. There was evidence of sexual confusion, as well as terrifying sadistic impulses. Edward employed obsessive–compulsive defenses along with denial, constriction, and passivity. He was fused with a powerful maternal figure who enraged him, leading to self-hatred. There were passive longings for a father, but these were not deemed constructive as they involved wishes to live without effort and responsibility. His utter interpersonal impoverishment was noted. He was seen as an emotionally shattered and despairing individual who compensated with a grandiose exhibitionistic facade. Both homicidal and suicidal potential were noted. Edward had a sense of doom about the future, as well as a belief that he possessed a strange and fearsome power. A neurological evaluation was unremarkable.

Treatment

Year One

I met Edward shortly after his admission. He was a thin, bespectacled young man with stiff posture and a pedantic quality, a caricature of politeness and courtesy. He spoke with flat affect, obsessing litigiously or philosophically, and his language was stilted, abstract, archaic, and replete with scientific terminology. He seemed to have some interest in debating with me or proselytizing about his beliefs. We agreed to meet three times per week, and I worked with him for a total of 1½ years.

In subsequent therapy hours Edward was increasingly bizarre and withdrawn. He did not seem to be in distress. He sat stiffly and talked in a flat voice, using words idiosyncratically and at times coining neologisms; his associations were loose. His response to my attempts to encourage him to translate into communicative English was to try to get me to debate with him in and about his language. The more I allowed myself to do so, the more confused I found myself becoming about what it was he meant. As time went on he made clear that his aim was not to communicate with me, but to use my responses to help him to perfect his own unique system of thinking and speaking. With at least partly conscious intent he was playing with words and with me. In one session, when I pointed out the contradictory nature of some of his thoughts, he left the meeting early, saying he guessed he had nothing more to talk to me about.

In his early meetings with me Edward shared his belief that others were controlling his thoughts and behavior. He said he was frightened of homosexual assault, but he did not seem anxious and his concern seemed to me to be more about loss of identity than about sexual issues. He talked intellectually about being angry at everyone and said he controlled his anger by being a vegetarian, as meat eating symbolized killing.

On the ward Edward was passive in everything but speech. On a ward filled with isolated, bizarre individuals he quickly gained a reputation for being someone who had no idea how to make or conduct a human relationship, as well as for his priggish, pedantic, pseudoscientific manner. He talked mostly to female patients and in a hostile, controlling manner, bombarding them with personal questions and moralistic judgments of their behavior. It seemed to me as though he were trying to debate with his own projections, and I wondered whether he might be caricaturing what he experienced as being done to him. While he felt alienated and was full of hostile thoughts about others, he simultaneously believed that he could tune into their thoughts and become intimate with them instantly. Responding selectively to some of what he told me, I attempted to reach some consensus with Edward that he had long-standing feelings of loneliness, sadness, and anger and to confirm my hypothesis that he withdrew into independent beliefs and preoccupation with words as compensation. His response, without much affect, was to tell me that his relationship with me was the most important one he had, a notion he continued to share with me from time to time, that, like many of his comments throughout the time I knew him, I sensed, but could not be certain, had some significant content beyond what was obvious. Edward went on to describe his parents as totally self-preoccupied, and to ask if I would communicate to them his loneliness and need for their understanding. At the end of the next hour, in which he was much more withdrawn and I had even more difficulty than usual making sense of his productions, he informed me that we had been trying to deal with why he was angry, but that he preferred to remove himself into what he called a world of simplicity, involving preoccupation with eating and sleeping. He added that he had been dreaming he was in hell. Punctuated by such disruptions, our sessions continued to include occasional communications that seemed meaningful, if laden with a puzzling and mechanical quality. Edward made apparently insightful comments—such as that he did not know how to relate to others except in terms of dominance and submission,—but at some significant level it did not sound as though he meant what he was saying.

After 6 weeks of therapy Edward's medication was switched to 50 mg trifluoperazine. Over the next month this was gradually lowered to 30 mg. During the ensuing 2½ months until my summer vacation, Edward became increasingly able to look with me at his thinking and behavior, and he seemed progressively less confused. Against a backdrop of withdrawal and preoccupation with eating and sleeping he developed an intellectual curiosity about our sessions and looked forward to them. He began to talk about his detachment and the reasons for it and about his underlying vulnerability. Gradually he began to acknowledge the bizarre, psychotic nature of his thoughts and behavior. He was clearly less confused but he remained detached, with intellectualized speech habits and flat affect, and I still did not sense that I was truly reaching him.

Edward talked with me about his anger and its relation to his self-esteem problem. As he did so he had to stand up and stand over me; he was finally able to admit, on questioning, that this was his way of righting the self-esteem imbalance he felt. In the subsequent hour he was more tense and walked out of the session early; in my notes I wrote that he "conveys the impression of someone who could become explosively and suddenly angry. That is why I am not making more of an effort to keep him in the room when he decides to leave early." Edward confided that he did not trust me and that I might be committed to an ideology and might ridicule him.

For the most part Edward acted in a way that made me feel dull and sleepy and frequently left our sessions early. He told me how lost, different from others, and envious he had felt in college when his peers would act enthusiastic about their lives and how, in compensation, he had begun to use drugs and had commenced his task of inventing a new language. He talked about how he had perfected a chronic stance of aloofness and boredom, of being an observer of the world, as protection against his fears of losing his identity and being destroyed psychologically. Had he delusionally imagined himself to be a genius, or was he actually one? For the first time he was able to entertain the proposition that this belief might have been the beginning of his sickness rather than the solution to his problems.

In an hour preceding a weeklong separation Edward acted as if things were meaningless. After making a palpably feeble attempt to convince me that he was ready to leave the hospital, he stared out the window, yawned, and spoke grandiosely about the important matters that were preoccupying his attention. On my return he brought up but a single thought—his disappointment that he had been unable to actualize some of his grandiose fantasy life—and then he sat back and waited, becoming increasingly upset that the meaningful interaction he had apparently anticipated between us did not ensue.

At the beginning of our third month Edward seemed more relaxed. He began to talk about needs and feelings and to show flashes of tentative warm smiling and interest in me. He talked of his mistrust of emotion, which he viewed as "an error in the machine," and he admitted his reluctance to talk about anything that was intimate and personal, which made him feel vulnerable. Trifluoperazine was lowered to 20 mg without return of gross psychotic symptoms. Edward joked with people, resumed playing his guitar, which he had given up some time prior to hospitalization, and told me about the sexual interest he felt in some of the female patients. But his participation in the ward community continued to be minimal. Although he stayed in bed as much as possible, he was given privileges by his hospital administrator to leave the ward and go off the hospital grounds, including to my office for some of his appointments.

Edward continued to spend much time in bed, often left our meetings early (after much yawning), and was preoccupied with food and sleep. He began to talk about his family and over the course of several hours painted a picture of parents who acted as if they did not have children, or as if their

children were already grown. Edward described his mother as either physically absent or sadistic. He said she was a self-centered woman who was
interested only in her extrafamilial activities and who seemed unaware that he
was a separate person with a valid mind of his own. He sounded uncharacteristically angry when he referred to her as a "schizophrenic bitch." As he
described her pompous, overbearing, know-it-all attitude, I cautiously called
his attention to the similarity to some of his own behaviors. He responded that
his father was a more tuned in, but physically absent or emotionally distant
person, one who was preocupied with his own work unless others made an
effort to relate to him. Edward yawned conspicuously and felt more detached
as he spoke of father's absences from the family. While Edward seemed softer
in manner—and there was more of a sense of continuity and focus to his
thoughts—he seemed confused about whose thoughts were whose, and believed that the thoughts of other patients were responses to his own concerns
and preoccupations. I wondered to myself how much of what he was telling me
about his parents was accurate and how much was projection of the behavior
he was enacting.

Edward made an effort to talk to his mother about some of his ideas about
the family; while he was pleased that she did not get angry at him, he was
dismayed that they could establish no consensus and that everything he said
seemed to get transformed and become a part of some issue of her own. He
seemed to be telling me she spoke her own private language. In our next hour
Edward spoke of how he controlled his feelings so as not to be vulnerable. He
told me that he could not remember me between sessions and that I seemed
like a new and threatening authority at the beginning of each meeting, a
danger he might then distract himself from by attentions to his body. This loss
of a sense of who I was seemed so natural to him that it had not occurred to
him to speak about it with anyone.

I informed Edward that I would be taking my summer vacation in about
a month, and he responded by telling me he was ready to leave the hospital.
When I suggested that he might be reacting to my announcement, he admitted
that it would be upsetting to him for us to be separated for so long and that he
found it necessary to think of himself as all grown up and able to cope with
anything. I pointed out that he was doing what he accused his parents of, that
is, denying his true self and presenting himself as totally self-sufficient. In the
next meeting Edward yawned, told me I was on the periphery of reality, and
talked about his wishes to go to bed and his readiness to be discharged from
the hospital. Toward the end he joked that he perceived me as someone who
was kicking him out of bed. He continued to enact his detachment and boredom. At times he was actually in bed when I came to the ward for his sessions;
in response I often found myself feeling detached and bored.

In the weeks preceding my vacation Edward alternated between his bored
yawning and a sense of increasing emotional vulnerability. But he was able to
perceive and talk about some of these changes in his state, particularly the
ways he attempted to become invulnerable—by being a know-it-all, making his

speech lifeless, staying in bed, crossing his legs, or averting his gaze. Then he began to talk about anger. When I sneezed he thought it meant I might be angry with him. He wondered about whether his sense of the hostility of others was real, or whether it might be what he termed a "flaw in my thinking." He admitted to fantasies of grinding people up and eating them, as well as to the belief that if he did not conceal such ideas there would be retaliation.

Edward began to use his privileges to leave the hospital grounds to smoke marijuana and to get drunk with an old college acquaintance. On one occasion he informed me that he and his friend had actually been involved in a minor theft. As our vacation separation approached, Edward became more detached, with flat affect, sparse and guarded speech, and frequent yawning. He seemed most interested in eating, sleeping, and smoking marijuana. During our last hour he overslept and was half an hour late; then he described himself as like a little baby who just wanted to sleep and to have someone take care of him. He told me that, on weekends during high school, his parents hardly seemed to notice when he would often stay in bed more than half a day.

During my month-long summer absence, at the end of 4 months of therapy, Edward's troublesome behavior escalated. In the hospital he avoided people, was increasingly apathetic, and spent much time in bed unless mobilized by staff. He used passes to leave the hospital as occasions to drink heavily. He acknowledged to ward staff that he was depressed because I was away. Despite the regressive, destructive, and depressive signs the staff did not contain him but continued to encourage him to plan for discharge from the hospital; his trifluoperazine was cut to 15 mg. Edward made plans to return to college and take a reduced course load in the fall, but the screening psychiatrist at the university could see that he was not well enough.

Edward's depression lifted somewhat when I returned from vacation, although he did not reengage with me. It was decided by his administrative psychiatrist at a review conference to continue a discharge-oriented program. Edward talked about his belief that he didn't need anyone, and he both recalled and began to enact the belief he had had before entering the hospital, namely, that he was the center of everyone's thoughts. He wondered if we should meet less frequently because our time was being wasted if the problem was his lack of emotional involvement. Edward brought me the part of his halfway house application I had to fill out. When I told him we needed to discuss the answers to the questions together, he was shocked. We reached a surprising consensus about the answers. He was clearly confused about two of the questions: his prehospitalization condition and his current condition. With regard to the first Edward felt that he had experienced thought telepathy and the ability to control others, but he also believed that he had been psychotic and out of control of his thoughts, with visual and auditory hallucinations. With regard to the second he believed that people need to make themselves emotionally vulnerable and take risks in relationships, but he also believed that human interactions could be instantaneous and magical, and that intimacy was preordained and did not need to be worked at. With Edward in this precarious situation his administrator chose to discontinue his trifluoperazine completely.

Edward seemed more fragmented, and he talked in a highly intellectualized way of a life of science and of his interest in finding a woman who would care for him in a motherly way while he was passive. I learned that he was continuing to use marijuana, and he began to report visual hallucinations, critical auditory hallucinations, and ideas of thought transmission and to tell me, with some exhilaration, about his ability to establish instant intimacy with others. At the same time, he was suspicious that others might be controlling him. At first I attributed his regression to the marijuana consumption, and while I urged his administrator to curtail his privileges, I did not yet suggest that he be placed back on trifluoperazine. After 6 months of therapy Edward was more clearly delusional and grandiose. He denied being ill and began to deny any need to see me. His passivity was consciously provocative; he made it clear that he wanted to force me to gratify his wish for someone to direct his life and take control for him. He was stubbornly silent and held me responsible for this, insisting that I was the disengaged person who would not become involved. In retrospect, as I reflect on my delay in responding to his deteriorating condition, I believe he was partially correct.

Edward became increasingly arrogant and articulated wishes to collect women and study them analytically, through a kind of therapeutic microscope. He lectured to me in a pompous manner. In the midst of one such lecture he startled me by casually asking if I knew that he had asked staff for trifluoperazine 2 days earlier. When I asked him about this he told me of his belief that he was telecommunicating with many students and faculty at his old university, but he articulated doubts about whether his thinking was unusually sensitive or psychotic. He forgot to attend his next appointment with me.

Around the end of the sixth month a 15 mg dose of trifluoperazine was reinstituted by Edward's administrator, again without informing me. Nonetheless, and despite feedback from me, the ward staff did not alter their perception of Edward as more isolated than psychotic, and therefore they continued to encourage him to get involved in rehabilitation programs and to make arrangements to move to a halfway house. Edward continued to find ways to drink when let out of the hospital. Waiting for me to take some action in therapy, he either feigned sleep or actually fell asleep. During one therapy session he dreamed that two girls were courting him. Edward was convinced that I knew the direction he should be taking but was withholding this information. He said he felt closer to me than ever, but I experienced him as aloof and contentious; whatever I said, he objected to. His description of his behavior on the ward sounded like a caricature of a sadistic therapist attempting to "break through" the problems of female patients. He was convinced his thinking had become clearer and more creative. As his administrator still did not restrict him despite my requests, I decided to take the only action available to me that would indicate to Edward my concern for him: I stopped seeing him at my hospital office, which was in another building, and resumed seeing him on his ward.

Gradually, Edward's paranoia and hallucinations diminished. He was more noticeably depressed, and he spent prolonged periods in bed. He seemed to recognize that he needed trifluoperazine and remarked that he might have to be on it for the rest of his life. He knew that the reason for this medication was to ameliorate his tendency to feel merged with his environment, a tendency that rendered him unable to live around others without becoming confused, and in addition led him to act aloof, withdrawn, and critical, in an Olympian caricature of a psychiatrist. But he could not decide whether these cognitive idiosyncracies meant that he was ill, or that he was an exceptional individual with extraordinary sensitivities who knew everything about himself that he needed to know—and more about the rest of us than we did. Edward could sense when he was more fragmented but considered the possibility that this might be a special ability—to be more than one person. In therapy he became intellectually compliant. He recognized that I thought he should talk about feelings and relationships, and he even brought a pad and pen in order to make an outline of our conversation, as though I were the professor. Edward talked about the detachment and denial he perceived in other members of his family, but it was clear his observations were being made from a position of omnipotence and omniscience. He was convinced of his superior intellect and knowledge, and believed that he could educate others but needed nothing from them.

Edward continued to spend much time in bed and to resist staff efforts to mobilize him into any kind of therapeutic program; in particular, staff members wished for him to get a hospital job. Their efforts met with what they referred to as his "authoritarian rigidity," as well as with his denial that he had any problems with which their help was needed. Edward acknowledged that he was lonely but went on to tell me that he could only relate to others who agreed with his point of view, and that in his opinion anyone who did not think he was well, including myself, had a simplistic and stereotypic way of thinking. His trifluoperazine was increased to 20 mg, but my sense was that the intent was to make him more tractable.

His family visited and, according to Edward's description, it was as though they had come for a college weekend of activities. They had no meaningful discussion. On one occasion, Edward said, he had attempted to discuss his mother's anger but she denied having any. Our hours seemed to become a bit more productive, and Edward once again began to acknowledge his own anger and how he expressed it through his aloof, judgmental position as pseudotherapist, a behavior that left him alone and separated from others. He felt his behavior was a response to the fact that everyone in his family pretended that everything was fine.

Edward seemed a bit more receptive to my input, but the gains were transient. Soon he seemed more fragmented and spoke of himself as a machine without feeling, then, without awareness of contradiction, he talked of all the feelings he had been having. When I pointed out the inconsistency, he told me he was convinced that machines were capable of love. He became quite grandiose about his powers of reason and perception, and made it clear that he was convinced he knew more about others on the ward than anyone, including the chief psychiatrist. He spoke sanctimoniously and condescendingly about the flaws of other patients, for example, the sadism of other male patients and the inability to love that he perceived in a girl he claimed to be interested in. He analyzed the delusional self-sufficiency of a male patient who was trying to leave the hospital against advice and who attacked any feedback he was given. Edward said this young man was confused, did not know himself very well, and tended to attack and devalue others. I pointed out that Edward was talking as though he were a psychiatrist, and I wondered if any of these issues might be related to his own. He agreed with the first proposition, and when I wondered what this meant for our relationship, he said that he thought I was an interesting person, but essentially superficial and superfluous, and that we could probably terminate immediately! In our next meeting he talked righteously about a meeting with his family in which his mother was narcissistic (his term) and would not accept feedback from him.

On the ward Edward openly expressed his belief that he was superior to and without need for anyone around him. In hall meetings conducted by the ward administrative psychiatrist he pronounced himself a kind of psychiatrist who was there to help others. At 7½ months the ward staff finally began to realize how serious Edward's problem was. They colluded less with his denial, began to accept the inevitability of a longer hospital stay, and stopped pushing him toward rehabilitative-discharge-oriented programs. Edward was restricted to the ward and his treatment reviewed. Trifluoperazine was increased to 30 mg.

In his objectless world, with his own language and his belief in his self-sufficiency, Edward used food, drink, cigarettes, sleep, and masturbation for stimulation. He was willing to admit that he needed trifluoperazine—but this, he said, was because he was an exceptional person. I suggested that it might be possible to acknowledge that he was psychotic and needed medication while retaining the right to reject any human therapeutic contact and help for his problems. The idea frightened him, although he argued that it was I who was afraid and that my fear was contagious. After this he became more confused.

Meanwhile, in their meetings with the social worker since their son's admission, Edward's parents had expressed much guilt and claimed they would do anything they could to help, if only she would tell them what to do. At the same time they adamantly denied any family problems whatsoever or any knowledge of what might be bothering Edward. When the social worker raised issues with them Edward's parents would promptly forget them. In stark contrast with his parents' blanket denials were the specific problems

Edward claimed various family members had, problems, the reader will recall, Edward had been telling me about from the very beginning. With Edward's permission I decided to meet with parents and social worker to obtain a firsthand impression. During the meeting I discovered that the thinking of Edward's parents was strikingly similar to his own. They felt it inconceivable that Edward's problems might in any way be related to other family members. They thought of Edward as an unreasonable and withdrawn person and found his behavior utterly incomprehensible. Of course they wanted to do anything they could to help, they said, but because they could conceive of no problem in which they were involved, we must tell them what to do. After this conference the social worker and I decided to begin conjoint family therapy, including Edward, his sisters and myself, his parents, and the social worker.

The family meetings began with denial of any family issues other than Edward's illness and alienation from the rest of the family. Edward was looked upon as some sort of anomaly. The first issues we struggled with included the parental myth of the happy family, which mother, in particular, seemed invested in maintaining, and the tendency of all members to gloss over unpleasant events. No one listened to anyone else; each member had fantasy projections about each of the others that compellingly overshadowed anything that person might actually say. Father was especially vocal about his conviction that our meetings were without purpose. He was unable to remember the topic of our previous week's discussions, and expressed open disbelief and disagreement regarding any comments made by the therapists that suggested the existence of causal interpersonal links of any kind.

At first Edward acted like nothing the others said or did mattered to him. But after a few meetings and some encouragement from me, he attempted to tell his parents of the serious feelings of despair and alienation he had experienced during high school. They were shocked and disbelieving, and countered with their conviction that he had been an active, productive, and self-confident person. Edward became angry at his parent's failure to believe his account of his adolescent suffering, and walked out of a meeting. The other family members hardly appeared to notice, much less to show any interest in why he had done it, and simply continued their conversation.

Edward's trifluoperazine was raised to 40 mg. During the ninth month, concurrent with the beginning of our exploration of family issues, he began to seem more alert and to show some new interest in what he might be feeling. I forgot one of his therapy hours and my unconscious enactment of the sense of unimportance of our relationship made me realize how profoundly his delusional omnipotence and self-sufficiency had affected me. As though in confirmation, Edward did not seem to notice my dereliction, but I called his attention to it and told him what I understood about how his attitude had engendered similar feelings in me. He was shocked to hear himself protest that our relationship was meaningful to him. He began to identify some of what for him were my positive characteristics. He realized how difficult it was for him to admit these feelings, even to himself, much less to share them. It dawned on him that he could not expect his parents to know him unless he made the effort to communicate his feelings and thoughts.

On a day when we did not have an appointment we had a chance encounter on the hospital grounds, during which Edward told me, excitedly, that he couldn't wait to see me the next day to tell me about a dream. But when the appointment came he questioned me about *my* feelings, as though I were the patient, and then asked me to look at outlines of papers about psychotherapy he was planning to write. I indicated my puzzlement about the discontinuity from the previous day's encounter, and about which of us he thought was the psychiatrist and which the patient. He responded by talking about his difficulty bearing his feelings and about his fear of emotions and needs for others, which he had experienced during a ward meeting the previous day. In ensuing sessions he began to be aware of the feelings of rage and hopeless depression he experienced in relation to his parents, and of his need to see me if he was to deal with these feelings.

Edward seemed both more emotional and, at the same time, more confused, distractible, and unable to focus his attention. We realized that he could appear more organized and focused only by maintaining a state devoid of awareness of emotions, needs, and relationships and by immersing himself in a world of eating, drinking, smoking, sleeping, and masturbating. We agreed that he was attempting to avoid the very disturbing experience of overwhelming rage and hopelessness with regard to his parents. This depressive despair involved a basic skepticism about the presence of helping human beings in the world. As Edward became more aware of how much his psyche was organized around avoidance of overwhelming pain, he also began to perceive the possibility of choice. An essential element in the choice was his awareness that he had never trusted that a human relationship might be able to help him with his feelings.

Edward alternated now between more emotional openness and his more customary aloof, obnoxious, grandiose attitude. In a rather moving exchange he told me that he felt he and his sisters were like the newborn turtles who race along the sand in an attempt to reach the protective safety of the water before they are dissected and devoured by frigate birds. In the process of describing the attack of the birds on the baby turtles he became more aloof and detached and even sadistic, and I was able to point out to him how his identification shifted in the middle of the story, just as he tended to shift roles from that of the vulnerable patient to what he conceived of as the dissecting, sadistic, all-knowing parent or psychiatrist. Edward responded that he had been reading Taoist scriptures, and that if our work was successful there might be three stages, the first involving an attempt to appreciate his real feelings, the second involving total immersion in them and a need for my help, and finally, achievement of some perspective. Subsequently, he recalled how he and his younger sisters ate many of their meals alone because father was absent and mother isolated herself in her bedroom. At these times Edward would imagine he was the parent and would act quite aloof and critical toward his sisters.

After a weekend separation Edward brought me a note, which read, in part:

> I feel so lost and alone . . . I feel desperately afraid. There is no just and righteous path for me to follow. Everything is shaped by internal pressure. My hands are cold, my heart trembles. I am an artist with no way to speak. I do not see, I cannot hear; I taste no fine wine; the subtle points are lost on me. I am a mute in a land of singers. Sometimes I wish for death . . . I feel an anger which would consume the material of the bonds which lie about me. Yet in its impotence my anger is redoubled.

Edward talked about his belief that feelings like this made him vulnerable to attack, and then he recalled a dream in which his mother was driving the car recklessly. He finally got her to stop, and she admitted that she had felt like attacking him. The dream seemed to relate to some efforts family members were making to talk more directly to one another in the family meetings.

In the tenth month trifluoperazine was decreased from 30 to 25 mg. The rest of the family took a vacation, and family therapy meetings were interrupted. Edward was angry with other patients on the ward for not making good use of their hospitalization. He felt that he could not possibly relate to people who were so much like statues and so unable to learn from what was said to them. Then he proceeded to be enraptured by his own thought processes and to tune out what I had to say to him about his own role in situations. When the issue of whether he heard what I was saying arose, he insisted he had and repeated, in essence, things he had been saying to me that I had disagreed with, as though they were *my* comments. It was quite discouraging.

In the 11th month, after being defeated in an election for the position of ward patient chairman and having a disturbing telephone conversation in which his middle sister told him she was upset, had withdrawn from school, and was seeing a psychiatrist, Edward became very upset. He began to share more directly and graphically the extent of his psychotic thinking, but continued to vacillate in his belief about whether it was abnormal or supranormal. He admitted that for at least 2 years he had been having auditory and visual hallucinations and that casual conversations and radio and television programs seemed to be directed toward him. He realized that at certain times his thoughts made no sense even to him. His speech at times was nonsensical and neologistic. He shared his confusion about what was coming from inside and what from outside himself. He had some awareness of his tendency to think that people had spoken to him when they had not and of how at times he did not understand what it was I had said while at other times he attributed all of his associations to me, as though they were my ideas. At times he was not sure if the external world was real or a figment of his imagination. His realization that he could not even rely on his own thinking, which he had turned to when he felt he had nothing else, frightened him. He admitted having withheld this information because he could not stand anyone to question his sense of reality. He wrote me a long note, which I quote in part:

> I continue to hear messages in the environment. I'm frightened by these un-explained events. I'm angry over the fact that these messages seem to occur everywhere . . . I can only hope to respond imaginatively and appropriately to the significance contained herein. . . . In the daytime I become someone else. . . . Only as I wait for sleep do I perceive reality as a tangible presence. There is no substance in my waking life, no truth . . . I have the feeling people don't clearly understand what they say. This is disconcerting for me. They are trying to say something meaningful, and instead express themselves in terms that are too general for comprehension, "Do you want to talk about it?"; "I don't know what you mean." . . . I have been having thoughts I can't decipher . . . Why should I tell people what I think? Does this make my perception of reality more thorough? Is it significant that I wish to retain my private conception of reality? . . . I want to do no less than develop an understanding of my perception of the world and publish it so as to share my completed synthesis of a world view.

Edward discovered that, if he went out of his room at bedtime when he was paranoid or hallucinating and made contact with someone, the intensity of the disturbing experience tended to diminish. He read *The Divided Self* by R. D. Laing and began to wonder whether his belief that he had extrasensory communication with alien beings was really a product of the fragmentation of his own mind. He began to wonder if I could help him to unify his mind. But he tended to talk of these things as though the observing self or commentator and the phenomenological or experiencing self were two separate people.

When Edward tried to confide more of his confusion about his thinking with his family in our joint meetings, he was greeted with responses not unlike his own: hyperintellectual questioning and personalized misconstructions. His parents expressed no surprise upon learning that he was hallucinating. Later Edward claimed that this was because his parents hallucinated too; he said his mother had told him that she had conversations with him, which she believed were real, when they were in their separate bedrooms. Then he became more agitated and depressed and shared with me various violent and suicidal thoughts. Even with encouragement he was unable to connect his mood change to what he had been talking about.

In our family meeting—and for the first time in the memories of other family members—father attempted to become an active emotional participant in family life. On several occasions—in the face of an obvious uncertainty which was markedly in contrast with the image of the all-knowing and totally competent business magnate he usually conveyed—he became vocal and tear-ful about his sadness and helplessness about Edward's problem and that of his daughter, who, it emerged, had a serious depression and anorexia (informa-tion Edward had long since told me and at a time when his parents were adamantly denying the existence of any family problems other than his). Seemingly in response to his father, Edward became more openly contentious and argumentative, and asserted that no one understood or respected him and that everyone was ineffective in their efforts to help him.

Edward began to fight more openly with his male administrative psychiatrist as well, but for the first time he revealed to him (as well as to other staff) his belief that he lived in two separate worlds; he also told about his extensive hallucinations, including children's voices; his delusions of thought transmission through public communication media; and his thoughts of suicide by cutting his wrists. Although he continued to spend much time in bed, Edward began a hospital job and became leader of the ward meeting group.

In the family meetings father realized with surprise that he wanted a response from Edward to his expression of concern. In a moving tableau he cried and reached out for his son, who remained stony and unresponsive. Edward subsequently told me of a dream in which father returned to an old house where they had lived and tried to talk with him about a mistake that he, father, had made. Then he was watching a bearded man on television whom he could not hear. And, finally, he was in his parents' bedroom wrestling with his younger sister, who turned into a green monster. He called for help, and his middle sister came out of the bathroom and sprayed insecticide at the monster but hit Edward with it instead. After telling me this Edward recalled how his father had taken him on a trip at age 5 and then left him alone in the car for a long time. Edward had become very frightened and imagined that his father had vanished in a puff of smoke. In response to my efforts to explore possible links between the dream and events in family therapy Edward denied that there had been any recent change in father's behavior, and he waxed eloquent about his mother's self-preoccupation and her constant use of the royal "we" when talking. When I disagreed with the accuracy of his perception about father, Edward responded that when I pointed out things he was not aware of, no matter how accurate they might be, this made him unable to think and, as a result, very angry. In subsequent hours he pontificated solipsistically about the contents of his hallucinations and delusions, and seemed to have little awareness of what was occurring in the family meetings. Edward began to smoke marijuana again, and we struggled over his confusion about whether doing so led him to attain greater clarity and capacity to communicate or whether it made him more forgetful, more fragmented in his thinking, and more suspicious, and was perhaps responsible for his concern that others thought him homosexual.

Coincident with father's increasing involvement in family meetings in the 11th month, mother began to act more threatened. She and father fought about the family therapy, and she was openly resentful of father's increased pressure to involve other family members. Then she missed the next two family meetings. On her return she denied that anything had happened. In marked contrast to Edward's response and that of his mother, Edward's younger sisters seemed to appreciate father's new role and the novel prospect of openness in family communication. They recalled how mother had tyrannized them during father's absences, getting physically and emotionally out of control and then declaring afterward that what she had done had not occurred or else that it was meaningless.

The family fragmentation and absence of communication was next acted out by episodic absences on the part of all family members except father. Attendance was unpredictable and inconsistent. It was Edward who finally began to express anger at the others about this, but, as was so characteristic, the family seemed to choreograph an elaborate dance in which when one member tried to be emotionally present the others all found ways to leave or deny it. Now other family members began to respond by becoming more consistent and accessible, but Edward once again regressed.

Meanwhile, ward staff—who customarily allowed Edward to be with-drawn, to sleep, and to wander about—placed pressure on Edward to become involved in ward life. In response he became openly paranoid and angry. After expressing some feelings of fear and hatred, mistrust that I might divert him from his sources of pleasure; and wishes to protect himself from assaults by others, Edward's speech disintegrated and at times he talked gibberish without concern. He told me that he was the center of the universe and of all com-munication and that he needed no one. He was cold and affectless. He hinted that another patient was helping him plan his strategies in what he perceived to be a war with me, and that he was planning to "use" his family for some mercenary purposes he would not divulge. He described his state of mind with what he said was the title of a popular song—"Comfortably Numb." In another hour, after giving me some of his latest grandiose writings and telling me of the pleasure he was getting from "analyzing" other ward patients, he told me of a dream of a ward that he described as a mirror image of this one and in which there lived three characters: an observer; another with face averted, whom he called the avoider; and another who was a sadist who was challenging the avoider and "putting the avoider down." Edward briefly stopped taking his trifluoperazine, now 25 mg daily, in order to test himself, and talked of having big plans. In another session he described a variety of feelings. At the end of the hour he told me that he thought he liked me and impulsively tried on my hat. But I was uneasy, even suspicious, about why he was telling me these things. In the following hour he explained that he was trying to construct a way of relating to me so that we could pretend we were working together.

Year Two

At the end of the first year of therapy, around Easter, Edward's delusions began to take on a more religious, messianic flavor, and for the first time he became assaultive. He attacked a staff member in response to his belief that God had told him to. As a result he had to be placed in a seclusion room, and trifluoperazine dosage was raised to 40 mg.

Both I and the social worker who was acting as co–family therapist planned to go on vacation in the 13th month of Edward's treatment, which meant interruption both of Edward's therapy and the family meetings. vacation time approached, Edward told me that he wanted my help, that he was aware that clinging to his ways of thinking was interfering with his treatment, but that he had no idea what to do. There were brief bursts of feeling. Edward, almost crying, told me he felt homesick, but he said he did not know how to talk about it because he had never experienced what it was like to have a family. He said that it was not his current family he missed, that he did not even know how to think about home and being homesick. After expression of genuine loneliness he attributed ridicule to me, and gradually he became more abstracted and fragmented. I commented that he did not seem to comprehend the idea of a family in which people talked with, listened to, and tried to help one another.

Then Edward withdrew completely into a belief that the problems were all outside himself. He ignored my presence as a separate person and denied his need for help. Nothing external seemed to register with him; he was preoccupied with his habits, smoking and eating, and he seemed to experience little distress other than some fears that something in his food might somehow change him. Because he was now episodically assaultive on the ward, our meetings were now sometimes held in the seclusion room. To put his behavior in some perspective, being assaultive and getting transferred to another ward was modal patient behavior on Edward's ward at the time, and those patients who indulged in it tended to receive much attention from the staff.

Before our last meeting preceding my vacation Edward assaulted another patient in what the ward staff described as a provocative, masochistic manner. He told me that he had been having ideas that he was Christ, and that he was responsible for all the crises in the world. He said he wanted to make fun of me, because that was what he felt I was doing to him. Then he engaged in a long self-enraptured soliloquy about how his thought process was that of a fine machine while biting viciously at his nails. Finally, I reminded him of our impending separation, which he had by then forgotten, and he told me he felt like he was losing his best friend. When I pointed out the discrepancy between this sentiment and his earlier belief that we were making fun of one another, he could not recall having said the latter and concluded that it didn't matter anyway.

While I was gone Edward had numerous episodes of violent behavior and was in seclusion and restraints much of the time. Ward staff felt there was a clear connection between my absence and his regression. Trifluoperazine was raised to 55 mg and then to as much as 80 mg. On one occasion he punched a nurse who entered the quiet room because he had been banging on the walls and screaming; he claimed afterward that his behavior was morally justified and was part of his treatment.

On my return at the end of the 13th month Edward's agitation briefly diminished and he was able to spend more time outside seclusion. He walked out of our first appointment after 25 minutes; during that time he was bizarre and fragmented, but before leaving he also made some surprisingly accurate statements. He said that there were three choices: if he remained in the hospital he would, he predicted, become increasingly violent to himself and others, because he could not differentiate himself from others, and would eventually be transferred to a state hospital. Or he could leave the hospital, but he did not believe he could take care of himself. The solution, he felt, was to take drugs. On further reflection he thought maybe he could try to learn to compromise and accept some of the ideas of others, particularly me, but he concluded that this was unlikely as he had always been uncompromising in his attitudes. As was so often the case, I wondered if I was not attributing more profundity and meaning to these statements than was warranted. The following hour Edward told me that he was firing me and his family and was leaving the hospital. He changed his mind during the hour, but he was very disorganized. He tried to keep one eye closed because he was convinced that doing so would clear up his thinking and make him less agitated.

His attendance at family meetings was irregular. Sometimes he refused to come, and at other times he was unable to because he was in seclusion. After a period of absence he decided to resume attending, but he behaved in a grandiose way, directing all the members in what to think and do, and acting as omniscient judge of what was right and wrong. Without qualms he interrupted and cut short the other members. Father began to object, and mother, who had never been directly and realistically confrontative despite her own history of tyrannical behavior, began to express her concerns about how unreasonable and unrealistic Edward was being. One of Edward's sisters tried to talk about herself, but Edward told her she could not as he was the sole arbiter of right and wrong. Father expressed anger and told Edward to be quiet. Edward's older sister joined the objection, but it was his youngest sister, barely adolescent, who observed how Edward's behavior was simply a caricature of what each family member did to abort dialogue and engagement with the others! Quite uncharacteristically, other family members began to acknowledge their patterns of withdrawal and nonmutuality by projection of their own beliefs and by their sadistic devaluation of opposing points of view.

After this meeting, Edward, in response to an auditory hallucination and to a sense that he had read her mind and was gratifying her wish, suddenly slapped a female patient. As a result, after 13 months of therapy he was transferred to a more disturbed ward. There his assaultiveness continued to escalate in frequency and intensity in response to auditory hallucinations commanding him to harm himself and others. Edward expressed homicidal ideas, and he made efforts to escape from the ward. Because of the evident danger he required frequent seclusion and chemical (chlorpromazine) as well as physical restraint. Trifluoperazine was discontinued and Edward was placed on a high dose of loxapine. He began to induce vomiting and pretended to swallow medication but later spat it out and saved it, and he initiated legal efforts to leave the hospital. When his behavior was discussed with him, he claimed quite openly that he had no control over it and justified what he did with messianic ideas of entitlement. He went so far as to predict that he was going to harm himself or others and warned that if staff wanted to avoid this they would have to take control. He consciously emulated the behavior of the most disturbed patients, claiming that they were the most normal and objective. He reported two dreams in which he was in the driver's seat of vehicles that were out of control and from which other people had been excluded. He claimed to recognize that this represented his own thinking and behavior. When we talked about whether he wanted help, he abruptly walked out of the session; he then returned, saying that he realized what he had done.

In the family meetings the others talked about their distress and fear about Edward's behavior. In response to the intractability of his illness and the stresses of family travel from another state for our regular meetings, they began for the first time to talk about the possibility of transferring Edward to a hospital nearer home. Because of the frequency of his assaultiveness and the need to keep him in seclusion, and at times in restraints as well, Edward's attendance at the family meetings became even more infrequent. He attended part of a meeting "out of politeness" in order to explain his reasons for signing a legal notice of intention to leave the hospital. But he would not respond to the concerns and questions of others and simply asserted his conviction that he was Christ or Christlike.

During the 15th month I requested consultation from a senior analyst colleague, and over a period of time he met with patient, family, and relevant staff members.

In the 16th month Edward voiced delusional beliefs that he needed to hit others in order to protect himself. He was almost continuously assaultive and required not only seclusion but also restraints. Family therapy went on without him, and focused increasingly on mother's role in the family as the absolute monarch or tyrant who controlled the children in ways that were often arbitrary and whimsical and punished whomever might disobey. Mother was shocked and distressed to learn about this, and it was clear that it was the first such feedback she had ever been aware of—and perhaps had ever been given from other family members. Then we began to approach the underlying marital schism that had allowed such a family system to flourish, and both parents become very agitated. Mother, in particular, became suspicious of me and my intentions.

Meanwhile, I continued to see Edward in the seclusion room, even though what little dialogue we had been able to have had by now more or less dried up. Now he expressed the wish to assault me when I said something he did not wish to hear, and on more than one occasion he actually attempted to do so. In his restraints he spent much time screaming and chanting; released from them he was assaultive. Finally, I suggested that if he did not wish to see me he could simply ask me to leave, rather than having to attack me physically, and I would do so. He responded to my suggestion by asking me to leave any time I challenged or tried to interpret his thinking in even the mildest of ways.

In the middle of the 16th month staff had a conference with the consultant, who emphasized the serious long term nature of the illness and the importance of continuing both individual and family therapy. He felt that father was depressed and that mother was grandiose and psychotic. He also felt it was urgent that something be done quickly to calm the situation. As a consequence a course of 30 electroconvulsive therapy (ECT) treatments was embarked upon. After 3 of these Edward was in somewhat better control and able to be out of restraints more, and for a time there was a guarded feeling of optimism on the part of the treatment team. At the same time Edward refused to eat for several days, claiming that he was too special for such a mundane activity.

At the end of the 16th month I went on vacation for 2 weeks. At that time the transient improvement we had attributed to the treatments seemed to come to an end, and by the middle of the 17th month, after a total of 16 treatments, no clear-cut change was apparent. Edward's medication was switched once again, this time from loxapine to chlorpromazine, 800 mg. (At the time of Edward's treatment, about 15 years ago, the palette of antipsychotic medications was more limited than it is today.) Now Edward claimed that he had the right to assault staff because he was a mental patient; he was especially sadistic and intimidating to female staff and patients. He proclaimed that he had his own master plan for his treatment. Chlorpromazine was raised to 1,200 mg.

Family therapy continued without Edward. While family members expressed a sense of futility and despair regarding Edward, mother began to change and to help her daughters to communicate and understand one another's points of view. In response, the daughters began to be aware of their anger at mother. There was discussion of how the wishes and needs of one family member were perceived as deprivations of another.

By the end of the 18th month, and despite 20 ECT treatments and a daily dose of 1,600 mg of chlorpromazine, not only was there no sign of improvement in Edward's condition but he had begun to deliberately urinate on his bed and would shout, hallucinate, and bang his head even when placed in restraints. Now Edward required more or less total and continuous nursing care, and staff began to find him increasingly intolerable.

In the 19th month of our relationship Edward tried twice to assault me. He continued to assert the completeness and omnipotence of his own thinking, but he talked about the annihilation he feared were he to engage in any kind of dialogue or relationship.

Father began to miss family meetings, ostensibly for business reasons, and then sisters began to do the same. When father was confronted with his behavior, he was able to talk about his being upset over family problems and business issues and his wish to withdraw. The family then began to talk about their distress about Edward's intransigent regressive behavior. Now, confronted with withdrawal and opposition from family, ward staff, and Edward himself, it was I who felt helpless, beleaguered, and without choice. I told Edward that, under the circumstances, I could not see that there was anything to be gained by continuing to try to work with him. This seemed to sober him. Family members and ward staff joined in telling Edward if he did not exercise more control he would be transferred to a state hospital. To emphasize a point he seemed unable to assimilate in words, that is, that he was not making constructive use of me and that there were finite limits to his treatment resources, I reduced the length of our sessions to 30 minutes.

After another brief hint of positive responsiveness, Edward became increasingly bizarre. He began drinking his own urine and defecating in the quiet room. Transfer to a state hospital was recommended and plans were made. Again, seemingly in response to the threat of transfer, Edward's behavior improved markedly, but briefly. While awaiting transfer, Edward made an unsuccessful attempt to kill himself by stuffing a sock down his throat.

Edward's parents could not tolerate the idea of sending him to a state hospital, and at the last minute relented and arranged for his transfer to another private institution, where he would be more comfortable but would not get intensive therapy. In our family meetings they began to grieve his seeming "death" as a member of the family. They used our final family meetings to define their marital difficulties much more clearly and recognized how father's passive acquiescence based on wishes for tranquillity meshed collusively with mother's neediness and difficulty tolerating another point of view. In this atmosphere of parental disengagement the destructive ways all the children had of getting attention were also clarified.

When Edward was transferred to the new hospital, which was not far away, he expressed a wish to see me again. When I went to visit him I found him for the first time in months not in restraints. He had forgotten the reason for our meeting. Not only was he unable to indicate goals or interests, but he was unable even to complete his sentences or pursue a train of thought. He was suspicious and looked as though he were continuously hallucinating. It was my impression that he would become violent were I to question or challenge him in any way. He said he would contact me in a couple weeks about meeting again but he did not, and after a time I wrote him to finalize our termination. Our effort at treatment had lasted about 1½ years. Father's last comments by letter to me included the following statement: "Surprisingly, I find myself missing the weekly family visit . . . I would like to thank you for your efforts . . . I know we have been helped greatly."

About a decade later, in the course of writing this book, I wrote to the family requesting a follow-up but received no reply.

Part III

Viewpoints on Schizophrenia: A Pluralistic Model

Chapter 6

The Perspective of Neuroscience

Two hypotheses, self-evident to our late-20th-century ears, have stimulated most of the schizophrenia research until relatively recently. These are the idea developed by Morel and Griesinger in the mid-19th century that insanity may be associated with the brain and with morbid heredity, and the implication of the frontal lobes in schizophrenia by Alzheimer (1897) and Kraepelin (1896/1919) around the very end of the 19th century, following the identification of this site as the seat of higher mental functions. Studies of the relative influence of heredity and environment continue to be actively pursued. Despite the failure to find gross lesions in the frontal lobes, researchers are conducting increasingly sophisticated searches for central nervous system abnormalities in schizophrenics and members of their immediate families. These searches might better be looked upon as efforts to understand the spectrum of different ways in which the brain can be structured and organized than as examples of the traditional quest for pathological lesions that clearly demarcate normal from abnormal subjects.

The Origin and Nature of Neurobiological Hypotheses

From whence do neurobiological hypotheses originate? One source is our as yet primitive but expanding knowledge of the complexities of normal brain functioning and of deranged function related to other conditions. The first hypotheses, as we have noted, were generated by knowledge of the association of the frontal lobes with higher-order mental functioning and by the simplistic conception of insanity as losing one's mind—a belief that, as we shall see in Chapters 7 and 9, may not be so unsophisticated as it appears.

Other hypothesis-generating observations include the discovery that neurosyphilitic psychosis is a response to microbial infection, the recognition that a schizophrenic-like psychosis can be induced by drugs such as LSD, and the discovery by Delay and Deniker (1952), Delay, Deniker, & Harl (1952), and by Laborit, Huguenard, and Alluaume (1952) of a reciprocal phenomenon, namely, that a drug, chlorpromazine, alleviates psychotic symptomatology. These observations led to the study of neurochemistry, to the identification and study of neurotransmitters, and to the discovery that effective antipsychotic medications all appear to be antagonistic to dopamine transmission (Creese, 1976). This discovery, in turn, has stimulated the search for dopamine receptor sites in the brain.

Some who have been impressed with the element of splitting or nonintegration in schizophrenia have seized upon the notion of a bicameral mind with specialized and lateralized cerebral hemispheric functions, and have considered the prospect of disrupted intercommunication between parts of the mind, as occurs in cases of pathological or surgically induced commissurotomy. Most recently, as we shall see, the fact that psychotic features (however atypical of schizophrenia most of these may be) are found in some instances of temporal lobe epilepsy and may be elicited by electrical stimulation of parts of the limbic system seems to be focusing attention, along with such new knowledge of brain function as MacLean's (1990) concept of the triune brain, on the function and malfunction of the limbic system. As investigations become more complex, however, neuroscientists are less able to use gross schizophrenic symptomatology as the epiphenomenal "smoke" potentially leading to the abnormal central nervous system "fire" and are becoming increasingly dependent on knowledge of sophisticated mental processes and functions in order to generate hypotheses. Some of the most respected hypothesis makers and investigators of brain function, such as Paul MacLean, readily acknowledge that a full appreciation of the subtleties of the psychological level of function is essential in order to generate useful neuroscience hypotheses.

The Genetic Hypothesis

There has been much speculation about the role of toxic, traumatic, and viral etiologic factors, both in utero and postpartum. Parnas et al. (1982) note that the schizophrenic offspring of schizophrenic mothers are more likely to have a history of pregnancy and birth complications than the normal offspring. Nonetheless, the only organic etiologic hypothesis currently supported by significant data is genetic. To place the genetic data in some perspective, Gottesman and Shields (1982) and Kringlen (1987) note that about 90% of schizophrenics do *not* have a schizophrenic parent, and that 81% have neither a parent nor a sibling who is schizophrenic. Nonetheless, there is a strong association between the magnitude of risk of developing schizophrenia and the degree of relatedness to a schizophrenic. The most powerful predictor of risk for the disorder is being an identical twin or a first-degree relative of a schizophrenic (Gottesman & Shields, 1982). Children of nonschizophrenic parents have a 1% lifetime risk for the disorder. With a single schizophrenic parent there is a 13% risk, and with two schizophrenic parents a 46% risk (Kinney & Matthysse, 1978; Kessler, 1980). According to the Gottesman, McGuffin, and Farmer (1987) report on the pooled results of European family and twin studies between 1920 and 1978, the statistics for the presence of schizophrenia among relatives of schizophrenic probands are as follows: 9.3% of children, 7.3% of siblings, 2.9% of half siblings, 12% of dizygotic (DZ) twins, and 44.3% of monozygotic (MZ) twins.

Gottesman and Shields (1982) and Kringlen (1987) have summarized twin concordance studies for schizophrenia, which have yielded the most conclusive evidence in favor of the genetic hypothesis. Concordance rates for schizophrenia among DZ twins range from 7% to 19%, averaging 10%, and MZ concordance rates range from 15% to 42%, averaging 30%. The MZ concordance rate is three times that of DZ concordance and 35 to 60 times that of the lifetime risk for schizophrenia in the general population. Kendler (1992) has summarized 11 major twin studies in which monozygotic concordance rates range from 31% to 78%. More recently, Torrey (1992) has conducted his own survey of these studies, and he estimates MZ concordance at 28% and DZ concordance at 6%. Striking as these data may be, approximately 70% of afflicted monozygotic twinships are discordant for schizophrenia, and 14% to 43% of MZ twins of a schizophrenic are entirely normal, that is, without any sign of mental illness of any kind. There tends to be a higher twin concordance for schizophrenia when the proband has a preponderance of so-called negative symptoms —flat affect, withdrawal and apathy, passivity, and the like (Berenbaum, Oltmanns & Gottesman, 1987). The classical schizophrenic subtypes do not seem to breed true (Farmer, McGuffin, & Gottesman, 1984), raising questions about the validity of such hypotheses. For example, the Genain quintuplets were concordant for schizophrenia but presented different clinical pictures (DeLisi, Dauphinius, & Hauser, 1989).

In interpreting the findings of twin studies the MZ concordance figure is generally considered to be the most revealing of the genetic component since MZ twins have identical genotypic constitutions. Since MZ twins also experience much similarity of childhood interpersonal environment, it is difficult to use these studies to separate genetic from environmental influences more precisely. Two studies, however, involving monozygotic twins discordant for schizophrenia, followed a handful of twins who were adopted and separated in early childhood, a condition that appears to enable a differential assessment of the effects of heredity and environment. Gottesman and Shields (1982) report twelve such cases, with a 58% concordance rate. Kringlen (1987) reports seven such pairs in which four were concordant for schizophrenia. The figures in these admittedly statistically insignificant samples are about the same as for MZ twins reared together, and the very tentative conclusion is that heredity and not simply environmental similarity is involved. However, Kringlen (1987) cautions us that the childhood psychological environment in the case of *each* twin in the concordant pairs in his study was "miserable" and stressful.

Adoption studies in which the fate of offspring of schizophrenic mothers or the origins of schizophrenic adoptees are investigated also seem to affirm the existence of a genetic factor. Heston (1966) reported a schizophrenia rate of 11% among children of schizophrenic mothers who were adopted and raised by other families, compared to no cases in the control group. Conversely, Rosenthal, Wender, Kety, & Schulsinger (1971) and Wender, Rosenthal, Rainer, Greenhill, & Sarlin (1977) reported no cases of schizophrenia in offspring of normal parents who were adopted and raised by schizophrenics. And Kety, Rosenthal, Wender, Schulsinger, & Jacobsen (1971, 1975, 1978, 1983) studied biological relatives of schizophrenic children who had been adopted and report that they are at greater than normal risk for schizophrenia.

The findings that a minority of MZ twins are concordant for schizophenia and that the vast majority of schizophrenics have neither a parent or a sibling who is afflicted strongly suggest that other factors in addition to genetics are involved. Studies of 24 MZ twin pairs one of whom was schizophrenic (Suddath, Christison, Torrey, Casanova, & Weinberger, 1990; Bracha, Torrey, Bigelow, Lohr, & Linington, 1991) have demonstrated that the affected twin has larger ventricles and diminished temporal-limbic substance. These investigators speculate that in the schizophrenic twin genetic susceptibility has interacted with fetal trauma. The role of early injury, toxins, and infection, however, remains almost entirely speculative. It seems likely that in most cases the etiologic element that acts in concert with genetic predisposition must be found in the early interpersonal environment (Holzman, 1975; McGue & Gottesman, 1989). Kringlen (1987) also suggests the possibility that it is not schizophrenia per se that is inherited but a predisposing personality structure. When the concordance rates of DZ twins are compared to those among nontwin siblings (when siblings have been raised in the same family), the rate is higher among the DZ twins. This also suggests the etiologic importance of the interpersonal environment, since while the genetic similarity between DZ twins is no greater than that between nontwin siblings, the DZ twins have a more similar interpersonal environment.

Heston (1970) found that about 10% of the offspring of schizophrenic mothers who were adopted in the first month of life became schizophrenic, and also found that this group of women produced a greater proportion of offspring with serious mental illnesses of all kinds than did a control group. The findings of Tienari et al. (1985 & 1987) are quite similar; in addition, they note that the odds for mental illness among children of schizophrenic mothers who are given up for adoption are significantly higher if the adoptive family is an emotionally disturbed one. Gottesman and Shields (1982) report that 20% of the discordant (nonschizophrenic) members of a MZ twinship had significant pathology.

How do the geneticists and genetic psychiatrists interpret these data? At one extreme a statistical geneticist has estimated that the relative contribution of genetic and environmental factors in the liability to develop schizophrenia is 70%/30% (Rao, Morton, & Gottesman, 1981). Plomin (1982), on the other hand, uses the MZ concordance figures to speculate that the environmental contribution exceeds 50%, and this is certainly consistent with the finding that even within MZ twinships with an afflicted member the other twin is not schizophrenic in more than two-thirds of the instances. Gottesman and Shields (1982) state that "the risk of schizophrenia to the relatives of an index case increases markedly with the degree of genetic relatedness ... even in the absence of shared, specific environments. The observed risks, however, are not compatible with any simple Mendelian genetic models" (p. 243). Tsuang, Gilbertson, and Faraone (1991) believe a multifactorial, polygenetic model of inheritance is most likely. Some doubts still remain, however, as to whether the family concordance statistics truly reflect a genetic predisposition for schizophrenia.

Another way to analyze the genetic data is to contrast it with our admittedly rudimentary knowledge of the genetics of other psychopathological entities. Recent family and twin studies suggest that some of the neurotic illnesses, particularly anxiety and obsessional states, also appear to have a genetic component. Pardes, Kaufman, Pincus, and West (1989), for example, note that the incidence of anxiety disorders is 9 times greater in first-degree relatives of patients than in the general population and that there is a 31% concordance rate for monozygotic twins—not so different from the schizophrenia studies! Torrey (1992) notes that the genetic predisposition to major affective disorder is twice that for schizophrenia. He contrasts twin concordance figures in schizophrenia with those for some other central nervous system conditions and observes that the genetic factor in schizophrenia is less than that in congenital abnormalities, poliomyelitis, and autism, and approximately equivalent to that in multiple sclerosis, a condition most of us do not ordinarily think of as genetic. Perhaps specific genetic vulnerabilities may be uncovered for all or at least most forms of mental illness (Pardes, 1989)—and even for so-called normal variations in temperament and personality as well. And perhaps the genetic contribution to schizophrenia is not so great as those on this most recent schizophrenia bandwagon have asserted.

I would like to present one more set of statistical data that appear to bear on genetics and schizophrenia, followed by some anecdotal information, before drawing some tentative conclusions. The statistical data bear on gender differences in the course and outcome of schizophrenia and suggest the possibility of sex-related genetic factors, although as we shall see further on, such data raise interesting and complex questions about the relationship of genetic factors, environmental factors, and neural plasticity. Goldstein and Tsuang (1990) summarize studies that demonstrate gender differences in the course and outcome of schizophrenia. Gittelman-Klein and Klein (1969), Flor-Henry (1978, 1990), Lewine (1980, 1988), Seeman (1982, 1985, 1986), Gur et al.

(1985), Nasrallah et al. (1986), Haas et al. (1989), Goldstein and Link (1988), Haas, Glick, Clarkin, Spencer, and Lewis (1990), DeLisi et al. (1989), and Angermeyer, Kuhn, and Goldstein (1990)—all have noted that the onset of schizophrenia is earlier and that its course, with regard to cognitive impairment, predominance of negative symptomatology, and response to neuroleptic medication, tends to be worse in male than in female patients. Goldstein and Tsuang (1990) and Josiassen et al. (1990) report that male schizophrenics are more withdrawn than females. McGlashan and Bardenstein (1990) report that female schizophrenics have more affective symptomatology, and Haas et al. (1990) write that schizophrenic females respond more favorably to family treatment intervention than do males.

Finally, I would like to add some anecdotal data. In their recent book, McGlashan and Keats (1989) review the cases of five schizophrenics treated at Chestnut Lodge. With due consideration for the insufficiency of family history data, they nonetheless remark on the absence of convincing family histories of schizophrenia. In each of the five cases I report in this book at least one parent probably manifested a primitive personality disturbance (borderline, narcissistic, paranoid or schizoid). With the possible exception of Celia, none of the patients had a schizophrenic parent or first-degree relative. In fact, there was but a single unequivocal instance of a schizophrenic relative in the entire group. These findings are quite typical of my broader experience of almost 30 years, which includes consultations, running wards, and coming in contact with large numbers of schizophrenics in a variety of settings. Reviewing a schizophrenic's family history is not like taking the history of a patient with a medical illness such as diabetes or glaucoma or breast cancer, where the genetic influence is usually evident. It is my subjective impression that unequivocal instances of family members with schizophrenia do not seem to emerge with much greater frequency in the schizophrenic population than in other patient populations. Furthermore, most of the schizophrenics I have observed in a private mental hospital that, in the past, specialized in long-term psychotherapy lacked not only any positive family history of schizophrenia but also any history suggestive of neurological trauma or illness; nor was there any contemporary evidence of neurological or neuropsychological dysfunction. It is my belief that in addition to genetically predisposed schizophrenias there may be pure psychogenic schizophrenias.

While the evidence implicating inheritance in the etiology of schizophrenia is reasonably convincing, not only do we not know whether nongenetic cases of schizophrenia exist but it would be difficult even to design an experiment to conclusively prove that they do or do not. Heredity is not the only factor predisposing to schizophrenia. In other words, a genetic predisposition toward schizophrenia may be necessary—we cannot be certain—but it does not seem sufficient. Even some of those most committed to the genetic hypothesis conclude that the early interpersonal environment must play a significant role (Holzman, 1975; McGue & Gottesman, 1989). Lacking proof that there are instances of schizophrenia without specific genetic predisposition, we must proceed on the conservative assumption that there is a constitutional predisposition in all instances of the illness. Quite possibly, heritability is not what uniquely distinguishes schizophrenia from other forms of mental illness. In consequence, even as neuroscience seeks to elucidate the constitutional underpinnings of character and personality, normal and abnormal, psychological theories may increasingly be called upon to take account of a variety of constitutional vulnerabilities and their influence on psychological development in the context of qualitative differences among parents and families and to help us understand the range of different outcomes, normal and pathological, that may ensue from any given genotype.

Neurotransmitter Hypotheses

The observation that all effective antipsychotic medications interfere with dopamine neurotransmission (Snyder, Banerjee, Yamamura, & Greenberg, 1974; Creese, 1976) has led to the search for dopamine receptors in various areas of the brain and for possible associated abnormalities. More recently, this hypothesis has been amended, and it is now speculated that the early stages of symptomatology and the so-called positive symptom complex may relate to dopaminergic hyperactivity in mesolimbic, mesocortical, or nigrostriatal areas, whereas negative symptom schizophrenia may be a product of diminished dopaminergic activity. These hypotheses have not been especially productive, although it has recently been noted that clozapine, which appears to be an unusually effective antipsychotic agent, acts selectively to inhibit the mesolimbic dopaminergic system whereas other and less effective antipsychotics are more generalized in their dopamine-inhibitory effects.

Central Nervous System Abnormalities

Let us turn from genetics to a small sample of the wealth of recent studies of central nervous system abnormalities in schizophrenics and their families, that is, studies of the perceptual apparatus and its developmental role in internalization and the genesis of thinking, of the frontal lobes, and of the temporal-limbic axis. Some of the findings and hypotheses may overlap. The search for central nervous system abnormalities generally employs four types of methodology. The most time-honored and familiar are postmortem neuropathological investigations. Studies of regional neural metabolism, as reflected by in vivo blood flow measurement techniques, computerized tomography (CT), and positron emission tomography (PET), and studies of brain structure by means of CT and magnetic resonance imagery (MRI), both depend on the new technology known as neuroimaging. Finally, there are studies of neurophysiology and psychophysiology that employ sophisticated EEG techniques as well as neuropsychological measures.

The Perceptual Apparatus

Constitutional impairment of the visual apparatus in schizophrenia may have a developmental role in the formation of the mental apparatus. Impairment of smooth-muscle pursuit eye movement or eye tracking (SPEM or SPET) has been noted by Diefendorff and Dodge (1908), Holzman, Proctor, and Hughes (1973), and Siever and Coursey (1985). Siever and Coursey (1985) report this disorder in 80% of schizophrenics. Along with Venables (1987), they note the presence of the impairment in a high proportion of first-degree relatives and twins of schizophrenics as well and suggest that it may be a biological marker for schizophrenia. Holzman (1987) relates these eye movement problems to impairment of automatic attention deployment in schizophrenia. He also notes disturbances in the early and late components of stimulus-evoked brain-related EEG potentials (ERP), reflective of impaired capacity to modulate stimulus input, and comments that the early component of the ERP is related to automatic attention deployment and the late component to selective, controlled attention deployment and attention span. In 1984 Dawson and Nuechterlein reported a variety of psychophysiological disturbances. Spring, Weinstein, Freeman, and Thompson (1992) describe selective attention impairment in the form of de-automation, distractibility, and inability to sustain controlled processes. Studies of the visual system have also indicated that early sensory-perceptual experiences are essential for structuring of the nervous system (Hubel & Wiesel, 1977). Piaget (Flavell, 1963) described how in infancy mental activity is initially undifferentiated from perception and action (the sensorimotor phase). Thinking as an "internal" activity—with mental representation, symbolization, and reflective awareness of feeling—evolves from this phase (Robbins, 1981a, 1983, 1989), and if the sensory-perceptual apparatus is constitutionally disordered it would not be surprising if one result is such a lack of integration and ability to attend and concentrate.

The Cerebral Cortex and Frontal Lobes

The very first investigations of possible brain abnormality in schizophrenia, dating back to Crichton-Browne (1879), Alzheimer (1897), Kraepelin (1896/1919) and Southard (1910, 1914), focused on the cerebral cortex, particularly the frontal lobes. Enlarged ventricles in schizophrenics were first reported by Jacobi and Winkler (1927). More recently a number of autopsy studies have demonstrated decreased thickness, size, weight and volume of cortex, and/or increased ventricular size. Changes have been noted in the cerebral cortex, particularly in the prefrontal and temporal areas, as well as in the subcortical basal ganglia, globus pallidus, thalamus and hypothalamus, corpus callosum, and limbic structures, including the cingulate gyrus, amygdala, and hippocampus (Stevens, 1982; Bogerts, Meertz, & Schonfeldt-

Bausch, 1985; Benes, Davidson & Bird, 1986; Brown, et al., 1986; Kirch & Weinberger, 1986; Parkenberg, 1987; Bruton et al., 1990).

The advent of noninvasive imaging techniques, including pneumoenceph-alography, and, more recently, computerized tomography (CT) and magnetic resonance imagery (MRI), has enabled studies that are less contaminated by the variables of old age, mortality, and other pathological factors that char-acterize autopsy studies. These noninvasive techniques have demonstrated enlargement of the ventricles, particularly the frontal and temporal horns, as well as an increased ventricle/brain ratio (VBR) and a decrease in the size of the cerebrum, the cranium, the frontal lobes, and temporal-limbic structures (Haug, 1962; Johnstone, Crow, Frith, Husband, & Kreel, 1976; Reveley, Re-veley, Clifford, & Murray, 1982; Reveley, Reveley, & Murray, 1983; Shelton & Weinberger, 1986; Coffman & Nasrallah, 1986; Crow & Johnstone, 1987; Roberts, Colter, Lofthouse, Johnstone, & Crow, 1987; Shelton, et al., 1988; Suddath, Christison, Torrey, Casanova, & Weinberger, 1990; Weinberger, Ber-man, Suddath, & Torrey, 1992). While most studies have focused on white-matter volume, an MRI study by Zipursky, Lim, Sullivan, Brown, and Pfef-ferbaum (1992) concludes that it is gray-matter substance that is diminished. Ingvar and Franzen (1974) report diminished regional cerebral blood flow (RCBF) in the frontal lobes of chronic schizophrenics. Gur et al. (1985), An-dreason (1988), and Buchsbaum (1990) note frontal hypometabolism. Buchs-baum's 1990 PET study of 18 never-medicated schizophrenics demonstrates hypometabolism in the frontal lobes, temporal lobes, and basal ganglia.

Andreasen et al. (1986), Venables (1987), Weinberger and Berman (1988), and Weinberger (1988) are among the many who have observed that these changes seem to be more consistent and pronounced in schizophrenics with "negative" or "defect" symptoms (dulled affect, passivity, withdrawal, lack of motivation, impairment of problem-solving ability), and Cleghorn and associates (1989) report increased frontal and decreased parietal glucose me-tabolism in untreated schizophrenics in the acute, agitated phase of the illness. Pearlson, Garbacz, Moberg, Ahn, and DePaulo (1985) find that the most severe instances of ventricular enlargement are found in schizophrenics with histo-ries suggestive of early brain damage. Reveley et al. (1983) report that schizo-phrenics with cortical atrophy are unlikely to have a family history of schizo-phrenia, suggesting that they may constitute a separate organically damaged group of patients.

Two interesting studies have utilized MRI and RCBF techniques to at-tempt to distinguish between schizophrenic and nonschizophrenic MZ twins. An MRI study by Suddath et al. (1990) reports that all but one of the fifteen schizophrenics in discordant MZ pairs had enlarged lateral and third ven-tricles and diminution of anteromedial hippocampal size. Weinberger and associates (1992) report that in their sample the affected twin had a smaller left anterior hippocampal and diminished dorsolateral prefrontal cortical RCBF during an intellectual task. These studies suggest the possibility that the schizo-phrenia in these patients may not be genetic in origin.

The findings of cerebral atrophy are difficult to interpret. Individually, they are rarely remarkable; the difference between schizophrenics and normal subjects is evident only when large groups are contrasted statistically. In cases of unusual individual deviation from the norm the diagnosis of organic brain syndrome is likely to be favored. Moreover, the finding of ventricular enlargement is not unique to schizophrenia, and the possible influence of long-term administration of neurotoxic neuroleptic drugs—or even of chronic environmental deprivation or lack of "mental exercise"—has not been ruled out. After next reviewing evidence for pathology of the limbic system, we shall suggest a possible connection between limbic and prefrontal atrophy via afferent thalamostriatal fibers.

The Temporal-Limbic System

Some of the most interesting and promising of recent research has focused on the temporal-limbic axis. Since this area of the brain (first noted by Broca and referred to as the rhinencephalon because of its intimate association with smell) is less well known both anatomically and functionally, I will review some of this knowledge before noting the findings and speculating about their significance. Not all investigators agree on what structures constitute the limbic system, but generally they include those tissues surrounding the brain stem, namely, hypothalamus, cingulate gyrus, hippocampus, amygdala, septum, temporal pole, and some thalamic structures. The area gained attention for its possible relationship to schizophrenia because of the psychotic symptomatology that frequently accompanies temporal lobe epilepsy and is also evoked by electrical stimulation. However, these symptoms do not bear close resemblance to those of schizophrenia.

The functional interrelationship among limbic structures and between them and other parts of the brain has been elaborated by MacLean (1985, 1990, and in many publications, dating back 40 or so years), Torrey and Peterson (1974), Isaacson (1982), Kling (1986), Aggleton and Mishkin (1986), Fonberg (1986), Rolls (1986), and Weiger and Bear (1988). MacLean's concept of a triune brain defined by the evolutionary and functional primitiveness of its parts is now widely referred to. In the middle are the early mammalian temporal-limbic structures and at the two evolutionary extremes are the protoreptilian brain stem and the evolutionarily more advanced neomammalian or primate brain (prefrontal-cortex and thalamic structures). The former lack direct sensory-perceptual access and are responsible for what MacLean refers to as the "R" complex—that is, the reflexive, stereotypic behaviors, derived from ancestral learning which sustain life and characterize the most primitive species. The latter processes sensory-perceptual input, as well as visceral and emotional input from the limbic system, but is not stimulus- or experience-bound and supplies elements of judgment and reflection in order to modify both reflexive and previously learned responses to stimulation and thus, paradoxically, acts to free the organism from emotional and visceral imperatives for more creative endeavors.

Our knowledge of the limbic system is based on studies of humans and laboratory animals afflicted with natural illnesses or man-made lesions, on experimental and therapeutic surgery, as well as on electrical stimulation experiments. Of its numerous functions perhaps the primary one, ascribable to the amygdala and hippocampus, is the generation of drives (oral, genital, maternal, aggressive) and affects. The limbic system also serves as modulator, volume control, or amplifier for the drives and affects, for sensation and perception, and for input from other areas of the brain. Among other things, it modulates the control of the primitive protoreptilian brain and allows for new learning, flexibility, and adaptation. The limbic system is believed to be responsible for simple learning patterns, both their establishment and their evocation in response to subsequent stimulation, and for the continuation of organized sequences of behavior. The relationship of the amygdala to aggression, which is reflexively structured at the hypothalamic–endocrine level in ways we shall examine in a moment, is complex. According to Fonberg (1986) there is a facilitatory or excitatory center in the dorsomedial amygdala and an inhibitory center in the lateral amygdala. The fact that the hypothalamus depends on the amygdala for its connection to the cortex and to the sensory-perceptual world suggests that intactness of the amygdala is crucial to continuity of learned control over emotionality. Amygdalectomy in male primates diminishes aggressiveness whereas in females aggressive assertive behavior is enhanced. If one thinks of this in terms of the learning function of the amygdala it might be more accurate to say that the female becomes less submissive (Haber, 1981) whereas the male loses some of his learned aggressiveness. Humans with amygdaloid lesions have generally diminished emotional responsiveness and flattened affect. Their loved—and hated—ones lose emotional significance (Marlowe, Mancall, & Thomas, 1975), a consequence that is comprehensible if one considers that the amygdala is responsible for emotional learning in the course of important relationships. The limbic system is also felt to play an important role in basic identity sense and self-awareness.

The hypothalamus is worthy of note insofar as it regulates the autonomic nervous system and is responsible for endocrine secretion. It is a generator of reflexive, stereotypic affective responses. As it lacks direct cortical sensory input, its linkage to sensation and perception and to the cerebral cortex is dependent on mediation by the amygdala. Most of the constitutional or innate sex related differences in brain structure and function with regard to emotionality and assertiveness may be traced to the hypothalamic-endocrine-autonomic axis and to the effects of sex hormones on the various areas of the male and female brain that selectively concentrate them, particularly the neocortex, amygdala, and hypothalamus. Swaab and Fliers (1985); Hanske-Petitpierre and Chen, 1985; Fuxe et al. (1988); Seeman and Lang (1990); and Kopala and Clark (1990) note the existence of sexually dimorphic nuclei in each of these areas, and Kopala and Clark report that they contain the brain's highest concentration of estrogen receptors. Lowered estrogen levels—in the late luteal phase of the menstrual cycle, postpartum, and in menopause—seem to have some general relationship to emotional disturbance, and estrogen is thought by some to be protective against affect disturbance and psychosis (Sherwin, 1988; Seeman & Lang, 1990; Kopala & Clark, 1990).

The literature on androgens (especially testosterone) and aggression is complex. In adult male primates, including humans, there is no simple correlation between testosterone level and aggressive behavior (Leventhal & Brodie, 1981). Experiments with neonatal female mice and rhesus monkeys given testosterone, and "natural" experiments with female human infants who for reasons of individual pathology or maternal exposure have sustained elevated testosterone levels, show that as these females grow they continue to be more aggressive than normal female controls (Bronson & Desjardins, 1968; Rose, Haladay, & Bernstein, 1971; Joselyn, 1973; Leventhal & Brodie, 1981). But aggressive adult males do not always have elevated testosterone levels, and administration of testosterone to adult females does not necessarily make them more aggressive, indicating that social learning also plays an important role. Studies of primates by Rose, Haladay, and Bernstein (1971) and by Mazur (1976) reveal a bidirectional correlation between testosterone level and social status. For example, subsequent to conflict resolution and social status change within the group, newly dominant rhesus monkeys show an elevation of testosterone levels, whereas those demoted to subordinate status show a diminution. Davis and Fernald (1990) have demonstrated that socially induced alterations in the dominance/submission patterns among male cichlid fish lead to alterations in hypothalamic neuronal size, which in turn lead to alterations in pituitary gonadotropin secretion and testicular size.

Thus far we have been describing the normal structure and function of the limbic system. Abnormalities have been reported in schizophrenics of both sexes. Studies have tended to concentrate on the left temporal-limbic area because it is part of the dominant hemisphere in most patients and hence part of the language center. It contains the planum temporale, which is language-specialized. Earlier I noted some of the reports of cortical atrophy based on postmortem studies and noninvasive imaging techniques. Stevens (1982) reports increased gliosis in the basal limbic system of schizophrenics, even those who have never been medicated. Left temporal hypermetabolism, consistent with the "positive" symptoms, has been noted by Gur et al. (1985) and Andraeson (1988). Tamminga et al. (1992) report hypometabolism in the hippocampus and anterior cingulate gyrus of actively psychotic, drug-free schizophrenics with deficit and nondeficit symptomatology. They note that the deficit group manifested hypometabolism in frontal, parietal and thalamic areas, as well. Psychophysiological studies by Broff and Geyer (1978), Adler et al. (1982), Liberman et al. (1984), Freedman et al. (1987), and Holzman (1987) suggest functional alterations consistent with a sensory gating defect related to the temporal-limbic area. Broff and Geyer note in schizophrenics an exaggerated acoustic startle response. Holzman (1987) and Liberman et al. (1984)

report that the skin conductance orientation response (SCOR) to innocuous environmental stimuli, which is an indicator of "gating" or modulation of incoming stimuli, is absent in 40% to 50% of schizophrenics, in contrast to only 5% to 10% of controls. It is more frequently absent in the most withdrawn and disorganized patients, and the SCORs of those schizophrenics who do respond tend to be abnormally high. Kopala and Clark (1990) report olfactory agnosia in approximately half of all schizophrenics; recall that the temporal-limbic area is otherwise known as the rhinencephalon.

Holzman (1987) reports diminution in variation and latency of the early components of stimulus evoked brain potentials (ERP), which suggests impaired modulation and inhibition of stimulus input. McCarley and associates (McCarley, Faux, Shenton, Nestor, & Adams, 1991, 1992) have investigated an ERP they call P300; a characteristic EEG spike 300 ms following a cognitive stimulus that they describe as an unusual event that requires the patient to make some alteration in his worldview. They discovered P300 reduction in the dominant hemisphere temporal lobe of 85% to 95% of unmedicated schizophrenic patients. MRI studies of these same patients show significant tissue loss in the dominant posterior superior temporal area, which includes the limbic system structures, and the extent of tissue loss seems to be correlated with severity of the patient's thought disorder.

It is possible that atrophy and hypometablism of the frontal lobes may be linked to the abnormalities of the limbic system (Weinberger, 1988). The limbic system appears to inform the more rational, judgmental, planful frontal lobes of the emotional significance of events through the afferent striatal connections, and to modulate the visceral, emotional, and sensory-perceptual information transmitted to it. Of course, this hypothesis raises another puzzling question, namely, whether secondary frontal hypometabolism and atrophy might be the result of primary limbic system pathology or the result of the mentally and often environmentally impoverished existences (meaning, lacking in sensory-perceptual novelty, human stimulation, and emotional imput) led by more chronic schizophrenics.

In Chapter 2 it was noted that the course of schizophrenia is more severe in males than females. And in Chapters 7, 9, and 15 the central role in schizophrenia of the complex variable that includes ordinary aggressiveness and assertiveness, as well as pathological rage, is explored. It is certainly possible that the combination of normal sexual dimorphism in the limbic system and neocortex, and primary pathology of this area of the brain in schizophrenia, may help account for gender variability in the severity of the illness.

Neuroscience and Psychology

We conclude this summary of the neuroscientific contribution to schizophrenia with a review of the rationale underlying neurobiological reductionism, and, in particular, the scepticism of many neuroscientists about conceiving of schizophrena as a psychological condition. It is both paradoxical and ironic that the very contemporary neurosciences, which have been used by some scientific materialists in their efforts to invalidate the psychological sciences and reductively consume the mental phenomena that constitute their data, have provided us with findings that suggest that experience—that is, the influence of the environment mediated through mental processes conceived of as independent variables—plays a critical role in schizophrenia and that the brain is a plastic organ, constantly in the process of modification as the person adapts to his life experiences.

Earlier in the chapter we reviewed studies of pairs of monozygotic twins, one of whom was schizophrenic, which demonstrated an average of 30% concordance in the other twin, even when the two were reared in different environments. While this is impressive evidence for a genetic factor, it is also true that approximately 90% of schizophrenics do not have an afflicted parent, 81% have neither a parent nor a sibling who is schizophrenic, and only a minority of monozygotic twins are concordant for schizophenia, findings which suggest that schizophrenia cannot be totally or even predominantly accounted for by organic factors. In fact, the genetic studies themselves suggest the etiologic importance of other factors, such as interpersonal and psychological ones: There is a higher concordance rate for schizophrenia between dizygotic or fraternal twins than there is among other siblings when both sibling groups have been raised in the same family. Tienari et al. (1987) studied a large group of adopted children, ten of whom became schizophrenic; in each instance the adoptive family was seriously disturbed. And Kringlen (1987) notes that the psychological environment, in each of the instances in his study of concordance for schizophrenia in monozygotic twins reared apart was "miserable" and stressful.

The neuroscientific evidence suggesting the importance of experiential psychological factors in schizophrenia is not limited to genetic studies. Evidence has accumulated in support of the hypothesis of neural plasticity (Vital-Durand, 1975), the continuing adaptative structural modification of the nervous system throughout life as a result of experience. At the cellular level, Kandel (1978, 1979) and Carew, Walters, and Kandel (1981) have demonstrated microscopic changes in single neurons of the marine snail *aplysia* during and after the learning of a conditioned aversive response; they suggest that this may be a simple neurological model for the changes evoked by psychotherapy. Kandel (1979) says "It is only insofar as our words produce changes in each other's brains that psychotherapeutic intervention produces change in a patient's mind" (p. 1037) (see also Levin & Vuckovich, 1987). Diamond (1988) reports animal experiments that demonstrate that experience can influence cerebral cortical thickness. Davis and Fernald (1990) have demonstrated that following socially induced changes in the dominance/submission status of male cichlid fish there are alterations in hypothalamic neuronal size. And Kolb's 1987 hypothesis that posttraumatic stress disorders are mediated by neuronal changes appears to have been confirmed by Ornitz &

Pynoos (1989) who have demonstrated in traumatized children inhibition of the startle response, which is a brain-stem mediated reflex. Thus, from the perspective of neuroscience, both the interpersonal or experiential causation of mental illness and the psychological treatment of it may have effects every bit as profound as those attributable to any physical process.

More accurately, from the perspective of neuroscience pathogenic and therapeutic psychological factors might better be conceptualized as physical processes. But when they are conceptualized as such, they lose their essence, that is, the ability to explain why a given interaction or set of events is experienced benignly by one person and traumatically by another. Observing the same sporting event may make one man ecstatic, another gloomy, a third angry, and may trigger a heart attack in a fourth. These crucial distinctions may be understood in no other way than through conceptually independent psychological theories of meaning and emotion. Earlier in this chapter we concluded that generation of meaningful neuroscientific hypotheses is highly dependent on an understanding of intrapsychic life; it is a search for physical and chemical system analogues or substrates in the brain to the psychological processing of thoughts, feelings, and behavior that we apprehend in ourselves and others. A sophisticated conception of neuroscience, paradoxically, requires us not to abandon psychology but to embrace it as a lens through which to study schizophrenia and to seek new forms of interdisciplinary collaboration.

The reader of the first section of the book, particularly Chapter 2, should be in a position to see that the entire debate about "the" cause of schizophrenia—whether causality may be imputed to organic or psychological factors or, going beyond either-or thinking, to a bit of each—is spurious. Understanding and explication must occur simultaneously at both levels—and others as well.

Conclusions

What conclusions can we draw about the current status of neuroscientific hypotheses and research into schizophrenia? First, it is noteworthy that the limbic system, which is the current focus of attention, is a primary generator and regulator of drive and affect in the brain. This suggests that the current descriptive dichotomy between schizophrenia conceived of as a thought disorder and the so-called affective disorders may be not only artificial but misleading. Schizophrenia may in fact be an affective disorder. Each of the five cases in this book demonstrates a profound affective disturbance.

The genetic contribution to schizophrenia may not be so great as many have believed, and interpreted in the context of growing evidence of a genetic substrate for all mental illness (and probably normal personality variants, as well), it may not even be what most distinctively sets schizophrenia apart from other conditions.

While the existence of a genetic factor in many, if not all, cases of schizophrenia now seems established and while the likelihood of subtle neurological abnormalities, particularly in the limbic system and its neocortical circuitry, also seems great, the current state of organic research is nonetheless fraught with uncertainty and doubt. Mesulam (1990) concludes: "It is currently impossible to distinguish primary pathological processes from secondary epiphenomena or idiosyncratic observations from those that are universal" (p. 844).

One of the current problems confronting neuroscience research into schizophrenia is that of differentiating among psychoses secondary to organic brain syndrome with tangible lesions, Kraepelinian schizophrenia defined as an organic brain syndrome without obvious lesion, the kinds of neural network variations in nervous system structure and function that differentiate one person from another and one personality type from another, and central nervous system abnormalities that are primary from those that are neuroplastic responses to the environment. Seidman (1983), for example, concludes in a review of neuropsychological studies of schizophrenia that

> there is considerable evidence that chronic or process schizophrenics, especially those with negative symptoms, manifest neuropsychological impairment . . . and cannot be easily differentiated from diffusely brain-damaged controls. . . . Neuropsychological impairment appears to be mild to moderate in severity and more likely to be diffuse or bilateral than focal. (p. 214)

Studies by Goldstein (1978), Heaton, Baade, and Johnson (1978), and Malec (1978) corroborate his assertion. This is not consistent with my own clinical impression, which is based primarily on a different population—patients in a major private psychiatric teaching hospital, who were often (at least in the past) referred because someone thought them candidates for psychotherapy and who were admitted in the more acute stages of illness. Some investigators (Donnelly, Weinberger, Waldman, & Wyatt, 1980; Golden, Graber, Moses, & Zatz, 1980; Rieder, Donnelly, Herat, & Waldman, 1979) go even further and identify an obviously brain-damaged sample of patients with CAT (computerized axial tomorgraphy) abnormalities and neuropsychological impairment and call these schizophrenic. Perhaps these conspicuously non-Kraepelinian psychotics might better be diagnosed as having organic brain syndromes.

In many, if not most, of the organic studies of schizophrenia to date the effects of other variables have not entirely been ruled out, particularly the possibility of cerebral atrophy secondary to the mental attitudes of negative-symptom schizophrenics and to the stimulus-impoverished environments in which some of these chronically institutionalized people reside. A neurological route for such atrophy based on the phenomenon of neural plasticity, has been hypothesized. Lidz (1990) suggests that diminution in frontal lobe metabolism might be the result—and not the cause—of schizophrenic withdrawal and reluctance to think and to feel. The effects of the neuroleptic medication most of these people have chronically received is also difficult to assess. It is difficult to find large groups of schizophrenics to study who have not been chronically medicated, and since most of the medications are known to be neurotoxic (causing, for example tardive dyskinesia), the reported neuropathology might be secondary to medication and not to schizophrenia.

Moreover, the norms have not been established for many of the variables on which schizophrenics are measured, hence their distribution in a normal population and in patients with other diagnoses is not well known. Organic changes that have been found to distinguish large groups of schizophrenics from controls with statistical significance are usually not sufficiently deviant in any particular patient to allow him to be classified as abnormal by an investigator who assesses him without the knowledge that he has been diagnosed as schizophrenic. In fact, most schizophrenics fall within the normal range on variables such as ventricular size, and some abnormalities, such as ventricular enlargment, are neither universal in schizophrenia nor specific to it.

I have outlined how psychological processes may be conceived of at another hierarchical systems level as physical variables operating causally on a plastic central nervous system. And we have seen how a sophisticated knowledge of psychological process is necessary for the generation of complex neuroscientific hypotheses. The first neuroscientists, who were simply searching for gross lesions, could afford to look upon the schizophrenic as someone who had "lost" his mind and to search his brain for the defect or lesion concretely representing this loss. They had little need to consider him as a psychologically complex personality, much less to think of the illness as representing the central nervous system structuring of a curious—and, at some level, socially and interpersonally adaptive—expression of that personality. As I elaborated in Chapter 2, such concrete defect theories of schizophrenia are not restricted to neuroscience but may be found in psychoanalysis as well. It seems more likely that schizophrenia is the expression of a cerebral variant, a differently functioning brain rather than a normal one with some discrete defect; an expression of personality rather than a figurative wart on, or hole in, or meaning-gap in an otherwise normal brain. Therefore, a knowledge of the psychological complexities of schizophrenia, beyond simple descriptive psychiatry, is essential in order to generate useful neuroscientific hypotheses. We may conclude by reiterating two of the fundamental premises of a hierarchical systems theory of mind: pluralism and interdependence. A sophisticated neuroscience perspective does not eliminate the need for an independent psychological perspective but validates it, and vice versa.

Chapter 7

Constitutional Vulnerability and an Epigenetic Model

I t is fitting to introduce the individual and social psychology of schizophrenia with a broad model of the course of development of the illness, the details of which will be fleshed out in subsequent chapters. The human mind is first manifest at birth, in a social and interpersonal context, as a simultaneous expression of organic and psychological processes. In instances where an individual's constitution (the innate, unique configurations or patterns; the genotype and phenotype) seems pathologically remarkable we speak of constitutional vulnerability, and we may do so in the languages of neuroscience, of psychology, or of social and interpersonal process. The constitutionally predisposed individual must attempt to negotiate the same developmental tasks and milestones, and respond to the same social and interpersonal stresses, as do others, but their *meaning* to him and his *mode of resolution* of them may differ because of the unique aspects of his central nervous system, which emerge as psychological characteristics of mind as the infant interacts with his primary caretakers, who not only are in varying degrees, styles, and configurations normal and pathological but also are responding in their own idiosyncratic ways to the stress of having to deal with an "unsual" infant.

Since the limited concordance for schizophrenia among monozygotic twins informs us that genetic factors alone do not inevitably determine the emergence of clinical schizophrenia, and since the existence of other congenital organic stresses and pathogens has not yet been documented, it is reasonable to hypothesize that in a substantial percentage of instances pathogenic or ameliorative interpersonal elements in the dyadic and familial environment, in concert with neural plasticity, prove to be the crucial determinants, in a constitutionally predisposed infant, of whether or not clinical schizophrenia will be the eventual outcome. While pathological parenting alone may not be sufficient to produce schizophrenia—contrary to what is implied in Fromm-Reichmann's (1948) unwittingly inflammatory concept of the schizophrenogenic mother—dedicated parenting, in many instances, can probably abort it. While the florid symptoms we refer to as acute schizophrenia usually appear for the first time in late adolescence or early adulthood, the basic elements of the illness appear to be in place long before.*

A Four-Stage Epigenetic Model

In those instances where some combination of constitutional vulnerability and interpersonal insufficiency and pathology lead to the commencement of schizophrenia, there appear to be four stages in the development of the illness: First, phenotypic (characterological) vulnerability emerges as some combination of deficit and abnormality in the context of primary parenting that is not good enough and that exploits rather than repairs the emerging mental manifestations of specific genetic weakness. Such parenting threatens or rejects the infant's more autonomous assertions, gives idiosyncratic and bizarre rather than socially consensual meaning to the infant's experience, and rewards the infant's consequent psychological primitiveness and self-destructive compliance with infantilization.

Second, the family exploits the constitutional vulnerabilities, using the child's configuration of psychological primitiveness to express, or represent, and to compensate for traits, problems and limitations other members do not acknowledge and have not processed in themselves (Lidz, 1973). The family simultaneously compensates for their child's limitations by a process of infantilization and then denies the very existence of those limitations, thus creating a state of pathological equilibrium that depends on the unique family constellation for its continuity. Expectable intrapsychic structural developments do not occur, and the child fails to learn socially consensual modes of thought and to develop essential interpersonal and self-care skills. Because his disability remains hidden from the scrutiny of an objective world, he is shielded from many of the ordinary social consequences of it.

Third, at the time of young adult separation from family, including efforts to establish intimacy with others and to assume grown-up responsibilities, the individual undergoes an adaptive disequilibration involving loss of the compensatory symbiotic cushion of the family, which has served to conceal the

---

*One interesting question, to which we shall return at the end of the chapter, is whether there are neurological "critical periods" for the development of certain structures and functions. This relates to some profound therapeutic questions: To what extent may the neurological substrata of constitutional vulnerabilities actually be repaired in the course of dedicated parenting or effective therapy? Is some kind of compensation for irreversible neurological structures the best we may hope for? In which instances may neither of these alternatives be possible? These subjects are explored in some detail in Chapters 9 (on the family), and 13 and 14 (on psychotherapy).

individual's manifest pathology from the scrutiny and expectations of more objective outsiders who may perceive his ways of thinking and acting as dysfunctional and bizarre. At the same time, the individual receives more realistic feedback about his ineptitude. Social pressures define the person he is and the way he functions as abnormal. Expectations and capabilities are hopelessly mismatched.

Fourth, the social and psychological skills acquired at home prove hopelessly maladaptive to this developmental crisis, and the only possible response is regression and further maladaptation (Fromm-Reichmann, 1948, 1952; Bion, 1959a, 1962a; Searles, 1965; Arlow & Brenner, 1964, 1969). Acute schizophrenia manifests itself. Lidz (1973) clearly describes Freud's (1924a,b) hypothesis of a weak ego that cannot adapt to reality but repudiates it and regresses:

> Meanings alter in the service of emotional needs; and when a person's acceptability to himself and others is threatened, when no way out of an irreconcilable dilemma may be found, and when all paths to the future seem blocked. . . . [O]ne can simply alter his perceptions of his own needs and motivations and those of others; one can abandon causal logic or change the meaning of events; one can regress, retreating to a period in childhood when reality gave way before the wish. (p. 10)

The model I propose enables collaboration between the neurosciences, individual psychology, family systems theory, and social psychology in ways I suggested in Chapter 2 and will elaborate in the remainder of Part III. This model differs radically from contemporary conventional wisdom, which is that schizophrenia is an illness that begins in early adulthood. I believe the dogma of adult onset reflects the near-ubiquitous family mechanism of denial and the way in which our society and culture attempts to maintain the integrity of family structure.*

Constitutional Vulnerability: An Overview

We begin the task of elucidating the psychological nature of the characterological vulnerability in schizophrenia with a bit of psychoanalytic history. Freud's speculations about weakness of object cathexes and of the ego, and the subsequent ego-psychological concept of ego defect, have encouraged a number of psychoanalysts to speculate about that certain something that sets schizophrenia apart from neurosis (Hendrick, 1951; Federn, 1952; Hartmann, 1953;

---

*From his perspective as a child analyst Greenspan (1988, 1989a) concurs. Arieti (1967) also proposed a multistage model to account for the seeming paradox of early adult onset in a condition presumed to be developing throughout infancy and childhood, but his rather romantic effort—which postulates terribly traumatic infantile experience, later childhood compensation leading to a precarious adjustment, and ultimate disruption by the demands of adolescence—is quite different.

Jacobson, 1953; Bion, 1959a, 1962; Rado, 1962; Meehl, 1962; Arlow & Brenner, 1964 & 1969; Gibson, 1966; Mahler, 1968; Wexler, 1971, 1975; Kernberg, 1972; Grinker, 1973; London, 1973; Stierlin, 1975; Holzman, 1975, Grotstein, 1977, 1989; Pao, 1979; Ogden, 1980; Kestenbaum, 1986). This conception is derived from a neurosis-centered view of the psychic universe, in that functioning which cannot be readily analyzed in terms of intrapsychic conflict of the Oedipal period, defense, and symptom formation is looked upon as a void or deficiency state. From the broader perspective of a hierarchical systems model, however, more "primitive" and pathological forms of thinking, feeling, and behaving are better conceptualized more abstractly, as qualitatively different from neurotic functioning, rather than concretely as the result of an absence, hole, or defect. It follows that such mentation possesses a developmental and adaptive rationale of its own, which is every bit as cogent as that which characterizes neurotic thinking.

No matter how sophisticated the infant's perceptual and cognitive capabilities at birth, as investigators like Stern (1985) have made us aware, distinctively human thoughts, involving meaning and the capacity for language and communication, emerge gradually and from an inchoate matrix as aspects of developing human relationships and socialization. I would like to suggest two basic areas of vulnerability to schizophrenia. As it has been difficult to find comprehensive names for these, each may seem like a collection of distinctive and heterogeneous processes, nonetheless each appears to be both fundamental and unitary from the perspective of early development.

The first of these I call organization-affinity, and it comprises aversion to contact with other human beings, or people aversion, as well as a deficiency in psychological differentiation and integration, which is one of the fundamental processes from which the uniquely human mind emerges. Although we tend to think of one of these, people aversion, as involving relatedness, and the other, integration-differentiation, as involving thought, a closer look suggests that each connotes a similar process. Integration and differentiation are facets of a single variable, as evidenced by the fact that elements or differentiated entities are the blocks that may be integrated into more complex units. Integration connotes affinity whereas its lack connotes repulsion, aversion, or at least lack of affinity.

The second vulnerability involves problems with intensity and regulation of stimulation, both external (sensation and perception) and internal (drive and affect). It includes particular problems with unsymbolized or unrepresented, poorly controlled rage or, to look at it differently, the failure to develop certain mental functions related to emotionality and self-control. I further hypothesize that these two core vulnerabilities, in the areas of organization and affinity and in intensity and processing of stimulation, combine to produce a third: nihilism, or a deep aversion to the basic mental work involved in thinking, feeling, and being responsible for the content of one's mind. After formulating these vulnerabilities I discovered that they correspond to what Greenspan (1988) has postulated represent some of the core processes and developments that characterize normal infancy, namely, reaction to stimuli and self-regulation; engagement with others; and capacity to mentally represent experiences, with their affective component, and to integrate and differentiate these representations.

Organization–Affinity

Vulnerability in the area of organization and affinity is manifest as the schizophrenic's aversion to other human beings and his related deficiency in skills of differentiation and integration. Aversion to others was first noted by Bleuler (1911) and called autism, a term we now generally reserve for a condition of early childhood in which the aversion is quantitatively even more severe. While, so far as I am aware, there is no direct neurobiological data bearing on the subject of people aversion in schizophrenia, evidence is accumulating that the syndrome of autism is genetically determined, is associated with organic changes, and is an extreme manifestation of a disorder that exists on a continuum of severity (Ritvo, 1983, 1985). Freud also alluded to this in referring to the condition as a "narcissistic neurosis" (1914) and in asserting that schizophrenics are incapable of transferences (1915b). Although we now know that his belief about transference was incorrect, one of the more apparent features of schizophrenia is the failure of the individual to actively involve himself in specific relationships with others. The absence of friends and the presence of a subjective sense of discomfort with peers and feelings of alienation or being different from others are regular anamnestic findings, and it is difficult if not impossible to establish any sort of bond with a schizophrenic in the phase of manifest illness, although one may be responded to as part of his delusional system. Rado (1962) suggests that there is a genetically determined "schizotypal" premorbid organization, and Meehl (1962) postulates an underlying "schizotaxic" genotype, one of whose characteristics is "aversive drift." With regard to other persons, Grotstein (1989) believes, as did Freud, that the basic problem is one of decathexis (or, as he puts it, divestment of meaningfulness from objects), but whereas Freud was not clear about whether he considered this to be a primary or secondary process, Grotstein postulates, as I do, a primary central nervous system problem that may predispose the individual to later withdrawal from relationships. One way to account for this is to postulate difficulties maintaining self–object boundaries, differentiation, or mental representations. Such a formulation suggests that people aversion and problems of integration and differentiation may stem from an underlying problem of affinity. Such a vulnerability might lead one to keep a distance from others and could produce during the florid psychotic phase the solipsistic thinking that makes it appear that the schizophrenic is not invested in other humans. Federn (1952), Jacobson (1953), Wexler (1971, 1975), and Burnham (Gunderson, 1974) have speculated about such a defect.

There is evidence in the case of the autistic child of very subtle but specific responses to the presence and absence of the mother (Shapiro, 1989b). Nor are schizophrenics totally unrelated to others; they make a global passive adaptation to the world that is similar to their primary object adaptation. Because of a variety of cognitive and behavioral deficits, including the absence of object-seeking behavior and adaptive interpersonal aggressiveness, inability to differentiate strange or nonparental objects from familiar ones (an extreme form of what psychoanalysts refer to as transference), and inability to conceptualize a symbiotic transference template and displace it onto new objects, the global adaptation of the schizophrenic is not readily transferable to a specific relationship. It is noteworthy that some of these deficiencies relate to differentiation and integration, whereas the problem of aggressiveness suggests difficulties related to affect and emotion which I group as a separate vulnerability.

The reader will recall that schizophrenia is a more severe illness in males. The predisposition in females toward connectedness or affinity (whether constitutional or arising from the primal identification) observed in all primate groupings, may mitigate against the fundamental and possibly constitutional predisposition of schizophrenics to disconnect emotionally from others, whereas the psychic organization of men around the socially distancing emotions of aggression and competition may reinforce schizophrenic alienation and aversion.

We have noted the possibility that constitutional boundary or differentiation weakness may lead schizophrenics to distance themselves from others, that they have difficulty differentiating strangers from intimates, and that in their primary relationships they do not seem to form an organized symbiotic template that can later be "transferred" to others (a concept that will be elaborated in Chapter 9). Difficulties with voluntary attention and concentration or focus, as well as deficient psychic integration manifested as loose associations, disorganized and readily fragmented thoughts, and readily disrupted concentration, are common among schizophrenics. Bleuler (1911) was perhaps the first to note the integrative disturbance. Meehl (1962) described a "schizotaxic" genotype, Kleinian theory of the paranoid-schizoid position is predicated on "splitting" of psychic functions or failure of the integration characteristic of the "depressive position"; and Kohut emphasized the presence of fragmentation and loss of self-cohesion in psychosis. Similiar ideas have been advanced by Bergman and Escalona (1949), Gibson (1966), Kernberg (1972), Clerk (1972), Stierlin (1975), Wexler (1975), and Holzman (1987). Kestenbaum (1986) believes that attention deficit is the neurological substrate of schizophrenia. These observations and data suggest the presence of a core disturbance in integration and differentiation, which Werner (1940) first noted to be an essential characteristic of primitive thinking and which others, such as Searles (1965), have related specifically to schizophrenia.

In infancy mental activity is initially undifferentiated from perception and action. Piaget called this sensorimotor thinking (Flavell, 1963) and postulated an initial sensorimotor phase of development. I have adapted his schema, based on the infant's interaction with his inanimate environment, to the realm of human relationships (sensorimotor–affective thinking; Robbins, 1981a), and postulate that the symbiotic relationship enables the first stage of integration and internalization, or connection between self–object undifferentiated aspects of mind. In other words, a primary affinity for others is a prerequiste for a recognition of the affinity of elements of one's mind for one another and a prerequisite for the development of mental organization. It is possible that the problems of integration and differentiation might be related to the eye movement disturbances in schizophrenics and their immediate family members, mentioned in Chapter 3, via a faulty mechanism of internalization. Studies of the visual system have demonstrated that early sensory-perceptual experiences are essential for structuring of the nervous system (Hubel & Wiesel, 1977). Since thinking as an internally experienced or reflective activity, with mental representation, symbolization, and awareness of feeling, evolves from this phase (Robbins, 1981a, 1983, 1989), it would not be surprising if a posited genetically disordered sensory-perceptual apparatus resulted in such a lack of integration and ability to attend and concentrate. Nuechterlein and associates (1992) note difficulties with attention span and with figure–ground discrimination or differentiation that persist beyond the acute phase of schizophrenia and into the phase of remission, an observation leading them to hypothesize that these difficulties are products of an underlying vulnerability.

Undifferentiation of self from object and absence of integration of mental content is also reflected in schizophrenic delusions and hallucinations, activities that suggest a fundamental failure of integration of thoughts and feelings. Freud asserted that hallucinations represent the beginnings of normal archaic thought and are the earliest form of mental representation in response to a wish, but it would seem that the hallucinations and delusions that characterize schizophrenia are the result of a deviant developmental pathway that begins with constitutional vulnerability in the realm of organization-affinity. Hallucinations and delusions in schizophrenia are a result of the failure to integrate cognitive, affective, sensory and perceptual experience as internally experienced elements of mind, around differentiated self and object representations. Of course, hallucinations are not genuine sensations and perceptions in the sense of being responses to the real external world, but since no sensory-perceptual experience exists independently of a mediating psychic apparatus, and since prior experience thus mediated may be encoded as memory, we cannot dismiss schizophrenic hallucinations as pseudosensory experience merely because the immediate external input appears to be minimal. We may consider them as inadequately internalized and represented affect-laden ideas and as constructions of sensory, perceptual, cognitive, and affective elements—in particular, of elements related to dependency and rage—that reflect the extreme failure to cognitively differentiate subjective experience from objective perception and to cohesively integrate aspects of the self and objects. The pseudodifferentiated, concocted self and object world of hallucinations and delusions substitutes for these failures and provides a sort of restitution, as many observers of schizophrenia, beginning with Freud, have maintained.

Parish (1897) noted that auditory hallucinations comprise a person's unnoticed thoughts. More than unnoticed, these thoughts are *undifferentiated* (from the object world) and *unintegrated* (with other aspects of a cohesive self). Gould (1948, 1949), in an interesting electromyographic study, demonstrated activation of speech musculature during the hallucinatory process, a phenomenon illustrated by Celia's hallucinations (see Chapter 21). Searles (1965) states that the "central difficulty in schizophrenia [is] the impairment of [the functions of] integration-differentiation" (p. 320), "which are but opposite forces of a unitary process" (p. 317). Gibson (1966) and Stierlin (1975) agree, although they view the impairment as a primary deficit whereas Searles believes it is a consequence of regression. Delusions represent more of the cognitive aspect of mind, and hallucinations the sensory-perceptual-affective aspect. The very separation implied by the classification of these psychotic manifestations into these two categories also reflects the schizophrenic's failure to integrate cognitive, affective, sensory and perceptual experience around cohesive and differentiated self and object representations.

Schizophrenic hallucinations and delusions reflect not only extreme undifferentiation and disintegration of mental content, but also alienation from other potentially thought-containing persons. Whereas the sensorimotor-affective thinking of the primitive personality (a thinking that is realized through enactment with others who are conceived of as unacknowledged uninternalized aspects of self) is loosely integrated with an archaic self-sense and is potentially precursory to a maturely internalized mental life, the hallucinations and delusions of the schizophrenic represent a failure of even the most archaic self-cohesion or self-integration and of differentiation, as well as the most archaic use of other persons. The underlying failure of integration and differentiation is reflected in the inability to recognize the disparate components of self and to discriminate the otherness of a potential symbiotic object and make active sensorimotor connection with the individual in an archaic precursor of mature internalized thought. In this extreme situation the integrative linkage of mental contents to one's psyche and to a realistically differentiated object is simultaneously lost. To put it simply, delusions and hallucinations represent lack of affinity with others and with one's own thought content and process.

Bion (1957, 1959a, 1962b, 1965) voices a similar idea when he contrasts the normal use of an object as a container to "metabolize" projective identifications, the beta element precursors of mind, into alpha elements, which comprise integrated and differentiated symbolic thought, with the schizophrenic failure of containment and the fragmentation and evacuation not only of the elements of thought and feeling but of the very experience of the perceptual and cognitive apparatus itself. Havens (1962) concludes that the spatial distance and placement of hallucinations corresponds to the extent of the schizophrenic's alienation from objects and from his affects; he notes that as hallucinations diminish in the process of successful treatment, real objects are allowed "closer," affect enlivens and is less flattened, and sensations of bodily discomfort are more apparent.

Intensity and Processing of Stimulation

The second postulated constitutional vulnerability involves intensity and regulation of stimulation, both external (sensory-perceptual) and internal (drive and affect), a vulnerability that particularly shows itself around problems of rage and its management. Some schizophrenics are hypersensitive to stimulation and are overwhelmed by what might seem to another person to be unremarkable perceptual input and emotional stimulation. In an investigation of schizophrenic children Bergman and Escalona (1949) postulated a weakness, either genetic or as a result of maternal failure, in what Freud had conceptualized as an innate stimulus barrier. Hartmann (1953) suggested an ego failure in neutralization of aggressive energy, and Gibson (1966) believed the ego lacks autonomy both from drives and external stimuli. According to Kernberg (1972)

> Schizophrenic patients may present lowered thresholds to perceptual input leading to information input overload and excessive arousal, and/or lowering of anxiety thresholds . . . leading to diffuse, massive affective reactions, and secondary cognitive disorganization. A biological disequilibration in autonomic reactivity may underlie both types of lowered thresholds (perceptual and affective). (pp. 237–238)

Schizophrenic hypersensitivity to stimulation has been noted by Torrey and Peterson (1974). Grotstein (1977) has elaborated a psychosomatic hypothesis in which such constitutional hypersensitivity leads to defensive projective attacks on perceptions and the very perceptual process itself: "The origin of the schizophrenic portion of the personality lies in (a) a constitutionally inadequate threshold barrier; and/or (b) a constitutionally precocious sensitivity to perceptions. " This results in a "failure of primal repression," and the resulting "perceptual emergency causes the infant to employ a desperate defensive maneuver . . . in which not only the perceptions or perceptual objects are attacked and projected out of awareness (via splitting and projective identification), but the very capacity to perceive the perceptual objects is attacked" (p. 448). Problems of focusing and attending to stimulation, which might relate to the processing end of the stimulus-intensity-processing continuum, were noted in Chapter 6. These ideas are compatible with the findings, also presented in that chapter, of abnormalities in the dominant temporal-limbic system.

I have observed the problem of hypersensitivity to internal and external stimuli in many of my own patients. It may well be a determinant of their reluctance to be actively involved with others. Emily, for example, did not appear to be especially sensitive during the acute phase of illness, when she had rather effectively walled herself off from feelings and from people, but once these barriers were resolved in the course of her psychotherapy and she relinquished her psychotic insulation and was attempting to lead a more normal life and to deal with things she had previously insulated herself from, she turned out to be exquisitely sensitive to stimulation of any kind. In a diffuse, nonspecific way, she responded to objectively unremarkable stimuli by jumping or cringing. She experienced a complex of vaginismus and associated back muscle spasms so severe that she required hospitalization at one point. She was unable to sleep if there was any surrounding stimulation, and at times she needed to limit stimulation by such maneuvers as clapping her hands over her ears, removing herself from bright light, or curtailing human contact. It turned out that she had a history of such hypersensitivity dating to early childhood. Her mother reported, for example, that she would run and hide from the noise of airplanes flying overhead when she was small. Detailed analytic investigation suggested that this sensitivity was generalized and did not appear to be of specific psychological (conflictual) origin. It is interesting that, after successful treatment Emily eventually became an artist. Might this sensitivity have involved activation of genetic potential? If so, it was not ameliorated by reparative parenting. Emily's father was a withdrawn, possibly schizoid man. In his relationship with Emily as a child he was rather insensitive to her needs and overstimulating in his physical contacts with her. Her mother was both neglectful of her needs and overprotective insofar as she did not encourage Emily to develop mature coping or adaptive skills and, instead, led her to believe that she would suddenly and magically become great if and when she decided to do so.

Celia (Chapter 21) struggled with a feeling of sensory "overload" when trying to deal with stimuli, and she attempted to deaden herself in various ways so she would not have to experience sensation and emotion. Rachel (Chapter 20), at her apparent healthiest, became very excited and overwhelmed when trying to negotiate more autonomously in a normal world, so that even with support and soothing she could not tolerate it for very long without becoming psychotic and withdrawn again. Edward could not tolerate being around others because, as he once told me, he became so overwhelmed that he could not differentiate himself from them.

Each of these patients seems to have had a basic hypersensitivity to stimuli. Moreover, since each grew up in an environment where they were not held accountable for knowing about and controlling their feelings, it is understandable how they might have felt overstimulation and aversion when called upon as adults to bear and regulate emotion, which is an inevitable product of stimulation. Incidentally, for those committed to understanding overstimulation phenomena in terms of the neurotic model, it is important to note that the capacity for aversive response to overstimulation is characteristic of the most primitive organisms and is clearly evident in neonates; thus, we have no need to postulate the existence of intrapsychic conflict and defense in order to understand it.

Rage: A Special Instance of Vulnerability to Stimulus Intensity and Regulation

A consideration of schizophrenic rage must play a part in any discussion of constitutional vulnerability related to experiencing and handling emotion. Numerous authors have made note of the remarkable and indiscriminately destructive core of rage in schizophrenics, beginning with Klein's (1948) articulation of the importance of the death instinct in psychosis (Winnicott, 1947; Fromm-Reichmann, 1948, 1952; Bion, 1959a, 1962a,b, 1965; Arlow & Brenner, 1964, 1969; Searles, 1965; Grinker, 1973; Grotstein, 1977; Ogden, 1980). The presence of schizophrenic rage is sometimes easy to infer from the content of hallucinations and delusions, from the destructive acts that often precipitate hospital admission (Tardiff & Sweillam, 1980; Craig, 1982; Rossi et al. 1986), and from acts of violence by hospitalized patients (Shader, Jackson, Harmatz, & Applebaum, 1977; Fotrell, 1980; Tardiff & Sweillam, 1982; Karson & Bigelow, 1987). Follow up studies have indicated a high rate of suicide among schizophrenics as well: 13% over a 15-year period in McGlashan's 1984 study; 10% in the more recent (1991) review by Carone et al., and somewhere between these two figures in a survey of studies undertaken by Caldwell and Gottesman (1990). McGlashan (1988) found the suicide rate among schizophrenics to be higher than that among those with bipolar affective disorder (0%) and those with unipolar disorder (8%). But most schizophrenic rage goes unrecognized as such by patients and observers because it is unsymbolized or unrepresented in mind and therefore unreported in language; instead, it is thoughtlessly enacted against the patient's very self-organization and his sentient and autonomous self; against the thoughts, feelings, and actions that constitute his unique mode of aliveness and self-expression, in a way that more or less insiduously undermines his self-care. Spotnitz (1976) has particularly commented on the turning against the self of rage that has no avenue of social discharge.

Schizophrenics, however innately intelligent, tend to be socially inept; lacking in adaptive assertiveness and aggressiveness in their daily lives, and personally disorganized. Often this is starkly reflected in the colorless docility characteristic of the more chronic schizophrenics, in the "negative" symptom-and-sign configuration that characterizes them. That this ineptness and disorganization relates to rage is usually not apparent until the rage becomes represented in thought and language and reported as such, which under the best of circumstances does not occur until well along in the course of effective therapy. At that time the presence and handling of rage may come to constitute the central problem in the treatment. When in the course of treatment schizo-phrenic rage is focused on—a development many, including Searles (1965) and Winnicott (1947), believe is essential if growth toward having a mind of one's own, as well as personal autonomy, is to occur—it is not readily con-tained within a constructive relationship so that it may become mentally rep-resented, comprehensible and maturely controlled. Instead, the schizophrenic may become a serious suicide risk or may actually become murderous toward the therapist. My mentor, Elvin Semrad, to whom this book is dedicated, used to say that schizophrenia was an alternative to suicide or homicide.

Bion (1959a, 1962a,b, 1965) has described, perhaps better than anyone else, the schizophrenic's hatred of and global attack on his mental aliveness, which includes not only a destruction of coherent thoughts themselves but an attack on the sensory, perceptual, and mental apparatus. Bion refers to this destructive phenomenon as (-K). It is his opinion that rage, along with an intolerance of frustration, make up the constitutional core of schizophrenia. Borrowing from Klein, Bion believes that the self-destructiveness is based on a malignant variant of the so-called normal processes of splitting and pro-jective identification so that these processes are employed not for communica-tion (what I call sensorimotor–affective thinking) but for evacuation and de-struction. The sine qua non of projective identification, a containing object, is missing. The result of such self-attack is deanimation and meaninglessness, a kind of psychic death, and an animated external world of hallucination and delusion, an idea we shall return to in discussing mental nihilism. Grotstein (1977), who is influenced by Bion, describes the self-destructive process as "mutilating attacks on the capacity to feel, to know, to experience the stimuli of awareness" (p. 437). Ogden (1980) similarly asserts that "the schizophrenic unconsciously attacks his thoughts, feelings and perceptions, which are felt to be an endless source of unmanageable pain" (p. 529); in a footnote (p. 516) he goes so far as to suggest that this propensity may be constitutional.

The extent of the schizophrenic rage that may become mobilized during the course of treatment is sometimes illustrated in dreams. In the first year of our work Emily dreamed of trying to get a tiger into a car in which therapy was occurring. In the fourth and fifth years of her treatment, when attempting to be more constructive in school than she had ever hitherto been, and while struggling against characteristic internal pressures to deprive herself of food and sleep, to avoid thinking, and to withdraw into passive grandiose fantasy, Emily first dreamed of being helpless while a madwoman attacked her, and subsequently, in the course of a therapy session in which we were discussing her conflict, felt an angry, tearing sensation inside and imagined a cornered rat, which she associated to her psychotic part, clawing and biting her.

A particularly vivid and meaningful dream was reported by Celia (Chapter 21) at the conclusion of her seventh year of treatment, after her exhaustive dealings with her diffuse, destructive enactments and our discussions of the unintegrated nihilistic and life-threatening part of her—which repetitively led to a destruction of her efforts to think, to relate, and to make a fulfilling life for herself—had made her much more self-aware. I quote her written description:

> I was searching for something but there was this demon following me around in the shadows killing people. It was like some robot that ripped the tops of people's heads off and ate their brains. Really gruesome! It ate people's hands, too [Celia's hands were her most alive and expressive part]. It crept around and I could never quite make it out but I saw it doing the killing. It was terrifying because I couldn't find anyone to help kill it because it kept killing everyone that I saw or talked to.

Reflecting on the dream she added:

> What a vivid picture of what I am doing! I can barely think about it because I get so scared thinking about myself and what a horror I am. The monster is obviously me and I can't kill it and you can't kill it because all it does is constantly try to kill you. I don't think that you really understand what a monster I am. You are the recipient of all its wrath. It is subtle and not as stupid as you think [I had often commented that, in its gross, indiscriminate and life-destroying aspect this part of her did not seem very intelligent]. I get you where it hurts. I get you to care about me and try to help and then kick you in the head over and over. There is a part of me that is getting kicked in the head as well.

Dreams such as this appear to be different from the sadomasochistic and paranoid nightmares and fantasies of being attacked and chased that are frequently reported, beginning early in their analyses, by primitive personalities. Years of work objectifying the rageful, mind-destroying psychotic part of the schizophrenic, developing new but dissociated constructive caring structures, and creating an attitude in which self-destructiveness is no longer syntonic must occur before the patient can dream the kind of dream Celia reported. Such dreams, then, represent not the basic illness, as in the instance of the primitive personality (i.e., the borderline, narcissistic, paranoid, and schizoid group), but substantial progress in the treatment, including the ability to conceptualize a hitherto inchoate and mentally unrepresented process. Katan (1954) and Bion (1957, 1959a) were among the first to call attention to the existence of psychotic and nonpsychotic aspects of the schizophrenic personality.

The problems with aggression, assertion, and rage that characterize the schizophrenic differ from those typical of primitive personalities. The aggressiveness of the borderline personality, for example, is interpersonally organized in the form of repeated verbal assaults on the current object of his special interest, assaults that are rationalized or disguised as caring and that are efforts to coerce that person into admitting that he, not the borderline, is the angry, uncaring, and rejecting person and into attempting to do something about it. In other words, the borderline personality maintains a weakly integrated sensorimotor–affective symbiotic linkage or affinity toward his own disquieting thoughts and feelings and uses an adaptable symbiotic object as a kind of projection screen on which to enact what he has not integrated into internalized thought. In contrast, the rage of the schizophrenic is self-destructive; a basic attack on his own sentient being. There is no adaptive connection with his interpersonal and social environment. The environment may suffer from the destructiveness of the schizophrenic, and may even be represented in an associated delusional system, but actual environmental elements seem interchangeable and nonspecific, and the environmental suffering he inflicts appears to serve no constructive, adaptive purpose for him.

Like all generalizations, the distinction between the global, non-object-specific, destructive adaptation of the schizophrenic and the active, aggressive efforts of the primitive personality to process rage in the context of a specific symbiotic relationship is is not entirely clearcut. In the cases of Rachel (Chapter 20), Edward, and Emily in particular, it can be seen that ineptitude, withdrawal, and destructiveness were used along with more or less evident grandiosity in a masochistic or passive-aggressive manner to force and control the environment to initiate limiting and infantilizing responses. However, I think there is a qualitative difference between this self-destructive activity and what I have described in the primitive personality. In his paranoia Edward may have appeared to exercise power and control, but it was neither interpersonally specific nor adaptively effective. There seemed no potential for a relationship to convert enactment into internalized thought or to assist in constructive self-care. The similarity between primitive personality and schizophrenia in this regard is that in neither condition is the rage or hostility represented as internal, reflected on, and controlled; instead, in both instances, it is enacted. A more comprehensive contrast between schizophrenia and the primitive personality disorders is to be found in Chapter 9.

It is unclear whether or to what extent the schizophrenic rage represents a constitutional excess (this is the Kleinian, 1948, view, rooted in the death instinct concept, and is embodied in the contemporary thinking of Kernberg) or deficits in mental representation and control mechanisms (Grinker, 1973; Robbins, 1988). Quite possibly it is some combination of the two. In any case, as we noted in Chapter 6, the temporal-limbic axis (specifically the amygdala) is important, both with regard to emotionality in general and schizophrenic pathology in particular. The fact that the hypothalamus, which appears to generate emotion, depends on the amygdala for its connection to the cortex and to the sensory-perceptual world suggests that intactness of the amygdala is crucial to the continuity of learned control over emotionality. The limbic system and the hypothalamus are also the major sexually dimorphic areas of the brain. Adding the evidence of pathology of the temporal-limbic axis in schizophrenia noted in Chapter 6, the numerous studies demonstrating gender differences in the severity of schizophrenia, and the evidence of the normal functioning of the amygdala in regulation of assertion, aggression, and rage, leads to the conclusion that the possibility of an organic, possibly constitutional, element underlying the problem of schizophrenic rage is worthy of serious consideration.

The relationship of schizophrenia and gender, aggression, assertion, and rage is a complex and interesting one. Males and females normally differ in the expression of emotion and, specifically, in the manner in which they regulate and express aggressiveness and are assertive. These differences involve complex and reciprocal interactions between innate factors whose origins reside in gender differences in the brain-stem–endocrine axis, and culturally encoded factors mediated primarily through the temporal-limbic axis. The typical psychic organization of men around the socially distancing emotions of aggression and competition (which primate research and brain research both suggest have a constitutional element) may reinforce the effects of schizophrenic rage, making the illness less severe in women than in men. As we shall see in Part IV on treatment, psychogenic theories of schizophrenia emphasize suppression of a person's alloplastic assertiveness and aggressiveness and a pressure toward extreme (and self-destructive) forms of compliant autoplastic adaptation. Such forces are much more unnatural and deforming to the male psyche, which is both constitutionally and culturally predisposed toward the alloplastic assertive discharge of aggressive elements, than to the female psyche. In the female, schizophrenogenic pressures toward adaptation and compliance, albeit extreme, are syntonic with normal constitutional autoplastic predispositions and cultural traditions. As a result, the pathogenic learning in the course of development may, under appropriate therapeutic conditions, have more growth potential for female than for male schizophrenics.

Earlier in the chapter I remarked on the compensatory or substitutive function of schizophrenic hallucinations. The absence of self awareness of core emotions suggests that hallucinations appear to function in lieu of appropriate psychic capacities for affect representation as well. In the hallucinatory experience inchoate and externally experienced rage also simultaneously performs a kind of self-regulatory function. Hallucinations articulate routes and patterns for impulse expression and control, usually but not always involving extreme self-suppression. Such mental activity does not seem to be a defense insofar as the concept of defense implies the presence of dynamically unconscious and conflicted representations of affect and ideas, but, rather, seems to reflect an adaptation. In Chapters 9 and 10 we shall examine the related role of the suppressive, attributing persons in the schizophrenic's family in providing him with a primitive introjective mode of self-regulation, a basic adaptive turning against the self which precedes attainment of affect representation and the capacity for intrapsychic conflict and defense. Some of what I am describing is illustrated in the case of Celia (Chapter 21), who appeared to have not developed unconscious representation of such affect states as aloneness, fearfulness, despair, and rage, representation that might have enabled her to institute defenses against awareness of these affects.

Mindlessness or Nihilism: A Product of Two Vulnerabilities

One regularly encounters, in the course of any systematic effort to relate to a schizophrenic, an urge toward mindless and emotionless states of mental oblivion and a powerful reluctance or aversion to mental and emotional work; both tendencies give meaning to the colloquial description of the disorder as "losing one's mind." Schizophrenics pursue a kind of anesthetic, narcotic, nirvana-like existence, the natural outcome of which is the set of "negative" symptoms, namely, withdrawal, passivity, flattened affect, and apathy or social impoverishment. In a sense they have learned to achieve a narcotized state without resorting to drugs. It is possible that this finding is related to the experimental findings of cortical atrophy and frontal metabolic hypoactivity (described in Chapter 6) and to the two hypothesized constitutional impairments we have just reviewed: in affinity–organization and in regulation of external and internal stimulation.

The hypothetical relationship between diminished cortical substance and aversion to cognitive, affective, object-related thinking cannot be a simple one, however. The five patients whose cases I present in this book, for example, were above average in intelligence and, with one exception, had completed at least some college before becoming incapacitated. Either specific pathways are involved related to affective, object-related thinking as opposed to more abstract thinking about things, which is consistent with recent data suggesting attrition of selected cells and fibers, or there is a specific neural mechanism underlying the aversion, related, for example, to the temporal-limbic system and its cortical projections, and the actual atrophy is secondary to disuse.

The mental nihilism that I am describing encompasses not only distressing emotions of fear, anger, and varieties of sadness and despair but also the more positive emotions of loving and erotic arousal. In the course of analytic therapy, rejection of the analyst and his attentions occurs partly because he makes the patient more self-aware and encourages mental effort including the bearing of intense emotion. This is one of the reasons why simplistic conceptions of empathy may be of limited value and may even be misleading in primitive conditions such as schizophrenia. The reader may recall the delusional and hallucinatory states of terror, hostility, or "love" patients experience, especially in the acute stages of illness; these states suggest great distress and suffering to the empathic nonpsychotic observer, who imagines how he might feel in the state of mind the patient is articulating and who may question my assertion that schizophrenics have an aversion to emotionality. However, on innumerable occasions patients in advanced but still conflicted stages of treatment have retrospectively described the psychotic state, especially the chronic one, to me as pain-free and therefore powerfully attractive in contrast to the painful state of self-awareness, thinking, and feeling they learned to tolerate in the course of treatment. Insofar as pain is actually experienced in the acute psychotic state, it seems, again judging from retrospective accounts, qualitatively different from a mature experience of emotional distress and, despite appearances, not nearly so troubling to the schizophrenic.

The process I describe is doubtless related to the oft-cited but still mysterious schizophrenic aversion to reality. However, a more precise conceptualization might be that it is not that reality itself is somehow relinquished or destroyed, or even that cathexis of it is somehow withdrawn, but that the schizophrenic mounts a chronic and destructive attack on his sensory-perceptual and cognitive capacity to perceive reality—as neo-Kleinians, including Bion (1959a, 1962a,b, 1965) and followers (Grotstein, 1977; Ogden, 1980), with their focus on epistemology have described—associated with his characterological predilection for the nihilistic nirvana state that is perhaps embellished by a delusional grandiose identity. Eigen (1986) reminds us that bearing thoughts and feelings about the self and others is not so easy as we, as reasonably functioning adults, may have come to take for granted:

> Thoughts are persecutory and depressing because they must be tolerated. One must suffer the buildup of tension for thoughts to become part of a genuine thinking process. . . . The discovery of thinking opens one to the siege of emotional truth, which has its own requirements and which may conflict with one's ordinary needs and wishes. (p. 115)

Celia, once again, is an excellent illustration of the aversion I am describing. She entered treatment with me in her late twenties after repeated hospitalizations and the experience of disabling psychotic symptoms, including hallucinations and delusions, since her early teens. Even after considerable success in treatment—when she no longer needed psychotropic medication, no longer hallucinated or was deluded, and held a responsible and gratifying job—this very intelligent woman preferred to use vague words (*weird, strange, awful*), catch phrases (*strung out, freaked out*) and explosive expletives to denote (and, I think, simultaneously attempt to rid herself of) complex emotional and cognitive states. She spent much time telling me that she had no thoughts or that she did not have any associations to what we were discussing or else that she could not remember anything. I gradually came to realize that these comments, which came rapidly and almost reflexively after important questions were raised, really meant that she was resistant to—even enraged at the prospect of—thinking in more depth about what she was experiencing. This was in striking contrast to the high-level thinking involved in her work, which sometimes involved thinking about the psychological processes and motivations of other people. Celia would report long periods of oblivion to her mental content and to the passage of time, during which she occasionally hallucinated and was usually somewhat more paranoid. She invariably experienced shock upon seeing me, which was expressed with expletives, avoidance of visual contact with me, and the wish to leave the office. We eventually concluded that what she experienced was the shock of coming in contact with an emotional and mental life that she was at other times unaware of—feelings such as depression, anger, caring, and the like. She said that when she saw me she experienced "overload." By the end of the therapy hour, when she had gotten more accustomed to what she was feeling, Celia would characteristically and with equal vigor state that she did not want to end the appointment and that she was afraid of her tendency to become lost and disoriented again once the hour was up. She once commented to me that the reason her face was strikingly youthful and unlined was because she had experienced so little feeling and showed so little facial expression! It is notable that her family of origin used denial and avoidance extensively. Celia was unable to recall a single instance of family members recognizing or communicating about anything of emotional importance! This was not simply distortion on her part; her family continued to act this way in the present, as I myself had several opportunities to observe. Her mother, whose psychosis and hostility were a matter of hospital records, had attacked Celia as a child for being a disturbance when she attempted to make her needs known. Not only was there no family support to think or talk about important matters, but on several occasions when upsetting things happened, Celia's father had actually sent her away, perhaps the most notable instance being when, in her early adolescence, he was dying of cancer and arranged for her to become a governess to children of a business acquaintance in a foreign country, where she knew no one and could not speak the language.

Another adult patient, whose case I have not chronicled in this book, became acutely psychotic during college. She experienced florid paranoid delusions and command hallucinations which led her to attempt suicide, and she became mute, refused food, and made serious efforts to bite off her tongue. She came to me after the failure of repeated hospitalizations in another city, as well as years of supportive psychotherapy and a variety of neuroleptic medications. After the more acute stages of illness were superceded by an adaptive symbiotic engagement (see Chapter 15) and over the course of several years she and I gradually concluded that she conceived of herself as a kind of princess awaiting her mythic prince, a relationship she constantly sought to actualize with those around her, including myself, often by means of a sexual relationship. She was to achieve an idyllic transmuting union with this magical personage, who would take such total care of her that she would attain an effortless, mindless, and emotionless state, which she conceived of as a vacation, leisure, or a romanticized marriage and career. She would winningly (but soon cloyingly) present to anyone who seemed to have the qualities she sought an endless account of her life and problems, cast in therapy language, and seek detailed advice and assistance with the moment-to-moment details of her life. This was invariably accompanied by an idealization of the person being called upon, which was most effective in stirring that individual's most grandiose fantasies, whether the situation be professional, romantic or whatever, and which was virtually impossible to resist—and usually even to question. If she met with resistance she might convey an implicit threat that if she were refused there would be a catastrophe for which the ungiving other would be responsible. Her attitude was reinforced by her family, who flattered and soothed her to her face but clearly viewed her as too fragile and incompetent to cope with ordinary adult responsibilities and expected therapeutic personnel literally to be her caretakers. Such a combination was particularly destructive in a hospital setting where therapeutic personnel almost invariably believed that by becoming very involved with this patient and attempting to provide her with endless attention, advice, and assistance they were not only doing their jobs but doing them very well. In fact, my patient was insatiable; the more she was offered, the more she seemed to relinquish responsibility for her own mind and her own autonomous life, resulting in a loss of self–object boundaries and self-control and eventually ending in suicidal preoccupation and psychosis. It was difficult to set limits with her, because she was so adept at turning from the frustrating person to others more gullible and more susceptible to her flattery, but when frustrated in her desires she would also regress, becoming disorganized, self-destructive, and frantic in what I eventually came to recognize as a covertly rageful, tantrumlike demonstration that she could not function. Such behavior served to coerce others to care for her. In one such state she made a nearly successful effort to bite off her tongue, and in another a near-fatal suicide attempt. My patient adamantly refused to think and reflect about herself, to feel, or, indeed, to take any personal responsibility. She could not tolerate delay or bear conflict, frustration, or distress. She openly preferred to pursue fantasy gratification rather than work for what was realistically attainable, which she was convinced was unsatisfying, a belief we eventually discovered, after years of slow and painful work, meant facing an infantile state of utter heartbreak, despair, and rage. At one point in our therapeutic dialogue when she was called upon to bear some distressing thoughts and feelings, she acidly characterized me as "a gnat in my paradise."

Rachel (Chapter 20), Emily, Joanna (Chapter 19), and Edward also illustrate the schizophrenic's aversion to bearing thoughts and feelings. Rachel preferred to be at a South Seas island beach in her imagination, in the state she called "marking time," waiting for the world of mental effort to vanish so that she might experience a state of untroubled perfection. The use of her mind for anything other than acting as her father's clone or duplicating machine had been systematically attacked and invalidated in her family, particularly by him. As a result, her mind did little adaptive work beyond forming fantasies and delusions that attempted to make sense of her dysphoria without facing its real causes and envisioning equally unlikely situations of emotional nirvana as solutions. Eventually Rachel made the conscious choice to continue this life rather than face the alternative prospect of learning to bear her thoughts and feelings, which, like those of the patient described in the previous paragraph, were heavily colored by despair and rage.

Emily attempted to break off her therapy with me after about a year, as we began to talk of things that felt to her emotionally distressing, particularly her growing attachment to me and her angry feelings about her mother. She refused to see me and spent a month in bed, "trying to get rid of the world," during which time she fantasized walking effortlessly and tirelessly through beautiful fields. Our work was far enough advanced, however, that she was able to realize that the nirvana she sought was not realistically attainable. During subsequent family therapy we learned that mother and patient shared the fantasy that it was mother's symbiotic responsibility to bear all of Emily's feelings and issues—and to take appropriate infantilizing action. Mother literally felt the physical pain from Emily's self-mutilation in the hospital (while Emily herself was anesthetic), although the two were separated by hundreds of miles at the time. The question of tolerating her feelings remained unresolved until the months preceding Emily's termination, when an episode of rage at me for my "crime"—of depriving her of the worry- and feeling-free state that she equated with her illness seemed to lead to an irrevocable decision to be responsible for her mental life.

Joanna (Chapter 19) struggled to become a feelingless machine, or to merge herself so totally with a man that he would take over her identity and she would not have to work, think, feel, or relate at all; she, too, was avoiding a core of despair and rage. At one point when I encouraged Edward to think more about what was troubling him, he told me that his favorite popular song at the moment was called "Comfortably Numb."

The division of hypothetical constitutional vulnerabilities to schizophrenia into two phenomena, organization-affinity and stimulation-regulation—with consideration of a third element, mental nihilism or aversion to the work of thinking and feeling, as a product of these two—must be looked upon as provisional. In concluding our discussion of constitutional vulnerability I would like to mention another reason why I have rejected the seemingly obvious conclusion that aversion to object relations and aversion for bearing feelings and thoughts about the self and others may be aspects of a unitary phenomenon. If we contrast the schizophrenic with the primitive personality, we find that many primitive personalities seem unable to bear and sustain emotion and seem readily overstimulated and emotionally volatile; I have therefore hypothesized that they have not learned to form and sustain affect representations (Robbins, 1989, 1993). Nonetheless, relationships, however disturbed, seem to be the major priority in their lives and are used, among other things, as symbiotic projection screens for noninternalized enactive or expressive forms of cognition and affect. In other words, primitive personalities appear to have turned away from owning and bearing emotions and their consequences but not from an affinity for compensatory symbiotic human relationships, which might serve as externalized mental precursors.

Critical Periods in Development

If we conclude that there is a constitutional predisposition in many if not all instances of schizophrenia—a predisposition that may be necessary but is not of itself usually sufficient to account for clinical pathology—and that an inadequacy and/or disturbance of earliest relationships is also required, it is logical to wonder about the role of critical periods in the course of central nervous system development. With regard to other phenomena,* there is experimental evidence that a quantitative or qualitative abnormality of environmental stimulation at particular periods may have structural neurobiological consequences and cause development to be arrested, leading to activation of specific forms of pathology in subsequent adult life. It follows that environmental and personal interventions prior to the conclusion of such a critical period may have different impact from those subsequent to it. In Chapter 14 we shall return to some of the implications of these ideas, including the likelihood that treatment of a neurologically rooted illness such as schizophrenia may involve rehabilitative or compensatory processes rather than reversal of pathology or resumption of arrested development.

---

*The phenomenon of imprinting in ducklings exemplifies the potential for a qualitative and irreversible abnormality of bonding (e.g., imprinting on the wrong species) in response to inappropriate stimulation at a critical developmental phase. Primate experiments have correlated absence of maternal stimulation at critical stages of infancy with both subsequent adult social impairment and abnormality (Harlow, 1958; Harlow & Harlow, 1962; Mason & Sponholz, 1963; Harlow, Rowland, & Griffin, 1964). The studies of Hubel and Wiesel (1977) indicate the critical nature in monkeys of certain kinds of visual stimulation at key points for adequate development of the visual cortical pathways.

A peculiarity of language acquisition also highlights the critical nature of appropriate input at particular developmental stages for subsequent normal adult functioning. If a second language is learned prior to age 5 or 6, it can be mastered without accent; when learned later it is characteristically tainted with the accent of the "mother" tongue. This may be because both cerebral hemispheres possess active language capabilities in the early years of life and a second language may be learned separately from the first by the nondominant hemisphere. After 5 or 6 years of age, however, the language ability of the minor hemisphere regresses (Basser, 1962); apparently, a second language must be learned via mediation of the mother tongue and in consequence will be tainted with its accent. This finding is of interest not only insofar as it provides a model for the interaction of constitutional and environmental factors in development but more particularly insofar as there is now preliminary evidence (Chapter 6) that an abnormality of the temporal-limbic system—which includes a language center, the planum temporale—may be implicated in schizophrenia.

Chapter 8

Introduction to a Psychoanalytic Systems Perspective

I n this and the chapter to follow I elaborate a psychological theory of schizophrenia: a holistic approach in which person and illness are considered as a meaningfully integrated entity. What I shall describe is not what is now typically meant when reference is made to the psychotherapy of schizophrenics or to a biopsychosocial model, which is that an otherwise presumably intact person is called upon to struggle with the stress of coping with the symptoms of an organic affliction and needs interpersonal support and instruction in order to do so. I would like to illustrate my meaning briefly by using as an example the problem of how one might approach a patient who is deluded and hallucinating. The contemporary psychiatrist is likely to be sensitive to the stress he believes is being imposed on an otherwise presumably normal person who is experiencing such harrowing but intrinsically meaningless experiences because of the malfunctioning of his nervous system, and to perceive it as his role to help his patient cope with them, perhaps even by teaching him to apprehend his hallucinations and delusions as nothing more than a disturbing side effect of his illness.

The holistic approach, by contrast, is that these phenomena represent repudiated and unintegrated aspects of the schizophrenic's mind: that they are messages from the self that are not being received and processed in a mature manner, and that their meaning must be comprehended and taken seriously. The fact that these messages are "transmitted" in this manner and not more straightforwardly is related to the idiosyncratic organization of the patient's central nervous system, attributable both to the interpersonal experiences of his early formative years and to his constitutional legacy. With this orientation the therapist helps the patient explore why these data are not integrated as ordinary thoughts and feelings and why they are not differentiated from perceptions of the environment, what their significance to the patient might be, and how he might be helped to perceive them as ordinary elements of thinking and feeling in ways that enhance his understanding of himself and his world and, hence, his ability to cope. Although elements of other psychological systems, including behaviorism, Gestalt, and cognitive psychologies, explicitly or implicitly enter into my approach, my discussion of the psychology of schizophrenia is grounded in psychoanalytic theory and uses the hierarchical systems viewpoint I outlined in Chapter 2. After a brief review of psychoanalytic contributions to the theory of schizophrenia I shall outline an intrasystemic approach to psychoanalytic clinical theory based on the hierarchical systems model.

A Cautionary Note About the Data

It seems appropriate to begin the discussion of psychoanalytic theory with a cautionary note: What I am about to present is based on data that are not clearly and precisely specified. I do not refer to the controversy about the validity of in depth clinical studies, which was reviewed in Chapter 3, but, rather, to the fact that authors of psychoanalytic hypotheses about schizophrenia only infrequently specify the sample from which their ideas are derived. In fact, many analysts think about schizophrenia and the neuroses from entirely different experiential bases. With the exception of the intensive exposure many psychoanalysts had to schizophrenia during their World War II military service, few have done significant work with schizophrenic patients beyond their own early, hospital-based residency training. Like Freud, who worked in his office with neurotics, not in mental hospitals with psychotic patients, most analysts have little clinical experience with schizophrenics. Gibson (1989) informs us that even Harry Stack Sullivan, the psychoanalyst whose work is most closely associated with schizophrenia, had no more than 4 years of direct clinical experience with hospitalized patients (p. 191)! Much to their credit, a few analysts have prefaced their ideas about schizophrenia with disclaimers about their lack of experience or have indicated what its limits are, including Eissler (1951), Jacobson (1971), and London (1983). For others, this has not been so. For example, Arlow and Brenner (1969) apparently rest secure in the belief that they have worked with schizophrenics, although examination of the limited case material they have offered makes it seem most unlikely (see Freeman, 1970). Two of the three examples in their 1969 paper were married, and the third, an unmarried woman, was undergoing a classical outpatient psychoanalysis and was said to be capable of loving.

It is no accident, then, that psychoanalytic theories of schizophrenia tend to be based on a few of the more blatant and eye-catching signs and symptoms of the condition, such as confusion of self and object, fragmented thinking, hallucinations and delusions, and withdrawal, rather than on a deeper knowledge of the personality structure of individual patients. Another symptom of the lack of direct intensive contact between theorist and patients is the conceptually abstract or rarified level of the theories, which rely heavily on metapsychological abstractions such as ego, cathexis, neutralization, and fusion, concepts that sometimes seem more like renaming than understanding.

Freud's Views

The scope of the clinical experience that served as Freud's base for his theory of mind was for the most part limited to his epochal self-analysis and his office practice. He had little experience with seriously disturbed patients and none with those in hospital treatment. Although he was fascinated by some psychotic individuals (for example, Schreber; see Freud, 1911) and did attempt to treat some patients we would now diagnose at least as borderline and in some instances as psychotic, perhaps he was not aware of how ill they were at the time he did so (Tausk, 1919; Reichard, 1956).

Moreover, Freud made numerous references to the limitations of his theory and to his belief that his method of treatment was only applicable to less seriously disturbed individuals. He concluded early in his career (1911, 1914, 1915b) that schizophrenic patients lack an ingredient essential to benefit from psychoanalytic treatment: the capacity to form a transference relationship. He speculated that schizophrenics, in contrast to neurotics, might be unable to maintain cathexis of object representations and that there might be related alterations of ego or self-cathexis. His theoretical position that schizophrenics could not benefit from his technique and his practical decision to devote his career and attention to the neuroses and the model of intrapsychic conflict and defense that characterizes them are certainly consistent. His major contributions to schizophrenia relate to his conception of developmental fixation and his hypothesis, now more or less discredited, of an initial autoerotic stage of development that precedes object libidinal cathexis and psychic representation. Freud speculated that schizophrenia might be distinguished from the psychoneuroses by a preoedipal fixation at this stage and a related weakness of libidinal cathexis of object representations and of the ego. He thought the schizophrenic process underlying the presumed inability to form transferences might involve a regressive withdrawal of object cathexes in response to adult conflicts (1911, 1914, 1915b). In this model projection of the feeling associated with libidinal withdrawal is responsible for the belief that the world is coming to an end; autoerotic reinvestment in the ego from erstwhile object cathexes is hypothesized to result in alteration of the ego, hence the clinical phenomena of megalomania and hypochondriasis. Freud postulated that this acute stage of illness, in turn, is then followed by hallucinatory and delusional efforts at restitution.

In some of his writings Freud (1894, 1911) emphasized the similarity between schizophrenia and the neuroses in terms of conflict and defense; elsewhere he (1915) emphasized the difference: the inherent weakness of object representational cathexes. He stated that "paraphrenics display two fundamental characteristics: megalomania and diversion of their interest from the external world—from people and things. In consequence of the latter change, they become inaccessible to the influence of psychoanalysis and cannot be cured by our efforts" (1914, p. 74). Later, Freud (1924a,b, 1940) suggested that whereas in the neuroses the ego makes compromises between wishes and the dictates of reality and of the superego, the schizophrenic ego is uncompromising and disavows reality. He (1940) concluded that "what occurs in all such cases [of schizophrenia] is a split in the mind. Two mental attitudes have been formed instead of a single one—one, the normal one, which takes account of reality, and another which under the influence of the instincts detaches the ego from reality" (pp. 115–116).

Freud's speculations about the special nature of schizophrenia have not deterred psychoanalysts of later generations from efforts to subsume schizophrenia within the neurosis model of intrapsychic conflict and defense. Others have been encouraged to develop new hypotheses about so-called preoedipal difficulties, which do not seem to rely on neurosis theory. But most analysts, following Freud's model, have turned away from psychoanalytic accounts of schizophrenia altogether and have left it to neuroscience to find causes and treatments.

This solution seemed to satisfy Freud until later in his life when he (1920, 1937) became aware of a set of problems, which we now subsume under the category of treatment failure and repetition compulsion, that made him wonder about the sufficiency of a neurotic conflict model based on libidinal wishes. He encountered difficulty trying to make a comprehensible formulation of predominantly self-destructive states, among which one could certainly include schizophrenia. Given his assumptions that mental life was founded on a "pleasure principle" and a dynamic of intrapsychic conflict, the problem of repetitive patterns of destructiveness and psychoanalytic failure inevitably led him to postulate an "x" factor. Freud (1920) eventually called this the death instinct, a concept that has since been a theoretical specter accompanying discussions about the limits of analytic therapy. This line of reasoning, along with the idea of disruption of object cathexis, placed certain conditions beyond the reach of analysis as Freud then defined it, namely, a search for truth by a mind that is capable not only of experiencing conflicting wishes and goals but of concealing the conflict from conscious awareness, a search that depends on certain elements that the analyst takes for granted: the formation of a collaborative relationship or alliance between patient and analyst, a relatively intact ego, and an underlying orientation toward pleasure or satisfaction, however tempered by the demands of reality and of conscience.

Contemporary Theories

In the limited time remaining to him Freud never got around to reformulating the problem of schizophrenia in relation to the death instinct concept. The first fruitful efforts to do so came from Melanie Klein (1948), who accepted Freud's implicit challenge that aggression, not sexuality, must be central to an expanded psychoanalytic theory. Klein's contribution is familiar in some respects, particularly her emphasis on a neurotic or conflict–defense model of normal development and of schizophrenia, a model based on the concepts of splitting of the ego and projective identification in defense against the postulated death instinct. It is novel in others, including her emphasis on the importance of dyadic relationships (although the infant in her theory is engrossed in solipsism and the object appears to be little more than a figment of its hostile imagining) and her emphasis on the role of integration and differentiation in development.

Klein's theory continues to evolve, thanks to numerous contributors, most notably Bion (1959a, 1962a, 1962b) and Rosenfeld (1965). Bion's valuable contributions include emphasis on the role of the mother in development and the relationship of maternal function to epistemology—the growth of the mind. Bion described how maternal containment of the projective identification of the paranoid–schizoid position, which under normal circumstances may be viewed as protocommunications of self, may lead to their "metabolism" from what he terms "beta elements" to the "alpha elements" of internalized symbolic thought (the "K attitude"). This process of integration and differentiation leads to achievement of the subsequent depressive position in which an intrapsychic integrated, differentiated "whole" object representation exists. In this position the infant is capable of experiencing ambivalence and guilt and of instituting active reparative efforts to compensate for the tendency to mentally eradicate the object with projected rage. Borderline personality is distinguished from schizophrenia in such a schema according to the extent of rage and frustration tolerance and according to the use of projective identification as protocommunication versus its use for evacuation and destruction of mind. In the case of the schizophrenic it is not possible for another person to "hold" or contain the infant's experience so that its "beta elements" may be "metabolized" by a process of integration and differentiation into "alpha elements." This pathological situation is what Bion calls the "(-K) attitude." It is characterized by a malignant rageful cycle of projection and re-introjection of rage, that manifests itself in efforts to evacuate and destroy not only the content of mind but also the very apparatus of perception and thought.

The model developed by Klein, Bion, and others is an extremely useful one, particularly in its emphasis on the centrality of impairment of differentiation and integration in the genesis and the shape of primitive mental states. What is problematic, and that I shall address in Chapter 9, is the apparent assumption made in their model that the differentiation–integration process is sufficiently advanced, both in the normal neonate and in the primitive personality and even in the schizophrenic, that there are stable mental structures, rudimentary symbolic operations, intrapsychic conflict, and primitive defenses, so that a neurotic or classical model of the mind can be applicable. The related idea, that there is a common developmental pathway in normal, neurotic, primitive personality, and schizophrenic development, is also problematic.

The classical psychoanalytic neurosis model of the mind, based on intrapsychic conflicts among dynamically unconscious mental configurations representing the drives, the superego, and the ego's perception of reality, and their resolution in the realms of character formation, symptomatology, and adaptation, and derived primarily from Oedipal conflicts of the 3- to 7-year-old child, has not only been applied directly to theorizing about schizophrenia but has influenced it indirectly as well. The mind of the Oedipal phase has become something of a benchmark or definition of normalcy and beginnings in psychoanalytic theory, like the birth of Christ in the construction of the Western calendar. Developments antecedent to it have never quite achieved theoretical legitimacy, and the result is an unfortunate tendency to dismiss them as pre-Oedipal or, worse, in examples of pathology to view them as instances of deficit or defect rather than as organizations in their own right. This is like labeling the mind of childhood as preadult or, worse, as a state of deficit by contrast to that of the adult. The primitive mental states to which I shall be referring throughout the book involve organizations based on early stages of integration and differentiation, including states developmentally prior to intrapsychic conflict and ambivalence; rudimentary states of internalization and mental representation; and the presence of an enactive or sensorimotor mode of thought. They have every bit as much cogency and validity as epigenetically later neurotic mental organizations, and they are certainly more fundamental.

Most contemporary psychoanalytic theories of schizophrenia, like most of Freud's contributions on the subject, are hybrids of the theory of neurotic conflict and defense that include the concept of deficiency or special vulnerability, a phenomenon whose origin is usually unspecified. This deficiency or vulnerability is said to create a preoedipal point of fixation to which intrapsychic function may regress in response to conflict. The deficit is also said to exaggerate and deform subsequent intrapsychic conflict (Grotstein, 1977, 1989; Pao, 1979; Ogden, 1980). Arlow and Brenner (1964, 1969) come closest to a pure neurosis-conflict hypothesis. Ogden (1980) utilizes Bion's notion, derived in turn from Klein, of an underlying war on thought, feeling, and meaning, but suggests that this conflict is qualitatively different from neurotic conflict insofar as one pole is not represented in the unconscious.

As for that essence that sets schizophrenia apart from the neuroses, Mahler (1968) and Searles (1965) believe, as did Freud, that there is fixation at the earliest (autistic and symbiotic) stages of the separation-individuation process, presumably due to excessively severe infantile conflict. (Searles's seminal contributions are outlined at length in Chapter 15, on the stages of treatment.)

Reflecting the ideas of Freud and Klein, many hypotheses about schizophrenia center around anger, either unusually intense for reasons reactive

(Fromm-Reichmann, 1948, 1952; Arlow & Brenner, 1964, 1969; Searles, 1965) or constitutional, for example, an excess of death instinct (as believed by Kleinians and those influenced by Klein's thinking, including Bion, 1959a, 1962a, 1962b; Kernberg, 1975; Grotstein, 1977; and Ogden, 1980), or else processed in faulty ways. Some of those adhering to the latter position were influenced by Freud's (1920) subsequent structural theory and by post-Freudian ego psychology (Hendrick, 1951; Federn, 1952; Hartmann, 1953; Gibson, 1966; Grinker, 1973). Hartmann's (1953) ego psychological view is that there is failure of the ego function of neutralization and that many of the observable abnormalities in schizophrenic thinking and relating are directly traceable to other ego defects. Gibson (1966) suggests that the schizophrenic ego is particularly vulnerable to disorganization and disturbed in its capacity to test reality and that it is relatively lacking in autonomy both from internal drives and external stimuli.

Some of the deficit theorists postulate faulty differentiation, or boundaries, or faulty integration. Federn (1952) suggests a decathexis of ego boundaries, by which he seems to include both boundaries between representations of self and object and topographic boundaries responsible for repression, resulting in a regressive revitalization of archaic ego states in the form of hallucinations and delusions. Some who stress differentiation defects utilize Hartmann's (1950) concept of mental representation. Jacobson (1953) suggests loss of boundaries and regressive re-fusion of self and object representations, perhaps due to an underlying constitutional weakness. Wexler (1971, 1975) believes there is an inability to maintain object representations. Burnham, Gibson, and Gladstone (1974) make an important distinction when they suggest that the pathological process in object relations is one of dedifferentiation rather than decathexis. London (1973) believes there is a deficit in the capacity for mental representation but does not take a position about whether it is a product of nature or nurture. Stierlin (1975) hypothesizes that there is a basic disturbance in the developmental process of psychic integration, and Gibson (1966) believes that capacities for both integration and differentiation are disturbed.

Finally, the psychoanalytic literature on schizophrenia includes hypotheses of deficient stimulus-processing. Kernberg (1972) postulates a disturbance in threshold function for internal and external stimulation, and Grotstein (1977) seems to agree. He also (1989) notes a primary constitutionally determined state of meaninglessness.

Not all the psychoanalytic contributions to schizophrenia can trace their lineage to Freud. Harry Stack Sullivan, arguably the foremost United States proponent of psychotherapy for schizophrenia, proposed what he called an "interpersonal" theory (1929). According to Sullivanian thinking the infant is not a Freudian cauldron of libidinal drives and constitutional phylogentic propensities, but a *tabula rasa*, impinged upon by an overanxious mother when he mainfests "oral dynamics." In response, the infant somehow becomes anxious himself, and as his anxiety increases he dissociatively reorganizes his self-esteem to avoid the menace, forming a "good me," split off from a "bad me," and eventually a "not me," encompassing sequentially feelings of awe, dread, and panic. Schizophrenic fragmentation and emergence of "not me" feelings along with loss of reality occurs as the adolescent, under the influence of "lust dynamics," attempts to achieve intimacy but experiences severe blows to his self-esteem, heightened anxiety, and weakening of his self-system. Schizophrenic thinking is viewed by Sullivan as an adaptive effort to restore security.

Use of a Hierarchical Systems Perspective to Expand the Scope of Psychoanalytic Theory

In Chapter 2, I elaborated the effects of monistic thinking on the relationships among psychoanalysis and the other human sciences, and proposed a hierarchical systems frame of reference which might enable better interscientific collaboration. In the remainder of this chapter I shall apply similar reasoning to psychoanalytic theory itself, in order to set the stage for a new psychoanalytic perspective on schizophrenia.

Within psychoanalysis the classical neurosis model continues to be the exclusive major paradigm for understanding and treating psychopathology. Yet it rests on basic assumptions which, while applicable to psychoneurosis and normal development, seem inapplicable to conditions such as schizophrenia. These assumptions relate to the basic postulate that the person has achieved a considerable degree of psychic integration and differentiation. More specifically they include: adequate mental representation of affective experience with others, be it conscious or dynamically unconscious; the capacity to maintain relatively constant representations of aspects of oneself and one's thoughts, which are also relatively well-differentiated from representations of others; a relatively clear differentiation of thought process from enactment, associated with appropriate elements of self-control; an integration of the various elements of the mental world into an organization based on intrapsychic conflict, defense and ambivalence, and a dynamically unconscious mind in which these elements are represented, which may be explored using the technique of free association. This mental apparatus has presumably issued from a psychological beginning similar for all persons, including both common constitutional factors and paradigmatic early interpersonal or familial configurations, and has evolved over a common course of development. The forms of psychopathology are determined according to idiosyncratic profiles of developmental arrest and fixation, or regression, and related conflicts and defense, along this common course. While it is true that different theoretical models have been proposed to account for more serious disturbances (Klein, 1948; Kohut, 1971; Kernberg, 1975), focusing on such elements as the dyad, aggression, splitting, and projective identification, and that considerable controversy exists between proponents of each and defenders of the classical model, on close examination, with the exception of Kohut's theory (and that of his predecessor Fairbairn, 1952), they share most of the basic assumptions of classical theory and are much less different than they may appear to be on the surface. As for Kohut's theory, it is truly predicated on a different model of mental function than the classical, but it is presented in the same terms, that is to say that one is called upon to embrace it monistically, to the exclusion of the classical model of the mind, or indeed any other. To the reader who wonders if I am overlooking the dynamic, evolving aspects of classical theory, for example, the contributions of ego psychology, or important contributions in the field known as object relations theory, I respond that the Fairbairn–Kohut model of the mind is the only existing comprehensive alternative to the classical model.

Psychoanalysis' classical monistic stance is not a problem so long as theorists and clinicians confine themselves more or less to neurotic patients, preferrably male, raised in Western European cultures by more or less devoted neurotic parents. The basic similarities among this population far outweigh the differences, and the differences may satisfactorily be accounted for by postulating relatively minor (but to the individual significant) differences in early experience or in wishes and fantasies. But there is no a priori reason to believe that such a model will suffice to account for more seriously disturbed individuals. The way in which psychoanalysis has dealt with this, for the most part, is to dismiss conditions such as schizophrenia as products of defect or deficiency, analytically incomprehensible and untreatable, and by default allow them to become the province of other human sciences, most notably neuroscience.

It is my contention that adequate psychoanalytic signification of conditions such as schizophrenia requires the development of new models based on different beginnings, both constitutional and environmental, new and different concepts and principles of organization, and recognition of interpersonal and cultural forces mitigating toward very different kinds of outcomes than in the case of normal or neurotic individuals. In this regard the intrascientific problem confronting psychoanalysis is intertwined with the interscientific problem of relationship among psychoanalysis and other sciences, for the findings of such disciplines as neuroscience and family systems psychology may suggest unique and differentiating effects on the nature and functioning of the mental apparatus, some of which I began to outline in Chapter 7.

It is possible to employ hierarchical systems theory intrapsychoanalytically in several different ways. The first, which is more familiar to us in the realm of modern physics, legitimizes simultaneous viewing of a phenomenon from different theoretical perspectives, for example, classical theory and self psychology. While for pragmatic reasons most of us probably do this every day in our clinical work, and will continue to do so, such usage has never gained the acceptance afforded, for instance, to shifts back and forth between wave and particle theories in contemporary physics, and I present it here only for the sake of completeness. A second use involves the dimension of time or development, and is based on psychoanalysis' epigenetic tradition. It may be useful to view individual development from the multiple perspectives of a transformational succession of mind models, in which earlier and more primitive organizations appear to be transformed into more complex or higher level ones, leaving little or no trace of their predecessors.

Gedo (1979, 1984, 1986; and with Goldberg, 1973), among psychoanalysts, is largely responsible for calling our attention to the potential of hierarchical systems concepts to assist in such an expansion of psychoanalytic theory. He has postulated five models on an epigenetic continuum, each organized around a major task or achievement: state regulation or homeostasis, a variable which was identified through infant observation; integration (or cohesion of the self), which might have come from Kleinian theory or from self psychology; self-esteem regulation including acceptance of reality and relinquishment of illusion and grandiosity, which comes from self psychology; intrapsychic conflict and defense from the classical model; and self-actualization beyond conflict, an Eriksonian notion. The supraordinate variable around which his hierarchy of models is organized is not the drive-based psychosexual maturation of the classical model, but cohesion of the self around aims and goals. His stages also have metapsychological parallels. Insofar as it is an epigenetic hierarchy Gedo implicitly utilizes the genetic viewpoint, albeit one in which organismic aims and goals replace the classical economic implication. The stage of state regulation is based on the reflex arc model, and that of intrapsychic conflict on the structural model.

Earlier I listed some assumptions of the classical model which are not necessarily true for persons whose pathology lies within the borderline, narcissistic, paranoid, and schizoid spectrum, whom I refer to as primitive personalities. Elsewhere (Robbins, 1981b, 1983, 1988, 1989) I have utilized the concept of a hierarchy of mind models in an effort to comprehend these apparently qualitative differences in mentation. I observe in these patients a basic failure of self integration and cohesion. The incoherent and pre-conflicted self (or selves) is characterized by extremes, contradictions, and pars pro toto thinking. There coexists an equally basic failure of differentiation, leading to an adaptive use of objects as externalizations of not-yet-internalized and usually intolerably dysphoric aspects of self. Rather than being internalized, thinking is largely enactive, or sensorimotor-affective. Emotions are not owned as internal predispositions but perceived as normal reactions to the current environment. There is frequently a radical disjunction between observed affect and reported emotion which is not due to defenses in response to intrapsychic conflict, but results from the fact that affects have not been internalized and represented to begin with. Because one's emotional predispositions are not adequately identified, emotional self-control is primitive and impulsive injudicious actions are commonplace. In Chapter 9 I propose a model for schizophrenic thinking and relating which is even more primitive.

If a different mind model or models are required to comprehend persons with more primitive mental function, whether primitive personalities or schizophrenics, how does it or how do they fit within the classical developmental schema? While the fallacy of isomorphism among normal and pathological development seems most egregious in Kleinian theory (Peterfreund, 1978), such a reasoning process is commonly assumed by almost all currently popular psychoanalytic theories, which tend to distinguish forms of pathology not so much by the road not taken as by where, along the only road that exists, the traveller has stopped or chooses to return to; that is, by a particular profile of fixation, arrest, and regression. This is not surprising considering that the classical model is based on the premise of more or less common beginnings and a single developmental pathway, and is a modal theory (Devereaux, 1978) presuming also a common developmental end-point. It is also to be expected considering that, until the recent interest in infant observation, psychoanalysis has tended to reconstruct normal infancy from analysis of pathological adults. The claim that a mind model may validly be constructed to account for primitive pathology which is qualitatively different from the neurosis model does not necessarily imply that these models nest in either the same epigenetic hierarchy or in different ones, nor does it tell us anything about whether normal and pathological development necessarily take the same general course.

However, efforts to define normal and psychopathological development and to relate the two, whether through infant observation or through reconstruction from analysis of pathological adults, both face the barrier which is the very rationale for a hierarchical systems theory, namely, the discontinuous nature of development with its succession of transformations and new organizations. Nonetheless I do find it heuristically useful to postulate a model of primitive mentation in normal development, albeit not necessarily the same one that characterizes more serious forms of psychopathology. In such a model the beginnings consist of a highly competent perceptual-cognitive apparatus which is nonetheless neither differentiated nor integrated in the adult sense, and is characterized by an enactive, sensorimotor-affective form of mentation such as Piaget described. Evolution, with the assistance of a symbiotic object, occurs along a continuum of progressive psychic integration and differentiation. This process involves increasing representation of and control over the affects, ideas, and self-states which are first perceived and enacted in the symbiotic world of the other but come to characterize the gradually discovered mind; development of the capacity for accurate differentiation between self and object; and the acquisition of an integrated capacity to experience both intrapsychic conflict and ambivalence. It eventuates, through a qualitative transformational process, in a mental apparatus which is self-contained, integrated, and internally regulated, and functions by a different set of principles, for example, involving intrapsychic conflict and defense, in a world of differentiated others.

As for the developmental line eventuating in primitive forms of psychopathology, it is not necessarily the same one which leads to the primitive mental states encountered in normal epigenesis. I have already intimated my belief that there may be significant qualitative differences between normal and pathological primitive mentation, and even in the mentation of individuals with different pathological conditions, for example, primitive personalities and schizophrenics. This brings us to the third possible intrapsychoanalytic use of hierarchical systems theory, to postulate different lines of development marked by different constitutional and social beginnings, and taking different hierarchical transformational paths to different end-points. In Chapter 7 we noted how interscientific employment of a hierarchical systems model might lead us to utilize neuroscientific data in conjunction with clinical observations to postulate constitutional predispositions or vulnerabilities to various forms of psychopathology.

To view the problem another way, while some of the mental and behavioral peculiarities which characterize patients with more serious forms of pathology such as absence of affect representations, or sensorimotor-affective (enactive) thinking, appear to have normal infantile counterparts, other elements may not. Pathological symbiotic relationships which compensate for developmental failures at pre-neurotic levels of function, for example, are not simply perseverations of developmentally normal symbiosis, but are unique configurations (Robbins, 1981a, 1989). Like Fairbairn (1952) and Kernberg (1975) I doubt that self-esteem vacillations from grandiosity to extreme and destructive shame and devaluation are normal in infancy. And, contrary to the belief of Kohut and Gedo, lack of self-cohesion or disintegration of aims and goals may not be a normal part of childhood, either. While psychological differentiation and integration may be rudimentary in early childhood (note again that I do not refer to neonatal organismic cognitive capacities which Stern has demonstrated, but to the the conscious and symbolic mind which arises only through socialization), that does not necessarily imply an antecedent state of disintegration or fragmentation. Certainly small children do not demonstrate the singularity of goal directedness and purpose which may characterize *some* mature adults, but can we truly say they are psychologically unintegrated and disorganized as opposed to Werner's (1940) view that symbolic psychological development normally proceeds from globality through less mature forms of integration and differentiation to more mature ones? The normal infantile mind is global, neither differentiated nor integrated (see also Fairbairn's 1952 concept of self), though possessing innate capacities to make distinctions. It is only as differentiation occurs that organization and integration can follow; in the global state disintegration is a meaningless concept. Perhaps the phenomenon of unintegration is encountered only in pathological situations.

To conclude, an intrasystemic application of hierarchical systems theory has the potential to enable us to create new models of the mind that are more suitable for describing primitive mental states, those encountered in both the primitive personality disorders and in schizophrenia. It is likely that such primitive mental systems cannot be situated within a normal developmental sequence of mind models, but that they belong in a model continuum characterized by different beginnings (constitutionally vulnerable phenotypes interacting with pathogenic forms of parenting) and pathological developmental pathways. We undertake a more detailed discussion of these issues in the next chapter, and continue them in Part IV, which is devoted to the treatment of schizophrenia.

Chapter 9

The Psychological System

Having reviewed psychoanalytic theories of schizophrenia in Chapter 8, I should now like to propose some of my own ideas and contrast schizophrenia with the primary personality disorders (paranoid, schizoid, borderline, and narcissistic) which I have written about elsewhere (Robbins, 1981b, 1983, 1988, 1989). In the ensuing discussion the concept of primitive mind or mentation refers to the psychological functioning of both primitive personalities and schizophrenics, whereas the concept of primitive personality organization refers to the specific group of personality disturbances noted above.

The intrapsychic pathology of schizophrenia, as with other primitive mental states, is inextricably intertwined with pathology of the dyadic relationship. While the content and structure of a person's mental life, having emerged in the context of human socialization, is inseparable from his formative relationships, in the primitive personality disorders and in schizophrenia the connection between mental life and interpersonal relationships is more concrete, immediate, and functionally obligatory. This is a consequence of the failure of the normally expectable developmental process of internalization, for having a mind of one's own renders a person relatively functionally independent of others, and free to choose how intimate with them he does or does not wish to be. In the primitive personality there persists an obligatory dependence on others for a sense of the completeness of mental processes and a sense of self, as well as for the adequacy of related self-care functions. In the case of schizophrenia, the capacity to utilize human relationships to create a functional, adaptive state of mind, however primitive, has not yet developed, leaving the individual in an extreme but adaptively and psychologically ineffective state of environmental dependency. In this chapter I shall describe what I conceive to be a unique psychic configuration that characterizes schizophrenia and contrast the pathological relationships formed by primitive (borderline and nar-

147

cissistic) personalities with the more or less complete inability of the untreated schizophrenic to actively enter into an adaptive relationship of any kind, however pathological, without extraordinary assistance.

Symbiosis and Related Disturbances

Winnicott made the profound yet commonsensical observation that, from a psychological vantage point, there is no such thing as an infant. The very existence of a psychologically competent infant presupposes the presence of a maternal caregiver, and the two function as inseparable parts of a unit, or dyad. Not only is this dyad essential for the infant's physical survival, filling the place capacities for mature self-care will eventually occupy, but the uniquely human capacities of mind hatch and derive meaning from these earliest interactions and could emerge in no other way. Aspects of perception, ideation, and feeling are gradually differentiated from the global mother–infant matrix, represented mentally, and symbolized, and these parts are progressively integrated or organized into functional units representative of aspects of the self and object worlds.

I have chosen Mahler's (1968) concept of symbiosis to represent the dyadic relationship paradigm that is central to normal early infant development, the primitive personality disorders, and schizophrenia, in preference to other extant terms such as container–contained (Bion) and selfobject (Kohut). Kohut's selfobject concept (1971, 1973) is restricted to the narcissistic (self-esteem) sphere. Bion's concept of relationship between container and contained (1959, 1962a) connotes a functional relationship but has unfortunate inanimate mechanical connotations. In its formal sense, symbiosis refers to an obligatory and incompletely differentiated self–object relationship that serves one party, perhaps both, in lieu of mature self-care capabilities, enabling physical and psychological equilibrium and adaptive functioning; and in lieu of a more mature awareness on the part of at least one of the members of the dyad of significant aspects of mind and of a sense of personal identity. It is a concept involving the boundary between the intrapsychic and the interpersonal. In a symbiotic relationship at least one of the partners is, and at times both are, unable (not reluctant, or unwilling—the obligatory component of the definition is essential) to function adequately without the other, and in that instance the other performs mental and at times physical functions that the more immature or disabled party is unable to perform.

Normal infants require a symbiotic relationship with a mother whose unique characteristics may be appreciated by the infant's innate neurocognitive capacities, but whose separate personhood is not comprehended at all. Mother anticipates and satisfies her infant's needs so it does not experience its extreme limitations before it has developed more mature skills and capacities to deal with the world. Although it is another person, the mother, who performs these essential homeostatic and growth-promoting functions and although the infant soon comes to smile with pleasure at the sight of its symbiotic partner, the mother and her functions are for some time perceived as undifferentiated from the earliest self-sense and are experienced as under "self-control" in much the same way the infant gradually comes to experience parts of its own body. Countless interactions between the primitive sensorimotor–affective thinking of the baby (Robbins, 1981a) and the special combination of symbiotic participation and reflective mirroring that characterizes the good-enough mother lead to the infant's progressive awareness and represention of its own thoughts and feelings. Through this process of internalization the infant develops what we think of as his mind. Progressive refinements of integration and differentiation lead in turn to the development of a cohesive self-system, which comes to include those aspects of self-care and regulation that the mother hitherto performed. Simultaneously, removal of the shadow of self from the mother (and from others), along with the capacity for love that has been engendered through the caretaking process, enables a new awareness and appreciation of the "real" characteristics of that person.

As for the good-enough mother, attending to and gratifying her infant becomes an extension of her own self-care, self-esteem, and identity sense. In most instances this boundary blurring is entirely volitional on her part and is readily reversible, albeit not without pain to her, as the infant becomes increasingly autonomous and independent.

Mahler believed that psychosis in children was derived either from fixation-regression pathology of the symbiotic phase or from fixation-regression pathology in what she believed to be an antecedent, normal phase of autism. She believed that in the normal autistic phase the infant maintains homeostatic activities with whatever assistance the mother may render, although the infant is as yet unable to perceive or to respond to the maternal presence. The schizophrenic lacks the capacity for effective symbiotic bonding, although a certain responsiveness to the environment is maintained. To say that the schizophrenic is autistic, in the sense Mahler employed the term, would be incorrect. Thanks to the work of many infant observers who employ the tools and methodology Mahler established, we now know that the normal infant is not autistic, but actively engaged with the world from birth. What is more, even autistic children are now known to be subtly responsive to the presence or absence of mother (Shapiro, 1989b). In other words, autism, as Mahler defined it, does not seem to exist in normal infants, "autistic" children, or schizophrenics.

Yet schizophrenics have not developed the capacity to form and sustain a symbiosis. Moreover, the symbiotic relationships of primitive personalities (paranoid, schizoid, borderline, and narcissistic) are quite different from those of normal infants. Therefore, it is necessary to explore the possibility of pathological variants of symbiosis. And for the schizophrenic state, which can be characterized neither as autistic nor symbiotic, I suggest the concept of protosymbiosis. Finally, the implication of these qualitatively different kinds of relatedness and pre-relatedness for a multilevel epigenetic or maturational hierarchy of systems of mental functioning remains to be explored.

Pathological Symbiosis of Primitive Personalities

A disturbed mother may initiate with her infant projective–introjective oscillations. In these she may attribute to the infant her own unconscious gestures, meanings, and agendas, and she may initiate complex associated sensorimotor–affective behavior patterns in the child. In the resultant interactions the infant may come to serve essential identity-stabilizing functions for its mother, much as the normal mother does for her infant, a development that impedes the process of further separation between the two. For this reason and in contrast to the normal symbiotic relationships of infancy, the symbiotic relationships of primitive personalities do not seem to foster growth. However, in contrast to the protosymbiotic situation of schizophrenics, which I shall shortly describe, they do permit a kind of adult adaptation and identity maintenance, however maladaptive this may seem to the observer, and they are transferable or displaceable from one person to another. In other words, the primitive personality is not obliged to remain dependent on its primary (parental) object, even though symbiotic objects are required by the primitive personality to maintain tenuous mental integration and to preserve both a sense of self and the illusion of autonomy. The linkage of mind to external object compensates for absent psychic structuralization. For this reason primitive personality organization is an interpersonal or adaptive as well as an intrapsychic disturbance.

I have called these pathological variants of symbiosis "possession configurations," after Winnicott's 1951 definition of a transitional object as a "not me possession" (Robbins, 1981b). One striking characteristic that differentiates the relationships of primitive personalities from those of schizophrenics is the tenacity with which they are held. This is because sensorimotor–affective thinking and nondefensive or precursory forms of projection and introjection provide the linkage between self and object at the same time that they reflect an early stage of integration of the subject's mind (Sandler, with A. Freud, 1983). In this primary sense, projection and introjection are both adaptive organizations of the self and its relation to the object world which are subjectively experienced as forces acting on the self. Two major possession configurations—always unintegrated (not defensively, in response to intrapsychic conflict)—or modes of relating which I call possessor and possessed may be found in primitive personalities, sometimes simultaneously and at other times in alternation. These are characterized by primitive, noninternalized enactive (using the sensorimotor-affective mode of thought) modes of relating, much like the thinking of the infant (Robbins, 1981a, b). Weakly integrated aspects of self and incompletely differentiated aspects of self and object are located in the object and processed through interactions with the other person, who is unwittingly enlisted to help process them.

In the possessed mode the primitive personality assimilates and relates to the world according to the dictates of a self-destructive introject. Pathological introjection (the mechanism underlying compliance) involves direction inward of unrepresented aggression, in the form of attacks on one's own thinking, feeling, and behaving, in conjunction with fantasies or delusions of badness and self-devaluation that are derived from and maintained by actual attributions from an object or from the subject's re-introjected hostile projections. Patients "possessed" require and readily adapt to persons who need to disavow and attribute to others hostility and other forms of "badness." Objects are sought out by the primitive personality in this perverse nurturant dependency to "feed" his self-destructive introject. The introjection serves to bind hostile, uncaring, otherwise undependable objects by providing a secure "fit" for these qualities, and it simultaneously provides the subject with a quasi-delusional sense of self (bad) and object (good). Self-attack is directed toward any autonomous emotional, cognitive, and behavioral agenda the subject might have that has the potential to differentiate and unlink him from the projecting symbiotic object, that is, any agenda that risks loss of the object. Such "possessed" individuals relate more "naturally" when they are used as receptacles and caretakers, and treated as though they are bad, than when they are cared for and attended to, for the latter state requires them to attend to and deal with both painful and autonomous thoughts and feelings that have not been subjectively owned and internalized. It could be said that this self-destructive relationship with the object serves a primitive self-regulatory or self-control function in lieu of more mature ego and superego functions related to affect awareness and impulse control, as well as being a regulator for self-esteem (devaluation) and, overall, a way of deriving a sense of self.

The reciprocal possession configuration, which I call possessor, emerges in sensorimotor–affective enactments with persons who are unconsciously selected because their attentive, caring qualities distinguish them from the primary objects. The interest of such persons is interpreted by the primitive personality, in the sensorimotor–affective mode of thinking, as potential aliment or nutrition, that is, as a source of the feelings of well-being and self-esteem that he is unable to represent and sustain for himself. He then aggressively seeks to control and manipulate such persons in a way that rapidly becomes openly hostile if they resist his attempt to deprive them of autonomy by attributing to them and then coercing them to process what objectively appears to be the borderline's own mentally unrepresented and uncontrolled dysphoric feeling state. The borderline seems to wish to be fed good feelings without limit and to have removed like waste products such painful ones as anger, hurt, rejection, and devaluation. In the case of the narcissistic personality, the goal is to have his dependency needs satisfied while maintaining his grandiose illusion of being superhuman, above ordinary mortal needs.

Alongside these magical wishes and beliefs is an unrecognized need on the part of the borderline to enact and process disturbing affects such as hurt and rage, affects with which he retains a weak integrative linkage in their pre-representational form of percepts, sensations, and related actions. Probably, the attention of a caring object who is not busy projecting and making attributions is both inviting and threatening; the longing for emotional nourishment and the need to attend to incompletely internalized aspects of mind, precursors of represented self-sense, is balanced by the threat posed by the potentially disturbing thoughts and feelings, not only because of their painful nature but because of their potential to make the primitive personality aware of conflict with the object of his primary (possessed) symbiotic adaptation, thus threatening the continuity of his relationships with others who exploit and abuse him. Possessor behavior is organized around nondefensive projection, a primary predefensive process (Sandler & A. Freud, 1983) related to sensorimotor-affective thinking in which dysphoric noninternalized aspects of self, especially the affects of anger and hurt and the narcissistic state of devaluation, are attributed to the object, who is coerced to process them, thus enabling the primitive personality to maintain a sense of completeness of self as well as a quasi-delusional sense of the object as bad, that is, as angry, hurtful, and devaluing. However inappropriate and maladaptive the projective possessor behavior may seem to the observer, it has growth potential if these cognitive-affective elements (which Bion [1962a, 1962b] denotes with the Greek *beta*) are adequately contained so that they may be "metabolized" into "alpha elements" (internally represented and controlled emotion and self-esteem).

A Different Line of Development: Protosymbiosis

For the remainder of the psychological discussion I would like to propose a qualitatively distinctive model for the schizophrenic mind, and a different line of development. The reader is referred to Figure 10.1 which schematically contrasts normal and neurotic development, primitive personality development, and schizophrenia. Let us look first at the nature of schizophrenic relationships. In so doing we move to a position beyond, or, more accurately, ontogenetically antecedent to a concept of symbiosis that is defined as requiring the active participation of both parties. Since Freud's contribution it has been commonplace to think of schizophrenics as withdrawn from the real world and unable to relate to others, a line of thinking that eventuated in Mahler's concept of autism. The beliefs of Freud and Mahler reflect our use of the concept of relationship to denote activity and initiative with respect to a specific and at least partially differentiated other. In writing his economic or energic concept of relationship (cathexis) Freud used the German term *besetzen*, which means investment. While some of us may doubt the value of energic concepts in psychoanalytic theory, the equation of relationship with active emotional investment is a commonsense one. In this sense the schizophrenic is certainly disengaged; he is unable to do much more than transiently and indiscriminately include another person—it could be almost anyone—in a

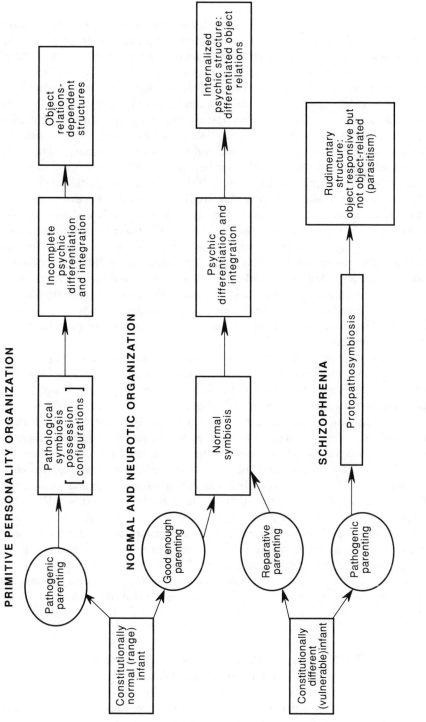

PRIMITIVE PERSONALITY ORGANIZATION

NORMAL AND NEUROTIC ORGANIZATION

SCHIZOPHRENIA

Object relations-dependent structures

Incomplete psychic differentiation and integration

Pathological symbiosis [possession configurations]

Pathogenic parenting

Constitutionally normal (range) infant

Internalized psychic structure: differentiated object relations

Psychic differentiation and integration

Normal symbiosis

Good enough parenting

Reparative parenting

Rudimentary structure: object responsive but not object-related (parasitism)

Protopathosymbiosis

Pathogenic parenting

Constitutionally different (vulnerable) infant

FIGURE I. Different developmental lines.

delusional landscape. Nonetheless, data from family therapy, analysis of ward behavior and retrospective reports from recovering patients suggest that schizophrenics remain responsive to some aspects of the world during the "out of contact" phase. They are passively compliant with some expectations—for example, those of their families or of hospital ward personnel, particularly unconscious messages that they remain disabled and allow themselves to be infantilized—while resistant and aversive to others, particularly ones requiring their initiative, mental work, and processing in dealing with internal and external reality. This passive, global, indiscriminate adaptation of the untreated schizophrenic toward others is best described as "protosymbiotic," in contrast both to normal symbiosis, which involves active emotional and cognitive engagement with mother and is predicated on selective discrimination (of mother's face), and to the pathological symbiotic bonds actively and discriminately formed by the primitive personality. Grotstein (personal communication) refers to this adaptation as "parasitism," a term which is descriptive but has other unfortunate associations. We now know that it is possible through active, skilled, dedicated efforts to engage at least some schizophrenics and that under these circumstances patterned transference configurations do emerge. While these bear some correspondence to the possessed configuration of the primitive personality, no processes corresponding to the possessor configuration are detectable.

The extreme passivity, absence of active relationships outside the family, and global indiscriminate way of relating to the world that characterize the schizophrenic all stand out rather starkly in the premorbid histories of Emily, Rachel, Edward, and Celia. Joanna (Chapter 20), in contrast, had some modest success in finding a boyfriend/mother substitute (Deeg), even though their relationship was constituted in a more blatantly shared delusional manner than the symbioses formed by primitive personalities. In the cases of Emily, Rachel, and Celia, a simultaneously grandiose and self-destructive symbiotic configuration, which combined elements of relationship with and introjection of the primary object, was eventually enacted in the transference. With Edward the element of self-abnegating compliance, that is, the destruction of feelings, needs, and personal agenda, had to be inferred from his history and ward behavior as he did not become sufficiently involved in treatment to be able to communicate it. Edward's needs, like Celia's, seemed to arise only when the object seemed safely unavailable or rejecting; otherwise, he enacted a grandiose, sadistic, self-sufficient repudiation of needs and rejection of caring persons.

The Mind in the Primitive Personality Disorders and in Schizophrenia

Let us go from these general descriptions of relationship patterns to a more specific description of some of the salient characteristics of the primitive mind, including similarities and differences between the primitive personalities, for example, borderline individuals, on the one hand, and schizophrenics, on the other. I would like to begin by stressing once again the importance in mental organization and maturation of the processes of integration and differentiation.* I think of differentiation and integration as aspects of a unitary process. As aspects of mind are differentiated from one another and from the caring persons who have attentively mirrored them back to their author, they may gradually be integrated or structured into complex patterned configurations. In turn, the configuration or organization of differentiated entities is part of their further differentiation from one another. The building of mental structures and complex representations establishes their separateness and distinctiveness.

Both primitive personalities and schizophrenics have problems of psychic differentiation and integration. This very fact makes it difficult to describe their mental functioning, for in so doing it is unavoidable that we resort to categorizing and systematizing (differentiating and integrating). However, to abandon the descriptive effort and to resort to a description of the primitive mind as monolithic and unified is equally unsatisfactory, for relatively enduring patterns and configurations do seem apparent to the observer. The problem posed by the paradox inherent in employing linguistic concepts to describe an unintegrated, undifferentiated state increases in direct proportion to the primitiveness of the mental state we attempt to describe, and it is a formidable obstacle to the comprehension of schizophrenia.

However disturbed and immature, the primitive personality possesses mental capabilities that are lacking in the schizophrenic and that enable him to be an active participant in a symbiotic possession relationship. The primitive personality manifests an active thrust to leave his family of origin. He is capable of exercising initiative in recruiting new objects for relationships. Although he is not consciously aware of what he is doing, he can distinguish among objects as either familiar (uncaring but attributing or using, like the primary object) or strange (attentive and potentially caring) and can engage selectively in behaviors "appropriate" to each. However, he lacks the stable, internal self-parenting (valuing and caring) structures that might enable him to separate. His disturbing affects (anger, hurt, rejection) and the elements of his self-esteem (or lack thereof) are inconstantly represented and weakly integrated with a sense of self. He lacks the capacity to sustain caring feelings about another. But he is capable of using sensorimotor–affective thinking to form poorly differentiated bonds with symbiotic objects that are adaptive (or from an adult perspective, maladaptive); these include projective enactments with the other person of loosely integrated and differentiated dysphoric mental

---

*Among the first to be aware of the importance of these processes was Heinz Werner (1940), who suggested that "the development of biological forms is expressed in an *increasing differentiation* of parts and an *increasing subordination*, or *hierarchization* . . . an ordering and grouping of parts in terms of the whole organism" (p. 41) and that "the fundamental law of development [is] increase of differentiation and hierarchic integration" (p. 44).

contents. The primitive personality has also developed a structured symbiosis-ready internal template based on introjection (possessed configuration), a template he is able to transfer to a "familiar" object in order to maintain a sense of identity while physically separate from his primary family. However maladaptive it may seem to the observer, restitution of a primary self-destructive relationship in a new guise is a route to leaving home concretely and establishing the superficial semblance of a separation.

The schizophrenic mind, in contrast, is extreme in its undifferentiation and unintegration, although this state may be masked by the pseudo organization and stability of delusional ideation. It is at the very opposite pole from the structured and internalized psychic organization of the neurotic mind, which is characterized by integration in the form of an overall organization, patterning, and control of often conflicting intrapsychic forces, as well as by mature ambivalence (the panoply of feelings are personally enriching rather than fragmenting, contradictory, and personally impoverishing). In schizophrenia, subjective components of mind are not differentiated from characteristics of other persons, and despite the seeming richness of delusional ideation, the schizophrenic conveys but little sense of awareness of the discrete "inner" components of his mind, especially the obvious ones that may be inferred from observation of his behavior and speech. Integration or organization of mental components under the aegis of a cohesive and relatively constant sense of self is lacking. Some characteristic deficits in schizophrenia—such as incapacity to differentiate the true strangeness or unfamiliarity of others, difficulties with state and tension regulation, incapacity to reflect about the self, extreme inconstancy of self-sense, aversion to others, and delusional and hallucinatory thinking—are probably also aspects of failure of integration-differentiation.

The schizophrenic is unable to differentiate the salient characteristics of others. Here I am referring not to complex or subtle differences but to the most basic distinction of vital characteristics of objects that normal infants make in the first months of life as either caring or rejecting, as either familiar (like parents) or strange; distinctions which primitive personalities are capable of. The reader may cogently object that, except in the most acute stages of illness, schizophrenics appear to have at least rudimentary capacities to discriminate others on the basis of name, sex, and the like, but of course I am not referring to the simple capacity to identify objects and to use the most formal aspects of language (although these too may be impaired in certain stages of the illness) but to more subtle psychological distinctions involving affect and emotion.

In schizophrenics there is no internalized mentally represented, abstracted, or conceptualized template or model of a symbiotic relationship analogous to the possession configurations found in primitive personalities. As a result the schizophrenic is unable to make a mental displacement or transference of a primary relationship pattern to other persons who are selected or discriminated in the ways just described, as others do. He cannot initiate a relationship with a person outside the family as can the primitive personality, either as a possession or as a possessor, that is, as one who actively invests that person with emotion (*besetzen*), endows him with loosely integrated projections of aspects of self, and induces him to become a symbiotic partner. Hence, the schizophrenic is unable to separate physically, much less psychologically, from his primary family.

It is widely held that primitive mental states represent fixations at or regressions to normal infantile states. Gedo and Goldberg (1973) maintain that the most primitive mental state is characterized by difficulties with tension and state regulation as well as by absence of integration; from this it follows that persons so impaired should welcome the therapeutic "holding" and soothing of a containing symbiotic object. But, in fact, schizophrenics act aversive to others. It is necessary to maintain at least a weak degree of integration of such aspects of self as unrepresented rage, as well as at least the rudiments of differentiation of self from other, in order to want and be able to use another person as possession or container for not-yet-internalized mental contents and processes, just as it is necessary to be attracted to others in order to learn to represent, symbolize, and regulate one's own mental activity. The schizophrenic's fundamental failure to own (differentiate) and integrate his mind is related to his equally profound repudiation of a facilitating symbiotic relationship with another.

Delusions and hallucinations are reflective of the extreme undifferentiation of self from object and the absence of integration of mental content that characterizes schizophrenia. They may superficially resemble the defensive projection of the neurotic or the more rudimentary nondefensive sensorimotor–affective projective enactment of the primitive personality, but their significance is very different, for the schizophrenic's mental contents are linked or integrated neither to a sense of self or identity nor to specific objects or socially adaptive activity; instead, they reflect a nearly total failure of differentiation of self from nonself and a profound loss of integrative connection between mind and self-sense. This can be illustrated by examining the fate of hallucinations in the course of psychotherapy: The hallucinatory state is succeeded by one in which the hallucinated elements are initially owned as aspects of self, although these are not integrated with other parts. And they are experienced as self only at certain times—for example, when the patient is aware of his enormous rage and destructiveness. At those times a sense of constructiveness and caring connectedness to others may be entirely missing. At other times the rage or destructiveness is looked upon with horror, as though it were the attitude of another person, even though the patient is capable of becoming aware—and may even remember, albeit without emotional connection—that the hallucination is an expression of self, much as we may look upon a nightmare. At this intermediate stage, when he no longer hallucinates, the patient seems more like a primitive personality. In the angry, destructive state the nonangry state does not seem to exist, that is, does not seem affectively real; reciprocally, in the non-angry state the destructive rage is intellectually appreciated but seems like an unreachable separate self. In other words, there is no capacity for bearing intrapsychic conflict. Eventually, the two states of mind can be experienced more or less in juxtaposition, a state of growth that, interestingly enough, these individuals first and invariably label as pathological, saying they are "confused" or have lost "clarity" of thinking and in some instances literally complaining of an accompanying "splitting headache." In other words, the process of therapeutic evolution of the schizophrenic hallucination suggests that it is both a deviant and a more developmentally primitive phenomenon than the oscillating self-contradiction that typifies primitive personality organization.

The therapeutic evolution of Celia's hallucinations (Chapter 21) illustrates these developments. One line of change occurred as her self-destructiveness came under progressive control, self-caring began to develop, and reconstruction based on memories and associations supervened. The function of her hallucinations in preserving her adaptive tie to her destructive mother and in preserving the form of self-regulation which that relationship had promoted became clear. Another line, not unrelated, involved the progressive integration and representation of rage, an affect that was entirely absent from Celia's conscious awareness and manifest behavior when I first made her acquaintance, except for what might be inferred from an occasional affectless fantasy (for example, of machine-gunning the world). As Celia began to own her rage the hallucinations diminished. First they became inner voices, which she could acknowledge as the nasty, hateful aspect of herself. Later she described the sadistically laughing, ridiculing, attacking part of her as being localized in the back of her head, as a kind of flexible skin that "kept after" her and could not be escaped from. Still later she told me that I had no idea how badly she wished the hostile part of herself were "out there" in the form of persecutory voices and ideas, for when it was she felt more of a sense of control whereas when she owned it as her own hostility she literally felt terrified of herself and unable to escape. Celia complained of a splitting headache along with her first integrated awareness of rage.

The second characteristic of schizophrenic mentation is global passivity. While passivity may seem a characteristic of behavior and not of mind, the schizophrenic mind is concrete and not well differentiated from the world of things and actions. This passivity may be obscured by the behavioral turmoil characteristic of acute episodes. It pervades all aspects of the personality, unlike the compliance of the primitive personality, which exists alongside an aggressive, adaptive possessor configuration. The schizophrenic makes little effort to actively and selectively recruit others into his life or to utilize aspects of the world around him adaptively in the service of actualizing some cognitive-affective schema, except, on occasion, in a personally indiscriminate manner as props for delusional enactments.

A third characteristic of schizophrenic thought is a lack of assertiveness or adaptive interpersonal aggressiveness. While this may be another aspect of passivity, what I wish to emphasize is the fate of the aggressive affective-behavioral spectrum, including anger, assertion, and the like. There appears to be no socially or interpersonally adaptive deployment of aggression, the closest manifestation being delusional elements that appear to lack reality-adaptive value. In place of the missing capacity to process aggression and hostility in an interpersonal relationship and concomitant socially adaptive activity, unrepresented rage is diffusely directed toward the workings of the schizophrenic mind (thoughts and feelings, nascent constructive components, and expressions of autonomous selfhood) as well as toward other persons whose attentions stimulate self-awareness. In this we note another aspect of the schizophrenic's tandem aversion to the attention of others and to the awareness of the workings of his mind. Instead of symbiotically bonding the schizophrenic to the attentive and mirroring object and enabling a rudimentary self-and-object sense, as in the case of the possessor configuration of the primitive personality, schizophrenic rage appears to destroy self-cohesion as well as to lead to assaults on and rejections of the other. The schizophrenic's anger is not well represented as an internal emotion or predisposition. Its presence and expression must at first be inferred from self-destructive behavior, absence of self-care, and the content of hallucinations and delusions. The powerful attacks the schizophrenic makes on the use of his mind, a deep-seated repugnance to thinking and bearing feelings about the self and the object world, which seems to represent a nihilistic urge toward mental anesthesia or death, and the associated aversion to other caring persons who would help him attend to himself are things that cannot be fully appreciated unless one succeeds in engaging a schizophrenic in an intensive psychoanalytically informed treatment process.

Schizophrenic hallucinations appear to serve functions in lieu of the actual and psychological presence of suitable objects related to self or identity maintenance and adaptation, as well as being a substitute for appropriate psychic capacities for affect representation and regulation, particularly of rage and neediness. Insofar as they articulate routes and patterns for impulse expression and control, usually involving extreme self-suppression but sometimes leading to shocking destructive actions, they constitute a primitive form of self-regulation that substitutes for mature identification and internalization. That is, these individuals have no more mature way to regulate their emotions and needs than to attack and attempt to suppress them or to explosively enact them. This perpetuation of an infantile adaptation to a mother-world that rejects or attacks autonomous expressions and functions in an all-or-nothing manner may also act as an anodyne to the experience of being separate and alone.

Celia and I, for example, ultimately came to believe that the harsh, depriving, admonitory voices she experienced that led her to attack the coherence of her thoughts and awareness of her emotions and to abandon constructive efforts to care about herself or anyone else and to put herself in abusive situations must have commenced shortly after her mother's prolonged mental hospitalization and absence from home. These seemed to represent her own unacknowledged rage, a global sense of her mother's person, and her mode of adaptation in their early relationship. As a child Celia tried every mode of nonexistence short of actual suicide so as to eradicate in herself any sign of life that might provoke her mother's bizarre and wrathful behavior and thereby stabilize the only relationship she had. As an adult she came to rely on this extreme deadening or selflessness as a form of self-regulation and control. Celia's schizophrenia was chronic, and much of the time she maintained a tenuous, albeit self-destructive social adaptation. While I have emphasized the schizophrenic person's minimal capacity to adapt, it is possible to view Celia's pathology from an adaptive standpoint more than the other patients in this book. She learned to function without the concrete presence of her mother, and she developed the most remarkable capacity to live in strange, objectively frightening, and dangerous environments, geographically distant from home, without experiencing any feelings of aloneness or fearfulness. These places were "like home" to her, particularly when their already threatening (and often actually harmful) quality was augmented by her delusions and hallucinations. So Celia's hallucinations and delusions provided her with a sense of familiarity and autonomy in strange places, as well as with a curious form of impulse control. The underlying sense of grandiosity and omnipotence that accompanied her extreme masochism provided her with a sense of identity as well.

Pao (1979) views hallucinations as defenses against dependency, a form of pseudo independence. In his view hallucinations represent the construction of a substitutive dependency, akin to Winnicott's transitional objects. It seems more likely that this process is not a defense so much as the perpetuation of a very early adaptation to a pathological relationship with a primary object and a primitive identification with that person as a form of self-regulation; a protosymbiotic adaptation or precursor of the possessed configuration but one in which no specific current object is required, even as projection screen. Among other things, the concept of defense implies unconscious and warded off configurations of affect and ideas, and it seems unlikely that Celia had developed sufficiently to represent aloneness, fearfulness, despair, and rage so as to institute defenses against awareness of these things.

The fourth characteristic of the schizophrenic mind, which may seem like another facet of elements I have already described, is severely impaired capacity for social and interpersonal adaptation, reflected particularly in an absence of the sensorimotor–affective thinking that characterizes normal infants and primitive personalities and in an incapacity to utilize what aliment the environment may have to offer either for maintenance of equilibrium or for growth. Sensorimotor–affective thinking is a characteristic of the primitive, incompletely integrated mind in which the physical activity of manipulating and eating is not yet differentiated from the mental processes of assimilation and learning (psychoanalytically the oral incorporative phase). * In this process loosely integrated aspects of mind are perceived as though they were

---

*It was first described by Piaget, and I have elaborated its application to affect development (Robbins, 1981a).

located in the environment, and thought is not differentiated from action. In ordinary infant development some of the actions resulting from such thinking, for example, grasping and mouthing, are crucial to adaptation and provide a concrete model for mental internalization and growth. The most primitive form of sensorimotor–affective thinking does not differentiate among objects (that is, anything can be aliment for the mouth-sucking schema), but through a gradual process of assimilation and accommodation the infant comes to have stable recognition representations of which objects will better serve as aliment for his ongoing cognitive schemata and which will not.

With this description of four characteristics of the schizophrenic mind—undifferentiation and nonintegration, global passivity, lack of assertiveness, and inability to adapt—we conclude our discussion of the psychological perspective. Our description has been shaped and limited by the undifferentiation and nonintegration of the schizophrenic mind. The very process of description implies linguistic sophistication; we must consider the consequences of our necessary use of concepts implying discrimination and organization (integration and differentiation) to describe a mental state characterized by undifferentiation and nonintegration. And we find that it is impossible to confine a so-called psychological discussion to the intrapsychic sphere, for one of the characteristics of primitive mentation is its incomplete differentiation from the interpersonal (dyadic) world.

Chapter 10

The Family System

I t is currently fashionable to dismiss psychogenic hypotheses and think of schizophrenia as an illness that develops rather unexpectedly in early adulthood in an hitherto relatively normal person who is a member of a family that is psychologically, if not genetically, relatively normal. An alternative hypothesis, which does not require us to jettison the idea of a genetic contribution, is that the psychological pathology elaborated in Chapter 9 crystallizes out of the constitutional vulnerabilities described in Chapter 7, in the context of inadequate or pathological parenting and a disturbed family structure, and is present from the earliest stages of life if only the observer takes the trouble to look and has the special expertise to do so. While at this stage of our knowledge we cannot chose between these alternatives with certainty, in this chapter I shall review a preponderance of evidence that the schizophrenic individual is an element of a disturbed family system and that schizophrenia may be defined and viewed at a family dynamic level as well as an individual level. I shall describe how the family simultaneously exploits, amplifies, compensates for, and denies the existence of the cognitive and affective characteristics of its schizophrenic members (which were described in Chapter 9), the net result being a fragile state of equilibrium that usually persists until the schizophrenic member is forced to try to separate and make his way in the outside world. As this viewpoint is currently out of fashion, I shall also examine some of the common objections raised against it.

Statistical Research on Trauma: Studies and Limitations

Some of the evidence for psychogenesis comes from clinical studies of families done in the 1950s and 1960s (Bateson, Jackson, Haley, & Weakland, 1956;

Wynne, Ryckoff, Day, & Hirsch, 1958; Jackson, 1960; Wynne & Singer, 1963; Lidz & Fleck, 1965; Alanen, 1966; Lidz, 1973), which tend to be discounted because of their psychoanalytic "bias." The Lidz and Fleck study (1965), for example, involved an intensive and prolonged investigation of 17 families of hospitalized schizophrenics against a backdrop of several hundred other families of hospitalized schizophrenics who were studied less intensively. Four of these families were actually selected because the referring psychiatrist believed they were normal. And it utilized a control group of families of depressed patients, who were found to be much different in their psychological makeup. Some of the evidence comes from psychiatric demographic studies, for example, M. Bleuler's (1978) retrospective review of a large group of schizophrenic patients from the Burghölzli, which concludes that psychogenic factors are at least as important in the development of schizophrenia as hereditary ones. Another such study is reported by Tienari et al. (1981), who abstracted 10 schizophrenics from a large group of adopted children and studied the adoptive families of these 10 in depth; they concluded that in each instance the families were seriously disturbed. Kringlen (1987) notes that the psychological environment in each instance of schizophrenia in one of a pair of monozygotic (MZ) twins who were reared apart was "miserable" and stressful. More recently, Greenspan (1988, 1989a,b) has authored some notable studies of infant and child development in which he lends support for the hypothesis that schizophrenia is an illness that develops gradually, beginning in infancy.

Not all studies comparing stress or trauma in the family background of schizophrenics to that in families of patients with other diagnoses have demonstrated a convincing difference, however. Severe trauma in the form of statistically enumerable family problems, such as disintegration of the home, presence of criminal behavior, child or spouse abuse, or drug abuse, is common in the histories of many who do not become schizophrenic, and in using such gross criteria of trauma many families of schizophrenics, at least at first glance, do not seem terribly disturbed. It is my impression that these apparently negative findings do not disprove the psychogenic hypothesis so much as they illustrate one of the limitations of the statistical experimental method, namely, that in order to define stress in a quantitative measurable sense as a linear variable one cannot possibly consider the sophisticated nuances and gestalts of parent–child interaction or individual psychological dynamics (see Chapters 2, 3, and 18). I shall attempt to demonstrate that the pathogenic agent in schizophrenia is not gross quantity of stress or trauma measured on a linear, psychological Richter scale, but rather a particular configuration of family dynamics, which may even derive some of its power to harm from its concealment from persons outside the family. Such "stress," if that is even a good name for it, is certainly imperceptible to the casual observer and to the quantitative experimenter with his straightforward checklist, and becomes visible only if one takes considerable time and pains to get to know the schizophrenic and his family in action.

The Psychogenic Hypothesis

I should like to review the psychoanalytic literature about the pathogenic role of the primary caregiver relationship and the nature of the family disturbance, including such topics as denial, shared distortion of reality and meaning, misattribution of thoughts and feelings, and the roles of love and hate.

Lidz (1973) has proposed a gender related family typology that seems quite applicable to the cases in this book, particularly those of Rachel and Edward. The fundamental problem he describes is the egocentricity of one or both parents, which remains confined to the family and is not apparent to casual observers. In "skewed" families, the pattern Lidz associates with male schizophrenia, beneath a superficial appearance of harmony mother is seductive and domineering and father is passive. In "schismatic" families, the pattern he associates with female schizophrenia, father is grandiose and seductive while the mother is devalued and aloof. In both instances the role of the child is to help maintain this equilibrium by alliance with the dominant parent.

Lidz, Cornelison, Fleck, and Terry (1957), Wynne et al. (1958), and Wynne and Singer (1963) describe family complicity to deny basic problems and assert a false harmony. The Lidz group refer to this phenomenon as "skew," the Wynne group as "pseudomutuality." Such families make implicit threats of expulsion toward the member who does not comply. Lidz (1973) states that "At times, the deviant or delusional ideas of one parent are accepted by the spouse and become a *folie à deux*, or when shared by all family members, a *folie en famille*" (p. 31). Wynne and Singer originated the concept of pseudomutuality to describe the use of shared denial to cover over irreconcilable conflict and related failures of communication.

Bateson, Jackson, Haley, and Weakland (1956) introduced the concept of "double bind" to describe a combination of suppression of autonomy and shared denial that forces the child to remain pathologically dependent. Disability and undifferentiation are rewarded, and there are subtle threats of attack and rejection of the schizophrenic member should he use his mind and sense of reality to attempt to achieve a degree of differentiation and autonomy; pathological reasoning and responses are labeled as normal, and vice versa. The most destructive element of the "double bind" is the unspoken injunction that the contradictions are to be denied and not talked about.

Searles (1965) describes the interaction of families with a schizophrenic member as one involving powerful boundary interpenetrations by projection. Being part of the family means accepting this "pseudomutuality" and a spurious sense of oneness and harmony; the alternative is to be rejected and branded as "crazy." An attitude of curiosity, questioning, or disagreement on the part of the patient is looked upon as a form of insanity (as the case of Rachel, in Chapter 20, vividly illustrates). In order to preserve the harmony, intensive one-to-one relationships outside the family (such as therapy), which might foster other ways of thinking, are discouraged. It might appear that family harmony is preserved entirely by means of explicit or implicit threats, but Searles also hints that there is gratification that come from acceptance of the status quo; what I refer to in Chapter 9 as infantilization, which is often accompanied by parental attributions of omnipotence and omniscience. This composite description of family pathology derived from the studies I have cited certainly fits most of the cases presented in this book.

The caregiver–infant relationship has been the focus of numerous studies. Lidz and Fleck (1965) and Bowen (1960, 1965) note that mothers of schizophrenics tend to have boundary problems and to confuse their own needs with those of their children by a process of externalization and that they keep these misidentified children from individuating in order to feel a sense of personal completeness. What is projected onto the child, according to Searles (1965), is parts of the mother and her relationship to her own mother. Hill (1955) describes a mother–child symbiosis in which the child's illness involves efforts to maintain the mother's sanity.

Searles (1965) also writes about the schizophrenic's sacrifice of autonomy to preserve maternal integration. He describes this as a combination of the child's perception of the mother's real fragility and of its fantasy: "The child's own desire for individuation may be experienced by him as a desire to drive the mother crazy" (p. 271). The schizophrenic's psychological effort is expended to take care of his disturbed mother, rather than to allow her (or anyone else) to take care of him. This is the origin of what I have referred to as the possessed configuration (Robbins, 1981b, 1983, 1988, 1989; also see Chapter 9). Searles adds, "This infantile-omnipotent relatedness between the 'sickest,' least mature areas of the parent's personality on the one hand, and the patient's personality on the other, constitutes the greatest obstacle to the patient's becoming well" (p. 268).

What is less a matter of consensus is the role of love and hatred in the child–parent relationships of schizophrenics. Searles notes the widespread opinion that the relationship between schizophrenic and mother is characterized by mutual hatred (for example, Johnson, Giffin, Watson, & Beckett, 1956). While he does not explicitly disagree, he stresses the importance of love as well, as manifested in the schizophrenic child's self-sacrifice: "The child's loving sacrifice of his very individuality for the welfare of the mother who is loved genuinely . . . with the wholehearted adoration which . . . only a small child can bestow" (1965, p. 220). I would argue that what Searles describes is not love, which involves an active wholehearted investment of positive emotion in the process of which one's identity flourishes, but an adaptive attachment based on desparation and the need to survive as an entity of some sort, even if only physical, at any cost, even if it requires the destruction of one's mind. I believe that Searles confuses love with the kind of adaptive necessity to which Suttie (1935) referred when he said "I would suggest that the psychoses are to be regarded as the vestiges (and their results) of the child's attempt to find a secure 'niche' for itself in the family circle" (p. 200) and which I have also written about (Robbins, 1988).

The question of rage in the schizophrenic and his family is an equally obscure one. Rage is certainly not apparent from casual observation of relationships between schizophrenics and parents; what one is more likely to see is solicitude and compensatory care for a disabled person on the part of family and a combination of disengagement and bizarre engagement on the part of the patient. If anything, families of schizophrenics often seem remarkable for the absence of manifest anger and conflict among members, which is one reason why quests for family pathology based on superficial observation and questioning so often come up empty. It is more likely that there is a parental failure of holding or containment, consisting of a combination of the parent's failure to perceive and accurately evaluate the infant's gestures and needs and a tendency to substitute an unconscious parental agenda or gestures or meanings instead (Bion, 1959a, 1962a,b; Winnicott, 1960 a,c). The extent to which parental rage underlies such a perceptual, cognitive, and behavioral problem will probably vary in individual circumstances. I do believe that parental hostility is enacted in an overprotective, subtly authoritarian scenario in which actual devaluation masquerades as caring and in which a shared, rigid set of rules about what constitutes reality and what things mean, which may be quite at odds with the perceptions of an outside observer, is established and enforced to the detriment of individual autonomy. As for the infant, his experience may well include, other than the basic organismic need to survive, a constitutional excess of rageful propensity and/or a deficiency in the mechanisms to control it (as suggested in Chapter 7). Once this propensity is developed along lines adaptive to family pathology, the schizophrenic result is that unrepresented rage is expressed in a diffuse, internalized, delusional, and self-destructive form (elaborated in Chapter 9), which poses no real threat to the pathological integrity of the family.

Objections to the Psychogenic Hypothesis and the Problem of Denial

Our review of the psychoanalytic literature on family disturbance in schizophrenia and its presumed pathogenic role has not yet laid to rest any of the objections to the psychogenic hypothesis on which the reports are based. The conclusions just cited about the pathogenic role of the family emerged from the post-World War II interest of psychoanalysis in schizophrenia and were hyperbolically typified by Fromm-Reichmann's (1948) controversial hypothesis of the "schizophrenogenic mother" (p. 265), a characterization that has hung in the psychoanalytic portrait gallery alongside Winnicott's "good enough mother" (1960a). When misused as synonyms for "bad" mother in discussions in which theory and hypothesis are contaminated by covert anger, guilt, and value judgment, such terms quite rightly elicit a storm of protest and repudiation, which, in turn, has reinforced current antipsychoanalytic sentiment almost as much as has the objection to Freud's concept of penis envy. The pendulum of reaction has now swung in the opposite direction, so that not only is it now unpopular to maintain that parents play a significant role in the schizophrenia of their offspring, but the schizophrenic child is actually felt to be the disturbing influence in his otherwise normal family. If the parents of a schizophrenic are disturbed, the reasoning goes, it must be as a consequence of the stress to which they have been subjected. This radical reinterpretation of family life leads to the curious conclusion that the disturbed child is capable of inducing pathological behavior in his otherwise normal parents, but not vice-versa. Since the contemporary heightening of awareness of the reality of child abuse has provided many with yet another antipsychoanalytic rallying cry, as they point to Freud's abandonment of his original emphasis on the reality of parental seduction and his emphasis instead on the role of fantasy, it may be that in time the contradiction in these two social critiques of psychoanalytic theory will become more apparent, but as I mentioned previously, the element of denial in schizophrenic families is so impenetrable that the more subtle form of abuse to which I allude is invisible compared to the physical violation of the abused child. Of course, there is no good reason why both ideas—that parents disturb children and vice versa—cannot be true, but it defies even common sense to maintain that adults are more susceptible to basic disturbance by others than are their children.

On rereading some of the writing of Fromm-Reichmann, I am led to conclude that the moralistic "misinterpretation" of her term may not be entirely a product of the vicissitudes of social fashion. The tone of her 1952 article on psychoanalytic therapy of schizophrenia, for example, is, at least to my ears, distinctly moralizing, blaming, and patronizing, although the target is not the schizophrenic's mother but the therapist who cannot understand his patient's communications and bond with him. Based on her assumption, commonplace enough in literature and history, that the schizophrenic patient is in fact a savant who, with an unusual access to the workings of his mind, may understand more of the meaning of his productions than anyone else, save possibly the most gifted therapist, Fromm-Reichmann reasons that "psychiatrists can take it for granted now that in principle a working doctor–patient relationship can be established with the schizophrenic patient. If and when this seems impossible, it is due to the doctor's personal difficulties, not to the patient's psychopathology" (p. 91). Fromm-Reichmann lists in detail all the "problems" most psychiatrists may have that render them unable to work with schizophrenics. And she concludes:

> This enumeration of the psychiatrist's potential difficulties in establishing a workable relationship with the schizophrenic does not imply that a psychiatrist who cannot overcome these barriers in his own personality should worry guiltily about responsibilities not adequately met. Guilt-feelings are an unconstructive, paralyzing luxury, which should be discouraged. . . . Instead, the psychiatrist should admit to himself, that—in his present state of personality development—he is not equal to coping with schizophrenics, if there is danger of burdening them with his own anxieties. (pp. 93–94)

The belief that the schizophrenic and the "good" therapist are a very special couple, each posssessed of the most remarkable capacities, illustrates a certain loss of reality sense on the part of the therapist and is related to archaic narcissism in the family relations of the schizophrenic, a topic I explore later in this chapter and in the chapters on treatment. Meanwhile, I suggest the possibility that, in the passage just quoted, Fromm-Reichmann might well have been describing a "schizophrenogenic therapist," which leads me to suspect that, from the start, the term *schizophrenogenic mother* was probably not a neutral concept.

As I employ the concept of pathogenic family, I do not mean to imply that family members do not care about the patient, although the concerns they express should not be confused with growth-promoting love. The families of my patients were willing to make considerable expenditures of time, effort, and money for the care of the afflicted member and were not grossly neglectful or abusive in the sense that might be recorded in a conventional statistical survey. They involved themselves in the treatment process, more or less and however reluctantly, often in the face of considerable difficulty in the form of geographical distance, work commitments, and expense. It was the quality of their involvement with the patient that was clearly abnormal; the symbiotic attachments in these families were, at worst, hopelessly destructive and, at best, a monumental impediment to the patient's growth.

Ironically, a fuller appreciation of the constitutional predisposition to schizophrenia offers us a way to view pathogenic parenting that is both true to the clinical data and not censorious in its intent. I should like to suggest another portrait to hang alongside Winnicott's "good enough mother" and Fromm-Reichmann's "schizophrenogenic mother": that of the *reparative* mother—or as Greenspan (1989a) describes her, the "intuitively gifted caregiver." It is an extraordinary challenge and stress to have the responsibility, with little respite, for the rearing of a child who cannot tolerate stimulation, is averse to emotional involvement and to sustaining a relationship, may be excessively irritable when aroused, and is innately disorganized and unfocused. These deficits may stimulate the mother's own vulnerabilities, psychological and constitutional. Thus, along with the question of how it is that some mothers interact with such an offspring to foster a schizophrenic predisposition, it is important to ask the following questions: "Why didn't the *other* MZ twin become schizophrenic? Why is it that no offspring from some genetically vulnerable lineages become schizophrenic? A reparative mother is a caregiver whose ministrations prevent activation of phenotypic vulnerability from schizophrenic genes, or compensate in such a way as to institute a reparative sequence of organic and psychological changes which prevent the emergence of clinical schizophrenia and in some instances foster growth into a healthy, productive adulthood. Where would the world be without these unsung heroines? Unfortunately for the vantage point of theoretical balance, analysts, by virtue of their focus on psychopathology, do not ordinarily encounter these individuals in their practice. This is one of the reasons why infant observation and longitudinal studies of development and outcome must play an increasingly important role in psychoanalysis. From a more balanced viewpoint, taking into account both constitutional vulnerability and early caretaking relationships, the psychological "cause" of schizophrenia might be hypothesized to reside neither in mother nor child exclusively but in the interaction of their unique and possibly shared vulnerabilities.

Another reason mothers have been unjustly maligned may be that it is easier to see what they *do* than what fathers do *not* do. In situations where the outcome is grossly pathological, the other parent (usually but not always the father) does not provide an effective alternative or counterbalance. The absent or passively harmful parent does not necessarily have to be the father, and the more actively harmful one the mother. This is well illustrated in the case of Rachel (Chapter 20), though my guess is that, had Rachel been able to involve herself more intensively in treatment, we would have discovered that there were more problems in relation to mother than were apparent. In the other cases I present in full, the father was more or less absent as an effective parental alternative.

Lest it seem that I am espousing the one-sided view that the schizophrenic is simply a victim of his disturbed family, in particular his primary parent (even if the idea is nonjudgmental and is balanced by recognizing that other children are equally influenced by unusually gifted and dedicated parenting), I should like to emphasize that in the disturbed family constellations I am describing other family members suffer too, and in ways qualitatively, if not quantitatively, similar to the suffering of the schizophrenic member, although their suffering may not be so symptomatically apparent as that of the schizophrenic and they may be quite unaware of it (until the balance of family dynamics shifts in the course of treatment). Most commonly, the expressions of upset related to the patient that I heard from family members early in the course of treatment bore little or no resemblance to what I came to understand in the course of family therapy as their real suffering—usually major constrictions, which they had not realized, in the scope and richness of their lives. The energy of Emily's mother, for example, was chronically consumed in her disability-sustaining role in the symbiotic fusion with Emily. She felt she was literally experiencing the pain of Emily's confinement and distress, and even the physical pain of Emily's self-mutilation. In fact, her marriage was being strained because she was so preoccupied with Emily that she had no time for or interest in her husband, though she was quite unaware of this as a problem until he mentioned it in the course of family therapy. She felt liberated and the quality of her life improved as the symbiotic bond dissolved and Emily got better. Edward's father, in particular, and his mother, to a lesser degree, became less depressed as they were able to let go of some of their pathological interactions with him in the course of family therapy, and their relationship with their other children improved substantially. Rachel's sister said that elucidation of the suppressive dynamics of their family enabled her to separate herself and become more autonomous.

The heated and total repudiation of family responsibility for the illness of the schizophrenic member is more than simply a reaction to psychoanalytic prejudice and covert blaming. Denial of antecedent disturbance in the patient or significant problems in the family is a characteristic of such families. The success of disclaimers on the part of family and casual observers concerning antecedent personal or family problems is at least partially responsible for the current popularity, even among psychoanalysts (for example, Willick, 1990), of the reductionistic contention that schizophrenia is an organic illness of adult onset, and that psychogenic and psychodynamic hypotheses are irrelevant. In the face of such effective denial, intensive and prolonged psychoanalytically informed investigation of the family may be required to uncover the pathogenic forces and patterns. Recently, Walker and Lewine (1990) asked experienced clinicians to view home movies taken in childhood of five schizophrenics. With 78% accuracy they were able to select the schizophrenic-to-be from his siblings. The most intriguing aspect had to do with the "pilot" patient who was initially evaluated to determine the feasibility of the study. Trained observers had no difficulty picking him as the abnormal member of the sibship from the home movies. However, his parents not only stoutly denied that there had been anything abnormal about him as a child, but they even believed that he had been the best adjusted of their children!

This extraordinary family denial is apparent in the cases in this book. For example, it was only after half a year of hospitalization of Rachel (Chapter 20), whose illness manifested itself when she attempted to leave home for the first time to attend college, that her family members acknowledged that they knew she had been hallucinating since her early teens. Though questioned on numerous occasions about such matters, they did not believe that there was anything about her behavior that was out of the ordinary; thus, to their way of thinking they had not observed anything abnormal. As it turned out, Rachel's hallucinating was unremarkable to her father, who claimed he also "hallucinated." It seemed likely that, in his poorly differentiated relationship with the patient, father could not distinguish his own habit of talking to himself from his daughter's hallucinations. Even when Rachel's psychosis was impossible for her parents to ignore because of feedback from hospital staff, her parents still viewed her as normal, and made such remarks as "Any of us would act the way she does if we had to be in a place like this, with all these crazy people!" Since this denial of manifest illness in their daughter had been accompanied, on their part, by compensatory infantilizing behavior whenever she manifested her disturbance, Rachel's parents (and Rachel herself) were not required to face and deal with the problem.

Edward's history was similar. Long after his hospitalization and his repeated efforts to tell his parents not only how unhappy but how patently socially maladapted he had been, they continued to insist that he had been a normal, happy, productive, and even unusually accomplished adolescent. The fact that Edward seemed to have no friends and had spent much of his weekends in bed, for example, had not struck them as remarkable. His mother often did the same thing, and his father, who tended to overlook family problems, was preoccupied with his career and usually not around to observe such behavior. In the course of his treatment Edward told me that his mother did not consider his hallucinating remarkable and that she had informed him that she often carried on conversations with him when he was not actually present!

The Schizophrenic Family

Having reviewed some of the literature and controversy surrounding the psychogenic hypothesis we turn next to a description of a typical schizophrenic family. The state of dependence of the adult schizophrenic is less obvious than that of the normal infant, or even of the primitive personality, for he makes no active effort to discriminate and sustain vital relationships, and the caregiving that is essential to his survival may no longer be the function of a specific individual but may be diffused among one or more agencies of society. The schizophrenic may not directly indicate that he is aware of the importance or even the existence of the caretakers. At the same time (provided his significant family members are alive), detailed scrutiny will reveal that he is an undifferentiated participant in a dynamic family system that is characterized by the incomplete functional and experiential self–object differentiation and integration of its members, so that aspects of incompletely owned and internalized self may be owned and enacted by other members and vice versa. Paul Weiss's (1969) assertion that general systems theory is the study of group interactions and the fact that the human sciences are ordered in a hierarchy of emergent reorganizations are both elegantly demonstrated by the observation that families of schizophrenics function as though the members represent noninternalized, nonintegrated parts of the psyche of other members. From a family dynamic viewpoint schizophrenia is an illness of family structure in which the family operates as a single entity from which the members are no more able to separate themselves than an individual is able to dispense with parts of his body. The most important dynamic elements of family structure are collectively unconscious but enacted through projective and introjective mechanisms. The cohesion of such an immature or primitive group mind is essential in lieu of more autonomous mental integration and differentiation on the part of each member.

The function of the family as homeostatic unit is well illustrated in the case of Edward. When one member of Edward's family reached out, demonstrating vulnerability and need, the others enacted denial, rejection, and sadistic attack. And roles would alternate. When Edward appeared to be improving, other family members decompensated, and vice versa. While it is tempting to believe that Edward's transient improvements were "real," it is more likely that they involved a temporary relinquishment or projective identification of the psychotic part onto another family member.

The schizophrenic member, more than any of the others, introjectively represents and enacts repudiated and attributed (projected) elements of the identities of other members so that little or no room is left for experience and expression of his separate autonomous self. He is an indispensable caretaking receptacle for the projections of other family members; someone who, as Searles (1965) has pointed out, keeps them from going crazy. His unreality serves the important function of protecting parents against confrontation with disturbing aspects of their own behavior, their marriage, and intrafamilial conflicts. Families of schizophrenics tend to be quietly totalitarian and controlling, suppressive of the autonomy and potential for separation of individual members. Subtle attacks are made on the perceptions and viewpoints of the patient, especially ones that happen to be in conflict with views of other family members. They are defined as bad, crazy, or destructive to others in the family, and the absence of validation and support for them is combined with equally subtle bribes or rewards for remaining disabled. In particular, such families leave no room for constructive expression of aggression from the schizophrenic member; possibly for this reason above all others, since aggression in its myriad manifestations seems an essential aspect of differentiation, adaptation, and coping, no pathway remains for normal development. Two favorite aphorisms of my teacher Elvin Semrad are appropriate here: The first is that schizophrenia is the sacrifice of reality to preserve life, or for purposes of survival; the second is that schizophrenia is an alternative to suicide or homicide. In schizophrenic families the most basic polarities of thinking and feeling about reality and fantasy, right and wrong, tend to be inverted, and just as normal thinking and acting are subtly proscribed, courses of behavior and thinking that are fundamentally inconsistent with growth, autonomy, and constructive thinking are prescribed and defined as normal.

Once again I should like to correct any misapprehension that matters are one-sided and that the schizophrenic is simply a victim. In reciprocity, family members perform for the schizophrenic member essential caretaking and stabilizing functions he is unable to manage for himself, without articulating what they are doing, without indicating it is in any way out of the ordinary, and without expecting the affected member to learn to take on those functions for himself. Moreover, they help him maintain an archaic sense of self based on bizarre beliefs about himself and the world, beliefs that would be untenable were he provided with more objective feedback. Archaic narcissistic splits abound in these families. In one sense the schizophrenic is clearly devalued and victimized; even objective studies of families, for example, one recently completed by Beiser (1992), demonstrate that relatives of schizophrenics use more devaluing terms to describe them than do relatives of persons with, for example, physical illnesses. However, from a different perspective, the schizophrenic is infantilized and exempted from having to grow up and be an independent adult, responsible for his own thoughts, feelings, and behavior and their risks and consequences. His permitted and even enforced state of disability is masked in the family not only by a shared denial of what is happening but often by idealistic, even grandiose, beliefs about him. From that perspective, he is a kind of omnipotent master or king. In other words, schizophrenic megalomania is an object related adaptation to parental projections and to a family role and not simply a consequence of withdrawal of object cathexes to the ego, as Freud postulated, or a phase of archaic narcissism, as Kohut might maintain. It is because the schizophrenic and his family fill such vital functions for one another that schizophrenics have such difficulty separating from their families and that the illness has its florid onset at the time of life such separation is culturally mandated.

Illustrations

Some of these themes are illustrated in the cases of Emily and Rachel. Emily's mother unconsciously looked upon her as worthless, able to subsist on nothing, and incapable of bearing her own feelings and functioning autonomously. She had little regard for Emily's capacities or her real needs, a fact she managed to conceal from herself with conscious beliefs about her daughter's exceptional abilities, and she did not seem to hear or take Emily seriously when she finally began to try to tell her about herself. Of course, I do not mean to imply that mother was grossly uncaring; she arranged for Emily's hospitalization, made frequent trips to participate in the treatment program, and seemed willing to support the program unconditionally. However, she seemed to expect little of Emily and to be content to infantilize her indefinitely. She even claimed to "experience" all the physical and emotional pain of Emily's self-destructive behavior, which Emily herself did not seem to feel, and the disruption of her own life by these concerns was quite apparent. At the same time as she clearly devalued Emily's autonomy and capabilities, mother rather openly entertained a grandiose image of her as one who was great, so competent that she did not really need to learn anything, and certainly capable of being the best at whatever she undertook if and when she ever tried. Emily's dreams, in turn, symbolized mother as queen and herself as princess, or mother as God and herself as Messiah. It was an important event in Emily's treatment when she was able to confront her mother in a more mature manner on some important issues and hear mother respond to her uncharacteristic self-assertion with accusations that she was crazy and incompetent.

In Rachel's family marital stability appeared to depend on an unstated understanding that each parent would have an area of utter psychic domination, one in which the other's will seemed not to exist. Mother seemingly owned the bedroom and her workplace, and father the family. In short, this was a family structure predicated on single-mindedness. As the youngest daughter, Rachel seemed to be assigned the family function of acting as a grandiose/devalued (superstar/crazy) symbiotic object for father, a substitute for his narcissistic deficits as well as a substitute for his wife as marital partner, that is, for his wife's deficits. In this way Rachel stabilized the marriage, her father's precarious grasp on normalcy, and her mother's career outside the home. It is noteworthy that during Rachel's period of health and autonomy her sister Nina lived at home and began to develop symptoms much like Rachel's; perhaps she was becoming a substitute. When Rachel regressed again, Nina was then able to move out of the parental home and do better. The relevant family dynamic appeared to be father's unconscious insistence that Rachel remain overtly disabled and mindless, a kind of clone of himself, at the same time that he covertly supported her regal and grandiose thinking. Rachel's sycophantic behavior was designed to further the grandiose fantasies of her father and maintain his omnipotent supremacy in the family.

Father allowed Rachel absolutely no breathing space as a human being with thoughts and feelings of her own. He was quite content with her and claimed to understand her perfectly well so long as she remained psychotic and disabled, but when she made efforts to have a mind of her own in the course of treatment and to differ with him, he had no compunctions about calling her crazy and incompetent. Because she was dependent on father's assessment of her and the world, Rachel, in response, would obediently obliterate her shaky sane sense of self and became "crazier" once again in order to regain father's approval and stamp of normalcy. Father seemed to have no real expectation that she would grow up, and he took care of all her needs in lavish fashion and without question, so long as she remained his unquestioning disciple. Reciprocally, father's life was centered around the idea that he was the coach of this great athlete (Rachel was in fact a track and field star prior to her illness) and that together they constituted a world championship tandem. In family meetings father successfully fended off efforts to engage him in recognition of his problems by calling the rest of us crazy.

Elizabeth Swados (1991) has written a gripping biography of her family, centered around the chronic schizophrenia of her older brother Lincoln, which illustrates much of what I have described, especially the central and remarkable role of shared denial. Its unique illustrative value derives from the fact that Swados is remarkably articulate while clearly still caught up in the pathological family dynamics. She describes her brother as bizarre, erratic, and disorganized from as early as she can recall. While it is evident that at the level of fact everyone in the family was aware of Lincoln's disturbance, at the level of meaning they refused to label it for what it was. Instead, they found ways to call the remarkable aspects of his behavior wonderful, gifted, and creative, rather than psychotic. Though he was never employed and spent most of his adult life in mental hospitals or as a street person, Swados entitles the section of the book devoted to him "The Cartoonist." It follows from the inability of the family to acknowledge the serious nature of Lincoln's behavior that they were unable to hold him accountable or responsible for it. Members made remarkable excuses or rationalizations for him, engaged in pathological self-blaming in response to his actions and predicaments, and with varying degrees of anger blamed outsiders (for example, his schools and his doctors) and their presumed failure to understand him. Swados summarizes the report of the private school that could not contain him and suggested institutionalization:

> He had a terrible problem with authority. He fought with and struck some of his teachers. He drew obscenities on the walls. He recited nonsense poems, interrupting other students and causing chaos in the classroom. He often came to class dressed in costume and wouldn't talk in his normal voice.... He sodomized several boys in the locker room. He ran naked through chapel.... He stole indiscriminately.

Even though she had observed Lincoln doing similar things at home on numerous occasions, Swados concludes, ingenuously, "I have no idea if any of these stories were true or merely frightened exaggerations" (p. 17).

The family not only rescued Lincoln from his innumerable predicaments, but they used their considerable wealth and influence to bribe, coerce, and threaten the world to conform to his thinking and to do likewise, in the process fueling his own grandiose and rageful sense of power and control. By the time of his college years their efforts to get society to conform itself to his idiosyncrasies and provide him with special treatment began to fail, but even after Lincoln was chronically hospitalized, an interval punctuated by periods of discharge in which his destructiveness escalated and his condition progressively deteriorated (until he finally crippled himself by jumping in front of a subway and then became a street person), the family continued to pretend nothing was wrong. The parents went so far as to lie chronically to Elizabeth about his whereabouts: "I was never really told how sick my brother was, so I continued to believe that his actions were rational and his word was law.... I felt it [his irrational thinking] had to be founded on some deep truth" (p. 44). Regarding his hospitalizations and the unsuccessful efforts to treat him, which utilized medication but are not otherwise elaborated, Swados states:

> Since the information on Lincoln's illness was so contradictory and convoluted with psychiatric terms that could only inflame the terror of a parent, the easiest way to understand his schizophrenia was to believe it didn't exist.... My true beliefs centered around my esteem for my brother's gifts. He was a difficult genius who would prove himself to his opponents. (p. 30)

In a remarkable convolution of reality she concludes: "I've come to be very proud of my brother's courage and tenacity. I find myself angry at the medical profession for their lack of solutions for his state of being" (p. 53).

While the family pattern appears to fit Lidz' "skew," it is not clear from Swados's description what family elements were projected into Lincoln. He did attempt to enact a kind of incestuous control over his sister, which might have had parallels in his relationship with his mother, which seems to have been characterized by a kind of infantilizing closeness from which father was excluded. In fact, mother committed suicide some time after Lincoln died. The shared family infantilization of Lincoln and conspiracy to exonerate him from personal responsibility, which involved introjection into themselves and projection onto society of destructive and devaluing attitudes and projection onto him of grandiosity, gave him unlimited sanction to enact his pathological grandiosity and rage.

The Problem of Reconstruction and Elaboration of the Epigenetic Family System Model

Personal observation in the course of family therapy, corroborated in some instances by the verbal reports of family members, suggests that the pathological interpersonal patterns I have described are both rigidly fixed and historically chronic, not, as some have suggested, recent effects of the illness itself on family members. This strongly suggests both the pathogenic role of the family structure, and its contemporary function as the glue or chronicity factor responsible for maintaining the pathology of the patient.

From an adaptive, hierarchical systems point of view we may ask ourselves what new elements are added to the individual psychology of schizophrenia at the level of family organization? The passive protosymbiotic personality of the schizophrenic is symbiotically complemented by the activity and adaptation of his family. Missing elements of self-care are supplied by infantilization rather than by extraordinary devotion which might be required to assist the vulnerable child to develop such capacities himself. An identity sense, archaic and narcissistic, is supplied the disintegrated individual through grandiose and devalued projections. Aversion to human relatedness is compensated for by the enactments of family members, using projection and introjection. Absent self-control in relation to emotion and action is supplied by autocratic suppression. And the family supplies the missing reality sense in the form of denial and inversion of reality. We might go so far as to say that in the course of its homeostatic efforts the family system is the symbiotic preserver of its apparently normal members and of the designated problematic member's schizophrenia as well.

If we are cognizant of the problems of prediction and reconstruction inherent in the transformational nature of hierarchical systems, we can but speculate about the degree of correspondence between the cognitive, affective, and relationship difficulties of the adult schizophrenic and his family and those of the infant and small child and his family. So I shall conclude the chapter with a very provisional elaboration of the model for development of schizophrenia in the context of a disturbed family, a model that I outlined in Chapter 7. There we speculated about some of the constitutional vulnerabilities to schizophrenia that might emerge in the context of inadequate or pathogenic parenting: difficulties with psychological integration and differentiation and a related aversion to people; difficulties managing external (sensory-perceptive) and internal (appetitive-emotional) stimulation, in particular, difficulty mentally representing and controlling rage and converting it to adaptive interpersonal aggressiveness; and aversion to the mental work of bearing and regulating emotion-laden thoughts. I hypothesized that preschizophrenic vulnerability must develop when a constitutionally compromised infant is unable to actively enter into a growth-promoting dyadic symbiosis. In the absence of attentive, caring parenting from unusually devoted persons, essential capacities to develop the internal representations and structures that comprise mind, and related capacities for self-care, regulation, and self-esteem, fail to develop. As a result the child is unable to extend the undifferentiated loving ambience that should characterize its earliest relationship into a capacity to care about himself and to perceive and to love others who might care about him. Without the assistance of such a relationship and such capacities constitutional incapacities cannot be repaired or ameliorated; instead they exfoliate or "develop" along characteristic pathological pathways.

The infant with preschizophrenic vulnerabilities such as I have outlined is doubtless a remarkably demanding and stressful burden to parents, requiring qualitatively and quantitatively unusual forms of intervention and support from its primary caregiver in order to maintain homeostasis and promote reasonably satisfactory growth. Such an infant will tax its mother's capacities to lovingly contain its mental processes; to mirror them in a useful way, such as Bion has described; to assist in their regulation; and to master her own anger, frustration, disappointment and discouragement in the process. Even the most mature of mothers might be sorely provoked to respond with inconstancy and frustration, to reject the infant's real needs, and to attribute to the infant the responsibility for her ill-feeling. In the process of such an infant-induced maternal regression mother might even come to depend on her disabled infant as a symbiotic receptacle to stabilize her at a more primitive level of mental functioning.

For a mother such as Winnicott (1960a) describes—whose pathological self-preoccupation limits her capacity to respond to the infant's true self, predisposes her to coercively and exploitatively substitute gestures, meanings, and an agenda of her own, and then leads her to infantilize her child in order to hold on to the relationship for her own purposes—it is easy to envision a possible course for the constitutional vulnerabilities: rage enhanced and turning on the psychosomatic precursors of a sense of self; adoption in its stead of meanings for its sensations, perceptions, and thought-and-feeling anlage that are compatible with those of its parents but at odds with consensual social reality; a turning away from specific attachments and relationships with others; advantage taken of the "disability compensation" unconsciously offered by the parents and the choosing, instead, of a state of mental nirvana and adaptive passivity, possibly compensated for with grandiose fantasies. Greenspan (1989a, pp. 608–610) has recently speculated that one precursor of thought disorder may be the combination of infantile constitutional difficulties processing sensation and affect with an environment that provides distorted meanings.

Of course, this earliest sequence of events must remain a subject for speculation until neuroscience has more unequivocally established the nature of the organic vulnerability and it becomes possible to identify vulnerable infants by such things as biological markers (for example, specific ERP alterations or eye movement disorders) and to study them intensively in their earliest interactions with parents whose personalities run the gamut of normalcy and psychopathology and monitor them as they grow into normal or schizophrenic adults.

Subsequent to the activation of characterological vulnerability in a constitutionally predisposed infant are two related processes: failure to learn ordinary self-care and social skills, and developmental deviation (not simply arrest) in response to pathologial family dynamics and the characterological limitations on which they impinge. The family tends not only to define the resulting psychological primitiveness as normal and desirable, and to reward it with compensatory infantilization, but also to require of the individual its perpetuation in exchange for psychological survival as a family member. Continued hostile suppression by the family of efforts to express and accurately label thoughts, feelings, and perceptions may come to be internalized as a primitive form of self-control and self-regulation, a self-destructive structuring that poses considerable problems during later efforts at psychotherapy. In other words, the vulnerable individual forms a very passive, undifferentiated, protosymbiotic relationship with other family members.

This psychological primitiveness is seldom defined as dysfunctional and pathological until, under the social necessity of trying to grow up, the individual makes efforts to leave home and undertake advanced education, self-supporting work, intimate relationships, and adult responsibilities. School systems typically go to great compensatory and remedial lengths with disturbed children unless they are grossly antisocial (and preschizophrenic children are usually not), and in so doing they may unwittingly be doing more to bolster pathological symbiotic patterns and familial denial than to help the disturbed child. But however the preschizophrenic may be able to "pass" as normal during his preadult years, his strangeness and ineptitude are usually incompatible with the accomplishment of late adolescent and young adult developmental tasks, which require both physical and psychological separation from home as well as the capacity to function in less forgiving social systems such as are found in the workplace or college. In attempting to separate from the family the adolescent at once loses his protective infantilizing cushion, and comes under the scrutiny and expectations of more objective outsiders who may perceive his ways of thinking and acting, which were so adaptive in the home, as dysfunctional and bizarre. I call this process, this loss of the pathological symbiotic patterns that have served to conceal the manifest pathology, adaptive disequillibration.

It is likely that adaptive disequilibration is compounded by regression, which I view as a secondary rather than a primary aspect of the eruption of manifest schizophrenia. Heretofore, the structure and function of the individual were compatible with some sort of existence, however compromised, within the microcosm of the family. Now society defines continuation of such a lifestyle abnormal; since psychological primitiveness makes the individual incapable of survival in the larger world, he faces an intolerable dilemma (Lidz, 1973).

I closed the discussion of genetic findings in Chapter 3 by remarking that, striking as the statistical evidence for an inherited predisposition to schizophrenia may be, relatively few of the many schizophrenics I have encountered have had schizophrenic or even psychotic relatives in the immediate branches of their family trees. I shall close this chapter on the family system with an analogous observation: When schizophrenic families are compared to the families of patients with other forms of primitive psychopathology, it is not clear that the family dynamics alone sufficiently differentiate the schizophrenics from the others. I have observed no convincing qualitative differences between the families of schizophrenics and those of patients with some of the more severe primitive personality disorders. It is certainly possible that there may be a difference in the degree or severity of suppression of autonomy and particularly of the expression of anger, but, in some instances of primitive personality organization I have treated, the pathogenic family configuration may even have been "worse" than in some instances of schizophrenia. And I have encountered some primitive personalities who are configured much like schizophrenics, with subtle but pervasive failures of reality testing, aversion to mental work, overriding tendencies to escape into fantasy, and autonomy-suppressing family backgrounds, but for some reason they are able to function productively, if not happily, in the world. Observations such as these return us to the hypothesis that the essential difference between the two conditions may be one of constitutional vulnerability.

Chapter 11

Society and Culture

T he modern conception and treatment of schizophrenia is the outgrowth of developments and trends over the course of the last three hundred or so years in France, England, and the United States. One of the most striking of these is the polarization and at times cyclical fluctuation between organic and humanistic conceptions. I shall utilize some of these historical events and trends as data in support of the hypothesis that the social–cultural definition and representation of schizophrenia and society's responses to persons designated as schizophrenic are far from objective. And I shall propose that the answer to the question of whether or not these responses are considered to be constructive and therapeutic depends upon whether one views them from the perspective of the development and autonomy of the individual schizophrenic (the psychological perspective) or from the vantage point of familial and societal stability. We shall see how the response of society and culture to schizophrenia might be viewed not so much as a reasoned response to it as a higher-level reflection, reorganization, and expression of and compensation for some of the very features of the illness that I describe at a family dynamic level in Chapter 10 and at an intrapsychic level in Chapter 9, and that, as I propose in Chapter 7, may have a constitutional basis.

The Social–Cultural Schism: A Historical Perspective

The historical schism in our view of schizophrenia embraces an organic-hereditary viewpoint, on the one hand, and a moral-psychoanalytic one, on the other. From an equally valid but much less flattering perspective, which focuses on what is missing in each viewpoint rather than on what is positive about it, Eisenberg (1986) refers to the contemporary version of the radical reductionist orientation of some neuroscientists as "mindless," and to psychoanalytic theories that deny the importance of an organic process as "brainless." Both views seem to have crystallized out of the chaotic, infernal, religious-penal view of insanity reflected in Hogarth's 1733 painting of the British madhouse Bethlehem (or, as it came to be known, Bedlam). The idea that aberrant behavior might reflect organic pathology of the brain was articulated in the 18th century by William Cullen and by James Gregory, who coined the term "nervous system." Early in the 19th century Benjamin Rush, the father of psychiatry in the United States, represented both organic and psychological viewpoints, apparently without integration: While he believed that insanity was the product of a circulatory defect, his therapeutic approach to patients involved attempting to understand and to work with their curious ideas and beliefs.

The so-called moral treatment movement, which represented the formal beginnings of the humanistic, psychological conception of insanity, was heralded by the work of Tuke in Victorian England and Pinel in France, also around the beginning of the 19th century. Pinel, working with male patients at the Bicêtre and with females at the Salpêtrière, classified mental illness into four types, one of which (dementia) was characterized by a thought disorder. He also appreciated the significant role of the passions (emotions). Treatment involved, among other things, establishment of a trusting relationship between caregivers and the afflicted individual, enhancement of his self-awareness through the use of behavior mirroring techniques, and appeals to his judgment which emphasized making him aware of the consequences of his behavior. Tuke, at the York Quaker Retreat, attempted to civilize patients and subdue their passions through work programs and a moralistic induction of guilt feelings.

By the mid-19th century Maudsley in England, Griesinger in Germany, and Morel in France had begun to articulate the organic viewpoint in their respective countries. Griesinger believed insanity was associated with cerebral anatomical pathology. B. A. Morel coined the term *dementia praecox* in 1856 to denote a condition of degeneracy related to morbid heredity. He appealed to the demented at an instinctual level, using techniques of fear induction and punishment.

The Twentieth Century: Kraepelin

During the 20th century both the organic (now neuroscientific) and the moral (now psychological) viewpoints have continued to flourish, but the element of oscillation or cyclical alternation between them seems more apparent. Kraepelin (1896/1919) and Alzheimer (1897) looked upon dementia praecox as an organic disease of the frontal lobes whose pathognomonic lesion had yet to be discovered, not unlike neurosyphilis. Kraepelin believed dementia praecox was characterized in all instances by a deteriorating course and an unfavorable outcome. Owing to the influence of Bleuler (1911), who believed that Kraepelin's syndrome was not monolithic and dementia was not always inevitable, dementia praecox was renamed the group of schizophrenias. The predominant organic approach, which had gradually brought the syndrome under the jurisdiction of physicians and the medical model, led to the employment of a variety of somatic treatments in the first half of the 20th century, including induction of focal sepsis; efforts to "shock" the brain back to a more normal state through malaria-induced fever or with electrical current, Metrazol (pentylenetetrazol), or insulin; and extirpation of the presumptive offending areas (prefrontal lobotomy). However, these treatments proved not only of limited value but also fraught with iatrogenic complications, and since no specific lesion or toxic agent was identified that could link them to an acceptable scientific rationale, the influence of the neuropathological school gradually waned.

Psychoanalysis

Meanwhile, in the early part of the 20th century Freud was expounding his revolutionary ideas about unconscious conflict. While he believed that schizophrenics were incapable of forming transferences and hence could not make use of his psychoanalytic method, at least three of the founding analysts—Jung, Abraham, and Brill—practiced in a mental hospital, the Burghölzli in Switzerland, and attempted to employ variations of his technique. Another handful of European analysts, including Ferenczi, LaForgue, Nunberg, Federn, Wilhelm Reich, Bychowski, Melanie Klein, and Garma, attempted to apply psychoanalysis to schizophrenia in the earlier part of the century. In the United States the moral treatment movement, which by then had a foothold in many mental hospitals, was gradually infused with a psychological and psychoanalytic element, first owing to the influence of such persons as Adolph Meyer at Johns Hopkins, with his concept of psychobiology, which resembles the hierarchical systems approach I have taken in this book, and subsequently owing to the work of Harry Stack Sullivan, who practiced at Sheppard and Enoch Pratt Hospital and taught at Chestnut Lodge in the decades between 1920 and 1950. Although Sullivan was an analyst, his ideas bear little resemblance to Freud's. Sullivan directly or indirectly influenced many of the analysts of the halcyon mid-20th century era of application of psychoanalysis to schizophrenia, including Frieda Fromm-Reichmann, Robert Knight, Elvin Semrad, Alfred Stanton, Otto Will and contemporaries such as Ping Nie Pao and Harold Searles, to name but a few. The conscription of many analysts into military psychiatry during World War II, where they were called upon to devise methods of treatment of patients with schizophrenia, a population they might otherwise never have encountered in their traditional office practices, led to a postwar fascination with schizophrenia by psychoanalysis and general psychiatry mirrored in such popular books as Robert Lindner's (1955) *The Fifty Minute Hour*, and Joanne Greenberg's pseudonymous account (see Green, 1964) of her treatment at Chestnut Lodge by Frieda Fromm-Reichmann, *I Never Promised You a Rose Garden*, as well as movies like *Spellbound* (1945). By this time the organic approach had reached a nadir, and it was widely held that schizophrenia is a psychological process, related to pathogenic child-rearing practices and entirely amenable to psychoanalytic intervention.

However, the traditional location of psychoanalytic teaching in institutes apart from universities and medical schools and of psychoanalytic practice in private office settings rather than in mental hospitals, where schizophrenics abound, impeded its potential integration with neuroscience and with the hospital treatment of schizophrenia. Nor were those analysts who worked intensively with schizophrenics especially effective in conceptualizing the theories underlying their activity and in writing about the results of their work so that such information might come to the thoughtful attention of the general scientific community beyond their circle of pupils. Their influence has tended to be cultlike, transmitted more by personal apprenticeship than by scientifically acceptable written words.

The Drug Culture

Once again, extremist thinking and related inflated expectations led to equally extreme disappointment. Although some gifted analysts seemed able to engage and work with schizophrenics in a way that resembled, at least in some respects, the psychoanalytic therapy of milder conditions, the initial optimism that a cure had been found was frequently not borne out by subsequent recovery. Meanwhile, the introduction of chlorpromazine (Thorazine) in the mid-1950s heralded the development of a variety of neuroleptic medications, of which clozapine is the most recent, that appear to ameliorate at least some psychotic symptomatology and offer the prospect of symptom remission, normalization of regressive behavior and patient resocialization. These drugs were greeted, as the "antibiotics" of schizophrenia, with the same extremism accorded therapies of the past, though once again, their effects, like those of the somatic therapies earlier in the century, have not as yet been convincingly correlated with a specific neurological abnormality, and the limitations of their efficacy have become increasingly apparent.

It is worth noting that serious investigation and use of antipsychotic medication followed the post–World War II fascination with psychosis induced by drugs such as mescaline and LSD and that these, in turn, were important elements in the culture of the "beat" generation of the 1960s, which also employed various prescription medications such as Dexedrine (uppers) and sleeping pills (downers) to alter mood and thought and even to pursue a contemporary religious version of salvation. With this underlying cultural sanction, scientific materialism has once again gained ascendency, with its view that thinking and feeling, which are the products of mind, are nothing more than the epiphenomenal manifestations of brain function.

When mentation is distressing or deviant from the norm, such as is the case in schizophrenia, it is now conceived of as a kind of toxic delirium lacking intrinsic meaningfulness, and medication is prescribed to control symptoms and bizarre behavior and to effect rapid replacement of the painful or unusual mental state with a more "normal" state of tranquillity, pleasure, or euthymia. Such social devaluation of the autonomous mind and the technological manipulation and control of the brain held accountable may be a realization of the fearful, dehumanizing, culturally regressive enterprise George Orwell (*Nineteen Eighty Four*) and Anthony Burgess (*Clockwork Orange*) envisioned. The contemporary conception and treatment of mental illness is based on the belief that distress is abnormal and ought to be rapidly and effortlessly eliminated. In response to this demand an entirely new subspecialty of psychiatry has emerged—psychopharmacology—whose task it is to find the right drug(s) to match the patient's complaints. This most recent organic swing of the pendulum has been further enhanced by the proliferation of studies of schizophrenia reporting organic abnormalities and a genetic substrate (Chapter 6).

The Medical Model

Meanwhile, psychoanalysis—the last outpost of a humanistic approach to schizophrenia—not only has been unreceptive to the new genetic and neurobiological findings and their potential theoretical significance, but in many instances has actually refused to acknowledge their validity. In fact, the classical psychoanalytic view of schizophrenia as being "all in the mind" led, not infrequently during the early years of the psychopharmacology era, to the unfortunate practice of withholding medication from patients who were refractory to psychological intervention.

The contemporary result of the disparate forces I have summarized is a broad social and psychiatric consensus that psychoanalytic hypotheses of schizophrenia represent archaic science. Schizophrenia is now generally believed to be an organic disease, like diabetes or cancer, whose mental and interpersonal manifestations are alien or external to the self, a kind of cancer on the personality, whose "victims" and their families are viewed as suffering from them but as having no psychological or interpersonal responsibility for them. Such a conception places schizophrenia squarely within the purview of medical psychiatry. The psychotherapy that is sometimes included within the scope of this organic medical model is not analytic; the disease process is not conceived of as being integrated with or in any way related to the psychology of the person and is therefore not the focus of therapy. Therapy is directed in the form of so-called support and education toward the presumably normal part of the victim, and is designed to assist patient and family to "manage" the illness, that is, control and cope with its effects. In fact, as I describe in Chapter 18, this approach is really somatic therapy in disguise because it is based on the so-called stress-diathesis model which views stress as a physical force.

Some of the contemporary change in our perception and treatment of the mentally ill results from a curious alliance between social liberals, neuroscientific psychiatrists, and insurance companies. It is an outgrowth of the crusade to extend the civil liberties of minorities, a crusade generated by the same 'sixties generation that legitimated extensive use of drugs to alter mental state and mood. The asylum movement has been traditionally associated with elements of incarceration of the mentally ill and sequestration of them away from a general community of others who tend not to want to come into contact with and see schizophrenics or to entertain the thoughts and feelings such contact evokes. It began with places like Bedlam in the 1700s and evolved in such diverse pathways as the back wards of state hospital systems, on the one hand, and enlightened moral treatment communities employing psychoanalytic and sophisticated rehabilitative measures on the other. The Community Mental Health Center Act of 1963 was an outgrowth of the increasing social awareness of the limited and equivocal evidence supporting the value of prolonged hospitalization and psychotherapy, the deprivation of patients' civil rights, and, in some instances, the lack of decent care associated with the widespread use of asylums. The act was the result of social commitment to the idea that even persons whose ideas and actions are socially deviant ought to be free to "do their thing." As payment for mental health care has gradually shifted to third party insurance companies, and as etiologic thinking has shifted from complex issues of personality change to simpler ones of mood and thought alteration via drug administration, there has been a popular movement away from prolonged, labor- and cost-intensive forms of treatment, including long hospital stays and analytically oriented psychotherapies, toward briefer, outpatient, symptomatic, and rehabilitative modalities.

Despite its humane and civil libertarian origins, the new medical-psychiatric treatment philosophy has significant qualitative similarities to society's familiar tendency to use banishment to the asylum to avoid contact with the schizophrenic and what he might be thinking and feeling. According to the medical-psychiatric model it is not necessary to get to know the person of the schizophrenic beyond what is required to make a diagnosis, prescribe suitable medication, and direct him into programs for symptomatic relief and social rehabilitation. Anything more is looked upon as, at best, financially wasteful and consuming of time and attention that might better be devoted to helping larger numbers of patients, and as, at worst, an attempt to ascribe significance to schizophrenic thinking, an attempt that is scientifically unsound, potentially regressive to the patient, and unnecessarily disruptive to family and hospital staff.

The Social–Cultural Response to Schizophrenia: Objectification, Understanding, and Treatment or Blind Enactment?

It may appear that I have simply been presenting a brief, selective, and perhaps biased historical review of the understanding and treatment of schizophrenia in Western culture. But my purpose is to present data in support of a social–cultural hypothesis about the nature of schizophrenia. Social–cultural attitudes represent not so much objective commentaries on an illness—or, to be more specific, objectification of the disturbed thinking of the schizophrenic and the pathological dynamics of his family—as hierarchical reorganizations, at a higher level, of the very thinking and acting that characterize the organic and psychological process of the individual schizophrenic and the dynamics of his family. Far from the sophisticated scientific theoretical and treatment position it is purported to be, much of our belief system about the etiology and treatment of schizophrenia is little more than a naive reflection of and support for such pathological processes.

Recall, to begin with, that historically one of the most impressive aspects of schizophrenia is its fragmentary, extremist, *pars pro toto* nature—a kaleidescopic shifting such that seeing of one part is accompanied by scotomata regarding others. Nor is the schizophrenic of today ordinarily perceived and treated as a whole person, mind and brain, functioning continuously within a family unit over the course of time; instead, he is viewed as a collection of symptoms to be normalized, symptoms that are unconnected to his otherwise presumably normal personality and equally normal family and originate in a malfunctioning portion of his brain. Our very failure to grasp the possibility of an integrated, pluralistic approach that includes organic, psychological, interpersonal, familial, and sociocultural levels appears to mirror the unintegrated, fragmented character of the schizophrenic mind, as well as a similar quality within his family. Scientific materialism, with its reductionistic belief that the richness and complexity of the schizophrenic mind is merely an epiphenomenon, reducible to elementary neural parts, appears to be a reflection both of the schizophrenic's difficulty with abstraction and symbolization and of his tendency to live in a concrete and fragmented mental reality.

Cultural attitudes also reflect the undifferentiation and primitive projection and enactment, resulting in a basic unconnectedness with important aspects of self, which are aspects of the failure of integration both in the schizophrenic and his family. Through his hallucinations and delusions the schizophrenic reflects the belief that he is the victim of persecutory forces in the outside world or within himself; his family similarly denies problems and projects attitudes and responsibility. In the broader culture such ideas are expressed in the commonly held belief that the schizophrenic is the victim of "external" forces (the organic illness) that afflict him and over which he has no responsibility or control.

A consequence of viewing the mental manifestations of schizophrenia as expressions of an organic disease entity separate from the personality of the sufferer, manifestations that are meaningless and incomprehensible even to the schizophrenic himself, is the direction of so-called treatment measures to expunge these with "tranquilizing" drugs and to persuade the patient to conceal his thinking, symptoms, and limitations from others and try to function as if he were normal. In fact, a currently popular belief is that intensive therapy that elicits emotional expression, interpersonal engagement, and conflict is not only inadvisable but may actually be noxious, regressive, and disruptive to schizophrenics and their families. But the preferred "treatment" of today mirrors and enhances the schizophrenic's basic alienation from others, and, regardless of the impression conveyed by his compliance, lends reality and substance to whatever mistrustful paranoid beliefs he may have that the world is a dangerous place and that others are basically inimical to his well-being.

The consequence of such social efforts at "treatment" is to invalidate and suppress the inchoate observations, assertions, protests, and conflicts within the individual schizophrenic mind—rather than attend to them, work to comprehend their significance, and help the patient to learn to express them in more constructive ways—and to buttress pathogenic family beliefs. In the guise of treatment such measures only abet the patient's already overwhelming tendency toward mental self-destruction.

It is interesting that treatment based on some of these principles is naively believed to be "supportive," but what these sociocultural attitudes reflect and support is the schizophrenic's aversion to others, aversion to his own mental life, failure of integration, and his turning of diffuse aggression upon undesirable elements of the self and against projectively defined external forces in a primitive effort at self-control. Of course, history is replete with evidence that "normal" people have always shunned or been averse to contact with schizophrenic persons and are overwhelmed by the thoughts and feelings (probably helplessness, despair, and rage) that close contact with such disturbed and destructive people characteristically evokes. Even those of us who have chosen to work in mental hospitals are well aware of these forces in ourselves; I experience them every time I walk onto a mental hospital ward! In this sense we all think like schizophrenics. The case of Celia (Chapter 21) is a particularly vivid illustration of this problem. Her repudiation of her disturbed thinking and feeling, an attitude modeled after family attitudes, and her capacity to act "normal," which she was able to do rather convincingly for periods of time, turned out to constitute perhaps the most malignant aspect of her psychosis.

The schizophrenic has been perceived throughout history in two related but extreme ways, sometimes concurrently. The first of these perceptions (accompanied by devaluation, condescension, and attempts to control) is of an alien, frightening, subhuman, and degenerate being. In the past the schizophrenic was punished and incarcerated, but in today's more subtle guise this response takes the form of managing, manipulating, directing, tranquilizing, and rehabilitating him as though he were a member of some lesser species for whom ordinary human expectations and responsibilities are irretrievably for-closed. The second perception is of the schizophrenic as a savant, an extra-ordinarily creative person, gifted with special access to parts of the mind inaccessible to more mundane beings. In this belief system schizophrenics are the clairvoyant individuals who see through the sham of our sick, conformist society.* Both of these perceptions reflect the schizophrenic's lack of integra-tion and the archaic narcissism (that is, the coexistent grandiosity and deval-uation) as well as the related combination of suppressive totalitarian control and infantile pampering that characterizes his family's treatment of him.

The radical social critique of the diagnosis of schizophrenia that looks upon it as a weapon of totalitarian social control used to suppress and expunge individuality and constructive protest and to induce conformity—and that sometimes goes so far as to assert that the schizophrenic is a victim of a sick society—may represent a displaced acknowledgment of the totalitarianism or suppression of autonomy within the nuclear family of the schizophrenic (de-scribed in Chapter 10) that is overtly denied both by families and by society at large.

In fact, powerful sociocultural forces of denial appear to mirror similar processes within the family. While it may appear that society is acutely aware of the problem of schizophrenia and the suffering of the family, much of our current treatment seems predicated on efforts to deny the underlying serious-ness of the psychological dilemmas faced by the schizophrenic and his family. In Chapter 9 we examined the schizophrenic's aversion to facing his own mind, and in Chapter 10 the ways family members avoid facing and acknowl-edging their problems and conflicts. The contemporary treatment culture reflects the belief that the schizophrenic, far from being a person who is disturbed in a meaningful way in response to forces and conflicts within his family, is an otherwise normal personality with an organic problem, an un-fortunate person who is part of a family that is also relatively normal, except for its response to the stress of his illness.

Denial also seems to function at a broader social level when it comes to facing the need for adequate treatment facilities and expenditures. Kirk and Thierren (1975), Bassuk and Gerson (1978), Scull (1989), and Andreasen (1991) comment that the culture of deinstitutionalization, symptomatic treat-ment, and rapid return of patients to the community has merely shifted the problem of schizophrenia from one segment of society (medicine) to others (social welfare organizations, the law). Andreasen (1991) states that "various sectors that formerly assumed responsibility for the economic and medical costs of schizophrenia are attempting to shift them elsewhere, ... because schizophrenia is so costly, no one [it seems] wants to bear its burden" (p. 475). Patients are treated symptomatically by brief hospitalization and medication and are then returned to the community—where they may look good so long

*The historical origins of such an idea include attribution of divine inspiration and sacred presence to schizophrenics: other-worldliness, visions, and delusional prophecies.

as one does not relate to them too closely or follow their subsequent course, which seems to involve recurrent episodes, chronicity, and deterioration, at least for the first 15 or so years (Chapter 1). The patient may be shunted from one agency to another within the medical subculture, and from medicine to other areas of society, including social welfare agencies, the school system, and the legal system. This is certainly a form of social denial, as pernicious in its own way as was the old segregation of schizophrenics in asylums outside cities so that society could avoid being reminded of their existence. As a result society is confronted with more problems: homeless street people in cities, many self-medicated with drugs both licit and illicit; violent crimes committed by psychotic persons; and the less obvious consequences of the denial, such as unemployment, child and spouse abuse, and the like. According to a joint 1990 report by the Public Citizen Health Research Group, led by E. F. Torrey, and the National Alliance for the Mentally Ill, four times as many schizophrenics now reside in jails and on the streets as in mental hospitals. Another way to look at it is that the fundamental social issue impeding treatment of the severely mentally ill may not be funding and construction of effective programs so much as failure to recognize the continuing reality and seriousness of the problems themselves.

Conclusion: The Hierarchical Systems of Schizophrenia

At the dyadic level of the systems hierarchy, we concluded, the primary parental caretaker might either confront and ameliorate her infant's constitutionally determined tendency to elaborate vulnerabilities into schizophrenic character traits and teach him more mature ways of coping, or she might unconsciously stimulate the efflorescence of these traits and help to create a state which is pathologically symbiotic for her and vegetative or parasitic for her child in which they are simultaneously exploited and compensated for. At the next higher family level of organization we reviewed the dynamics of the schizophrenic's adaptation to particular pathological elements in his family, and the family's active, reciprocal symbiotic exploitation of and compensation for his constitutional weaknesses. Switching the magnification of our viewing instrument once again, we apprehend the sociocultural level of the human systems hierarchy. In describing society Rousseau (1762) likened it to the human body, prone to illness, aging, and death. From this vantage point we are less aware of the unique needs of the individual schizophrenic and more aware of him as a disruptive element in a family system. Intact family structure is the single most essential element of the social fabric. From a social Darwinist perspective society must maintain homeostasis in the face of entropic forces. That is, if a choice must be made, the survival of the family unit must take precedence over the autonomy of its individual members, especially if that autonomy is experienced as potentially disruptive, as Rousseau's aphorism, "A cancer on the body politic" suggests.

Therefore, it is hardly surprising that throughout history societies have tended to be more dictatorial and autocratic than supportive of individual freedom of expression. Because the recognition and validation of certain elements of genuine thought and feeling within the schizophrenic and his disturbed family have the potential to disrupt family structure should they come to light, and hence pose threats to the stability of society, society appears to enact and support the totalitarian forces within the family designed to suppress and deny them.

Viewed in this light it is not difficult to understand the myths of the happy marriage and the happy family that pervade middle-class American culture. People unfailingly tend to be surprised, even shocked, when evidence of marital and familial unhappiness surfaces among friends and acquaintances. Until recently, the idea that a marriage might be bad enough to justify divorce was generally unacceptable, and the existence and prevalence of physical child abuse and incest were generally denied. The need to deny the more subtle forms of child abuse, which those who work with primitive personalities and schizophrenics encounter with regularity, is cut from the same cloth.

Society devotes much concern and effort to finding "care" for the disabled schizophrenic, but avoids contact with him insofar as possible; looks at him in bits and pieces, sees him as the victim of mysterious external forces; denies the inherent validity of his mind and encourages him to do likewise; and at times denies his very psychological existence as a human being. The broader problem may be the existence of inherent conflict between the individual psychological level, at which development, autonomy and self-actualization are valued, and the sociocultural level, at which society must preserve the integrity of its critical component, the nuclear family, in the face of potentially rending conflicts among its individual members. The fact that the larger culture perpetuates and supports the individual and familial pathology of schizophrenia by enacting its elements in the guise of objectivity and treatment and by supporting the family's response to the disturbed member, be it in the era of the asylum or the era of deinstitutionalization and civil rights, may constitute the ultimate truth of the radical social critique of the schizophrenia concept. Nonetheless, it is important to remember that the radical social critique is inherently biased insofar as it is reached from the perspective of the individual psychological system, not from that of the social system. The moral and ethical issues involved in making the myriad decisions that stem from these seemingly antithetical perspectives appear formidable and daunting. We turn next to some of them in the section on treatment.

Part IV

The Treatment of Schizophrenia

Chapter 12

Evaluation and Treatment Planning from a Systems Perspective

T he clinician who employs a humanistically oriented systems view of schizophrenia does not reject the mind of the schizophrenic as a meaningless epiphenomenon and attribute meaningfulness exclusively to the organic level but begins with efforts to comprehend it as a meaningfully disordered system functioning in parallel with other systems ranging from the organic to the sociocultural. From this starting point the clinician views the myriad problems of schizophrenia from a variety of systems levels and perspectives that are presumed to be equally valid and meaningful. Such an approach lends a powerful sense of orderliness and direction to the evaluation of a patient and to the initial planning of treatment, as well as to its subsequent review.

The Flowchart

The accompanying flowchart (Figure 2) illustrates some of the more important branches of the decision-making tree. Application of the hierarchical systems model creates a three-dimensional decision-making process, which is difficult to diagram on a two-dimensional chart. Not only is there a linear course or progression from one issue to the next, as the flowchart suggests, but at each point there is a depth of levels or dimensions from which the particular point on the map may be viewed. Our efforts to maintain or equilibrate treatment around the person may, from a humanistic psychological viewpoint, necessitate that we move "higher" (family, social structure) or "lower" (organic) in

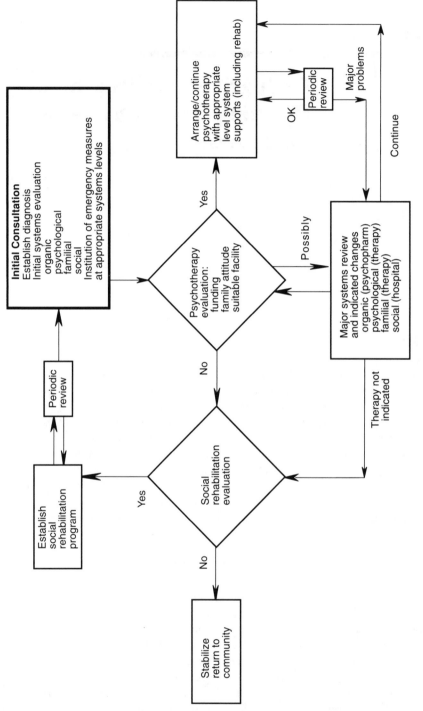

FIGURE 2. Planning treatment.

the systems hierarchy for assistance. In each of the five cases in this book many such decision points were encountered, where it was necessary to decide whether, for example, to introduce or to discontinue medication, to employ family therapy or alter its focus, or to hospitalize the patient or to alter the limits, programs, and interactional dynamics within the hospital in order to assist a flagging psyche to maintain a minimal constructive adaptation to the world and a productive therapeutic relationship with its primary representative, the therapist. In some instances the therapist will find it impossible to establish a meaningful psychological relationship with a schizophrenic, even after appropriate intervention at higher or lower levels of the systems hierarchy, and it may become necessary to abandon a psychological interpersonal treatment focus and make the sociocultural and/or organismic levels the primary focus of the therapeutic endeavor, a decision leading to such things as a program of rehabilitation or even simple stabilization using medication and social support, at the highest possible level of thinking and adaptive functioning.

To return to the flow of the decision-making process, it is first necessary to establish the diagnosis of schizophrenia, taking especial care to rule out manic–depressive psychosis and organic brain syndrome. It is less essential to differentiate schizophrenia from severe primitive personality disorder in the early stage of planning, as the initial treatment intervention in both instances is more or less similar. Appropriate neurological examination and neuropsychological testing should be performed at this time. As the initial evaluation is often conducted under emergency circumstances, following a chaotic and destructive failure of social adjustment and performance, it is often necessary to administer medication and/or arrange for hospitalization. (Considerations with regard to employment of these measures within the psychological frame of reference suggested for the initial evaluation, rather than as primary treatment modalities, are elaborated in the chapters to come.)

In brief, at this initial stage, unless it is abundantly clear that there is no realistic possibility of psychotherapy, the goal of medication is to facilitate a bare modicum of functioning and human relatedness, not to alleviate symptomatic distress and normalize thinking and behavior. The decision for emergency hospitalization of a schizophrenic is usually based on the conclusion that he is unable to care for himself in at least a marginally constructive way, including whatever additional assistance may be rendered by family and/or therapeutic groups, activities, living situations such as halfway houses, and antipsychotic medication. It may also be made in order to facilitate commencement of an organized treatment effort, centered around either rehabilitation or psychotherapy, for a patient who may be able to function marginally in the community may have little energy, motivation, and organized capability left to undertake a treatment program as well.

Once the initial evaluation has been completed, the next phase involving longer-term treatment planning commences. This includes ascertaining whether the patient is a candidate for psychotherapy, for a social and occupational rehabilitation program, or for both, either of which may involve, but does not necessarily have to begin with, a substantial period of hospitalization; or whether the best that can be hoped for is psychological and social stabilization at the highest level attainable in the short-term, which is followed by the patient's return to the community, possibly with some new social supports. Such an assessment begins with the attitudes and expectations of the family as well as with economic considerations and the availability of treatment facilities and personnel. Complex programs for treatment of schizophrenia, psychotherapeutic or rehabilitative, require, at least in the early stages, the expertise of a specialized treatment institution, not simply a general hospital ward. Sometimes the question of transfer to another city or state where appropriate treatment facilities exist must be considered, particularly in the present era, in which institutions that conduct the kind of person-centered treatment of which I write are nearly extinct. The possibility of transfer might not be as disruptive to the schizophrenic as it would be to one with a milder form of mental illness, since the former usually has few meaningful familial and social roots in the milieu in which he is found.

Few hospitals, at present, are philosophically predisposed or practically equipped to undertake the psychological treatment of schizophrenia, given the prevailing attitude that it is not only without positive value but also potentially detrimental to the patient and economically wasteful. Most treatment programs are predicated on symptom relief, functional stabilization, and rapid return to the community; some offer more or less sophisticated programs in social and occupational rehabilitation. The specialized knowledge of psychological, family, and institutional processes, pathological and therapeutic, that some institutions acquired in the decades following World War II has in most instances been lost.

Even with the best of intentions and a maximum of sophistication, it is difficult to conduct psychologically focused treatment of some patients and treatment of others based on stabilization, training, and rehabilitation, on the same hospital unit or ward, because of the very different attitudes about the relationship of mind or personality and illness involved in each. Part of the problem often encountered in efforts to conduct effective psychological treatment is that staff recruited to do so may be more or less consciously committed to a medical model of schizophrenia and the equation of illness with meaninglessness that it represents. I have little doubt that the reverse may be equally true, namely, that staff intent on probing for feelings, thoughts and psychological meanings may retard or disrupt the progress of rehabilitation programs. (These matters are further elaborated in Chapter 16, on treatment in the mental hospital.)

Economic Considerations in Treatment Planning

A discussion of economic issues may seem unnecessary or disruptive in a chapter devoted to optimal treatment planning, but economic considerations have always shaped society's response to serious illness, and perhaps in no area of medicine have the social forces and tensions been greater than in the treatment of major mental illness. In the remarks to come I can only speak with authority of the situation in the United States, where most mental health professionals, as well as the insurance companies that subsidize most health care, approach the idea of individual psychotherapy for schizophrenics, and the prolonged hospitalization often necessary to support it, with the conviction that it is certainly too expensive even to contemplate. The question of expense is frequently confused with doubts about efficacy. While expense would seem a sensible consideration in planning treatment of any kind, attention to it is carried to an extreme in the case of psychotherapy and prolonged hospitalization for schizophrenia; the potential treaters are called upon to prove the value of the contemplated treatment in advance, probably to an audience of confirmed skeptics, whereas in other fields those proposing relatively expensive forms of treatment for very serious illnesses are not required to meet such stringent criteria. Undergirding the doubts to which I allude are two related beliefs, both of which I have attempted to lay to rest throughout this book; first, the old Kraepelinian idea that schizophrenia is inevitably a deteriorating disease and, second, the specific conviction that psychotherapy of schizophrenia is not efficacious. The power of such beliefs is striking when they are juxtaposed with the successful treatment of a patient like Emily, an outcome that leads skeptics retrospectively to rediagnose the patient as having had a less serious disorder despite the fact that the original diagnosis satisfied the DSM-III-R criteria for schizophrenia.

Even if one accepts the potential value of psychotherapy in selected cases, there is social pressure to deny such treatment to one person both because it cannot be made accessible to everyone, and because it is inconceivable that it could solve the enormous schizophrenia problem that confronts society at large. Here it should be noted that despite passionate rallying cries to "cure" cancer (or heart disease or diabetes), few treatments ever meet such expectations. Treatments that lead to radical cures of serious conditions typically involve illnesses of viral or bacterial origin. Perhaps medicine's unusual success treating (and, in some instances, eliminating) infectious disease with antibiotics and vaccination leads people to have exaggerated expectations of treatments for other illnesses.

As for the ethical issues related to the allocation of scarce resources, the decision not to use them in any case is not only a poor solution but one that is not resorted to in most other comparable situations. Some will object that psychotherapy of schizophrenia is vastly more costly than alternative treatments. Before commenting on this argument in the abstract sense, I would like to offer some facts about the cost of the three successful treatments summarized in the book—the cases of Emily, Joanna, and Celia. The therapy of Celia consisted of approximately 1,200 fifty-minute appointments at a frequency of four times per week, and another 1½ years of weekly (or less frequent) sessions. Joanna and I met approximately 1,100 times, and Emily and I approximately 900. In each instance there were miscellaneous family meetings and conferences as well and, of course, the single prolonged hospitalization for each patient. Assuming an analytic fee of $100 per hour, the cost of each of these three successful therapies of schizophrenia, exclusive of hospitalization, was about $100,000. While this is substantial, when the magnitude of the illness itself and the question of gain or loss of a productive life is measured against the cost of treating similarly serious diseases, the cost may not seem so great. Moreover, the cost of the single prolonged hospitalization must be balanced against the cost of the repeated hospitalizations that are typically required in untreated cases, and which in the long run total months or years.

In contemporary general medicine, in fact, the labor cost is the least expensive part of treatment. Most of the cost is due to the high technology used for diagnosis and treatment—and to the profitable industry that has grown up around it. For example, CAT (computerized axial tomography) scans and MRI's (magnetic resonance imaging) currently cost approximately $1,000. And a new diagnostic machine, the PET (positron emission tomography) scanner, costing $5.5 million, has recently been introduced, expensive not only of itself but additionally in terms of the people and facilities necessary to operate it. The usefulness of the information it gathers has yet to be determined, and a single evaluation with it will cost $2500!

More specifically, we might compare psychotherapy of schizophrenia with the treatment of analogous major illnesses, such as catastrophic pediatric and geriatric cases involving multiple severely compromising difficulties and deficits or the total failure of vital organs or devastating chronic diseases in people in the middle or later stages of life. In instances of such major illnesses the choice lies between palliative treatment and acquiescence to the idea of a lost life, either in terms of concrete mortality or general productivity and satisfaction, or the employment of expensive (and in some instances experimental) techniques whose long-range benefits are often questionable. I have just had occasion to read about one such treatment in the newspapers—the transplant of a portion of liver from a living donor into a child suffering from biliary atresia. Not only was the cost of the surgery alone estimated at over $300,000, but the procedure endangered the life of the donor, and it was admittedly and clearly experimental. Yet it was done, and a prominent Boston surgeon was quoted as saying, "I personally wouldn't wait [for more data about the benefits of such surgery] if I think there is a technology that will save a life" (Knox, 1989). What a different attitude from that of most people on the subject of psychotherapy of schizophrenia, and how ready the reader is to perceive this doctor as an intrepid innovator! If the same quote were a statement by a psychoanalyst referring to treatment for a schizophrenic who might otherwise commit suicide, become a street person or be condemned to a back-ward existence, the reader would think him a fool or worse!

And yet I think there are some obvious distinctions between the treatment of schizophrenia and many of these situations in which society seems fearlessly (and possibly even foolishly) eager to intervene, distinctions that make the risk/benefit ratio in schizophrenia far more favorable. In seriously medically compromised individuals, life may be prolonged by employing heroic measures, at great cost, but its duration and quality remain, in most instances, significantly limited. Without the treatment, the afflicted individuals would in many instances die quickly and be little additional drain on social resources. By contrast, if treatment is successful the young schizophrenic may become a productive, contributing member of society, rather than a chronic drain on resources if he is untreated or treated palliatively. The population of schizophrenics potentially amenable to analytic therapy tend to be late adolescents and young adults, usually in good physical health and often with evidence of latent talent and ability. The ones with whom I have been most successful, not surprisingly, have already evidenced some of this talent, or have been able to begin higher education.

Without treatment, if they do not kill themselves, which happens in approximately 10% of cases, schizophrenics will most likely be economically and socially burdensome and destructive to society for much of their lives, by becoming street people, committing crimes, and requiring extensive and prolonged support from a variety of social agencies. This is to say nothing of the loss of their potential for social productivity. It may be myopic and misleading to believe that alternatives to psychoanalytically informed treatment are less expensive. Even the cost of medication may be great, as the families of patients given clozapine are protesting even as I write this. Moreover, it is easier to be horrified by a significant immediate expense than it is to look at what the personal and social costs of refusing to incur this expense might be over the life span of the patient in question. Over the long run, as the discussion of schizophrenia's typical course in Chapter 1 indicates, recurrences of florid psychosis and progressive disability and chronicity may require that the treatment that may have appeared successful when viewed myopically, needs to be repeated over and over again. Gunderson and Mosher (1975) assert that the economic cost of the loss of productivity of a given schizophrenic patient far outweighs the costs of psychotherapy. I would put it more positively: The gain in productivity of a successfully treated patient may more than justify the costs of analytic therapy. The result of such treatment may be profound, both for the patient and for society. While Rachel (and probably Edward, if he does not commit suicide) will likely be a continuing drain on social resources for the next 50 or more years, Emily, Celia, and Joanna have already become important and contributing members of society, and show every sign not only of continuing to do so but of expanding their contributions. The "ripple effect" of healthy, productive individuals like Emily (who is an accomplished artist), Joanna (who works in human services, is a musician, and has raised a family), and Celia (who has become a respected educator, influential in the larger community as well as in her particular school) on their families, the community, and generations to come may be difficult to assess because their contributions really begin when treatment ends, and if we terminate effectively with our patients, in a way calculated to promote their autonomy, we are likely to learn little about them. From an overall socioeconomic perspective, schizophrenics treated with intensive psychotherapy and necessary hospitalization may in the long run give back much more than they received.

Before leaving the discussion of economics and turning to the question of how one evaluates a schizophrenic patient for individual psychotherapy, I would like to comment on a more specific financial issue. Nowadays medical payment is increasingly synonymous with health insurance. Virtually all policies are issued to adults and their preadult children; coverage usually terminates around college age. Since most young adults of this age are relatively healthy and do not need extensive insurance coverage until they are able to become wage earners with policies of their own, this situation is not ordinarily a problem. But this transitional period of young adulthood is precisely when most cases of schizophrenia erupt; thus, many of the most eminently treatable young schizophrenics fall between the cracks, so to speak, and are not covered at all (and this is quite aside from the topic of the extreme and questionable limits most policies place on mental health coverage).

Evaluation for Psychotherapy

As my particular training and expertise is in the psychotherapy of schizophrenia, I would like to conclude this chapter with a discussion of the more specific question of evaluation for psychotherapy. Such screening is not a neat, technical process; in fact, it is difficult to differentiate some aspects of the evaluation from the psychotherapy itself. Not infrequently, a year or more of evaluative effort may be required.* Because the boundary between evaluation and treatment is fuzzy, I shall comment on some of the more formal aspects of evaluation here and continue it in the discussion on treatment in Chapter 15.

First, there is no doubt that the prognosis for therapeutic success is much better if the intervention occurs in the early stages of the illness, before schizophrenic ways of thinking and acting have acquired entrenched significance as social adaptations and as a secondary form of identity, as Pao (1979) describes. This means that age is a factor in the evaluation, as are duration of symptoms and extent of disability, facts that are not always so easy to ascertain as one might think, given the extent to which patient and family are typically committed to denial.

---

*Once again, those who doubt the efficacy of psychoanalytic therapy in general and of such treatment of schizophrenia in particular may be shocked, but I do not think the rather open-ended process to which I refer differs in principle from the enlightened clinical trial method that characterizes work with a patient with a serious medical illness. Risk and uncertainty are part of the human condition, and the fact that one cannot always identify with certainty the factors that differentiate those who will benefit from a treatment from those who will not does not ordinarily deter the curious and dedicated practitioner from making his best effort to conduct the treatment, so long as he has good reason to believe that *some* patients with whom he is working are capable of benefiting from the methodology he is employing.

Second, a history of some accomplishment or achievement—most commonly in the form of education but sometimes in the form of a special skill or area of expertise—is a good sign. If the patient has completed a bit of college it suggests he may have skills for verbal, abstract, reflective therapeutic dialogue and motivation for socially constructive effort.

Finally, there is the question, which concerns the very core of schizophrenia, of motivation and capacity to relate to another person, to tolerate feedback from that person, and to join with him in a task that involves bearing and thinking about distressing feelings rather than seeking avoidance or immediate relief of pain. It is important that the schizophrenic have sufficient energy to persevere, and that he be in a sufficient state of distress or suffering to want to work to gain relief. By suffering I do not mean bizarre behavior or symptoms that the empathic observer, by putting himself in the shoes of the patient, reads as suffering, but a consciousness of pain and a wish to do something about it, and by relief I do not mean surcease from the experience of emotion. It is for this reason that it is important to use medication sparingly and judiciously during the initial evaluation period, for a rapidly "tranquilized" patient may lose whatever motivation he may have had to seek human help for his distress.

Sometimes one is not certain whether to undertake therapy with a particular patient, and may elect to focus treatment on one or more other levels first, and then, perhaps after the environment is stabilized and some modicum of personal coherence and control has been reestablished, review whether the patient seems more motivated and capable.

Research has provided some support for the importance of motivation in treatment outcome. McGlashan (1984) believes the surprisingly positive outcome of the patients in the Vermont sample was because the rehabilitation program that selected them did so on the basis of their high level of motivation to learn work skills in order to make a living. The Chestnut Lodge group, whom one might naively have expected to do well because of their more educated backgrounds, in fact did relatively poorly, a fact McGlashan attributes to the protection their privileged socioeconomic status gave them against having to take personal responsibility for their lives.

In Part III I showed that the ways we tend to view and conceptualize schizophrenia at each level of the human systems hierarchy involve successive transformations of recurrent structures and themes and tend to repeat and enact the disease process in the guise of objectification. In the remainder of this section (Part IV) I shall demonstrate that the same can be said of most of what passes as treatment of schizophrenia, and I shall propose what I believe to be a more objectified approach.

Chapter 13

Studies of the Efficacy of Psychological Treatment and a Summary of My Own Experience

T he hierarchical systems approach to the treatment of schizophrenia begins with assessment of the patient's capacity to form a therapeutic relationship. But in the preceding chapter our discussion of economic considerations in treatment planning led us back to the current atmosphere of skepticism about the value of psychologically focused modes of treatment. Torrey (1988), for example, states that "to practice [psychoanalytic therapy] today on a patient with schizophrenia could be considered malpractice" (p. 162). Drake and Sederer (1986) write that because intensive psychotherapies of schizophrenics "provide or encourage intense relationships" they are "analogous to pouring boiling oil on wounds" and "overstimulating, intrusive, and produce strong negative affects" (p. 314). To introduce the chapters on psychotherapy I would like to survey of some of the literature on the efficacy (or lack thereof) of psychotherapy with schizophrenics. At the conclusion of this survey I summarize my personal experience treating schizophrenics. Constructing adequate studies of this subject is a formidable undertaking, and those in the representative sample I shall cite, while thought-provoking, are all significantly flawed and should satisfy neither advocates nor skeptics of psychotherapy. In Chapter 3 I argued that careful clinical case studies such as those presented in this book may be the best evidence in favor of the potential value of psychotherapy.

Psychotherapy Outcome Studies

To place the problem in its proper context, the failure to document the efficacy of psychoanalytic therapy through statistical surveys is by no means limited to schizophrenia. There are, regrettably, few outcome studies of any kind in the psychoanalytic literature and not many in the general psychiatric literature. Wallerstein (1986) reports a 30-year follow-up study of 42 patients, with diagnoses ranging from neurosis to paranoid and borderline personalities, approximately half treated with psychoanalysis and the other half with psychotherapy. The results in the two groups are roughly comparable: about 40% solid improvements and about 25% failures, with the remainder falling somewhere in between. In the 12 patients with serious personality disturbances treatment was an almost complete failure. Kantrowitz, Katz, and Paolitto (1990) have conducted a 5- to 10-year follow-up of 17 patients who underwent control psychoanalyses by trainees at the Boston Psychoanalytic Institute. Their percentages of improvement and failure are almost identical with those of Wallerstein. In addition, an intermediate group of 6 patients had deteriorated following analysis, but their gains were restored by subsequent psychiatric treatment. Thus, those who require, as an article of belief, statistically unimpeachable experimental studies still have legitimate grounds for doubting that psychoanalysis is of value even for treating psychoneurosis, much less schizophrenia!

Studies of Psychotherapy with Schizophrenics

Surveys of psychotherapy with large groups of schizophrenics have also failed to generate significantly positive conclusions. Studies conducted by Eysenck (1965), May (1968), and Grinspoon, Ewalt, and Shader (1972) all failed to document that schizophrenics improve with psychotherapy. In the May study patients assigned to drug groups, with or without psychotherapy, did better than patients treated with psychotherapy alone; however, the therapists were novices, therapy sessions were infrequent, and the study lasted but a single year. The Grinspoon study contrasted the effect of medication with and without psychotherapy; the therapy was conducted twice a week for 20 months by experienced senior therapists, some of whom were analysts. Karon and VandenBos (1981), who were influenced by Rosen's (1947, 1953) "Direct Analysis" technique, report the only study that claims that the psychotherapy of schizophrenia is beneficial. Experienced therapists treated or supervised treatment of patients for 20 months, and the psychotherapy proved useful.

But most of these studies have justly been criticized as inadequate for drawing any conclusions about psychoanalytic psychotherapy for one or more of the following reasons: use of unskilled and inexperienced therapists, insufficient efforts to define and control the nature of the therapy, therapy that was insufficiently intense or frequent, therapy that was much too brief to be expected to make a difference (in this regard see my discussion of motivation and engagement in Chapter 15 as well as the case reports), and inadequate methods of assessment of therapy results. In short, when one hears the commonplace assertion that none of the studies has been able to document the efficacy of psychoanalytically informed therapy, it is not possible to draw conclusions beyond listing the methodological flaws of the studies themselves.

Two investigators have done follow-up studies of patients treated at their institutions. McGlashan (1984) examined the long-term outcome of patients treated intensively at Chestnut Lodge, which is psychoanalytically oriented, and included patients treated by some of the most gifted therapists on the staff. He discovered that two-thirds continued to be ill or were only marginally improved at the time of follow-up; presumably, one-third were better. Stone (1986) traced the outcome of schizophrenics treated by psychotherapy at Columbia and concluded that psychotherapy is ineffective.

Probably the best-designed and conducted prospective study of psychotherapy of schizophrenia to date was conducted by Stanton, Gunderson, Knapp, Frank, Katz, Vanicelli, Frosch, Schnitzer, and Rosenthal, and reported in two parts by Stanton et al. (1984) and Gunderson et al. (1984). They compared the results of two kinds of psychotherapy, reality adaptive-supportive (RAS) and exploratory insight-oriented (EIO), over a 2-year period. RAS therapists focused on the present and on symptom management, whereas EIO therapists focused on the past as well as the present, utilized insight as well as support and limit setting, and were attentive to the vicissitudes of the therapeutic relationship or transference. Only one-third of the patients completed the 2-year study. In this group of 22 EIO- and 20 RAS-treated patients there were few differences in the outcome that correlated with use of one or the other of the two forms of therapy; RAS proved slightly superior with regard to recidivism and role performance, and EIO was slightly better with regard to ego function and cognition. Even this study, however, is flawed in terms of the standard for training of the EIO therapists, the brief duration of the treatment effort, the small number of patients followed even for this short period of time, and the large number of patients lost to follow-up. Parenthetically, the two treatment failures I report in this book, Rachel and Edward, each of whom was in therapy less than 2 years, were included in the Stanton and Gunderson study, apparently constituting 10% of the EIO population on which their conclusions are based!

Unfortunately, there are few reliable ways to differentiate "good" from "bad" therapists or to ascertain whether therapy is really a quantifiable entity like, for example, a dose of neuroleptic medication. Most of the studies I summarized made little effort to deal with these variables beyond utilizing rough measures of training, seniority, and experience. Even the most rigorous of the studies, moreover, did not employ psychoanalytically trained therapists exclusively. It is difficult to fault the studies for these omissions. After all, what training do we take into account? And are years of experience or seniority working in a mental hospital, or even completion of psychoanalytic training, any guarantee of skill? And since there has been little detailed study of what therapists, even with statistically similar dossiers, do in the privacy of their consulting rooms, it is doubtful that similarities in training and background are any indication that therapists approach their patients in ways sufficiently similar to postulate a monolithic entity called psychotherapy, much less to add therapist A's work to that of therapist B in order to reach conclusions.

The Experience of Individual Therapists

Although one might safely assume that there is more standardization in the nature and content of an individual therapist's work from one patient to another than in studies employing multiple therapists, there are very few studies of the outcome of the work of particular therapists. A handful of analysts with interests similar to my own have written, with varying degrees of specificity, that they experienced significant degrees of success treating schizophrenics (for example, Rosen, Sullivan, Fromm-Reichmann, Knight, Searles, Boyer, and Pao). Unfortunately, even fewer have published statistical summaries of their experience. Still others, including some of the finest clinicians, such as my own mentor, Elvin Semrad, never published their work and ideas about schizophrenia in any form. Once again, this state of affairs is by no means peculiar to schizophrenia; Gedo (1979b) is one of the few analysts to statistically quantify and publish the results of his psychoanalytic work.

Although it may seem so self-evident as not to deserve mention, it is vital to know about the nature of the sample on which the therapist's experience is based in order to interpret the significance of accounts like the ones that follow. Freud's remarkable contributions to the study of neurosis came from a combination of his office practice and his self-analysis. When it came to schizophrenia, however, he was on shakier ground, as he did not work in a mental hospital and had little firsthand contact with such patients. Wisely, he refrained from more than speculation about this condition. As psychoanalysis has remained an office-based treatment modality, only a minority of psychoanalysts since Freud have had extensive experience treating schizophrenics, and most psychoanalytic writings on the subject do not specify the clinical sample on which the author's experience is based and do not present case material in any detail. In fact, a surprising proportion of those who write about the condition do not even work with schizophrenics. Although I offer these observations as grounds for selective skepticism about psychoanalytic theories of schizophrenia, I would like to emphasize that, telling as these observations may be, they do not necessarily separate psychoanalysts from others who present themselves as authorities on the subject. Few of the experimental psychiatrists who search assiduously for an organic substrate work intensively with schizophrenics, either. For example, one of the most noted psychiatric contributors to the organic literature on schizophrenia, who also happens to be a psychoanalyst and clinician, informed me when consulting on a hospitalized schizophrenic patient of mine (Rachel) that he never treats schizophrenics!

Rosen (1947, 1953) claimed that he cured 37 of the approximately 100 patients with whom he utilized his direct analysis technique, which involves nurturant and aggressive efforts to engage the patient during the initial "out of contact" phase and to interpret to him the presumptive meaning of his psychotic productions. However, Rosen's cases were followed up in two studies—by Horwitz, Polatin, Kolb, and Hoch (1958) and Bookhammer, Meyers, Shober, and Piotroski (1966)—and both concluded that his long-term results were actually quite poor.

Sullivan (1962) claimed that he treated 100 schizophrenics at Sheppard and Enoch Pratt Hospital with psychotherapy, and that 32% of those with insidious onset and 61% of those with acute onset improved.

In Robert Knight's preface to Harold Searles' (1965) book on schizophrenia he recounted Searles' experience until that time, which appears to be remarkably similar to my own. Possibly, Searles undertook to work with a more difficult and chronic group of patients; much of his work was done prior to the broad use of phenothiazine medication, and it appears that his criteria for improvement are less stringent than my own. In any event, he reported work with 18 schizophrenic patients, with the average treatment lasting 9 years and the range of duration being from 6 months to 26 years. These patients had been previously hospitalized for periods up to 9 years, averaging 2.3 years; this statistic must be interpreted in light of the much greater acceptance of prolonged hospital stays in the post–World War II era and does not necessarily reflect the severity of Searles' patients' pathology. All but one of his patients had had prior psychotherapy. Searles reported 13 of the 18 "remarkably improved"; however, 7 of the 13 remained hospitalized at the time of his report. In other words, 6 of the 18 were able to leave the hospital; of these, Knight did not report how many were able to terminate therapy and lead productive independent lives. One or more of Searles' patients were the subjects of the cases reviewed in McGlashan's 1984 follow-up study; unfortunately, these were not identified by either author so we are unable to compare assessments.

Boyer and Giovachinni (1967) wrote about their experience treating schizophrenics outside a hospital setting and reported significant improvement in 14 of 17 patients treated for periods ranging from 2 to 10 years. Their group included 10 patients they diagnosed as schizophrenic (the basis for diagnosis of schizophrenia was not elaborated) as well as 7 they called borderline (probably using Knight's criteria of state, rather than personality, organization). Although some of those Boyer and Giovachinni called schizophrenic would have satisfied DSM criteria, judging from the brief vignettes, Meissner (1985), in reviewing Boyer's 1983 book, points out that most of them were probably characterological borderlines. For example, one of the two patients Boyer presented was a panphobic woman who had graduated college, was married, and held a job; another woman, more clearly schizophrenic, was also married. Seven of Boyer's patients had been hospitalized just prior to commencement of treatment; he saw these patients four times per week, had them use the couch, and encouraged free association. He did not use medication or communicate with relatives. Only two required hospitalization in the course of treatment.

Recently, McGlashan and Keats (1989) published an interesting study of psychoanalytically oriented psychotherapy of schizophrenia based on case reports from Chestnut Lodge hospital records and their own follow-up interviews; however, detailed and continuous records by the therapists themselves are lacking. They present four cases, two of which they classify as good outcomes and two as poor ones. It is my impression that only one of their cases (Joanne Greenberg, the patient of Frieda Fromm-Reichmann who made her treatment the subject of a novel and who is considered to have had a good outcome) could truly be said to have had an adequate psychotherapeutic trial. Ben, the second of their positive outcome cases, received treatment I would describe as supportive and rehabilitative rather than intensive and psychodynamic. An outcome similar to his might have ensued in any containing and supportive environment, so that this report tells us little or nothing about psychoanalytic psychotherapy. As for the two poor outcomes, Betty was not really given the opportunity for intensive psychotherapy until her illness was clearly chronic; by then she had sustained so many losses, interruptions, and rejections in the course of her hospitalization and treatment that the poor outcome of the belated treatment effort is hardly surprising. And Mark was allowed to leave Chestnut Lodge before any substantive dynamic issues were addressed in his therapy. At each point at which substantive pathological issues might have been joined and worked on, he and his treaters appear to have colluded in such a way as to avoid confrontation and to reconstitute a chronic psychotic equilibrium; the result was that Mark's therapy never progressed beyond a superficial level. Thus the capacity to benefit from therapy of this bright and vigorous but seriously disturbed young man was never adequately tested.

My Experience

I have spent approximately 25 years (excluding the years of my psychoanalytically oriented residency training, when I began to do this kind of work) in intensive (usually four times per week) psychoanalytic psychotherapy with several schizophrenics at any given time. Most of these persons required prolonged hospitalization, up to several years at a stretch; I have worked with some for 15 or more years. One of the reasons I have continued this work is that I have experienced significant success, so striking in some instances that it has provided a measure of professional satisfaction not to be found in work with less severely disturbed patients. This satisfaction, in turn, has compensated for the more commonplace and painful experiences of failure, of which I shall present some instructive examples.

I estimate my work with schizophrenics constitutes approximately 10% to 15% of my intensive therapeutic and psychoanalytic practice. Since completing my own psychiatric training, I have made significant therapeutic efforts (at least 6 months, at least three and usually four times per week) with a total of 18 patients who satisfy the DSM-III-R criteria for schizophrenia. As it is often difficult to find the line of demarcation between schizophrenia and particularly virulent forms of primitive personality organization, namely those characterized by rare hallucinations, ideas that seem delusional in their strangeness and tenacity but are masked by more "reasonable" beliefs, and major life dysfunction, I have resorted to hospital diagnosis in questionable cases, and I have attempted to take into account such ancillary sources of information as psychological test reports.

The 18 patients of my sample (Figure 3) include 5 males and 13 females. The reason for the gender difference (which I have already alluded to in Chapters 1 and 6) is that in my experience, which is consistent with that of others, male schizophrenics tend to be more refractory to intensive interpersonal psychological intervention than females.

These patients ranged in age from adolescence to early adulthood (from approximately age 16 to the late twenties) at the time treatment commenced. Two were of precollege age and eight had completed at least some college, in most cases meeting their functional Waterloo in the process of doing so. One had a professional school diploma, six had completed college, and one of these had a graduate degree. The woman with a graduate education was also atypical insofar as she came to me after completing a psychoanalysis in a manner satisfactory to her analyst, who was then in his own psychoanalytic training. In retrospect, the presence of delusional material and a delusional transference could be inferred in that analysis, and the turmoil the patient experienced at the time of termination—which was against her express and fervent wishes but was instigated by the analyst ostensibly for therapeutic reasons but probably as a countertransference enactment of his preconscious fear of her delusional attachment—heralded the florid emergence of her psychosis. At the time treatment commenced, only one of the 18 had been able to marry or form any sort of intimate adult relationship; the woman who married was also the only one with children.

In all instances the need for treatment was precipitated by major failures of adjustment at work, school, or relationship. Five patients commenced treatment with me as outpatients; of these, all were subsequently hospitalized. (In

Treatment Duration and Outcome of My Experience in Treating Schizophrenia

Duration (years)	Positive outcomes (9)			Negative outcomes (9)		
	Complete					
	Very successful	Moderately successful	Incomplete	Chronic hosp.	Deteri- orated	Unknown
½–1				3		1
1–2				3		
2–7	4	1	1		2	
7+	2	1				
Totals (18)	6	2	1	6	2	1

FIGURE 3

one case this meant the end of my effort to treat the patient, for she was taken home to a distant city by her family). In the other 13 cases, treatment commenced in the hospital. In 12 of my cases there were either multiple hospitalizations over a course of years or a single chronic hospitalization lasting many years.

In four of the 18 cases treatment efforts failed after less than a year—or a protracted evaluation proved negative, depending on one's outlook. Of the four who failed in less than a year, three went on to become chronically hospitalized schizophrenics, and one left the hospital against advice (I have no follow-up data about him). For three other patients treatment failed during the second year, and each of these remained chronically hospitalized. (The cases of two of these patients, Rachel and Edward, are described at length in this book.) In other words, of the seven patients whose treatment failed after 1 to 2 years, six are known to have become chronically hospitalized schizophrenics, and I have no information about the seventh. Of the remaining 11 patients, eight were in treatment with me for periods ranging from 2 to 7 years. One of this group of eight continues in her fifth year, and is doing well, functioning out of the hospital for a longer period and more autonomously than ever before in her adult life, and working in such a way that I anticipate a positive outcome. Two others of the eight experienced chronic deteriorations, and it gradually became clear that they had no real motivation to achieve an autonomous functional state; one of these was the aforementioned patient who came to me after difficulties she experienced terminating her psychoanalysis. Another of the eight made slow but steady growth and eventually transferred to another therapist when it appeared that we were unable to resolve a psychotic transference she had formed to me. The four others in this group of eight had strikingly successful treatment outcomes. (I give case histories in this book of two patients from this group, Emily and Joanna; a third has been reported elsewhere [Robbins, 1969].)

The outcome of each of the three treatments that lasted longer than 7 years was quite positive. One patient, the woman who was married and had small children at the time treatment commenced, was leading a satisfying, productive, and seemingly normal life when we terminated almost 14 years later. The treatment of another patient occurred in two courses, each lasting approximately 4 years, separated by a 10-year span; as a result of the first course of treatment the patient was able to leave the hospital, complete her education (including an advanced degree), marry, and have children. The second course was initiated because of problems she experienced as a mother, including an inability to experience pleasure and satisfaction, and serious depressive suicidal preoccupations. She did not require rehospitalization, and the outcome was partially satisfactory. The third case (Celia) was recently terminated with considerable success, as the reader will see.

In summary, four patients could be said to have undergone prolonged evaluations that proved them to be unsuitable treatment cases, at least with me. The remaining 14 patients had the opportunity for significant treatment (longer than 1 year). Of that group, eight are completed, with good to excellent outcomes, including relinquishment of all antipsychotic medication, achievement of functional autonomy, personal productivity in work or career, formation of reasonably satisfying intimate relationships, and cessation of all psychotic symptomatology (except in the case of the patient who had to be transferred to another therapist in order to resolve her psychotic transference). One patient remains in treatment and is doing very well; it seems likely that she will experience a positive outcome.

In the best of the completed outcome cases, the treatment lasted between 5 and 7 years. The better-outcome cases involved persons with significant manifest affect, whereas the failures often manifested elements of catatonia or hebephrenia, extreme and rigid paranoid features, and/or a chronic, flat, dead quality. This finding is consistent with the general belief that patients with so-called positive symptoms do better than those with "negative" symptoms (inhibition, constriction, passivity, apathy, and diminution of emotion and motivation). Nevertheless, the presence or absence of these negative elements was no more than suggestive, and by no means predictive, of the success or failure of treatment.

One might conclude from this brief summary that I have failed in my effort to establish the value of a psychological approach to schizophrenia. After all, I have only made sustained and significant treatment efforts with 18 schizophrenics, and I have had good results, in varying degrees, with only nine patients, a drop in the metaphorical schizophrenic bucket. Two of these positive outcome patients continued to have significant problem areas, albeit not psychotic ones, and with another who remains in treatment much progress has been made but the final outcome remains to be seen. And it is not entirely accurate to calculate the successes and failures as percentages of 18, for there were numerous instances in which I met with patients for less than 6 months, sometimes for no longer than one or two appointments, and I or they or both of us concluded that nothing was likely to be gained from further efforts. Whether this represents an ethically, socially, or economically efficient way to use energies and talents is a question that I leave the reader to decide.

Chapter 14

Psychotherapeutic Technique and Process

While the establishment of at least the rudiments of a working relationship can more or less be taken for granted in the psychological treatment of patients with other diagnoses, the first challenge in the therapy of a schizophrenic is to establish a relationship of any sort. Success in such an endeavor is at best a relative matter, for all that can be hoped for is a pathological symbiosis without growth potential. If such a relationship is established it is subsequently necessary to determine whether it is possible to convert it to a growth-promoting symbiosis. In this chapter I would like to consider the art and technique of relating to a schizophrenic person in a potentially therapeutic manner.

To set the stage I would like to quote from two very experienced therapists of schizophrenia, Otto Will and Theodore Lidz, on the subject of the therapist's personality. According to Will (1973):

> The therapist should have or acquire certain abilities, among which are the taking pleasure in the growth of another person; tolerance of attachment, dependency, and the inevitable stress of separation; the strength to set limits and yet permit another person to live in a way of his own; and the capacity to cooperate with members of a team, enduring the accompanying envy, jealousy, competition, anger, and affection. Finally, he should be able to accept the often slow pace of growth. (p. 155)

According to Lidz (1973):

> A major requirement for the therapist concerns the ability to care and refuse to give up while not needing the patient or his devotion. The therapist seeks to convey that even though he wants very much for the patient to improve and will go a long way and make personal sacrifices to foster such improvement, he pursues this goal neither for the parent's sake nor because he needs a therapeutic success. (p. 104)

I agree with Lidz in principle, but in Chapter 15 I shall elaborate the idealistic nature of this goal and the practical consequences when it inevitably falls short of realization.

The term *technique*, which is generally employed within psychoanalysis to denote the theory and practice of therapy as contrasted to the theory of psychopathology, has unfortunate mechanistic implications and may suggest to some a separation or nonintegration within the therapist of personality and process that parallels the fragmentation (noted in Chapter 11) characteristic of the sociocultural level of expression of schizophrenia. A technician in the narrow sense is not a good analyst of any patient or condition. However, a good therapist is simultaneously scientist, with a keen appreciation of theory, both of the nature and etiology of the condition he is called upon to treat and of the treatment process itself, and artist, using his own personality, which he has come to understand sufficiently through his own training and experience, as a tool to implement understanding and change in his patient. As each personality is different, so each therapist will implement theory in a unique and idiosyncratic manner. This makes me reluctant to write about technique at all, for doing so cannot help but foster the illusion that it can be taught didactically from a book or a lecture and lead to confusion between personal style and theory. From observing another therapist's successful style one may expect to learn about what constitutes style, but one cannot expect to learn a style of one's own. It is particularly hazardous to try to copy the style of a mentor, which may fit the student like a poorly tailored suit of clothes.

After asserting the importance of the therapist's unique personality and style I hasten to disassociate myself from the popular but substantively shallow belief that theories of psychopathology and of technique are entirely superfluous, that a good therapist is nothing more than a warm and wonderful sage, hoary with wisdom and common sense, overflowing with the caring his patient has presumably lacked, and guided unerringly by his supranormal intuitive and empathic capabilities; if nothing else, a cursory inspection of how some of us who may be good therapists do as parents should be enough to disillusion anyone of that belief. Nor do I subscribe to the related idea that therapists and patients can be matched successfully by a superficial observation of their personalities; or, worse yet, that an observer can decide who is a good therapist by looking at his apparent political and social skill in conducting his manifest social and professional relationships.

In other words, a good therapist is the product of an indissoluble marriage of personality and technique, artist and scientist. While he may always experience a creative tension between these ways of looking and being, they remain inseparable.

Critical Elements of Psychoanalytic Therapy

Since my psychological approach is fundamentally psychoanalytic, I would like to consider the knotty question of what constitutes psychoanalysis and whether the treatments I describe in this book do or do not fall within its parameters. Much of what differentiates psychoanalysis from other forms of treatment may be traced to two of Freud's discoveries: the unconscious mind and the transference. Freud described how the apparent irrationality of human behavior has lawful unconscious determinants, and he taught us that in an attentive human relationship in which the therapist, who imposes no significant emotional agenda of his own other than his wish to help his patient to understand himself, becomes a stage, projection screen, or microcosm, these determinants, both the impulses and the barriers to growth and change, will unfold like the staging of a drama. In this setting these unconscious elements may become amenable to identification and conscious awareness; then, through the process of interpretation, comprehensible with regard to their dynamic, adaptive, and genetic aspects; and, consequently, potentially alterable. In this way (to rephrase Freud's classic comments about replacing id with ego), where obligatory, irrational, maladaptive repetition once was, enlightened choice may come to be.

What most essentially distinguishes analytic therapy from other forms of treatment is the assumption that there is more to the patient's problem than what is obvious, commonsensical, and capable of simply being unlearned by a conscious instructional process, and that it is the shared task of patient and analyst not just to talk about a third entity "out there," known as "the problem," but to study and attempt to comprehend what transpires within the context of their interpersonal relationship. This broad definition of psychoanalytic therapy does not include as critical defining elements such specific technical propositions as free association or even, to be more concrete, use of a couch and proscription of eye contact, and it receives support from analysts such as Gill (1984) and Gedo (1979a, 1988).

Limitations of Classical Models of Technique

If we contrast the broad definition of psychoanalytic therapy I have just proposed with the classical technique of analysis we may see that the latter is dependent for its effectiveness on elements of the more or less normal and neurotic personality, which schizophrenics lack. In the remainder of this chapter we shall inquire as to what technical modifications might enable us to treat schizophrenics within a framework that retains the values and advantages of psychoanalysis, especially its respect for the unique potential of each individual.

Others have asked these questions, beginning with Eissler (1953), in his classical discussion of parameters, and including Winnicott (1960c), with his emphasis on the holding environment, Kohut (1971); and, more recently, Gedo (with Goldberg, 1973), with his concept of an epigenetic hierarchy of mind models and his suggestion that typical analytic interventions may need to differ depending on a patient's immediate level of mental functioning, and may range from pacification or soothing, which might be appropriate to the stage of inability to regulate tension; through unification, in the stage of disintegration; disillusionment, in the stage of unreality; to, finally, once the stage of intrapsychic conflict and defense has been attained, interpretation. Gedo has emphasized the role of learning in the analysis of deficits (apraxias), which characterize more archaic modes of thinking. Elsewhere, I have also written about interpretive and educational interventions in instances of cognitive and related adaptive pathologies in the treatment of primitive personalities (Robbins, 1989). (The reader is referred to Chapters 7 and 8 for a more comprehensive discussion of this subject from the perspective not of technique but of theory of psychopathology.)

The classical therapeutic posture that evolved through work with neurotic patients has, at best, limited value with schizophrenics, and may actually be destructive. While the associations of the neurotic tend to be centripetal in relation to his conflicts except when resistances, which may be analyzed, are encountered, in the case of the schizophrenic they are centrifugal, tending toward further loosening of integration and differentiation of mind and withdrawal from others. The procedure of sitting behind the couch where the patient reclines, out of eye contact, and waiting expectantly for relevant material to emerge is not merely a waste of time in the therapy of schizophrenics but tends to promote in the patient still further decompensation. It is a wonder that so many analysts have mistaken the schizophrenic's fragmented products for remarkable revelations of the unconscious mind. The capacity to associate freely but productively is a high-order cognitive accomplishment involving integrative linkages, a differentiated other (the analyst), and a sense of self, as well as the ability to reflect on the thinking process, monitor obstacles to it, and purposefully report the result to another person for his scrutiny as well, things schizophrenics require assistance to learn to do.

However, the most obvious alternative to encouragement of free association—the use of intervention techniques including confrontation, interpretation, and perhaps instruction—assumes in the patient a more or less integrated, differentiated mind with intact capacity for mental representation, the experience of intrapsychic conflict and ambivalence, and self-awareness of important cognitive and affective configurations. Without a prolonged period of preparatory cognitive work most intervention techniques at best influence but a segment of the schizophrenic mind, which is unintegrated with other parts, while fostering the illusion that this segment represents the whole person, and at worst are likely to be experienced as a form of assault, whether or not the patient is able to articulate this fact (since interventions may reflect things that the therapist observes but that the patient has not at all integrated and differentiated as elements of his own mind). Thus, active therapeutic interventions either foster a docile, lifeless compliance or else may serve as vehicles for the patient to externalize hostility. If the patient is a bit less disturbed, such interventions may simply be experienced as the therapist's significant failure of empathic understanding and validation.

Efforts at empathy gone awry are responsible for some of the most significant problems encountered in the effort to treat schizophrenics. Kohut's self psychology has led many contemporary therapists to place extraordinary emphasis on this way of knowing and relating without necessarily increasing the general level of sophistication about its attendant problems. In order to be effective empathy depends upon a qualitative similarity between the mental workings or structure of therapist and patient. But because the mind of the schizophrenic functions so differently from that of the therapist (as outlined in Chapter 9 and as recovered schizophrenics themselves inform us), his subjective experience is very different from what the therapist is capable of imagining, however hard he may try. An even more significant problem is that our assumption that we understand, particularly in the early stages of treatment, may unwittingly lead us to think like our patients, in circumscribed psychotic ways. Kohut (1971) himself cautioned that "the reliability of our empathy, a major instrument of psychoanalytic observation, declines the more dissimilar the observed to the observer, and the early stages of mental development are thus, in particular, a challenge to our ability to empathize" (p. 37). I am not suggesting that an empathic attitude is without value any more than I am rejecting the importance of well-timed interpretation; I am merely pointing out that in applying these familiar concepts to the unfamiliar mind of the schizophrenic we enounter new issues and problems. To some of these we shall return in a moment.

If such traditional elements as free association, confrontation and even interpretation may be potentially harmful, and even if such modern nostrums as empathy prove problematic, what do we focus our attention on in their stead and how? If we find alternatives, do they preserve the broader goals, intentions and values of psychoanalysis or do we find ourselves inexorably directed toward very different forms of treatment that, being less well studied, are replete with hidden pitfalls of their own?

Interpersonal Relatedness or Contact

The establishment and maintenance of a developmentally constructive form of human contact—symbiosis—in an individual ill-equipped to meet the therapist halfway, is the foundation without which psychological therapy of schizophrenia cannot effect change. In the absence of relatedness, genuine analysis of content as part of a joint therapeutic enterprise is an impossible exercise. Eye contact as well as a modicum of interactive responsiveness is required to establish contact, just as it is with an infant. It is not constructive to employ the therapeutic format of classical analysis, with use of the couch, which was recommended to minimize external interferences to the process of introspection, and a general posture of unresponsiveness so as not to interfere with the associative sequence. Therefore, I prefer to sit face-to-face with patients, and it is sometimes necessary to be involved with them in other more concrete and physical ways as well, either in person or by proxy.

If the patient does not speak of our relationship directly—and schizophrenics usually do not—I try to draw his attention to any suggestion of unusual relatedness or unrelatedness to me and encourage discussion of it. Eye contact is an especially important index of relatedness, both to the "true" cognitive–affective self and to the other person, and breaking or absence of such contact is an almost unfailing indicator of withdrawal or detachment from the other and/or from one's feelings. Disengaged or unintegrated states are characteristic of schizophrenics and tend to pass unnoticed unless commented on by the therapist. Use of the couch not only fosters such states, as mentioned earlier, but deprives the therapist of one of his most reliable clues to their presence.

Every constructive human relationship involves delineating areas of agreement and disagreement, and therapy with a schizophrenic is no exception. It is difficult and challenging to hew a pathway between a relationship of apparent total harmony based on pacification or placation and the equally extreme and distancing or alienating posture of opposing and challenging the schizophrenic's manifest bizarreness and unreality at every turn. As a consequence of their inability to establish a helpful dyadic relationship, schizophrenics live in a psychological world where mutual survival is felt to be impossible. Although confrontation and opposition are unavoidable in treatment, I look for every opportunity to join with the patient, rather than to confront, and to find other ways to draw his attention to issues that seem refractory to reflection. Disagreements, particularly in the early stages of treatment, tend to have a lethal or relationship-ending connotation, whether or not this is immediately evident, and often lead to a premature cessation of treatment.

But never noting and emphasizing differences and even going to the extreme of attempting to maintain apparent agreement with all the patient says and does will leave both patient and therapist alone in solipsistic universes. The external world that the therapist represents, exclusively in the earlier stages of treatment, will remain a psychologically undiscovered entity, covered over by the patient's undifferentiated and unintegrated mind. While there are some who believe such selfless compliance on the part of the therapist will ultimately lead to the patient's decision to trust and to value him, in my experience this is a futile endeavor, and what passes as trust is no more than the perpetuation of a psychological cocoon, with the addition of the therapist as an active, albeit mentally undifferentiated, participant. The trick is to be differentiated without being in opposition, and one way to do this is to emphasize playful elements in attempting to build a dialogue, as one would do with an infant.

Dialogue

Establishment and maintenance of dialogue is an essential aspect of any constructive human relationship. In the treatment of less disturbed patients who have at least achieved the capacity for symbiosis and, often, have gone beyond it into various stages of autonomy and mutuality, however intrapsychically conflicted, one takes this capacity for granted. With a schizophrenic it is an achievement to be worked at. Moreover, it may be through dialogue with the schizophrenic, analogous to the free association and self-observation of the neurotic, that the unconscious elements of his mind are revealed both to himself and to the therapist. An effective dialectic between therapist and patient may serve both to provide and articulate the elements of integration, reflection and monitoring whose existence we assume in a less disturbed patient. Earlier we noted that the mental content of the schizophrenic is not well integrated or differentiated and that he is not an effective sensorimotor–affective thinker who can readily employ a symbiotic relationship in the process of developing these capacities. To facilitate the sensorimotor–affective thinking of an infant the caregiver instinctively tries to establish a relationship involving sensory-perceptual contact, particularly eye-to-eye, and then to reflect, in a playful manner in which both parties elaborate meaning, both the themes of and the variations on the infant's expressions and productions. Something similar is called for to assist the schizophrenic to organize and identify his own mental contents. He needs visual contact with an attentive, active mirroring person who creates an external analogue of the undeveloped inner capacities for attention, containment, mirroring, organization, and control and for reflective self-awareness and who gradually assists the patient to develop and sustain these mental capacities himself. I believe Winnicott (1971) must have had something similar in mind when he devised his "squiggle game" for interacting with patients.

Insofar as possible—and no matter how bizarre or antisocial the patient's productions—the therapist respectfully attempts to understand what the patient is experiencing and how he sees things, and then tries to rephrase these to him both in order to check their accuracy and in order to provide some small elements of novelty from his unique mirror reflection that might stimulate the patient's self-awareness and elaboration along with the ambivalently and gradually received awareness that the two are separate individuals. By rephrasing what his patient has said the therapist is also assisting him to develop a language that is not so idiosyncratic and obfuscating but is more of a communicative map of his mind, how he sees himself and the world. At the same time that the patient is encouraged to use language in more precise ways, for example, to avoid fusing a special meaning with a common one, the therapist also learns something about the schizophrenic's idiosyncratic language usage. In his efforts to comprehend his patient the therapist might draw some speculative inferences from what the patient is telling him, checking these with a "You mean . . . ?" question. In the early phases, in particular, there are innumerable instances where I believe I have understood my patient only to discover subsequently that I did not.

In my attempts to understand my patient I may perhaps note that additional material seemingly relevant to a subject emerges subsequently in an unintegrated mental fragment, or perhaps I discover that patterns of thought and affect he has been convinced belong to others in the world actually seem more characteristic of his own psychological state or that he has been using common language to express private meanings. In each instance I bring what I have observed to my patient's attention and suggest some appropriate amendation of his views.

In other words, in his efforts to empathize with his patient the therapist inevitably, repeatedly, and often unknowingly dips into a subjective sharing of the patient's undifferentiated world and then reemerges into a more objectified or external stance. Patient and analyst together traverse a succession of approximations and corrections as they get to know the patient's mind better, sometimes making discoveries that are shocking and disturbing to both of them. In this process the mental apparatus, but not the mental content, of one of them—hopefully, the schizophrenic—will become more like that of the other.

Although I am respectful of what the patient tells me—and of his assumption that I understand or that I do not (frequently, the patient is indifferent to my degree of understanding of his verbalizations)—one of my most useful and commonplace interventions is to protest my ignorance of what he means or of what is going on at the moment. I am quick to tell my patient when, as is often the case, I do not understand what he is trying to tell me and quick to encourage him to educate me further, for this is an important element in making him aware that we are separate individuals. Similarly, though my patient in his solipsistic world may objectively seem lively enough, if I feel persistent boredom or disengagement I may remark about it. My patients often come to look upon my state of puzzlement, incomprehension, or drowsiness as a useful index or mirror that something within themselves is unclear or disengaged or disintegrated. By using my own lack of understanding and feelings of disengagement as therapeutic tools I encourage the patient's attention to accompanying aspects of himself, such as posture, gesture, inflection, particular words or ideas, that seem to me inconsistent, incongruous, or simply unrelated to what he claims to be telling me. My intent is to stimulate the use of attention in new ways, and to introduce the idea of reflection, curiosity, inquiry, and integration of disparate or unowned aspects of self. A common consequence of such a dialogue is that the patient discovers he is not so sure of things as he thought, and the foundation for a joint therapeutic inquiry or journey of discovery beginning with our mutual ignorance, has been laid down.

I try to ascertain when my patient's productions are reflective of work toward self-understanding and when they represent avoidance, of contact with others and/or important issues, as well as fragmentation of self. This is especially important as avoidance of his inner life and of others is such a central characteristic of schizophrenia. I do not mean to imply that I attempt to direct the topics of conversation, but I do look upon meaningful associations in a broad context that includes attention to the often subtle vicissitudes of the patient's attention and involvement with me as well as to the content of what he says.

This approach is not so different from classical analysis as it may at first glance appear. Freud's posture of respectful listening to the fantasy, dream, and associative material of his patients in order to traverse with them the "royal road" to dynamic unconscious conflicts did not simply translate into passive listening. First he demonstrated to his patients how to associate (Freud, 1913), and when he judged that resistances were emerging and associations were no longer "free," he then actively intervened and interpreted. Such identification of resistances inevitably involves the analyst's exercise of judgment about when his patient is or is not associating freely as well as his active intervention, which, hopefully, is consistent with the spirit of neutral inquiry. The forces of dis-affinity, of undifferentiation and disintegration, play a role in schizophrenia analogous to that of dynamic resistance in the neuroses. The fundamental difference between resistance and disaffinity is manifest in the nature of the associative process, that is, the associations of the schizophrenic tend to be centrifugal. Relevant elements of mind are not linked, and without linkage there can be no comprehension. By contrast, the associations of the neurotic are centripital; important unconscious linkages are approached until the path is blocked by resistance.

When I encounter primitive cognition (more about this in a moment) and lack of understanding of the analytic process, I become educationally active, supplying ideas and functions that I hope the patient will eventually learn to produce for himself. While this activity expresses some values (maturation to a higher level of function, at least sufficient engagement and involvement with other people to make a minimal social adaptation, persistent reflective attention to one's inner life), it avoids others with regard to choices of meaning, outcome of conflicts, and other life decisions. Moreover, while I attempt to help the patient develop latent therapeutic capacities, I am not trying to be a substitute parent or to demonstrate superiority to his existing family.

In the course of the playful dialogue I am suggesting, meanings and understandings characteristic of the patient's mind are conjointly developed. In retrospect it is often difficult to sort out how exactly they were arrived at and who contributed which elements. I agree with Spence's (1982) perception of the treatment process as the development of a shared narrative, though I do not subscribe to his pessimism about whether the resulting narrative reflects a construction of the patient's world, past and present, that contains some basic truths.

Readers of the case reports in this book may feel frustrated in their efforts to know exactly how particular meanings and positions were arrived at, but from the technical description just offered they will, hopefully, understand some of the reason why this is so. I cannot usually say that the patient arrived at a new idea by himself, yet it is equally unlikely that it came through my interpretation of totally unconscious material, and I would certainly object to the idea that my patient was simply acting as a sponge for my own beliefs. A productive dialogue is one in which the analyst helps the patient elaborate his thoughts at the same time that he maintains another perspective on the cognitive and affective processes and the genesis and adaptive consequences of his way of thinking. Such a dialogue assists the patient to differentiate and to integrate so that he can simultaneously hold in mind two ideas, have perspective and be reflective. This state is difficult to achieve and is readily lost, at least until well along in the course of treatment. I view a therapy session as a creation, a work of art. Each therapy session has a theme (or themes), productive or destructive, and, ideally, both parties should share some understanding of that theme when the hour is up.

Aspects of Dialogue: Play and Humor

As I have intimated, play is an important element of therapeutic dialogue. Melanie Klein (1948) intuitively grasped this fact when she designed her technique for analysis of children, and Winnicott (1971) subsequently wrote about it more formally. That play is important in the therapeutic dialogue is especially true with schizophrenics. It is helpful to adopt a playful attitude toward the therapeutic interchange, recognizing that a drama is unfolding, trying on the roles and their complements that the patient seems to be assigning, and experimenting with meanings. In using the term *play* I am in no way suggesting that the enterprise lacks seriousness; play, even when accompanied by humor, and certainly drama are very serious matters and require work, though the assumption of a playful attitude may make the work seem more like fun. Humor helps to leaven the grimness of the enterprise and to promote reflection and self-observation. It involves experimentation and creativity, and it helps to objectify and defuse narcissistic, egocentric attitudes.

For example, I was supervising the work of a young colleague with a very disturbed, though probably not schizophrenic, patient. He was vexed because his patient openly refused to explore the nature of and reasons for the intense discomfort she experienced prior to therapy sessions; he wanted to confront and admonish her that her conscious wish to talk instead about "trivia"— which she repeatedly attempted to implement, much to his frustration—was "not therapeutic." Indeed, she seemed to resist all his direct efforts at "analysis" and instead, had an agenda all her own for the sessions, an agenda that in other situations, with my help, he had tried to explore with her. On this occasion I suggested that he might help her dramatize her wish to avoid discussion of the painful feelings he thought were important by exploring with her whether he could participate in finding trivial issues, or whether it could in some way be a joint endeavor, in the hopes of seeing what new meanings and understandings this approach might lead to. This more or less forced the patient to take on, with humor, some of the analytic task she wished to exclusively ascribe to and repel in the therapist, as well as to objectify and reflect upon what she had been doing.

As psychotic patients often lack some of the cognitive capacities necessary to appreciate humor—particular, abstract ability and the capacity to view a topic from two simultaneous but integrated perspectives—there is some danger inherent in this enterprise (meanings often have to be clarified) but also some potential for cognitive growth. Most patients have at least a latent capacity for humor, and its cultivation in the course of the treatment goes hand in hand with the development of higher level cognitive skills, including mental integration and the capacity for therapeutic alliance and self-reflection, and usually signifies progress in the work.

Work with Primitive Cognition and Affect Precursors

Insofar as the therapeutic capacities I refer to require more mature thinking than the patient is initially capable of, it is necessary to point out to him aspects of his cognitive limitations as they arise in the course of the therapeutic dialogue (Gedo, 1988; Robbins, 1989; see also Chapters 7, 8, and 9). These include lack of integration (seeming inconsistencies and contradictions; separation or incongruity of thoughts, feelings, and actions; tendencies toward extremist black-and-white thinking); difficulties bearing emotions associated with perceivable affects; difficulties differentiating external from internal, past from present; egocentricity of thought; mental inconstancies (difficulties maintaining constancy of ideas, emotions, and people); and tendencies to deny, distract, and disrupt rather than to focus on the task at hand and elaborate relevant perceptions, affects, and thought processes. It is useful to call attention to omissions as well as commissions, things the patient seems unaware of or unconcerned about, including the state of his emotions and his body and the nature of his relationships with others, however negative.

Dialogue and the Formal Structure of the Therapeutic Situation: Provision of a Holding Environment

Extrapolating from our experience with less disturbed individuals, who have progressed beyond sensorimotor–affective thinking, acquired the capacity for internalized thought, and are ready to communicate with more or less differentiated others, we may be too ready to equate concepts of analysis and of dialogue with verbal interchanges and to dismiss action as antithetical to analysis. However, even with less disturbed patients the central role of enactment in the analytic situation is increasingly being recognized, giving rise to new concepts, such as the holding environment, that are not always and entirely reducible to words.

Especially in the early phases of treatment of a schizophrenic, the twin elements of absent self-care and inability to communicate verbally may require the therapist to provide elements of dialogue that are concrete and physical. Whereas during the analytic process a neurotic patient may be expected to conduct his life in a reasonably autonomous and satisfactory manner, so that the task of the analyst remains confined to assisting him to comprehend the unconscious elements of his mind that represent significant areas of conflict, the schizophrenic cannot be counted on to take reasonable care of himself or even to comprehend the issues that are involved. Moreover, his actions express unconscious elements of his mind that are destructive and maladaptive and that need to be channeled into words and into the confines of a therapeutic relationship where they may eventually be analyzed and understood. In order to help the patient differentiate perception from cognitive–affective process and thought from enactment, a primitive dialectic response that includes physical containment, mirroring, and counteractive limiting or caretaking may be required. Treatment of schizophrenia usually necessitates a variety of interventions that are not classically psychoanalytic, including physical restraint, the use of psychotropic medication, and intervention within the family system. These may be conceptualized as primitive environmental equivalents of the elements that are missing in the patient, elements that would, if present, enable verbal dialogue and, eventually, free association and self-observation.

The therapist may have to provide, particularly in the early stages of treatment, what the patient cannot articulate a need for, namely a holding environment and caretaking functions that may be quite tangible and physical. It is not as if I am eager to undertake the task of regulating my patient's life. Doing so raises moral dilemmas about autonomy and freedom of choice and can quickly become a consuming vocation quite different from the verbal psychotherapy most clinicians prefer. It may also interfere with the patient's capacity to see the therapist as relatively neutral with regard to meanings and as differentiated from others in his life who have infantilized him. The functions of exploration and understanding of a self-destructive phenomenon, on the one hand, and of caretaking in the sense of trying to limit and control that phenomenon, on the other, are to some degree antithetical until the patient is able to differentiate actions from verbalization of thoughts, feelings, and fantasies and to restrain the former and concentrate his expressive and reflective efforts on the latter. In my own work I am able to tolerate a good deal of destructive behavior before intervening in my patient's lives; for example, I try not to involve myself in struggles over such issues as self-starvation or self-mutilation, which often seem to cry out for engagement in conflict and to be exacerbated when it is provided. On the other hand, at times when I judge that serious risk to my patient's well-being or to the continuity of the therapeutic enterprise is involved, I make this clear, and I am willing to act, if necessary, to reduce it. During virtually every treatment of a schizophrenic with which I have been associated, and despite my intentions and best efforts to maintain a more mature posture of nonintervention, I have found that exigencies arise in which continued abstention seems to signify either an inhumane indifference to the patient or else a complicity through denial with his self-destructiveness. In order to minimize role confusions and conflicts it is better for the therapist, wherever possible, not to take on these holding and caretaking functions himself. For this reason, and because basic failures of self-care and serious self-destructive activity are characteristic of untreated schizophrenics, it is difficult if not impossible to treat a schizophrenic in the acute phases of illness without the assistance of a third party, such as a hospital, including such prescriptive actions on the part of hospital staff as limit setting and various forms of intervention into the physical life of the patient. (These matters are discussed at length in Chapter 16.) The relative separation of functions that hospitalization affords gives the therapist opportunity to devote maximum time and energy to what he does best.

I do not mean to imply that my more concrete or primitive dialectic responses are always intentional and planned. An example of an unwitting response, which at the time I considered to be a significant therapeutic gaffe, was my expression of shock and horror—probably with a mild expletive, when I came onto the ward for a therapy session with Emily and found that, because she had been uncontrollably destructive, she had been placed in restraints, in the quiet room, in a position that seemed to me quite degrading, and then had to decide whether or not to try to conduct the planned session with her under those circumstances. Years later it became apparent that the elements of my response, ultimately crucial to her self-care, had been missing in her own mind and that both my impulsive expression of concern and my remaining with her had been very helpful to her. Had I "controlled" myself better and made a rational comment, or perhaps cancelled the appointment because of the unpropitious circumstances, I am certain it would not have been nearly as effective.

Dialogue and the Psychoanalytic Method: A Reprise

The analytic stance with a schizophrenic, then, is more active than with a neurotic, involving engagement to compensate for the patient's disengagement, and dialogue with a verbally mirroring and at times physically active (in person or by proxy) therapist in lieu of the patient's missing capacities for self-care, delay, thought, and self-observation.

To those who object that such a posture is not neutral and therefore not psychoanalytic, I respond that it is now more generally accepted that the psychoanalyst is not simply a neutral observer who occasionally speculates about the meaning of things and that he should not aspire to be (Gill, 1984; Gedo, 1988; Levenson, 1989). Provision of face-to-face interaction, including visual contact and mirroring dialogue in lieu of encouragement of associations, not only does not alter the traditional position of analyst in relation to patient in any fundamental way but actually enables the analyst to achieve a kind of contact with the schizophrenic that is roughly analogous to the partnership with a neurotic patient, if psychologically more primitive.

Empathy, Dialogue, and the Danger of Therapist Insanity

Such experienced therapists of psychosis as Searles (1965) and Winnicott (1947, 1960b) believe that in the process of treatment the schizophrenic attempts to drive the analyst crazy. I look upon this elaboration of the psychoanalytic concepts of transference and countertransference as one of the more profound contributions to our understanding of therapy with schizophrenics. It is no accident that there are relatively few analysts who work intensively with schizophrenics, for willingness to attempt empathic involvement with such individuals brings with it the threat to the therapist of unrecognized loss of his sanity. I use the term *unrecognized* advisedly, and despite its possible redundancy (for it is a characteristic of being crazy that one is unaware or but dimly aware of the fact), and I think that many therapists who work with schizophrenics experience encapsulated psychoses in the relationship for greater or lesser periods of time. I shall return to this issue repeatedly throughout the remainder of the section on treatment, as I believe it is one of the major elements in the stalemates that seem to characterize so many efforts to work with schizophrenics.

The remarkable states of disturbance I experienced early in Celia's treatment—when first she insisted she had never hallucinated but was simply deceiving me and then later, and with equal conviction, asserted the opposite—illustrate my own efforts to maintain my sanity. In Chapter 15 I cite instances when I discovered I had been unwittingly collusive with patients for long periods of time and thus began to emerge from encapsulated psychosis.

The analyst is bound to respond to his patient's often convincing presentation of fragmented, poorly differentiated, distorted material by attempting to make sense of it. The schizophrenic's lack of psychic integration leads him to present *pars pro toto* thinking instead of intrapsychic conflict and ambivalence, resulting in an ever-changing sense of reality, as well as affect, ideation and motoric expression, which appear unlinked with one another. His absence of psychic differentiation leads him to present to the analyst, as if it were real, a concocted world, not simply one with ordinary expectable distortions but one with wholesale substitutions or inversions of subjective and objective elements, often convincingly rationalized. His sensorimotor–affective or enactive mode of thought leads him to speak in action language and to place pressure on the analyst to participate. The therapist's wish to be empathic and helpful, combined with reflexive efforts to avert a disturbing subjective experience of chaos may lead him to take his patient's experience at face value and to rationalize away or forget the more bizarre aspects. Therapists whose empathy leads them to this form of shared insanity often tend to see their patients as relatively normal, perhaps even exceptional, and to wonder why others do not share this perception, a not uncommon source of disagreement on hospital wards.

An apparent alternative to the insidious slippage from reality that I am describing is for the therapist to reject his patient's productions as making no sense at all. Such rejection may be overt or may take more subtle forms such as labeling the patient as "crazy." Were such rejection direct and final little harm might be done, but when the therapist maintains the outward trappings of psychotherapy, the results may be more subtle and harmful (and reminiscent of the familial double binds described in Chapter 10). Efforts to separate the presumably normal patient whom the therapist can care about from the frightening state of insanity that must be rejected involve the therapist's looking upon the illness as an affliction by a bizarre and incomprehensible "it." Seemingly innocuous therapeutic questions such as "Do you still hear voices, and what do you do about it when that happens?" may have the effect of fostering disintegration of mind. The aim of such treatments is that the patient develop a socially compliant adaptable facade. While this kind of therapy, based on the belief that the patient is suffering from an external disease process, is currently looked upon with favor by many, it may involve a circumscribed area of avoidance, due to thoughtlessness or defensiveness, within the therapist who allows himself to view reality as the patient does, that is, from the perspective of nonintegration, instead of attempting to help the patient view reality from an integrated perspective.

Finally, the therapist may counterattack the psychotic patient and attempt to control him with his own presumably superior mind, as, for example, in the case of respected analysts like Rosen and some of Klein's followers, who have tended to present themselves as deities or gurus, pontificating interpretations of the deepest recesses of the mind after the briefest of contact with their patients and firing their interpretive six-guns from the hip as soon as they can see the figurative whites of their patient's eyes. However factually correct the interpretations, such activity too readily fits schizophrenic undifferentiation, manifestly expressed in beliefs about mind reading, and stimulates in the patient passivity and compliant introjective acceptance of attributions, setting the stage for pathological symbiotic forms of collusion, or, as Winnicott termed it, analysis with the false self. Mythology about the ready accessibility of the schizophrenic unconscious notwithstanding, and judging from the many years and innumerable wrong turns it usually takes me to get any reliable, consistent sense of what my patients are about, I think in most instances these fragile interpretations are probably inaccurate. If by chance they should be accurate, they are mere words, delivered defensively (or offensively), without the achievement of a deeper emotional attunement between patient and therapist or of a capacity on the part of the schizophrenic to reflect meaningfully about what is said to him. What such therapists may in fact be doing is to circumvent dialogue and to present themselves to patients who inhabit solipsistic, undifferentiated psychic worlds in an almost equally solipsistic manner, backed by the power and authority of the society and institution they represent. This solipsism represents the therapist's responsive insanity and serves to maintain schizophrenic undifferentiation while substituting some of the therapist's mental content for that of the patient.

This problem of well-intentioned empathy or defenses against the threats posed by empathy, which, unrecognized, progresses not in the direction of therapeutic working through but rather toward a folie à deux and a masked circumscribed area of psychosis within both patient and therapist, is not readily addressed by prescriptive technique. Invariably, particularly in the early stages of any relationship, silences, ambiguous comments, and even seemingly clear statements alike are imbued by both parties with poorly differentiated meanings that are not readily clarified. I try to keep in mind that because of my patient's primitiveness or lack of integration and differentiation my sense of what is going on with him at any given moment (and his sense of what is going on with me) are probably both incomplete and inaccurate in fundamental ways. Thus, I am naturally suspicious about the experience of feeling perfectly attuned with my patient to begin with, and when such a feeling is abruptly disrupted, and I feel shocked, tricked, confused, or even a bit crazy, I am, hopefully, not quite so distressed as I might otherwise be. For example, a patient may abruptly and dogmatically assert a set of beliefs and feelings utterly contradictory to those uttered only moments before (or perhaps contradictory to those on which he and his therapist have been basing their work for some time) and then act as though nothing were amiss. Or he may suddenly inform the therapist that the latter attacked or rejected him when the therapist feels he has been most understanding.

Somehow, the therapist must remain sufficiently flexible to bear and reflect upon the resulting disturbance in his own sense of a coherent, cohesive self—an incipient micropsychosis, if you will—and perhaps selectively to comment about it to the patient, without gullibly and totally believing his patient's perceptions, enacting his own disturbance in some gross way, or defensively rejecting the experience (a) by counterassaulting the patient and telling him that he is crazy, (b) by distancing himself from the patient's experience by referring to the "craziness" as an "it," or (c) prematurely and rigidly organizing it into some theoretical system. He must even consider the possibility that the micropsychosis was the previous state of apparent harmony and that the disruption represents the patient's effort to restore sanity. Throughout, the therapist must retain a genuine and lively curiosity and must remain willing and able to tolerate not "really" knowing, being at turns surprised and even shocked, and struggling to reorganize his own comprehension. In this important way he provides a model for the patient, who will similarly be called upon to question and reorganize his own mind in ways that may retain its idiosyncracy as it becomes more personally constructive and socially adaptable.

The purpose of this activity on the part of the therapist is, of course, to gradually develop a shared or empathic perspective from which he can begin to address his patient in a more useful way. Perhaps at times he will recall relevant aspects of his patient's mind that the patient has temporarily "forgotten" and be an informed or expert participant-observer in his patient's inner life, one who understands how the patient thinks and feels and why but at the same time can suggest some additional perspective or vantage point having to do with the difference between conditions of the past and the present or between adaptative or maladaptive consequences of certain ways of thinking and behaving. Such truly empathic activity is by no means always welcomed by the schizophrenic—as it is in Kohut's reports of his work with narcissistic personalities—because it may involve bringing to the patient's attention potential aspects of his psyche that are unintegrated or undifferentiated and that he is fundamentally averse to knowing about, bearing and assimilating.

I would like to conclude this section on technique by reiterating that because therapy involves art as well as science and because the artists in this case—the therapist and the patient—have unique personalities, there is no single "correct" way to approach the treatment of a schizophrenic. One may learn general principles but not cookbook recipes. Many of those who have reported success with schizophrenics recommend different approaches. Sullivan, for example, apparently avoided eye contact with his patients. While Giovachinni (1983) and Boyer (1983) believe as I do that schizophrenia involves structural defects or deficits, they approach their patients in an inactive, adaptive, tolerant manner very different from my own, and have them use a traditional analytic couch so that eye contact is not possible. Pao (1979) reported success with what he described as a seemingly limitless, unconditional approach to treatment, regardless of motivation and realities of time and resources, in which the therapist seems satisfied by whatever the patient has to offer in response to his efforts, however minimal or insignificant this may seem to the observer.

After describing typical phases and issues in the therapeutic process in the chapter to follow, I shall return to the issues of process and technique for a final comment on the question of whether what I am describing may be considered psychoanalysis.

Chapter 15

The Psychological Perspective: Stages of Therapy

Beginning with what I have referred to as the protosymbiotic configuration of the schizophrenic mind, the therapy of schizophrenia proceeds as follows: engagement in pathological symbiosis, disengagement from pathological symbiosis, engagement in more normal symbiosis, and disengagement from symbiosis of any kind, meaning that mental processes and necessary self-care and adaptive functions have become sufficiently internalized so that termination of therapy is possible. The process is diagrammed schematically in Figure 4 on page 259.

Motivation

We concluded the discussion of evaluation and treatment planning in Chapter 12 with the proposition that it is motivation, more than any other single factor, that distinguishes schizophrenics who can be treated successfully using a psychological focus from those who cannot be treated. Now we may add that it is in the initial phases of engagement in pathological symbiosis and subsequent disengagement from it that the role of motivation is most apparent, and that these determinations of treatability are made.

In introducing the discussion it is sobering to admit that today we do not know much more about why some schizophrenics can benefit from treatment and others cannot than we did many years ago. For example, one of the best known contemporary statements about motivation—Strauss, Carpenter, and Bartko's 1974 prognostic distinction between so-called positive and negative symptom patients—is but a rebottling of the century-old wine of Hughlings Jackson (1931–1932). Federn's (1934) assertion of nearly 60 years ago, that "psychotic patients are accessible to psychoanalysis . . . first, because and in so far as they are still capable of transference, secondly, because and in so far as one part of their ego has insight into their abnormal state, and thirdly, because and in so far as a part of their personality is directed toward reality" (p. 210) is as applicable now as it was then.

Our initial assessment will enable us to exclude as untreatable by therapy which has a psychological focus that group of patients who, despite manifestations of bizarre and disturbing mental life and behavior, seem to want only stereotypic object-interchangeable interactions with the environment along with basic caretaking; who present a preponderance of the "negative" symptoms of apathy, withdrawal, passivity, and flatness; and who demonstrate total disinterest in integrating and differentiating their thoughts and feelings. These persons are candidates for treatment consisting of medication, prescriptive limited living arrangements, and rehabilitation, in proportions to be determined according to the treatment planning schema of Chapter 12. Those in whom we elicit motivation to get relief from distress through an interaction with another person, that is, to move from protosymbiosis to an active, albeit pathological, symbiotic engagement or collusion, may potentially benefit from our further efforts.

The Initial Phase of Engagement: A Historical Perspective

As an introduction to the discussion of engagement in a symbiotic relationship, I would like to survey and comment on some of the various ingenious efforts that have been made to engage schizophrenic patients. Commentary on the iatrogenic complications consequent to some of these methods will serve as an introduction to an elaboration of the idea that the symbiotic relationship that is the outcome of successful engagement of a schizophrenic is necessarily both pathological and collusive on the part of both participants.

The effort to engage schizophrenics in a constructive relationship dates back at least to the era of moral treatment, to its standard-bearers, Tuke and Pinel. Mothering or remothering forms of treatment were among the first techniques and consisted of attempts to supply the patient with friendship, caretaking, wish gratification, freedom from stress, and the like, all of which were believed to be missing ingredients. When Nunberg (1921) and Federn (1934, 1952) emphasize the importance of preserving, or not interpreting, the "positive transference" and of avoiding rage or other "negative" and disruptive emotions, they seem to mean more than eschewing interpretation of so-called positive elements of patient feeling toward the analyst. Some of Federn's patients actually lived with him, and he gratified their oral wishes by such things as feeding them candy. In the early phase of her career Fromm-Reichmann (1939) perceived the schizophrenic as especially delicate and in need of coddling. From her own pre-self-psychological perspective she employed a permissive, emotionally giving approach and discouraged stressful confrontation. Schwing (1940), a pupil of Federn, and Sechehaye (1951) carried this philosophy of treatment to its most extreme form by encouraging patients to express their dependencies and then attempting to gratify them. Schwing offered her patients love, deliberately acted motherly, and provided food, grooming, and kisses. Sechehaye asserted that schizophrenia is the result of deprivation of maternal love, and she practiced a form of gratification therapy that she called "symbolic realization"—a somewhat misleading term, for while she acknowledged that it was impossible for her patients literally to return to infancy to obtain what they had allegedly been deprived of, she attempted to supply them with the best possible substitute she could devise. Some of the "symbols" she offered them were compellingly concrete and immediate, particularly to a schizophrenic (for example, pretending an apple is a breast). Sechehaye (1951) wrote, "It was necessary to go again through the entire evolution, beginning by obliterating the effect of the original traumata. This could not have been done without a transference to a new mother, who brought 'gifts of love' . . . by the substitution of a giving (loving) mother for a depriving (hating) mother" (p. 142). Whitaker and Malone (1953) utilized her technique and literally treated their patients as though they were infants, providing bottle-feeding, rocking, spanking, and the like, activities that were even accompanied by the sharing of fantasies (or perhaps delusions?) that these elements are, in fact, part of a parent–child relationship. Reading these accounts I am impressed by their authors' conceptions of good mothering, which seem to me more like extreme indulgence.

It is ironic in light of current psychiatric repudiation of such ideas, based on the belief that they are regressive, that this point of view is insidiously achieving credibility within popular psychiatry once again, this time cloaked in neuroscience data (such as those presented in Chapter 7) suggesting that schizophrenics may be uniquely unable to modulate and control incoming stimulation and need somehow to be protected or sheltered and tranquilized or soothed. Such activities are theoretically compatible with Alexander's advocacy of the value of "corrective emotional experience"; with Kohut's (1971) position that developmentally prior to the achievement of self-cohesion the psyche is fragmented, and that what is needed is a selfobject relationship within which cohesion may occur; and with the view of Gedo and Goldberg (1973), and Gedo (1979a) that because the most primitive form of pathology stems from failure of tension regulation, the prescribed form of intervention may be soothing or pacification. While in some instances such an approach has been successful, sometimes strikingly so, the patients are in fact adults, and the cost of the indulgence necessary to achieve engagement may be the fostering of a regressive transference–countertransference replication of the infantilization, with simultaneously grandiose and devalued identity attribution (described in Chapter 10), that is typical of the pathological family response to the schizophrenic member. In other words, this may be another example of so-called treatment that under more careful scrutiny turns out to be a reenactment of the disease process.

Rosen (1947, 1953) employed some of these re-mothering techniques in an approach he called "direct analysis," whereby in the acute phase the therapist might spend several hours a day feeding, bathing, and grooming the patient. There is no question that Rosen and others who utilized his methods also had some unusual successes in engaging patients. Rosen claimed to have cured 37 of almost 100 patients he treated with this method, in periods of time averaging 2 to 3 months! But direct analysis is best known for elements that seem, from their very authoritarian and even assaultive qualities, antithetical to the approach of therapists like Schwing and Sechehaye. Scheflen (1960), a student of Rosen, attributed his success to a combination of aggression and promises made to the patient that he would be released from the hospital as soon as he became able to care for himself. Follow-up studies of Rosen's cases by Horwitz, Polatin, Kolb, and Hoch (1958) and Bookhammer, Meyers, Shober, and Piotrowski (1966) indicated that the long-term results were very poor. In fact, Rosen was not interested in the working-through phases of treatment that followed the engagement he was able to make: after his patients emerged from the out-of-contact state, he would typically transfer them to his students for continued treatment. I am not surprised at the failure of his method to provide lasting change; it seems likely that his patients were at least in part responding compliantly and self-protectively to psychic trauma, perhaps accompanied by seduction, and then subsequently to disappointment and abandonment. Such a method is more likely to solidify their underlying beliefs about the harmful and solipsistic or nonmutual nature of human relationships than it is to provide a foundation for further constructive object relatedness. The capacity of schizophrenics to mobilize themselves, transiently, in response to trauma, is well known. A colleague recently told me an anecdote from his psychiatric residency training years. He was on a ward composed of regressed patients when one set himself on fire with a match he had been given to light his cigarette. My colleague and the other mental health professionals on the ward remained paralyzed with shock and horror, but another regressed patient rushed over to put out the blaze, remarking as he did so, "Are you guys crazy? Why don't you do something? This guy is burning up!"

Eissler (1951) wrote an interesting review of the various approaches to engaging the regressed schizophrenic, approaches he characterized as ranging from more or less permissive and "loving," through stringent and limit-setting, to shocking and psychically assaultive. He was intrigued with Rosen's direct analysis technique but was cautious about endorsing it; instead, drawing on his limited experience treating schizophrenics in the military service, he advocated firm limit setting.

In 1952 Fromm-Reichmann altered her position. While she continued to believe that schizophrenics were very special people in terms of sensitivity and insightfulness, she now said of her previous advocacy of protective care and coddling, that "this type of doctor–patient relationship addresses itself too much to the rejected child in the schizophrenic and too little to the grown up person." (p. 106). She added that "understanding of that which has been done to the patient in his early years sooner or later must be followed up by the investigation of what, in turn, the patient has done to his environment" (p. 106). Implicit in her statement is the idea that schizophrenia is not simply an instance of arrested infantile development or absent parenting; that the schizophrenic is not an infant inhabiting an adult body. Now, for the first time, she advocated setting limits to patients' violence, she respectfully declined to offer them love or even friendship, and she addressed her therapeutic comments to the adult part of the personality rather than to the hitherto imagined child within. What she said in her 1952 paper, which I believe is important in any psychoanalytic treatment but critical in the therapy of schizophrenia, is that treatment "must be accompanied . . . by a consistent scrutiny of, and alertness to, the vicissitudes of the state of relatedness to the patient in which the psychoanalyst is involved" (p. 93). It seems that Knight (1953), Sullivan (1956, 1962), and Searles (1965) would agree that what the therapist has to offer is not love or mothering but a particular form of sensitive responsiveness to the vicissitudes of the patient's state of awareness and relatedness. Sullivan, for example, was active and confrontational; he told his patients some of his feelings about them, and he gave them corrective feedback about their cognitive distortions of reality.

Searles (1965) used some of Melanie Klein's contributions in formulating what has been perhaps the richest description of what he called the "out-of-contact phase" and its treatment. According to Searles, the schizophrenic has regressed to an infantile state of self–object undifferentiation and lack of integration. In this state his behavior is bizarre, he is alienated from others, and he lacks feeling, though he is enacting hatred. Because his sense of identity is invested in the psychotic state, therapeutic contact threatens his sense of individuality. Searles advised a neutral investigative analytic attitude and suggested that the analyst feel free to fantasize, read, and otherwise occupy himself when his patient is disengaged.

At this juncture I would like to digress briefly to examine two beliefs about schizophrenics that critically affect the stance of the therapist in the phase of engagement. The first of these is the belief of Fromm-Reichmann, Searles, and others that schizophrenia is the manifestation of regression to infantile mentation. If it is correct, then perhaps there is reason to model therapeutic behavior after good parenting—which, by the way, entails much beyond caretaking and indulgence; if not, some of the therapeutic efforts to engage patients, modeled after a caricature or fantasy of good parenting, may have unexpected untoward consequences. In formulating a technique of engagement it may be more useful to examine the unique elements that constitute primitive schizophrenic mentation. While there are superficial similarities between the infantile mind and that of the schizophrenic, such as the presence of undifferentiation and the absence of a cohesive self, schizophrenia is not ordinary infancy in disguise but a state of disability comprising unique sensory-perceptual, cognitive, affective, behavioral and relationship problems. Good treatment must make a clear distinction between the two.

A second belief with which I differ is that the schizophrenic, in contrast to the heavily defended neurotic, has an extraordinary access to and understanding of his unconscious mental life (Fromm-Reichmann, 1952). As I have indicated previously, I think that the schizophrenic is severely cognitively and affectively impaired and that the conviction that he possesses special understanding of the workings of his mind is part of the subtle grandiose investment therapists who work successfully with schizophrenics tend to make in their patients, which replicates the kind of investment made in them by their families (see Chapter 10).

While such beliefs may serve to motivate the therapist during the phase of engagement by romanticizing or idealizing his work, they constitute the therapist's contribution to the resultant pathological symbiosis, which we shall shortly examine, and they stand as impediments to eventual disengagement.

The sobering conclusion that emerges from decades of experimentation is that radical departures from a basic analytic attitude are largely ineffective, and that even in those instances where they appear to facilitate a relationship they introduce into that relationship obstacles so formidable that further therapeutic work may be rendered impossible. What all these methods of engaging patients seem to have in common is the unconscious therapeutic collusion with, or participation in the primitive mental world of, the schizophrenic, which I described in the previous chapter as a pitfall of efforts to be empathic.

Some Proposals to Facilitate the Phase of Engagement

To begin with, the prospective therapist of a schizophrenic should be alert for any sign his patient may convey that his solipsistic universe is unsatisfactory, any evidence of distress sufficiently great that the patient may be open to real assistance. While it is the patient's subjective experience of distress that is at issue, I must emphasize that the distress to which I refer is not equivalent to his symptomatic clamor; it is an example of the naive empathy I discussed in the preceding chapter to infer therapeutic motivation and a wish for help simply from the presence of a bizarre whirlwind of symptomatology and behavior, including self-destructive activities. Judging from the retrospective reports of patients, who have informed me repeatedly that the acutely symptomatic state was not nearly so disturbing to them as it appeared to be to others, it is misleading to assume that the pain experienced by the naively empathic observer is a measure of the patient's motivation. In fact, the symbiotic partner of the schizophrenic may experience the distress that the patient does not seem to feel; this was the case with Emily's mother, who even claimed that she felt the pain of Emily's slashed wrists, which seemed to bother Emily not at all.

Considerations of how one understands the schizophrenic's overtly disturbed state, and how one determines motivation, lead to the need to review the commonplace practice of heavy medication of newly hospitalized schizophrenic patients, with the goal of symptom amelioration and "euthymia." In Chapter 11 I made the point that from a social systems perspective the disease process and its treatment may not be as different as we wish to believe. The failure to differentiate the treating person from the patient, which leads to unconsciously determined overmedication in order to minimize the suffering of the treaters, is an example. It is becoming increasingly difficult to convince anyone in a position of responsibility in the average mental hospital of the reasonableness of tolerating a ward of patients who are manifestly more disturbed than they might otherwise be if full advantage is taken of the "state of the art" of psychopharmacology. Heavy tranquilization may reduce disturbance but it leaves patients in an indifferent, unmotivated condition. The question of whether to medicate during the evaluation process is not unlike the medical problem of differential diagnosis of an acute abdomen; one's empathic senses cry out for the administration of a narcotic, but one's diagnostic acumen responds that this would be the worst possible thing to do. These issues are elaborated in Chapter 18.

In taking inventory of the patient's wish for help from another person it is also important to distinguish stereotypic repetitive patterns of approach to others which consist of enactments of delusional scenarios and are not psychologically differentiated from those that take note of specific people and elements of the potentially therapeutic environment. Schizophrenics often engage in stereotypic, repetitive pestering or nagging patterns that have the superficial appearance of requests for dialogue or for help. In these instances the identity of the object—and in this instance the analytic term is quite apt—is completely interchangeable. Edward, for example, looked for a debating partner, ideally a woman to enact one or another side of his own unintegrated, projected contradictions, whom he might then "analyze," and almost anyone would do. Judging from his conversations with me, I believe nothing such a person might have said would have made an iota of difference in Edward's thinking, nor did any of these antagonists ever achieve anything approaching a separate identity in his mind. The therapist must look instead for manifestations of a desire on the patient's part for something more differentiated and scarce than what an interchangeable other can provide, something the patient may be willing to work to acquire and to retain. The resulting interpersonal tension is the context and the fuel for an initial and provisional therapeutic contract in which the therapist offers to try to help but, from the start, assigns the patient a working collaborative role. Emily was in this kind of distress; she could discriminate people who seemed to "understand" her and to have the potential to relieve her from those who did not. In retrospect, she really wanted from another person more of the infantilizing narcotic her mother had offered; this want was basically an aspect of her passive symbiotic collusion with mother; nonetheless, she was discriminating in her choice of a person with whom to re-enact this scenario. Rachel also seemed to want help with self-esteem and assertiveness, and while, for a time, it seemed as though she could discriminate me from others, retrospectively it seems people other than father were interchangeable. In both these instances the apparent capacity for some specificity in a relationship enabled the start of a pathological symbiosis. In contrast, to the extent I responded to Edward's agenda I only found myself becoming more confused and disorganized, and no dialogue was ever possible.

Medicated or not, some patients seem fixed in or content with their situation and repel human contact in any form. One of my supervisors in residency training was fond of likening the art of relating to such "sealed-off" (or what we would now call "negative symptom") schizophrenics to sitting perfectly still on a park bench, waiting and hoping that the squirrel gamboling about might eventually come and feed from your hand. Implicit in his metaphor is the presumption that the withdrawn schizophrenic has a more or less intact capacity to distinguish others from himself and to differentiate helpful from harmful others, as well as an intact curiosity, an innate desire to relate, and a cognitive capacity to learn from experience, all of which capacities, given time and patience, might mitigate against his presumed fearfulness and mistrust. But imputing such capabilites to a schizophrenic is not consistent with the intrapsychic and interpersonal features of the illness outlined in Chapters 7 and 9. Schizophrenia is not simply a manifestation of exaggerated timidity or unfamiliarity; such a belief is another example of the pitfalls of overreliance on empathy as a mode of understanding, a belief that might be corrected by recourse to a hierarchical systems theory of mind.

In Chapter 9 I described the protosymbiotic state that characterizes the untreated schizophrenic in his initial encounters with a prospective therapist. In contrast to the primitive personality (who engages with another person readily if pathologically), the schizophrenic lacks the capacity for assertive, aggressive, object-seeking and engagement; lacks object relation configurations that can be represented, transferred, and sustained, and does not seem to differentiate among persons. The initial phase of engagement with a schizophrenic involves work with some of his basic cognitive and affective problems toward the following objectives: differentiation of familiarity and strangeness, integration of externalized elements, development of stable internal representational templates and a degree of self-constancy, mobilization of bonding and social initiative, and mobilization of aggression and rage, which have hitherto been expressed primarily in unrepresented, nonsocial, delusional, and self-destructive ways. For example, all of the patients in this book were initially unable to perceive me as strange or unfamiliar. Even Joanna, who had the most unusual perception of me as a robot, turned out to perceive everyone similarly—as machines. The most differentiated response came from Emily, the patient with the best outcome, who seemed to believe that I understood her better than her previous therapist, although at the same time she showed no stranger anxiety on meeting me, and in retrospect probably did not differentiate me from her mother, who in turn was not well differentiated by Emily from herself.

While it is doubtless true that other cognitive and affective problems, including development of the capacity for intrapsychic conflict, affective ambivalence, and object constancy, must be worked out in succeeding stages of treatment (and we shall return to these later in this chapter), some of the most fundamental issues must be confronted at the very beginning and, paradoxically, in the context of the most tenuous of human alliances. This focus on pathology of cognition and affect, in the context of pathological object relations, characterizes my approach to each phase of the psychotherapy of a schizophrenic. While it has been commonplace to speak of the schizophrenic's withdrawal from reality (Semrad taught that schizophrenia is the sacrifice of reality to preserve life), my view is that basic normal cognitive and affective capacities are undeveloped; that, in accord with Bion's view, their anlage undergo constant self-destructive attack; and that the early adaptation which led to such an ongoing self-attack is responsible for other significant cognitive distortions. I am also in agreement with Bion, in contrast to another widely held view, that insight (I would call it learning about oneself) is an essential ingredient in the recovery process.

Contrast the cognitive and relationship disturbance encountered in the first phase of treatment of a schizophrenic with that in the treatment of a primitive personality. There the initial problem for the therapist, particularly if the patient is a borderline, is one of disengagement from a powerfully possessive patient who clings aggressively and makes active efforts to reduce the therapist to an object without a life of his own, while simultaneously and self-destructively re-introjecting projectively distorted aspects of the therapist's behavior and thinking and attempting to comply with them. While the absence of such a socially directed and aggressive possessor configuration makes engagement with a schizophrenic difficult, it may also be responsible for my observation, which violates common sense, that once the patient is engaged, the outcome of treatment may be both better and quicker for the schizophrenic than for the patient with a primitive personality disorder. The schizophrenic may manifest less fixed and virulent object-specific hostility and projection, whereas the transference of the primitive personality may be dominated for years by the destructive activity of a possessor configuration. Affects may be easier for the schizophrenic to own and internalize. And the basic relationship template of the schizophrenic, the compliant possessed configuration, may ultimately prove to be socially adaptive, particularly in females, as the cases of Emily, Joanna, and Celia illustrate.

If the therapist is successful in engaging the schizophrenic in a relationship it will not be a normal growth-promoting symbiosis but a pathological one, characterized by unconscious collusion by both parties to repeat the patient's early experience. While problems associated with the initial phase of engagement have garnered most of the attention in the therapeutic literature, the achievement of engagement far from guarantees the success of the enterprise. This hitherto silent problem of symbiotic collusion accounts for the fact that in so many instances therapy of schizophrenia becomes chronically stalemated. Little has been written about the problem—or, for that matter, about subsequent stages of therapy—so that most therapists feel satisfied if they are able to form and maintain chronic relationships with schizophrenics and relatively few seriously expect the process to eventuate in a successful termination with a relatively mature and independent individual. Many therapists who have repeatedly met with the same experience of stalemate eventually turn to other kinds of work. In other words, the problems of the second stage of treatment have been enacted much more than they have been verbalized; in fact, the very existence of the problem of pathological symbiotic collusion on which much of our attention in this chapter will be focused, has hitherto not been clearly recognized. An examination of pathological symbiosis and collusion will help us to comprehend more about what it is that motivates schizophrenics to become involved in a therapy relationship to begin with.

The Symbiotic Stage: Searles's Contribution

In a moment we shall review the second stage of therapy, pathological symbiosis, but first I would like to review and critique some of the work of Harold Searles (1965), who synthesized the work of Margaret Mahler and Melanie Klein and first applied the concept of symbiosis to the psychological treatment of schizophrenia.

Searles shares Mahler's belief that schizophrenic pathology involves regression to a normal developmental phase of infancy, symbiotic or autistic. Searles divides the symbiotic development of schizophrenics in the course of therapy, following their successful engagement, into three parts: a stage of what he calls ambivalent symbiosis,* characterized by unintegrated, contradictory, projected expressions of hatred and love that are mirrored in the therapist's equally extreme and variable countertransference responses; a stage of full, or what he calls "pre-ambivalent symbiosis," in which patient and

---

*Searles appears to use the terms *ambivalent* and *pre-ambivalent* in a somewhat idiosyncratic way. It is my impression that he derives his usage from Bleuler (1911), who defined ambivalence as the simultaneous existence of contradictory affective predispositions and considered it to be one of the fundamental characteristics of schizophrenia. In this usage both Searles and Bleuler emphasize the schizophrenic's characteristic lack of integration of elements, which I noted in Chapters 8 and 10; Bleuler stresses their simultaneous manifestion, Searles their alternation. My personal experience is that the latter form of absent integration (the alternation or oscilllation) is more common in primitive personality organization and in the more chronic phases of schizophrenia and the former is more common in the more acute phases of schizophrenia. My own definition of ambivalence differs from that of both authors and is more consistent with the current glossary of the American Psychoanalytic Association, *Psychoanalytic Terms and Concepts* (Moore & Fine, 1990), the Kleinian position, and ordinary dictionary usage. In this way of thinking ambivalence refers to simultaneous

therapist enjoy a nurturant experience that is happy and blissful for both of them, presumably like that of the infant and its good mother; and a stage of resolution of the symbiotic attachment, which concludes with termination.

Searles's formulation seems to combine elements of Klein's intrapsychic theory with Mahler's interpersonal theory of the normal symbiotic phase of infancy. His first two phases, ambivalent and pre-ambivalent symbiosis, correspond approximately to Klein's paranoid-schizoid and depressive positions, respectively. I agree with Searles and Klein that rage and hatred play an important part in the schizophrenic's mental life and in the most primitive stage of his relationships. Searles has attempted to reconcile this fact with the development of a blissful, anger-free relationship with his patients in the course of therapy. In order to view this latter configuration as progress he has likened it to Mahler's normal infantile stage of symbiosis. He maintains that effective therapy enables the patient to progress from a paranoid-schizoid part-object position—which is characterized by what he terms ambivalence and Kleinians call pre-ambivalent splitting, that is, inconstant and contradictory extremes in which the therapist is repeatedly psychically annihilated with rage—to a depressive or what he calls "pre-ambivalent" whole-object position (which Kleinians would call "ambivalent"), where the object representation of the therapist is preserved at the cost of the patient's internalization of and control over his painful emotions of rage and guilt.

In its all-good experiential quality, however, the full, or pre-ambivalent, symbiotic position that Searles describes differs from Klein's depressive position, in which the integrity and continuity of the relationship with the love-object is always threatened by the subject's anger and envy, which have begun, precariously, to be internalized. In Klein's theory, as a consequence of having to deal with his anger, the normal infant's struggle to maintain a state of positive object feeling about mother depends on a growing capacity to experience guilt and the wish to make reparation; thus, the depressive position is one of struggle and angst, not a state of bliss. Mahler's normal infants do not have to deal with excessive and prolonged experiences of rage, and Klein's normal infants in the depressive position do not experience unmitigated bliss. Therefore, it is not clear what Searles's schizophrenics who experience a

---

awareness of conflicting emotional positions, with some integrative capacity to reflect and mediate between them. It is a more mature position than either of Searles's positions (ambivalence or pre-ambivalence) for there exists a mediating integrative capacity and a consequent intrapsychic awareness of conflict. Because of the borderline's higher level of integration—in which large units of thinking and feeling, identified with self, exist unintegrated with similar but contradictory units—he presents an illusion of meaningful self-directness but, in fact, repeats cyclothymic oscillations, whereas the schizophrenic, particularly in the more acute phases of illness, is so fragmented that his simultaneous unintegrated contradictions may leave him literally paralyzed or blocked. If I were to describe Searles's phases in my own language, I would say that a stage of pre-ambivalent symbiosis or splitting, which is not a normal developmental analogue, is succeeded by a more normal stage of ambivalence. So as not to further confuse matters, in the subsequent summary of Searles's views I shall adhere to his terminology, and later return to my own usage.

blissful relationship with him have done with their rage, which, after all, is what distinguishes them from Mahler's normal symbiotic infants to begin with. Perhaps Searles provides a clue when he notes that the bliss of the relationship may make hospital staff hostile to the therapist–patient dyad. We may ask, Is their response normal jealousy of a blissful mother–infant dyad, or is it that the rage has not been internalized and integrated in the person of the schizophrenic, and contained in his relationship with the therapist, but is split off and projectively enacted with members of the hospital treatment team so that they are, in fact, responding to the patient's subtle devaluation of them? Searles also describes how in some instances what he calls a "paranoid symbiosis" may masquerade as a pre-ambivalent symbiosis. In these instances a folie à deux based on an illusion of being lovingly at one is an aspect of unresolved defensive splitting.

Searles writes that the therapeutic stage of "pre-ambivalent" symbiosis is followed by a third and final stage, which he calls resolution of symbiosis, in which the participants lose a sense of their individual specialness and the specialness of their relationship. The patient is able to relinquish his grandiose illusion of responsibility to make the therapist feel special and to make him better (perhaps this is the equivalent of the "reparation" of the depressive position). The therapist, in turn, is able to relinquish his grandiose illusion of being the central and indispensable figure in his patient's life, an illusion in which he supplanted even the parents, with its associated, albeit subtle, investment in keeping this special source of narcissistic supplies ill and therefore chronically enthralled to him. In a moment I shall elaborate some of these issues, and the problems they pose for disengagement from symbiosis, from a slightly different frame of reference.

Searles's phenomenologic descriptions are remarkably perceptive, and both his application of Mahler's concept of symbiosis to the relationships formed by schizophrenics and his application of Klein's ideas about rage in infancy are extremely useful. But the attempt to combine both theories poses formidable problems. The first is that Searles is attempting to reconcile two very different models of normal infancy, one based on the presumption of a core experience of rage and defensive mental disintegration and the other on the presumption of a core experience of blissful oneness with mother from which mental differentiations and integrations gradually emerge. Although contemporary infant research clearly indicates that the infant is neuropsychologically capable of sophisticated mental activities and discriminations, I am inclined to believe a model like Mahler's is the more accurate one. It assumes that mental representation and symbolization, differentiation, and integration are gradual developments from a more or less inchoate state of mind and that normal infantile experience is not filled with rage. The second problem is the assumption, which Searles shares with Klein, that normal and pathological development are more or less isomorphic and may be represented on a single epigenetic continuum progressing from defensively unintegrated part-object relations based on projection to whole-object relations. In such a schema psychopathological development is differentiated from that which is normal by the presence of fixation points and susceptibility to regression. I do not think such a model is an accurate portrayal either of the mind of the schizophrenic or of that of the normal infant. It is not consistent with the developmental model I outlined in Chapter 7 or with the portrayal of the schizophrenic mind in Chapter 9. Moreover, it leads to a model of treatment in which the relationship with the therapist resembles the symbiosis of normal infancy and therapy is, in a sense, a re-parenting or new beginning. This makes for blurring of critical distinctions between the adult schizophrenic and the normal infant, and related significant confusion between therapeutic technique and normal parenting during infancy. In fact, a point of view such as this, which tends to confuse the role of the therapist with that of the parent of an infant, also tends to promote some of the elements of the narcissistic collusion that characterizes the phase of pathological symbiosis, which we shall examine next.

Narcissistic Collusion of Everyday Life

The unconscious collusion between schizophrenic and therapist that characterizes the phase of pathological symbiosis is but an extreme version of the narcissistic collusion that is more or less ubiquitous in human relationships. In almost any initial encounter we search for some special qualities in the other (idealization) and some way in which he seems of potential use to us (valued for a service, not as a whole person), and it makes us feel good (grandiosity) if the other party imagines he sees something similar in us as well, although we may not often stop to think that perhaps we ought not to allow ourselves to be so flattered simply because another person has developed the idea that we may be of use to him. Narcissistic collusion is an important force as early as the bond between mother and infant: The mother perceives her newborn, no matter how unappealing it may seem to others, as the "apple of her eye," the one who is going to make her dreams come true, and the infant, in a less calculated and symbolic fashion, exploits mothering qualities that are not yet perceived as differentiated from itself. Narcissistic collusion also characterizes the initial infatuation phase of adult love, and it encompasses the more mundane relationships in our lives, in which we select people to perform various functions for us, ranging from electing our president to choosing our own doctors and tradesmen. In all these relationships eventual disillusionment is commonplace, leading, for example, to strained and often accusatory relationships between parents and their young adult offspring, to divorce, and to the firing of hired help and the search for others to service our needs.

The commencement of psychotherapy of any sort is a fertile field for unconscious narcissistic collusion. Patients usually search for a therapist with whom they experience a special rapport, and the initial choice of a therapist may be based, at least to some degree, on an idealization or a sense of transference familiarity that may even be part of the problem for which the patient seeks help.

While it is the avowed purpose of analysis to examine such fantasies, the very process of consultation for therapy may not only encourage such illusions but promote an unconscious collusive enactment of them that may have significant impact on the subsequent course of the treatment. Prospective therapists are in the business of trying to offer something to their patients. Particularly in the initial stages they are not always aware when they are conforming their behavior in some respects to a prospective patient's fantasies and desires, but there is obvious though subtle pressure to do so in order to cement a therapeutic relationship with him.

Pathological Symbiosis and Narcissistic Collusion

If the schizophrenic patient can be engaged in a relationship with a therapist, like any other patient in analytic therapy, he will form a transference relationship to the therapist, albeit a primitive one. That is, he will enact and repeat the passive and disabled state (outlined in Chapter 9) that characterized his primary relationships and that exacerbated his constitutional vulnerability and assisted him to become schizophrenic to begin with. And he will subtly encourage the therapist to unknowingly collude with him. In other words, a pathological symbiotic beginning is an inevitable consequence of success in the initial engagement stage of treatment. This unconscious collusion is a potent one, providing much of the initial motivation or fuel for the two to relate. It is the fate of this unconscious collusion, perhaps more than any other single ingredient, that will determine the ultimate outcome of the treatment. If therapeutic progress is to continue beyond pathological symbiosis then the fact of collusion must be made conscious to both parties, and a process of analysis, disillusionment, and modification of the nature and assumptions of the relationship must transpire.

But the special nature of the symbiosis poses several obstacles to this process. First, as we shall see, the therapist will also initially be unconscious of his part in the collusive process, however much he may have been trained intellectually to suspect its existence. So he must be capable of some sophisticated self-analysis as therapy progresses. Second, the patient must possess the capacity to confront the feelings and problems that lead him to maintain such a maladaptive relationship as well as the motivation to undertake the work necessary to make a developmentally more constructive form of attachment, and the bond that he has formed with the therapist must be sufficiently positive to encourage and support his efforts to do so. But it is not only the patient's motivation that is at issue: The final and, in many instances, key variable is the capacity and motivation of the therapist, not only to become aware of the pathological element in his own participation, but to renounce and relinquish the satisfactions that continuation of it affords him.

Let us examine in greater depth the structure of the pathological symbiotic configuration which ensues if it has been possible for the therapist to engage the patient. The schizophrenic's unrepresented rage is diffused toward his nascent thoughts and feelings. He requires an invalidating, misattributing, devaluing person to help him redirect the unrepresented rage feelings diffusely toward elements of his potentially autonomous self. Or, if such a person is not available (and, hopefully, the therapist does not meet these specifications), what is required by the patient to maintain his pathological equillibrium is a person who tacitly acquiesces when the patient projects and re-introjects his own hostility. While the schizophrenic has not been actively searching for a special partner in the same way as the person intoxicated with the idea that springtime or Paris are for lovers or the mother who eagerly anticipates the birth of her baby, nonetheless he is adaptively predisposed by his family experience to assume that the therapist will want and make use of his compliant, disabled, self-destructive state, and in return will exempt him from the work and responsibility of thinking, feeling, relating, separating, and growing. Once engaged in therapy the patient naturally makes a self-destructive and disabled, albeit overtly harmonious, form of adaptation to the real or imagined agenda of the therapist, in exchange for the therapist's real or imagined special approval and for what he hopes is the therapist's continuing infantilization of him in the form of exempting him from ordinary personal and social responsibilities and expectations. Insofar as such a process is enacted in the therapy, overt elements of mutual admiration between patient and therapist, as well as special gestures on the part of the therapist that masquerade as caring and caretaking but are based on an unconscious perception of the schizophrenic as irredeemably disabled, covertly devalue the schizophrenic and his capabilities and, less obviously, the therapist as well.

What differentiates this initial transference of the schizophrenic from the transferences of persons with other forms of psychopathology, in addition to its very primitive nature, is the unconscious collusive participation of the therapist; the sole responsibility cannot be laid at the doorstep of the patient. The therapist's narcissistic overvaluation of his patient, which may interfere with his capacity to assist the patient to grow, may come from the therapist's idealizing fantasies about the special creativity of schizophrenics or from a conception of his patient as a helpless victim in need of rescue from "bad" parents or others. Early psychotherapists of schizophrenia, such as Fromm-Reichmann, portrayed the schizophrenic patient not so much as a disabled person as one with special sensitivities and abilities, with a special access to his mind and a special creative coloration to his thoughts. The presence of such fantasies is understandable, for the professional identity of the therapist depends on his work with hospitalized schizophrenics, who are not only personally irresponsible and unable to care for themselves or to relate to him in anything approaching a mature state, but may be personally offensive in their behavior as well. If the therapist is to find his work meaningful he must make such a dubious undertaking seem more than simply economically worthwhile.

The therapist can expect much difficulty and little in the way of tangible reward, other than satisfaction of his intellectual curiosity, for a long period of time. This makes the patient a prime target for the therapist's unconscious hostility and devaluation and, in his helpless, compliant state, a potential source of compensatory satisfaction for the therapist's inevitable longing for approval and flattery, which may take the form of grandiose notions about his capabilities as a therapist or as a caretaker (he may have a wish to be recognized as a better parent than he perceives his own to have been) or of a quest for a perfect relationship.

Rosen's "direct analysis" approach to patients and a qualitatively similar approach too frequently (but not always) found among traditional Kleinian analysts illustrates another collusive pitfall. This is the formulation and promulgation from the very earliest stages of treatment of seemingly profound, authoritative interpretations about conflicts and defenses related to earliest infancy. In my opinion such conduct is unwarranted in all psychotherapy, but especially in a condition like schizophrenia, which is so arcane and opaque to understanding, and is based on the analyst's aggrandizing conception of himself as a kind of godlike omniscient figure. Some of the most popular techniques of engagement described earlier in this chapter, including fostering of "positive transference" (Nunberg, 1921; Federn, 1934, 1952), the various forms of what was believed to be love or re-mothering practiced by Federn, Schwing (1940), Sechehaye (1951), and others, and even the special handling advocated by Fromm-Reichmann earlier in her career, implicitly promote the mutual narcissistic illusion of a special child-patient and a wonderful therapist-parent. It is to be hoped that the therapist of schizophrenics does not require the idolization of a cult of chronically sick patients in order to shore up a defective sense of self-esteem and feel good about himself professionally, but unfortunately such a situation is not as uncommon as we might wish.

All of the elements I have described may find a place for mutual unconscious enactment masked by superficial compliance with the formal requirements of the therapeutic situation. The therapist's participation in the collusion may be quite subtle; for example, he may not bother to disillusion his patient when the latter presents grandiose and idealizing beliefs about him, and he may rationalize this lapse as a wish not to disrupt a positive transference. Or he may marvel at the pseudo-profundity of the patient's uncensored thoughts. The therapist may be overinvested in and uncritical of the profundity of his own interpretive insights as well—easy to be when the recipient is too disabled to argue back coherently and rationally. Lidz (1973) cogently advises us that "the therapist [of a schizophrenic] may also need to remind himself of his limitations. The patient's overvaluation of the therapist, together with the intensity of his desire for all-encompassing care, can lead the therapist tacitly to promise more than he can provide" (p. 109).

In responding to these covert therapeutic pressures the patient is reciprocally treating the therapist as though he were disabled, as well, and is undertaking the task of making the therapist feel as special in his role (and as dependent on the patient for continuation of that state) as he wishes the therapist to make him feel. This almost inevitable collusion insulates the patient from awareness of responsibility for his disabled state, as well as from his rage at the therapist for not remediating it. Equivalently, it insulates the therapist from having to bear the full brunt of the patient's thoughts and feelings, as well as from having to face his own limitations in being truly able to make a difference in that person's life. In other words, neither party has to face the reality of his own limitations as a separate person or of the limitations of the relationship. Searles alludes to this phenomenon when he asserts that in the course of resolution of symbiosis the patient must relinquish the responsibility he has unconsciously assumed for making the therapist feel happy, competent, and special, and the therapist must relinquish some of his investment in holding on to a very special patient, that is, one who must remain ill (but who, in fantasy, is always getting better) and therefore exclusively dependent on and idolatrous of him.

The concept of an essential initial mutual seduction or narcissistic folie à deux between therapist and schizophrenic patient may account at least in part for the commonplace therapeutic disposition made of these difficult cases to a young, inexperienced but eager, and perhaps secretly grandiose psychiatrist-in-training who has not yet been disillusioned by failure, who hopes to rescue the world, and who is still sufficiently youthful to imagine he has limitless energy to devote to the difficult task. It is commonly observed that such a zealous but inexperienced person may do better, at least in the engagement stage of the work, than a more knowledgeable and senior therapist. The issue may not be the boundless energy of youth versus the jaded disillusionment of age so much as the lack of self-awareness, the inexperience with life in general and this kind of work in particular, and the narcissistic fantasies associated with youthful omnipotence and with becoming a therapist of the very ill, all of which may make the young psychiatrist, at least at first, more susceptible to whatever special blandishments the patient may offer and, in return, more willing to provide fuel for the grandiose and self-devaluing beliefs of the patient that are associated with maintenance of his disabled state. Young practitioners and schizophrenic patients often form some sort of bond or attachment that is not progressive. Because the pathological narcissistic elements predominate the two have little sense of the working part of therapy and are unable to take the subsequent step of mutual disillusionment. Whereas the experienced therapist—whose grandiose and omnipotent fantasies may have been dealt mortal blows by the vicissitudes of life—may be less willing to expend the energy needed to enter into a relationship of mutual illusionment with his patient than the younger therapist, and therefore may be less able to engage the patient, the younger therapist is less likely to be able to recognize his countertransference participation in a collusion and to help the patient face conditionality, separation, and growth.

My contention that unconscious therapist participation in an initially collusive process is a ubiquitous part of the successful treatment of a schizophrenic may shock some and may confuse others who long for simple black
and white, right-and-wrong distinctions between correct and incorrect therapeutic conduct, distinctions that are impossible to make when one enters the
twilight zone of insanity. In concluding I want to reiterate that the vast majority of therapists struggle in their therapeutic role to be as realistic as possible. In each of the cases in this book the eventual awareness of my own
narcissistic enmeshment came as a considerable shock and a source of chagrin. What differentiates more from less effective therapists of schizophrenics
is not the presence or absence of the narcissistic agendas and fantasies I have
noted, for they are ubiquitous, but the ability, at some point, to stop enacting
and commence reflecting upon them.

An Illustration of Symbiotic Collusion

Emily fired her first therapist, a person of some stature. After I saw her twice
she flattered me by informing me, in all sincerity, that she felt I understood her
in a way that her first therapist had not. This led me to work hard to continue
to live up to her expectations, which, we later discovered, were that I provide
for her precisely the kind of infantilizing relationship her mother had fostered.
Emily and I were both unwittingly trying to actualize our dreams, and both of
us had to face disillusionment repeatedly throughout her treatment, beginning
around the end of the first year when it became evident to Emily that I did not
plan to infantilize her as her mother had done. At that time she refused to meet
with me further, although she was apparently unwilling to fire me directly. She
spent a month in bed trying to eliminate me from her mind and her life, but her
effort was unsuccessful and we eventually resumed our work. By the end of the
treatment Emily had formed and accepted a more realistic and mature idea of
what would give both her and me narcissistic gratification. However, judging
from her follow-up letters to me after the eventual termination of her treatment, Emily's the wish for a "narcissistic" relationship with me never dis-
appeared; it simply became a more mature part of her adult psychic makeup,
which is simply another way of reiterating that such agendas are a normal part
of all human relationships.

As the therapy—or the evaluation, depending on one's point of view—
may come to a premature conclusion during the effort at disengagement from
symbiotic collusion, I would like to address briefly, before considering the
subsequent phases of treatment, the question of whether one does harm by
trying to treat a schizophrenic patient and failing, a question raised explicitly
or implicitly by many who are opposed to the psychotherapy of schizophrenia.
Certainly, the constitutional aversion of the schizophrenic to thinking, feeling,
and relating to others, and his difficulty tolerating and modulating external
and internal stimulation, create some risk that misguided or ill-informed ef-

forts to encourage him to do these things may lead to an eruption of symptomatology. But any treatment can be done poorly. The two treatment "failures" in this book were probably no worse off for the effort. Edward seemed to lack any motivation to grow and change. One might make the case that the effort to engage him exacerbated the severity of his condition, but it is difficult to believe he would have been better off without it and it is important to note that the variety of somatic treatments he also received seemed to be no more helpful.* As for Rachel, with whom the issue of disengagement from pathological symbiosis was actively joined in the form of a poignant dialogue about alternatives, she seemed to make a conscious choice to remain ill and to interrupt her work with me rather than forgo the known gratification of being infantilized and flattered by her father for an unknown future to be discovered through exploration of her autonomous thoughts and feelings and through taking responsibility for the decisions and consequences based upon them. Rachel seemed no worse after our contact, and she still maintains an occasional relationship with me by letter, which on her part is characterized by a mixture of delusion, gratitude related to her belief that she grew during the course of our brief acquaintance, and sadness that she ended it prematurely. If harm is done in the course of unsuccessful efforts either to engage a schizophrenic or to resolve a pathological symbiotic engagement, I suspect it is by those therapists who unwitting collude with their patient's pathological agendas and engage in endless relationships that masquerade as therapy but that bear more resemblance to primary family pathology. The related question of whether intensive psychotherapy and hospitalization promote regression will be addressed later in this chapter, and again in Chapter 16.

The Phase of Disengagement from Pathological Symbiosis: Conditionality and Choice

It may may be as much as a year or two subsequent to successful engagement in pathological symbiosis before the second and last stage of assessment of motivation is completed, and it is possible to predict whether a particular patient–therapist pair are able to disengage themselves from the pathological symbiotic collusion I have described by agreeing to undertake the work of transforming it into a more normal, growth-promoting symbiosis or, alternatively, by agreeing to terminate after ascertaining that no further work is possible. This, to be sure, is a long period of evaluation, but it is probably not that much longer than the time it takes to ascertain whether analytic therapy is likely to be effective with other kinds of patients, particularly those with more serious forms of illness.

By the time the decision point has been reached, the preliminary work

---

*The spectrum of antipsychotic medications was more limited 15 years ago; perhaps he might have benefited from one of the newer medications such as clozapine.

should have laid bare for mutual scrutiny such issues as the patient's deep aversion to facing and bearing feelings, to thinking constructively, to making and sustaining warm human contact with persons who might enhance his self-awareness, and to separating himself from the deadening security of destructive forms of parental care. It will also have become more apparent that the patient expects the therapist to actively take care of him as others in his life, particularly parents, have done, enabling him to maintain the mentally irresponsible and adaptively disabled state to which he has become accustomed. The nihilistic or narcotizing quality of the schizophrenic solution will have been made apparent to the patient, as well as some of the consequences of it for his life both past and future, and perhaps he will have come to appreciate glimmerings of more lively and pleasurable alternatives. The patient must then chose either to continue to do what is familiar and easy, and thus part company with the therapist, who, after all, is not there simply to reenact with him a familiar scenario, or else to take the path that is strange and unfamiliar and requires a guide (the therapist) as well as mental work. Of course, the decision is not clear-cut and often both "choices" continue to coexist in the unintegrated psyche, each equally powerful and compelling when it dominates consciousness, until well along in the treatment process, when integration eventually occurs or compensatory processes bring the pathological part under control. This is illustrated particularly well in the case of Celia and can also be seen in my work with Emily.

It is not only the patient who must confront a difficult decision. The therapist, who will have made a considerable investment of actual time and effort and hopes, as well as his own therapeutic narcissism, also needs to be able to adopt a conditional attitude toward his patient and, if necessary, to relinquish the patient and whatever gratification he has hitherto been afforded by their relationship.

Conditionality rears its head when the patient gradually realizes that the therapist's goal is eventual separation and mutual autonomy for both of them. While the therapist hopes that the patient will elect to grow and get better, one way or another the two will eventually separate, either later, because the patient does the therapeutic work that will eventually lead to a termination, or sooner, because he declines to do it. It comes as a blow to the patient to realize that the therapist believes that each of them ought to learn to manage without the other. At this crucial point the patient must make the first conscious choice of the therapy (and I view psychoanalytic therapy with patients, regardless of diagnosis, as the provision of choices where hitherto none appeared to exist), either to take the active and unfamiliar course of caring and working toward an eventual goal of separation or else to repudiate what the therapist has to offer and thereby opt for the more immediate termination of the therapeutic relationship. It is at this stage of symbiosis that the two are able to establish some consensus about the nature of the problem and the probable consequences to the patient either of further therapy or of termination. The decision to continue, which Emily, for example, made after attempting to manage for a month without me while she remained in bed, floridly psychotic, signifies the commencement of a more normal symbiotic relationship, one with growth potential; the decision to stop, which Rachel made after an experimental period during which she seemed to get much better, leads to an end to the therapeutic relationship and, in many instances, as it did with Rachel, to chronic hospitalization.

In this critical phase of conditionality and choice it is the task of the therapist to help the patient to imagine the possible outcomes with and without further therapy and to recognize that both of them must make a real choice at this point about whether to continue. Many therapists are handicapped at this juncture by at least one of two tendencies: to confuse working with a schizophrenic with the parenting of a neonate, which is, of course, an unconditional commitment, and to employ the medical model of dedicated, unconditional caretaking which is learned by many therapists, particularly American psychoanalysts with medical backgrounds. Physicians are generally trained to believe that the job of the "good doctor" is to continue to strive to heal, no matter what, even to redouble his efforts as the patient seems more disabled. It is a bad doctor (the moral emphasis is intentional) who would leave his sick patient, no matter what the reason. Both of these mind sets mitigate against assumption of a conditional posture and play into the pathology of the schizophrenic and his family. Many therapists of schizophrenia continue unconditionally and indefinitely, through thick and thin (and in such circumstances it is more commonly thin), with regressed schizophrenics as though they believe their provision of unconditional care concretely supplies an important need of the patient. They fail to understand that if treatment is to be other than one which supports and resonates to the psychotic elements of personality, it is necessary that the patient internalize some of the caring responsibility. This overprotective orientation may prevent the therapist from helping the patient to choose between more normal life and psychosis, and thus to take the consequences of his choice.

The schizophrenic will require special assistance to envision such things as the rewards of autonomy, intimacy, and work—or even to understand the meaning of chronic hospitalization with gradual self-destruction, progressive disability, and indiscriminate relinquishment of control over his very life to faceless others. For his part, the therapist must struggle with the dilemma of whether he feels psychologically capable of continuing his professional life without the patient in whom he has made a narcissistic investment and on whose unqualified admiration he has come to depend, regardless of whether this loss occurs immediately through the patient's choice of chronic disability and mind-deadening security, as in the case of Rachel, or in the future, when the growth process that ensues leads to the patient's capacity to obtain gratification from loving other people and to obtain gratification from work, as in the case of Emily.

Disillusionment and Rage

A discussion of schizophrenic rage is appropriate at this point, for confronting the elements that constitute the pathological symbiotic bond of the second phase of therapy both liberates rage and provides it with a less diffuse and self-destructive form. That is, the opportunity arises to identify rage, its causes, and the adaptive and maladaptive roles it plays in the personality of the patient.

As already noted, poorly differentiated, integrated, represented, and controlled rage plays a significant part in untreated schizophrenia. Searles believes that the therapist must endure, contain, and not reject or be destroyed by the unmitigated force of the patient's rage if the patient is to progress to pre-ambivalence and object constancy (which is the equivalent of Klein's depressive position), and this places him in the tradition of Winnicott, the Kleinians, and the later writings of Fromm-Reichmann. If the therapist fails at this task, then the disintegration—or what Kleinians call splitting and Searles calls ambivalence, which is characteristic of this phase—is enhanced, and may lead to splitting between therapist and hospital staff as well. Another possibile outcome, which I have witnessed in cases where anger is collusively avoided, is that the patient remains withdrawn while displaying a compliant and docile, if lifeless, social facade, which, at least for a while, may fool observers who do not look too closely.

On the other side of the question of how to handle schizophrenic rage are Federn (1952), Hill (1955), Sullivan (1956), and the group mentioned earlier who advocate re-mothering, including Sechehaye (1951), Whitaker and Malone (1953), and Schwing (1954). No doubt self psychologists would be in this camp if they could find some way to subsume schizophrenia into a theory that at present has no room for unintegrated, incoherent states.* Those analysts who maintain that schizophrenic rage is potentially regressive and must be avoided have contemporary allies among psychiatrists who believe that schizophrenia is an organic illness and that relating to a schizophrenic in a manner that is calculated to elicit affect is "analogous to directing a flood into a town already ravaged by a tornado" (Torrey, 1988, p. 222) or to "pouring boiling oil on wounds" (Drake & Sederer, 1986, p. 314).

There is no doubt that those who look upon schizophrenic rage as disruptive are correct (as I have indicated in Chapters 7 and 9), but I think their conclusion is unfortunately narrow and nihilistic. The schizophrenic is especially vulnerable to disruption by the intense affects that accompany intimacy. For those patients who possess some capacity to develop their human potential it is precisely the role of analytic therapy to assist them to learn to handle feelings, including rage, so that these may become a comprehensible aspect of a sense of self and lead to adaptive forms of self-assertion. In the case of rage

---

*Kohut (1971) considered rage to be a meaningless fragmentation by-product of loss of self-cohesion.

this means that it is the function of therapy first to assist the patient in the containment and identification of rage and in the development of self-control, and then to help in the development of appropriate interpersonal and social aggressiveness. Should we not take this position we are explicitly or implicitly acquiescing to the belief that the schizophrenic not only is, but must remain, disabled and different from others; we are also encouraging the continuation of the intrapsychically unintegrated and undifferentiated state that characterizes the illness itself, as well as the schizophrenic's conspicuous inability to be constructively aggressive. Of course, in situations where individual therapy is not appropriate, and the aim of treatment is to assist the patient to adjust to his "disability," then the judicious use of medication and environmental manipulation to avoid anger is entirely justified (as we noted in Chapter 12 and return to in Chapter 18), although the outcome will most likely be a dependent and relatively lifeless and unassertive individual.

The origin of schizophrenic rage has generally been thought to be constitutional excess, regulatory problems, infantile frustration, or some combination of these. While emergence of rage as a palpable problem in the treatment is a consequence of the therapist's attentions both to the patient's aversion to thinking and feeling and to his subtle attacks on sustaining a constructive cognitive–affective process, it is also a major consequence of the therapist's first efforts to disillusion his patient of his assumption that he will be infantilized and considered special as long as he remains disabled. In other words, schizophrenic rage usually becomes a predominant problem at the stage of disengagement from pathological symbiosis. Those treatments in which rage between therapist and patient is not an issue most likely have not progressed that far. Until now the patient's participation in the relationship, his efforts to comply with what he thinks the therapist wants, and to get better or at least make a socially acceptable simulation of doing so, has been contingent on his belief that he would not have to become responsible for himself but would be permanently cared for by the therapist. Exposure of this reasoning process may lead the patient to believe he has been seduced under false pretenses into a relationship he has begun to depend on and to value, and is certainly an occasion for powerful rage, which cannot initially be held or contained within a constructive therapeutic alliance. It is directed not only toward the patient's own self-awareness and against the disturbing contents of mind that the therapeutic process is bringing to light, but sometimes against his very life. It is directed not only toward the attentions of the therapist but at times toward his very being as well. Such diffuse rage has many of the characteristics of a temper tantrum. This makes the stage of treatment in which a pathological symbiosis is converted to a more constructive symbiosis extremely difficult and challenging; it is often fraught with worrisome suicidal and homicidal fantasies and impulses, and at times with destructive behavior. Homicide potential emerged in the treatment of Emily, Joanna, and Edward, and while suicide potential is less well illustrated in these particular cases, it is most apparent in the treatment of Celia.

Unbridled expression of schizophrenic rage may at times require, in addition to interpretation, containing action on the part of therapist and hospital. The willingness of the patient to struggle with it and to question its direction toward his own mind, his awareness of thoughts and feelings, may be an important determinant of the ultimate outcome of treatment. The cases of Emily, Celia and Edward form a continuum in this regard. While the therapeutic requirement to think often enraged Emily, and while she made it clear that I made her aware of things about herself she would rather not know, implicitly she conveyed that she was willing to make the effort to think about them. The struggle between thinking and rageful obliteration was a continual one in Celia's treatment. And during one of our infrequent periods of communication, Edward told me that when I pointed out things about him that were true but that he had been unaware of, it made him enraged and literally unable to think.

Conversion of Pathological Narcissism to More Normal Self-Esteem, and Emergence of a More Normal Symbiosis

One fundamental reason schizophrenics remain psychotic and pathological symbioses become chronic stalemates is that the primitive self-esteem or narcissism of each party of the therapeutic dyad is not under his autonomous control but is dependent on collusion with the other. At each succeeding stage where the therapist encourages the patient to think, feel, make active choices, and accept responsibility for their consequences rather than comply with others in a passive, mindless, self-destructive way and hold the others responsible for the outcome, the therapist is also choosing to help the patient eventually dispense with his services (though not with a valued inner image of the relationship) and negotiate a more autonomous and satisfying life. If the therapist is incapable of doing this and remains hooked into the infantilizing model, he will unwittingly foster in his patient a chronic pathological (not simply infantile) dependency and the treatment will become interminable.

But the expectations on the part of the patient which constitute his contribution to the pathological symbiosis, do not die easily. Gedo has described the process of "optimal disillusionment," which characterizes the resolution of elements of grandiosity and which he relates to Stage III of his developmental schema. Even after repeated workings through of the disillusionment–rage sequence related to the ideas of having been seduced into conditionality, choice, work, and a goal of separateness, patients continue to feel that they are complying with the therapist's agenda not for their own self-esteem, self-satisfaction, and eventual autonomy but to enhance the narcissism of the therapist in return for his endless infantilizing care and attention, coupled with more or less subtly grandiose and devaluing attributions. That is, the patient continues to convert the data of autonomy and separation into the fantasy of symbiotic disability.

The patient seemingly endlessly reiterates his insistence that his fate and that of the therapist are permanently and inextricably intertwined. When disillusioned and frustrated he may reiterate this belief in a negativistic guise, namely, by regressing and destroying his apparent gains and progress in order to deprive the therapist of his presumed narcissistic gratification and self-esteem, to devalue him in the eyes of his colleagues, and to force him back into an unconditional caretaking posture in order that the therapist regain a more primitive form of self-esteem. Of course, in outlining typical therapeutic sequences such as this, I am not implying that the patient is conscious of his intentions without therapeutic work of the sort I have outlined many other places in the book.

If this issue is not thoroughly worked through, the patient's progress will never be self-sustaining because he will never internalize the capacity for obtaining mature narcissistic gratification from his own accomplishments. In other words, in the unanalyzed state, each step the patient takes that from one perspective has the quality of "getting better," of being a personal accomplishment and a source of more mature self-esteem, is from another perspective an insincere gesture of compliance with the therapist's narcissistic agenda, compliance based on the illusion of reflecting glory on the therapist and receiving infantilization in return. The therapist must help the patient take credit for his accomplishments, just as he previously helped him take responsibility for his problems, and the therapist cannot do so unless he can take responsibility for his own career satisfaction and self-esteem. Eventually, the patient may "get better" in a more realistic way and grant the therapist the real narcissistic pleasure of simply having done his job well and of watching his patient create, as a result, a meaningful and separate existence. These developments are well illustrated in Emily's termination. When these matters finally become clear to both parties, patient and therapist will have no further business together, other than to say a loving good-bye, and will look to their separate futures.

What is at issue here is our understanding of the pathways of narcissistic maturation, which must be experienced by both parties in the therapeutic dyad. The schizophrenic must traverse the path from bizarre states of grandiosity and devaluation based on disability and compliance with the therapist as transferentially recreated parent to more normal self-esteem related to his own adaptive accomplishments, and the therapist must undergo and recover from an encapsulated regression in which states of personal grandiosity and more covert devaluation are experienced in a dyadic relation. The kind of collusive relationship I am describing between schizophrenic patient and analyst is different from the archaic narcissistic transferences that Kohut wrote about insofar as the beliefs of the schizophrenic about self and object are more palpably bizarre and delusional and are self-destructive, whereas the selfobject transferences Kohut described contain developmental potential. Moreover, the mutative factor in work with schizophrenics is not so much quantitative and exclusively intrapsychic, as in the optimally timed frustration of the wish for merger with an empathic selfobject, as it is qualitative and partly interpersonal, involving interpretation of the pathological symbiotic configuration and direct limit setting, not only with the patient but with regard to the therapist's own inevitable countertransference response.

The transformation of a pathological symbiosis into one that is more nearly normal and certainly maturational and that may eventually lead to relative autonomy, a transformation that includes the analysis of collusion, the working through of conditionality, and the containment, control, and constructive transformation of rage, occupies much of the subsequent phases of the treatment, in counterpoint with identification, genetic and dynamic analysis, and remediation of related cognitive and affective deficits.

More Normal Symbiosis: Object Relations and Narcissistic Maturation Impeded by Global Rage and Despair

But what is it that makes the patient want to grow a self (pardon the teleology) and eventually to separate from a caretaker? One important element, from the narcissistic sphere of development, has already been alluded to, namely, the conversion of a pathological symbiotic narcissistic state, in which each of the parties is responsible for primitive precursors of self-esteem in the other and which is dominated by states of grandiosity and devaluation utterly unconnected with one's personal activity and initiative, to a state in which each party assumes responsibility for his own state of well-being and in which the patient can begin to experience a feeling of self-satisfaction and self-esteem directly related to his own efforts. The other element, from the unfortunately named object-relations sphere, involves development of the patient's nascent capacities to care about himself and to care about and selectively love others, consequent to the apparently novel experience of being attended to and contained in a need-satisfying manner, while simultaneously being encouraged to be responsible for his own mind and actions.

The presence of two powerful affective elements serves to distinguish the *normal* symbiosis of infancy, in which self-development fueled by object love and narcissistic maturation proceeds relatively unimpeded, from the *more normal* symbiosis that supersedes the pathological configuration of the second phase of therapy with a schizophrenic. In the former, elements of caring and love predominate. The growth of the schizophrenic, in constrast, is a much more erratic, regression-prone, and hazardous process because of the presence both of poorly integrated rage and of global despair. The presence of these primary unconscious affects and the threat of their entering awareness and demanding to be borne (represented) has much to do with the schizophrenic's aversion toward the prospect of being responsible for the contents of his mind (loving himself) and his aversion to the caring attentions of the therapist. For a long time being attended to by the therapist is by no means a wholly positive and love-fostering experience.

As we have already attended to the affect of rage, I shall turn for a moment to the state of despair that arises in concert with his renewed efforts to care and to work. I use the term *state* rather than *feeling* advisedly, for at first it is a global marasmus-like state of being and only with much effort can it be represented and identified as an emotion. Life in the present and prospects for the future are believed to be bleak, so much so that suicide may seriously be contemplated and not infrequently committed. The overwhelming despair seems related both to the patient's more realistic awareness of his developmental limitations and of how out of phase he is with others in his age cohort and, more insidiously, to the emergence of the primary prerepresentational (and therefore unrememberable) situation of earliest infancy in which further efforts at caring and constructive self-expression must have been abandoned in favor of self-destructive compliance. It is almost as if the patient would have killed himself if, as an infant, he had possessed a more mature mental apparatus; instead, lacking both the knowledge of this possibility and the capability to do it, he did the nearest thing—destroy his nascent capabilities to perceive and to think.

The Healing Power of Love

Successful treatment of schizophrenia requires not only development in the patient of the capacity to bear, integrate, reflect upon, understand, and control the rage and despair, but also development of the mitigating capacities to tolerate feeling cared about by another, to love one's self, and eventually and selectively to love others. The therapist cares about his patient but does not fall in love with him in any adult sense of the term. If that were to happen it would create unmanageable ethical and professional problems. Moreover, to become infatuated with so disturbed a person would indicate a significant area of immaturity in the therapist. But the patient who recovers must discover the capacity to love. Self-love and related self-care is initially undifferentiated from the love relationship of patient for the person whose attentions have helped him to grow—his therapist—much as the infant's initial object love is an undifferentiated component of learning to love himself. In this phase the therapist assists the patient to develop and express his loving capacities to the fullest, first within the therapeutic relationship—while tactfully limiting behavior, if necessary, to forestall a regression-fostering physical gratification between the two parties. While I have sometimes employed hand holding and even hugging in earlier stages of the treatment, as with Joanna (Chapter 19), in the phase of more normal symbiosis, involving development of the capacity to love, any kind of physical involvement usually introduces complications, consequences, and responsibilities ranging from encouragement of identity-undermining merger fantasies and related passivity to replacement of the old destructive symbiotic interdependency with a new version. There is a crucial difference between, on the one hand, helping the patient learn to depend on his inner resources to "make love" and to sustain this capacity even in the absence of the therapist's active participation, which takes work on the part of the patient but promotes object constancy and the ability to manage separations, and, on the other hand, acquiescing to or actively participating in physical activity which is gratifying for either party and prevents the patient from developing and internalizing independent capacities and renders him concretely dependent on physical contact with the therapist in order to experience caring feelings (at the same time perhaps that the therapist more or less consciously comes to depend on the patient).

The love that emerges in the course of therapeutic symbiosis poses problems for society, for the family, for the patient, and for the therapist. In the curious age in which we live it is perfectly acceptable for a physician to influence the emotional states of another person with chemical medication and technology, but the notion of doing so with nature's organic remedy, love, is looked upon with suspicion as potentially destructive, evil, and perhaps illegal. For this reason in writing this chapter I cast about for other terms to describe what I think Searles was also describing in his phase of "pre-ambivalent symbiosis," but I could not find any that did not also trivialize and obfuscate the process. Certainly there are risks that if this critial stage of treatment is poorly handled exploitative entanglement may ensue, or chronic and disabling dependency may be fostered. But it is also true that these fears are yet another example of the social enactment of schizophrenic thinking and family attitudes. They reflect the threat that development of the patient's ability to love and to care, and hence to separate, poses for a family bound together by suppression of these qualities. The fears also arise from projection onto the therapeutic relationship of an awareness of the personally dangerous, exploitative, and growth-stultifying nature of the patient's family relationships.

Patients also have difficulties with the phase of loving symbiosis. Their incomplete mental differentiation, sensorimotor–affective or enactive mode of thinking, and aversion to work and responsibility may lead them to demand concrete physical and verbal demonstrations of affection and gratification from the therapist, and may lead them not only to become enraged when these are not forthcoming, but to experience the pessimistic conviction that any loving investment they might make without actual physical consummation will turn out to be nothing more than an experience of intolerable frustration and deprivation, feelings reflective of the state of infantile despair previously alluded to. Moreover, the experience of loving satisfaction usually highlights, in a manner initially poorly differentiated as memory, awareness of what was missing in the patient's life, so that patients may initially believe that caring actually produces their rage and despair.

The love that characterizes this phase also poses problems for the therapist, problems that complicate and amplify those pre-existing from the stage of pathological symbiosis. While the engagement phase of treatment requires both creativity in the use of his personality and perseverance on the part of the therapist, it requires much less sophistication and comprehension of the schizophrenic psyche and of symbiotic relationships and much less in the way of technical therapeutic skills than does the task of disengagement of therapist and patient from the combined impact of narcissistic collusion and the emergence of object love. It is my impression that Searles was attempting to describe this problem in his description of the phase of "pre-ambivalent symbiosis." To be loved without reservation by a schizophrenic and to be told fervently that one is special without precedent in the life of the other is an intoxicating experience, not ordinarily a part of the therapist's life after earliest infancy, except perhaps in the throes of romantic love or when his own children are infants—and, of course, not all therapists are fortunate enough to have had all these experiences in their own lives. Intoxicating substances readily become addictive. The therapist's natural response is apparent to anyone who listens to his comments about his special patient at a midtreatment hospital conference. But mutually gratifying as this relationship may be, it cannot meet the mature needs for physical gratification and commitment of the therapist any more than it can for the patient, because it is limited in terms of time, action potential, and one-sidedness. From its very inception treatment of schizophrenia requires the therapist to demonstrate his ability to deal with things the patient is unable to deal with, as when he indicates that he can contain and process the thoughts and dysphoric feelings the schizophrenic is neither willing nor able to. In the disengagement phases of treatment the therapist must demonstrate how he deals with his own loving and narcissistic needs, fantasies, and wishes and that he is capable of setting limits, differentiating himself from his patient, and dealing internally with resultant feelings of disappointment, frustration and loss. In eventually allowing a person who has become an important part of his self-esteem system to separate and eventually to terminate treatment, he is setting a growth example for his patient.

In the face of the patient's reluctance to depend and to love based on his disastrous experiences in the past, his unfamiliarity with emotional intensity in the present, and the social stigmatization attached to this element of therapy, it never ceases to amaze me (as well as my patients) how emotionally satisfying they eventually find it to be able to cultivate and indulge their loving fantasies and feelings toward the therapist in whatever way they can, without behavioral consequences, and at whatever level of maturity (more infantile and more adult levels are often present in close proximity). As with the processes of learning to hate and to be angry, and to bear and contain feelings of despair, patients experience a sense of freedom to discover that it is possible to love to the fullest extent they are capable of without disrupting the constancy, dependability, and basic goals or purposes of the relationship. As the relationship proves strong enough to contain and sustain the patient's hatred, his despair, and his love, he becomes mature enough to contain and cultivate these basic parameters of a sense of self. It is, after all, our inner sense of whom and what we love and hate and our capacity to bear joy and disappointment and sorrow that orients and sustains us under the most difficult circumstances and traumas life may deal us. And love is the best "medicine" to combat hatred, depression, anhedonia, emptiness, and meaninglessness.

The loving attachment characteristic of this phase of treatment provides the indispensable fuel and support for the following remarkable changes: disengagement from the pathological symbiotic relationship; gradual assumption of more adult responsibilty; overcoming of active aversion to thinking, feeling, and reflection; taming and controlling the rageful psychotic core; identification and comprehension of the adaptive as well as genetic significance of cognitive and affective apraxias (Gedo, 1988); and development of new and more constructive capabilities for self-care and regulation. Psychic differentiation and integration gradually supervenes, and love becomes transformed into a silent but sustaining inner reservoir of feelings of security and self-esteem, as in normal development when children are able to use the good feeling residue from their relationship with parents as fuel to go forth in the world.

Cognition and Affect

In the life of the schizophrenic pathological symbiotic relationships have served to insulate him from basic learning in the areas of self-care and self-esteem and in integrating parts of the mind and differentiating them from external percepts, bearing and regulating the expression of thoughts and feelings, and using judgment and self-control. As we have seen, the awareness of conditionality and development of the capacity to love in the relationship of patient and therapist are powerful motivating forces. The kind of cognitively oriented approach I have proposed (Robbins, 1989) for the treatment of primitive personalities to deal with their problems of affect representation and constancy, integration and focus, enactive (sensorimotor–affective) thinking, and inconstancy of self and object representations is for the most part equally applicable to the treatment of schizophrenics in the stage of more normal symbiosis and disengagement from it.

Differentiation and Integration

To summarize, what transpires in the course of treatment of the schizophrenic is an evolution from a protosymbiotic configuration, an initially unintegrated and undifferentiated mental state, to a pathological symbiotic relationship comprising several nonintegrated configurations. These include an active attempt by the schizophrenic to recreate the role of being the disabled narcissistic possession of his family and a rageful configuration directed at his emerging mind, thoughts, and feelings and at the relationship, both intrapsychic and interpersonal, with the therapist, who not only attends to these things but attempts to disillusion him of his belief that he need not take responsibility for them. A third initially unintegrated part of the personality, based on loving and caring, also emerges and provides the fuel for the patient's efforts to sustain

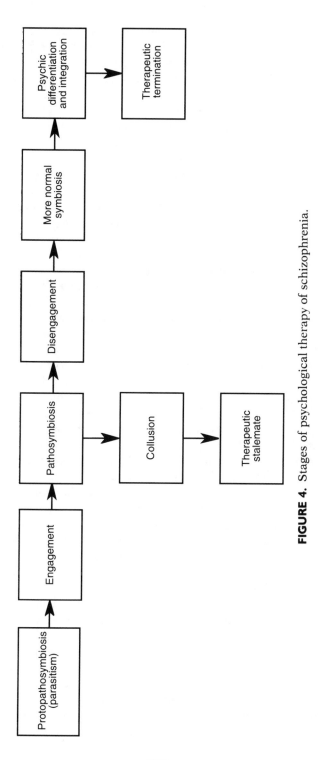

FIGURE 4. Stages of psychological therapy of schizophrenia.

disillusionment, to work to be responsible for his thoughts and feelings, to comprehend and repair cognitive and affective deficits, and eventually to be more responsible for his life. For some time these aspects alternate and oscillate as more or less separate (unconflicted) personas. (The case of Celia [Chapter 21] illustrates this development particularly well.) As the participants face and resolve the stage of conditionality, the pathological symbiotic relationship is gradually superseded by a more growth-promoting symbiosis. For some time the patient presents himself as unintegrated subpersonas: caring, rageful, possessed, and illusioned. Active intrapsychic conflict slowly and eventually develops between the caring and destructive attitudes; in successful cases the global self- and other-destructive, part is progressively brought under compensatory control of the caring part of the personality and diminishes in importance. While some may maintain that this process is nothing more than the attainment of mature ambivalence, the capacity for intrapsychic conflict, and a whole-object relationship (Klein's depressive position), I am not convinced that there is any true parallel to it in normal infant development. The presence of disintegration, unconscious rage and despair, and unusual cognition, to say nothing of the underlying constitutional vulnerabilities, make it unique. The process comprises evolution from protosymbiosis to pathological self-destructive symbiosis to pathological growth-promoting symbiosis to eventual disengagement, resolution of symbiosis, and achievement of relative autonomy, and it involves compensatory processes and structures (such as I described in Chapter 7 and elaborate further at the conclusion of this chapter).

It is interesting to note apparent fluctuations in psychic structure, integration, and differentiation over the course of treatment. Because Celia's characteristic state of fragmentation and undifferentiation was effectively masked by her false self and by the distance she kept from others, no one had a clear picture of what was going on in her mind. In therapy not only was this chaotic picture revealed, but gradually and intermittently Celia achieved another level of organization, superficially resembling "splitting," in which she oscillated between two seemingly unconnected configurations: one that attacked her mental apparatus, feelings, needs, and attentive, caring relationships and projected and introjected extensively and another in which she experienced her needs and painful affects along with wishes for a satisfying relationship. It may be that the concept of splitting as it is commonly employed in understanding borderline personalities is not appropriate here, for Celia's needy caring self emerged in the course of treatment as a novel development in an otherwise globally destructive personality whereas the more "positive" element in so-called normal splitting is thought to be present from earliest infancy and splitting and projective identification are thought to be secondary defensive developments to sequester and protect the good feeling state. The third and highest level of organization Celia attained resembled intrapsychic conflict over these contradictory attitudes; she developed a capacity to keep the destructive part of herself relatively well contained by a combination of self-control and maintenance of a certain interpersonal distance, particularly through the avoidance of the kind of intimacy that might develop out of intense caring, loving feelings. When Celia became capable of experiencing conflict, this development did not seem to supplant the unintegrated configurations, which from time to time continued to manifest themselves.

Emily's treatment is a good example of the evolution of symbiosis I have described. Emily viewed our initial contract and the relationship that ensued in passive terms, claiming, in retrospect, "You seduced me into it!" She meant that because my special attentions to her had allowed her to believe or maintain the fantasy that I would give her what mother had, the narcotic combination of infantilization and grandiose beliefs about herself, she had become "hooked" on me and had proceeded to make it clear that I was very special to her. What seduced me? It was an intoxicating experience for me as a middle-aged man the dimensions of whose personal life were more or less established to be looked upon by this attractive and intelligent young woman as the one and only person she could relate to, and to be the recipient of her admiration and gratitude for having assisted her to emerge from the psychotic abyss.

As Emily and I began to face the extent of our shared illusion (she in her musings to me and I in my private reflections), she expressed rage at me associated with the belief that I was now "making" her do the work of thinking, feeling, and acting responsibly, work she had never envisioned and that also began to disrupt her comfortable "disability insurance" agreement with mother.* She realized that she could not reject my expectation without also rejecting our relationship, which had become very important to her. She was then confronted with the first choice of her treatment: to try to relate to me differently than she had to mother and to grow rather than remain passive and infantile. That is, she could begin to differentiate herself from the narcissistic union with her mother, or she could fire me, face the loss of our relationship, and maintain the status quo with her mother. The first of our many critical struggles occurred after about a year of therapy, when Emily became extremely destructive and then took to her bed, refused to see me, withdrew into fantasy, became mute, stopped eating, and tried to ascertain, in the face of the beginnings of an attachment to me, whether she could do without me and continue as she had been before. It is important to note, however, than even when she decided to relate to me differently than she had to mother, and to try to bear her thoughts and feelings and be more active and constructive, she was still relating to me in the passive possessed mode she had, in fact, used with her mother. This transference mode would continue, alongside others, for some time to come.

It was only much later—after she had developed a loving relationship with me, had made significant progress in her own life, and had begun to experience powerful and in some respects competing loves in the outside world so that she might begin to contemplate termination and a life of her own—that

---

*While I use the term metaphorically, schizophrenics not infrequently petition the therapist to endorse their "disability insurance" applications. It is apparent why I almost never agree to do so.

Emily was able to make the decision to own her progress and take credit for it and to decide that this was her agenda, and not part of a symbiotic partnership in which she could blame what she was accomplishing on me, and I would ultimately reward her by exempting her from further responsibility. Much rage was involved over having to relinquish her mindless and narcotizing symbiosis. Emily was so successful working out her part of our collusion that, during the termination phase, she was able to point out to me unresolved elements of my countertransference collusion that I was more or less unaware of, namely, my reluctance to let her go that was based on my own need to have a disabled patient reflecting back to me flattering images of my professional skill and on my fantasies of having a fuller and more satisfying relationship with her when she "grew up."

It is my retrospective impression that as Rachel made some rapid and impressive changes, and as we basked in the glow of our special work together, she was really complying with what she perceived as my therapeutic agenda with much the same cultish enthusiasm she had shown toward her father's unconscious agenda, without either of us fully realizing it despite our intermittent discussions of her father transference. Finally, she found herself in a situation of significant emotional choices and of consequences so novel and distressing that the loss of symbiotic gratification from father and the possibility of an alternative emotionally based relationship with me and perhaps with others became more apparent. This possibility terrified her and held little real interest in comparison to the more familiar, secure mindless babying by her father. What had hitherto motivated her to do so well in therapy was the same thing that made her comply with her father, namely, the wish to be rewarded with a state of psychic oblivion or nirvana in which she would be taken care of and would share in grandiose fantasies; when I failed her in this enterprise, Rachel became enraged and returned to the original object and relationship. Of course, I represented both relationships, father and therapist, in the transference, and Rachel's treatment may have failed because she was willing to do anything (even look and act quite normal, which was, in a way, a testament to some of the innate capabilities of this chronic schizophrenic woman) in order to remain enmeshed in a narcissistic symbiotic partnership with me. I suspect that, along with the continued infantilizing seductions and coercions offered by her father, it was my failure in her therapy to deal adequately with the collusive aspect of her relationship with me that caused Rachel's sudden and devastating "crash" from her wonderfully high-functioning state to a regressive condition from which she never recovered.

At the beginning of this chapter I noted that disproportionate attention seems to have been paid to the engagement stage of therapy with schizophrenics. I suspect that is in part true because relatively few therapies of schizophrenics progress further. Many therapists work zealously with schizophrenics early in their careers and then "burn out" or become disillusioned, not, unfortunately, so much with the pathological narcissistic assumptions that characterize relationships with schizophrenics, attention to which might constitute a constructive phase of professional and personal development, but with the whole process of treating schizophrenics, who, for reasons which remain mysterious to them, seem to illustrate the destructive compulsion to repeat, no matter how promising the beginning of treatment may appear to be.

Termination

We cannot end a chapter on stages of psychotherapy of schizophrenia without at least a word about termination, the result of the final stage of resolution of symbiosis. Much of what must be dealt with in resolving the stage of more normal symbiosis is implicit in what has already been written, and need not be reiterated. Moreover, I think the case reports are instructive, as are the data presented in Chapter 13 from the relatively few studies of psychoanalytic psychotherapy of schizophrenia and from ordinary psychoanalysis. In general it seems possible to approach the psychotherapy of schizophrenia with the same kinds of overall expectations one has with patients of other diagnoses, but it seems important not to become mesmerized by grandiose notions of achieving a perfection of mental health and human relatedness. I would like to emphasize that such an attitude does not necessarily represent a dilution of standards so much as it involves a certain realism about the possibilities of the human condition, as some of the studies of psychoanalysis of patients who are less disturbed also suggest. On the other hand, when successful, the treatment of schizophrenia does not necessarily take longer than similar treatment of other disorders. As I have noted elsewhere, the duration of treatment in each of the three relatively successful cases in this book was approximately one thousand therapy hours, or 7 years.

The Nature of Change: Resumption of Development or Compensatory Process?

Does the fact that, in treating schizophrenia, we are dealing not only with psychological primitiveness but also with vulnerabilities based on constitutional organic abnormalities that have been exploited and elaborated into psychopathology mean that the therapeutic technique and process of psychological intervention differ in some respects from the analytic treatment of neurosis? Have I been describing something different from "ordinary" psychoanalytic therapy? The most general response is that this is a naive question that reflects a monistic approach to the human being and not one that would arise in the context of the hierarchical systems approach. From that vantage point, all psychological treatment deals with unusual elements of the brain as well as of the mind, and all psychological states are at one level manifestations of unique organic configurations. And, as I elaborate in Chapter 18, psychological interventions may be conceptualized as physical events that initiate organic alterations in structure and function, according to the principle of neural plasticity. Furthermore, resumption of normal development and employment of compensatory processes may be complementary, not mutually exclusive, pathways.

Perhaps, however, we have something to learn from the field of neurological rehabilitation of central nervous system injury, as well as from studies of the role of critical periods in the development of the nervous system, about when psychological interventions tend to "normalize" the abnormal nervous system and when their organic effect is to assist development of effective compensatory structures and processes that are just as abnormal as the originals in the sense of having no ordinary developmental parallel. Perhaps we have been naive in assuming that neuroses are "purely" psychological conditions and that ordinary therapy of neurotic patients, that is, provision of insight and resolution of conflict, has, when successful, no significant effect on the brain other than to restore a "normal" state or, as this idea is sometimes applied to the treatment of more primitive personalities, a "new beginning" (Balint, 1965). In much of what passes for ordinary psychoanalytic therapy I wonder to what extent we are reversing pathological processes and assisting resumption of normal development and to what extent we are fostering development of organically based compensatory processes and structures that, in the long run, may prove to be as serviceable as the naturally evolving structures might have been. Working with a more primitive population than ordinary neurotics, Gedo (1979a) has begun to consider related issues, and I have written about this as well (Robbins, 1989).

In describing the psychotherapy of schizophrenia as a kind of cognitive–affective rehabilitation based on development of compensatory processes, I am not referring to learning therapies based on behavioral manipulation and designed to teach the schizophrenic patient to conceal from others blatantly psychotic elements of his thinking, symptoms, and behavior and to conform to social norms. As noted in Chapter 12, there is certainly an important place for such therapies with patients who are not psychologically apt and motivated or in situations where funds and facilities for more ambitious therapeutic efforts are not available. But it is important to realize that the choice that is being made is to selectively reinforce such elements of schizophrenic pathology such as disintegration, concealment, false-self behavior, and suspiciousness of and alienation from others and not to delude ourselves into believing that we are undoing the pathological process.

The kind of therapy to which I refer, by contrast, is based on the premise that pathological elements of cognition and affect have become dynamically structured into the personality via early infantile adaptations and associated learning processes. In order for these elements to be modified it is first essential that the schizophrenic patient become conscious of their presence as they manifest themselves in the therapeutic relationship and in other areas of his life, and that he be helped to appreciate their self-destructive consequences in his life. These early adaptations to a pathological environment, which have become structured into adult forms of cognition, affect, and behavior that are maladaptive, are not dynamically unconscious (repressed), as is the case with the neurotic patient who developed capacities for mental representation and intrapsychic conflict and defense prior to the pathogenic events of his childhood. Rather, they have never been consciously represented to begin with. They may become the subject of intrapsychic conflict if the patient is able to perceive them as inimical to the personal aims and ambitions of a more constructive self, one he may have developed through long contact with the therapist—and by this I do not mean compliance with the will of others. The schizophrenic patient may then develop curiosity to explore their genetic roots and adaptive significance, and may develop compensatory mental structures and processes to satisfy an internal motivation for self-development, and not simply modify his behavior in response to external pressures and demands.

It is in the integration and control of the "psychotic core" of mental nihilism, specifically, the grandiose and rageful attacks on thinking, feeling, and relationships, that the notion of development of compensatory processes and structures motivated by new feelings of caring may be especially applicable. Successful therapy seems to help these patients develop a caring, attentive, thinking, and feeling part of the personality alongside but not integrated with the psychotic core. This development is particularly well illustrated in the treatment of Celia. This process seems akin to the gradual transition, during normal development, from more primitive modes of function to more mature aspects of judgment and control, except that in ordinary circumstances the seemingly new and reorganized areas of the psyche seem to supersede less mature ones whereas in the treatment of a schizophrenic the two elements first alternate in dominance; when one element is in ascendancy the other is either not present in awareness at all or is experienced as though it belonged to someone else, e.g., the therapist, if it is constructive, or a hallucinated voice, if negative. Very gradually, the caring and more mature part of the personality manages to approach and assimilate and control the psychotic core, just as an amoeba surrounds and eventually encapsulates a foreign substance. But it is not clear if the pathological organization is ever truly resolved, as contrasted with being thoroughly identified, controlled, and effectively compensated for. In Chapter 7 on constitutional vulnerability I illustrated this struggle with dreams and fantasies from the treatments of Emily and Celia. These dreams parallel the new development of a caring segment of personality, the conceptualization of hitherto unconsciously enacted self-destructiveness as a menace to the self, and the heroic intrapsychic conflict to control it. Previously frightened of presumed craziness in the world, the patient becomes more realistically frightened of the craziness within himself.

The hypothesis that schizophrenia represents a pathological line of development with a distinctive neurobiological substrate, and the related therapeutic concept of compensability, raise some perplexing questions: Are there critical periods for the normal development of specific functional human capacities, as there are, for example, for imprinting in ducklings, for development of social behavior in primates (Harlow, 1958), for development of vision in kittens and monkeys (Hubel & Wiesel, 1970, 1977), for development of sex role behavior in animals (Hofer, 1981), and for language acquisition in humans (Basser, 1962), such that functions not developed at these times cannot be reversed but may subsequently be compensated for? Where the original pathological organic changes are not reversible in what instances can alternative processes of compensation and control, which are ultimately organic and structural, be learned and activated? How can psychological forms of intervention help uncompromised parts of the brain "quarantine" the malfunction of more compromised parts and take over their functions? When do organic pathological changes become so extensive that they can be neither reversed nor compensated for?

What Is This Therapeutic Process to Be Called and What Are the Prerequisites of the Therapist?

The reader may have noticed that throughout the book I have vacillated between employing more general terms like *psychological* and *psychotherapy* and using the more specific term *psychoanalysis*, though I have tended toward the former. There have been several reasons for this: In part it has been a conscious effort to avoid unnecessarily burdening my argument with spurious elements from contemporary social controversies involving neuroscience and psychoanalysis. In part it has been an effort to avoid controversies within the field of psychoanalysis itself about the similarities and distinctions between psychoanalysis and psychotherapy, which might arise were I to assert that the treatment in the book is (or is not) psychoanalysis. And in part it represents a genuine uncertainty on my part as to what, exactly, I am describing. I do believe that the approach is basically psychoanalytic and owes more to that discipline than to any other. Though I am not prepared to argue the matter, I believe that if we view psychoanalysis in the broad sense as a therapeutic modality designed to assist growth and mastery, promote psychic differentiation and integration by making conscious to the patient that which he is not conscious of (whether dynamically or adaptively), and as a modality based on an examination of transference that is designed to provide insight and calculated to impinge minimally on mental autonomy, then what I have described qualifies as psychoanalysis, or at least modified psychoanalysis.

If it is a kind of psychoanalysis then it stands to reason that, insofar as possible, psychoanalytically trained persons should do it. Moreover, considering the central role of unconscious collusion as a stumbling block in the treatment, it also follows that success in the treatment depends upon attitudes and techniques of therapist self-analysis, which are a unique aspect of psychoanalytic training and practice.

Chapter 16

Treatment in the Mental Hospital

Because of his inability to care for himself and his fundamentally self-destructive bent, as well as the socially disruptive nature of some of his symptomatology, it is inevitable that the schizophrenic will spend a significant portion of his adult life in a mental hospital. Despite the age of deinstitutionalization, in which society's efforts to close hospitals, shorten hospital stays, and substitute a variety of day-care and halfway-house facilities have led to the renaming of many schizophrenics (as street people or criminals) and the shifting of social responsibility to the legal, welfare, and school system, the mental hospital remains the primary socially sanctioned institution designated to deal with the schizophrenic. In this chapter I would like to outline how hospitalization of the schizophrenic may be either a means of maintaining homeostasis within social, familial, and personal systems or an instrument of change, reorganization, and higher level functioning within the schizophrenic psychological system, and perhaps his family system as well. While these alternatives would at first glance appear to be freighted with moral judgment, and hence represent no choice at all, I shall continue the argument (begun in Chapters 11 and 12) that if both the needs of society and those of the individual are considered from the broadest possible perspective there is a real choice to be made, depending on the unique characteristics of each situation.

The Potential of Social Systems for Homeostasis or Change: Factors Indigenous to the Illness Itself

Before proceeding to describe the structure and function of the mental hospital both in ordinary and ideal situations, I would like to contrast the treatment and prognosis for the various conditions on the psychopathological spectrum with regard to the variable of sociocultural and familial "fit" or adaptation between the psychological structure of the patient and elements of his environment: The neurotic patient suffers from symptomatic distress but he is a more or less self-contained, autonomous, well-integrated, and differentiated individual in a more or less satisfactory adaptation to a relatively normal environment. His work and relationships may be problematic but usually not seriously so; most commonly, he is unable to derive maximum satisfaction from them or make the changes that would make them more satisfying. The pathology is autoplastic; that is, the issues and changes he contends with are, for the most part, internal, and the environment usually provides some support for or responds positively to the external adjustments he may make as a consequence of treatment. In other words, of all the disorders to whose amelioration a psychoanalytic therapist may apply himself, psychoneurotic pathology is the least severe, and because the patient is relatively well differentiated from a relatively normal environment to begin with, change is easiest to effect.

Primitive personality pathology (borderline, narcissistic, paranoid, and schizoid subtypes), in contrast, represents a disturbance of adaptation or, to be more precise, the establishment of pathological symbiotic forms of adaptation (Chapter 9, and Robbins, 1989). The relationships and work of the primitive personality represent an inadequately differentiated and integrated dramatization of aspects of his inner life. Despite the evident destructiveness and maladaptation it is very difficult for the primitive personality to change because the stability of his identity, as well as that of the persons with whom he is most intimately involved, depends on maintaining the status quo. His special network of relationships is experienced as vital to his survival. As a result, in primitive personality pathology, intrapsychic change in most instances will require or be accompanied by major and voluntary life changes, including disruptions or alterations of important relationships and perhaps of work, changes that have the additional connotation of loss of aspects of self, and are usually resisted by the environment as well. In summary, in primitive personality disorders pathology tends to be more severe than in the neuroses, and because the sense of personal identity is undifferentiated from essential interpersonal adaptations, both the patient and others in his intimate environment resist change. Successful treatment may be very difficult, with frequent illusions of success within long-term maintenance of the status quo.

In most instances the schizophrenic has failed to achieve even the social illusion of autonomy and independence from family, and has failed at even the most rudimentary efforts at self-care. As a result, treatment efforts usually commence in the hospital or very quickly lead there. Certainly from both an intrapsychic and an adaptive standpoint the schizophrenic's pathology is the most serious of the three groups, but the disruption occasioned by hospitalization is nowhere near as great as with the primitive personality, nor is it resisted as strenuously. If the treatment is not simply palliative, the patient must confront just how maladaptive and destructive his life is. He cannot remain in the hospital forever, and it usually becomes clear in the course of treatment that recovery involves a significant separation from his primary family and a new beginning to develop an identity, a lifestyle, work, and relationships. The family network is the major interpersonal obstacle to these changes, but family attitudes can at times be worked with in family therapy (as the cases of Emily and Edward illustrate, and I shall elaborate in Chapter 17) in ways that are usually impossible in the office treatment of primitive personalities so that the hospital may serve as a stepping-stone into a very different kind of identity and life.

In summary, in schizophrenia the pathological maladaptation is most severe, but neither the patient nor his extrafamilial environment have as active an investment in perpetuating it as is the case with the primitive personality. Thus, paradoxically, the very severity of the maladaptation in schizophrenia usually leads the patient to be removed to a hospital, a development that has the potential to lead to efforts to identify and encourage the major changes that are required to alter the status quo. This way of looking at things enables me to begin to account for my experience that schizophrenics, who by all our psychological measures are more severely disturbed, sometimes change more rapidly and dramatically than do primitive personalities, who typically promise change but actually improve with painful slowness and seemingly endless pathological repetitions; it suggests why the role of the mental hospital is so important.

For the remainder of this chapter I shall consider how the mental hospital, which is the designated representative of the social system, may function either to maintain homeostasis or to facilitate change. In the next chapter I shall view the family system from the same perspective.

Homeostatic Forces Within the Mental Hospital as Reflections of the Social Sytem

Asylum, the original name for the mental hospital, has diametrically opposite connotations that suggest some of the contradictions and paradoxes inherent in our attitude toward the schizophrenic and our efforts to treat him. The schizophrenic comes to the attention of society for diagnosis and treatment when his efforts to separate from the family and live more normally lead first to disequilibration of the now maladaptive patterns of adaptation he has established within the family and then, because he has nothing to replace them with that is more constructive, to further regressive decompensation. Society ordinarily verifies the reality of the beliefs of patient and family (such as that he is being acted on by external forces) and the associated denial and projection (nonintegration) of family conflicts. Society expresses not only a thinly disguised aversion to the person of the schizophrenic but a fear and aversion to his thoughts and feelings, including efforts to deny their meaningfulness and to suppress them and, in effect, to get the schizophrenic out of sight as quickly as possible. As I have suggested in Chapter 11, the average hospital is little more than a mirror of prevailing social definitions and attitudes and, as a consequence, is designed to effect an expedient social homeostasis by reorganizing and compensating for the basic elements of the disease process itself.

The average mental hospital tends to approach the patient not as a person whose illness and personality are meaningfully intertwined and need to be more intimately comprehended but as a person whose psychological normalcy will be restored once the physical illness that has disrupted his mind has been treated. This is the medical hospital model for treatment of physical illness. The schizophrenic's symptoms and bizarre behaviors are not considered susceptible to integration at a psychological level; instead, they are to be studied, labeled and recorded with symptom and behavior checklists and altered prescriptively and mechanically with medications and behavior modification programs. This is to be accomplished as rapidly as possible so as not to cause the patient to "regress," which might offend economy-conscious third-party payers or social critics concerned with individual civil liberties.

Such a view leads hospital staff to ordinarily take no more cognizance of their personal, or nonrole interaction with the patient than they would on a medical ward, where they would consider issues of personality and relationship more or less irrelevant to the treatment. From the individual psychological perspective this approach serves to encourage in the schizophrenic patient denial of the reality and meaning of his distress, disintegration, and undifferentiation. Why then, does it seem to work if viewed from a superficial social perspective in the short run? Probably because the chemical measures and tendencies within both the patient and his posthospital environment support a false-self reorganization. It is most likely that the hospital will return the schizophrenic to his primary family (or to other social agencies in the community) tranquilized and in a less overtly disturbed and more compliant state but inwardly more or less unchanged. This approach makes for a more socially effective schizophrenic, without requiring that any member of society make the disturbing effort to get to know him. It is also palliative, and its effects are not likely to be long-lasting.

My intent is not to imply that this course of action, though structured along the lines of the pathology itself rather than along the lines of its remediation, is always incorrect, for the decision to reinforce the status quo often is the best that can be done. The treatment I outline (described more fully in Chapter 12) may be offered knowingly and planfully because alternatives are not feasible, or reflexively and in ignorance, rationalized as treatment in situations where more intensive personal contact with the schizophrenic is too threatening, is not perceived as a possibility, or both. Unfortunately, the existence of this choice is often not appreciated, so that the selection and implementation of so-called therapeutic measures, in or out of hospital, tends to be blind and reflexive.

Since the supportive and rehabilitative approaches to schizophrenia are generally well-known and not in need of further elaboration here, the remainder of this chapter will focus on problems and potentials related to use of the hospital as an essential holding and sustaining resource for psychotherapy and family therapy oriented efforts to modify the schizophrenic system intrapsychically and within the primary family unit.

Role of the Mental Hospital in Implementing Psychological Treatment

I have not found it possible to engage a schizophrenic in a substantial psychotherapeutic relationship or to work through the issues involved in disengagement from pathological symbiosis, with the attendant disillusionment, conditionality, and rage (see the preceding chapter), without the support of a mental hospital for some substantial period of time. I believe therapists who claim they are able to treat schizophrenia on an outpatient basis from start to finish are either not treating patients with schizophrenia (for example, the cases described by Arlow and Brenner, 1969) or are subtly limiting the scope of the therapy so that pathological symbioses are maintained, rage does not overtly emerge, and the patient thus remains significantly disabled. Boyer's claim (Boyer & Giovachinni, 1967) of success working with schizophrenic outpatients is most unusual. Meissner (1985) contends that most of the patients in Boyer's sample were not schizophrenic, and Boyer agrees with him at least in some instances. Furthermore, Boyer (1983) emphasizes that he will not undertake such treatment without the assistance of a patient "manager." While in some instances the family may profess willingness to take on this responsibility, it should be clear from the previous discussion of family dynamics that such an arrangement probably effectively precludes any possibility of change (see also Lidz, 1973). In the past some therapists, including such notables as Federn and Winnicott, have taken patients to live in their homes for periods of time. But even if one should be so inclined as to wish to devote that much of his life and efforts to a single patient, as though adopting a child, or to take on the responsibilities of a hospital as well as those of therapist, it is likely that there is a basic confusion (and thus incompatibility) between the caretaking and psychotherapeutic roles, a confusion I have already indicated contributes to the maintenance of a pathological symbiotic collusion between patient and therapist. From the standpoint of the patient such an amalgamation provides a confusing actualization of his wish for a primary infantilizing and caretaking object, and makes it almost impossible for him to see the therapist in a more mature, collaborative perspective—to say nothing of the encouragement it provides the therapist to treat the patient like a disabled infant instead of an adult. The caretaking demands of a disabled and destructive patient, both explicit and implicit, will, at least some of the time, be so extreme and exigent that no time or energy remains to the therapeutic pair for the kind of investigative understanding that characterizes exploratory analytic work. The therapist will also experience role conflict insofar as he is aware that a possible outcome of expressive therapeutic exploration of emotion-laden issues is that the patient will become manifestly more disturbed and make trouble for him in his other role as caretaker.

The duration of hospital treatment designed to facilitate the psychotherapy of schizophrenia need be no greater than the amount of time it takes for the patient to engage in a pathological symbiotic psychotherapeutic relationship, develop the capacity to hold and contain the disturbing thoughts and feelings that arise without engaging in grossly destructive behavior, achieve the capacity for a modicum of constructive functioning, come to appreciate the existence of conditionality and choice, indicate that he has made the basic choice to work to develop a more constructive symbiosis, and demonstrate some capacity to face the disillusionment and rage that this task requires. Therapy can then continue outside the hospital, perhaps with the assistance of medication, partial hospital or halfway house programs, and family work. The hospital provides limits and structures designed to protect the patient from the consequences of unfettered poor judgment and behavior, to channel destructiveness into therapeutic dialogue, to foster instrumental learning, and to reward more mature patterns of thinking and acting. Nonetheless, hospitalization is often lengthy; it is no accident that the figure of 1 to 2 consecutive years, which is typical in my experience, is roughly the same amount of time it takes to determine the patient's motivation and suitability for psychotherapy. Once that has been accomplished, the functions served by the hospital can usually be superseded by the holding action or normal symbiotic element of the therapeutic relationship. However, in contrast to patients treated by so-called supportive methods, who require multiple brief rehospitalizations during the 15 or so years that characterize the unstable and often deteriorating phase of the illness, my patients, once they are discharged, rarely need to be rehospitalized. Lidz (1973) states that "brief hospitalization not only neglects the patient's need for a socializing and reeducational setting, but also usually returns the patient to his family without any change in the family situation" (p. 115).

What is required of the hospital that is devoted to bringing about real change in the organic, personal, dyadic, familial, and social systems that constitute schizophrenia? To begin with, it must maintain an anomalous position: As an official representative of society and an aid to the family system, it must simultaneously encourage a degree of expressiveness and autonomy in the patient that society and the family system have unwittingly suppressed. The hospital must respond to the disorganizing forces within the schizophrenic and his family by containment, reflection, and verbalization, rather than by adopting the reverberating, enacting, pathologically compensatory responses that emanate from the family and characterize our culture. This curious position makes the hospital a kind of unwanted social critic and social corrective at the same time that it is an important agent of social stability, and what the outcome will be very much depends on the manner in which these functions are carried out and how they are perceived, that is, as either adversarial or caring.

Effective hospital treatment of schizophrenia includes five related elements: (1) Efforts must be made to engage the patient and family members in whole, not fragmented or partial relationships; and to contain or hold their enactments, projections, and fragmented elements, by linking or integrating them and to foster goal-directed cohesion and constructive intrapsychic conflict. In this process patient and family require (2) assistance in realistic differentiation of personal boundaries and identification of those parts, often angry and primitively narcissistic, that are projectively and introjectively interchanged between patient, family, and members of the treatment team. (3) It is necessary to confront denial and archaic narcissistic ideas, be they grandiose or devaluing, and to provide disillusionment where appropriate. (4) Efforts must be directed to encourage genuine self-expression in a nonauthoritarian way while taking reasonable measures to control and contain it short of overt destructiveness. (5) The hospital must expect of the patient that he assume responsibilities and functions consistent with his age and ability and must not sanction disabled and infantile forms of behavior. Finally, (6) efforts must be directed to convert action language into verbal communication.

Regression

Before proceeding to outline some of the problems the mental hospital typically encounters in trying to effectively treat schizophrenia, I would like to address an article of contemporary belief that is at best a half-truth, namely, that extended periods of hospitalization, particularly hospitalization accompanied by intensive psychotherapy, inevitably cause dangerous regressions in otherwise well-functioning persons.

In fact, most regressed schizophrenics live outside hospitals; for every regressed schizophrenic who is hospitalized there are a myriad living in the community who are wandering the streets in a disabled state, abusing drugs, committing acts of violence, and being sustained marginally by social agencies. However much we may seek to deny their existence or the significance of their plight or, out of a misplaced respect for civil liberties, to romanticize it as individual idiosyncrasy, these individuals probably deserve hospitalization and treatment, provided there are sufficient funds and facilities. To do so in the manner I describe—far from being the authoritarian interference with personal autonomy some social critics maintain it is—may be the only opportunity to develop a degree of autonomy these persons ever get.

It is also probably true that the average mental hospital which is consciously organized around the medical model and regression avoidance has at least the same number of regressed, chronically dependent hangers-on, who are affiliated with a variety of partial hospital programs, require recurrent hospitalizations, and are more or less chronically disabled, as does the hospital that is oriented around long-term treatment. Perhaps the chronicity, regression, and dependency of the former group is not noticed or taken seriously, because hospital personnel working with these patients themselves come and go; because these patients move from program to program, from one group of mental health personnel to their successors, from one institution in the community to another, or remain chronically regressed at home, without enduring human ties; and because, adhering to a Kraepelinian model, no more is expected of these people. In summary, the simplistic notion that hospitalization induces regression requires us to believe that schizophrenic patients enter the hospital in a state of more or less psychic intactness and maturity, an idea that taxes credulity (and that I have addressed repeatedly throughout the book, most notably in Chapters 7 and 9).

Given these facts, then what are the historical and contemporary reasons for the commonplace equation of long-term hospitalization with functional regression? First, if the preexisting problems have been denied and the family tends to project, there may be a powerful collusion to look upon the hospitalized member as normal and to interpret any disturbance that becomes apparent during the course of hospitalization as new and indicative of a hospital-induced regression. The conviction of Edward's parents that he had been a relatively normal person until his hospitalization, even when he tried to tell them otherwise, is an illustration of this; Edward was certainly regressed and withdrawn in the hospital, but he had apparently spent much of his adolescence, when not actually attending school, isolated in his room at home. Any hospitalization that does not lead to an immediate and effective concealment of symptoms, then, is automatically susceptible to being viewed as regressive.

At one time, in the post–World War II era, purposeful induction of regression was considered by some to be an essential aspect of hospital treatment of schizophrenia. Regression was accomplished by prescribing indefinite hospitalization and proscribing personal freedoms and contact with the outside world, including family. Patients were forced to relinquish effective instrumental control over their lives and were placed in a relatively unstructured environment in order to create a state of cognitive and perceptual deprivation. A state of helpless, infant-like dependency on the hospital and its therapeutic representatives was induced, consistent with the belief (which I have taken issue with in Chapter 15) that effective treatment begins with a so-called normal infantile state. Such a state was felt to be necessary for a therapeutic new beginning, consisting of efforts to re-mother or love the patient, and was often accompanied by an attitude of overindulgence and failure to set limits on physically destructive manifestations of rage. Fostering such a presumably therapeutic regression was believed to be the hospital equivalent of the use of the couch in office psychoanalysis. While some excellent treatment occurred in this context, much needless deterioration of function was also fostered.

Clearly, this purposeful induction of regression is not the kind of treatment I am suggesting. However, regression is a complex and confusing concept. For example, equating prolonged hospitalization, overt disturbance on the part of the patient, and acknowledged dependency of patient on therapist with regression and equating rapid discharge, the use of tranquilizers, and denial of dependency with high-level functioning is simplistic, inaccurate, and misleading. Regression can be defined as the reversion to or reemergence of earlier, more primitive forms of mental organization associated with states of extreme dependency. A regressed patient is unable to achieve minimal standards of constructive care for himself and may be significantly destructive. But maturity is not necessarily synonymous with tranquillity, and regression may be present in instances of what seems like socially adaptive compliance and passivity, whereby the patient is more or less overlooked because he is perceived to be no trouble at all and therefore presumed to be more or less normal. In fact, probably the most commonplace (as well as the most overlooked) instance of regression is the patient who lives at home or the hospital, in a quiescent, even tranquil state (with or without medication), making no trouble for anyone, but on closer examination is found to be functioning at a socially and intellectually retarded level in relation to achievement of his human potential.

In the course of a therapeutic uncovering of the issues and affects related to the manifest illness, hitherto inoffensive (but disabled) individuals may manifest disturbed behavior and create social disruption. In fact, such disturbance is bound to occur in any environment that mobilizes the issues which the schizophrenic must learn to deal with if he is to grow and change. Good hospital treatment involves a certain degree of tolerance for disturbed behavior and thinking in addition to providing containment and protection of the patient during this phase, a function that depends on the ability to differentiate upsets that are truly regressive from those that entail reorganization of the personality and are potentially constructive.

I do not mean to imply that overt disturbance on the part of the patient is never an indicator of regression. It is critical and often very difficult to differentiate disturbance which reflects uncontrolled disintegration, undifferentiation, and loss of control from the chaotic and sometimes transiently destructive transference configurations which are an inevitable part of the treatment process. In order to make this distinction accurately it is necessary for caretaking staff and therapist to be in close and frequent communication. A state of regression may be said to exist when the patient manifests overtly destructive behavior and psychotic thinking which is not being actively and constructively worked with in the psychotherapy.

Another common misunderstanding both families and hospital staff are prey to is the belief that, when the patient who has been successfully engaged in therapy comes to articulate an extreme dependency on the therapist, he has regressed. (Societal suspiciousness about love in the therapeutic relationship was examined in Chapter 15.) This equation of therapeutic dependence with regression is usually accompanied by denial of the patient's previous and extreme aversion to others and equally extreme disability and de facto destructive dependency. The acknowledgment of dependency is indicative of the formation of a symbiotic bond, which may be pathological in its early stages but is growth-promoting in later ones, without which effective therapy cannot occur.

Problems of Hospital Treatment Consequent to the Nature of a Mental Hospital

Ideally, the mental hospital ought to be capable of intervening with the schizophrenic patient and his family in a manner qualitatively different from what his family and cultural conventions might dictate. But what sort of social organization is a mental hospital? The answer cannot help but be disquieting, for the mental hospital is a maturationally primitive organization; it is a heterogeneous collection of elements with, at best, limited internal coherence and integration and relatively fluid psychological boundaries between its elements, features that make it susceptible to internal projective–introjective oscillations and enactive processes among its staff in lieu of thoughtful problem solving. The average mental hospital is probably better organized to enact schizophrenia (or, more accurately, a kind of borderline organization) and to rationalize it than it is to treat it. The result of efforts at psychological treatment may be either a mutually destructive resonance and reverberation of primitive systems—that of the hospital, on the one hand, and of the patient and his family on the other—or possibly some significant change. Prospects for the latter depend on whether the hospital (and I refer to the functioning staff organization) can find a way to be self aware and to treat its own primitive tendencies first. The reader will note that this is very similar to the demand made on the therapist in the stage of pathological symbiosis. In other words, elements of collusion masquerading as treatment of schizophrenia are characteristic at the social as well as psychological level.

What is meant by characterizing the mental hospital as a primitive organization? Like systems at every hierarchical level—from the organic, the psychological self, the family, and society at large—the first task of the mental hospital is survival or maintenance of homeostasis. This translates into such practical considerations as maintaining commercial popularity within the community it serves, making money, and satisfying the wishes of external groups such as families, governmental agencies, and the insurance companies that ultimately subsidize it, groups whose interests reflect their own private concerns and values, which often have little to do with understanding or caring about what is in the best interests of the schizophrenic. Moreover, the attitudes of these groups (outlined in Chapters 10 and 11) may be an enactment of the illness process itself.

Problematic as this survival orientation may be for the treatment of schizophrenia it is not the reason I characterize the hospital group as primitive, except insofar as the hospital has difficulty adapting itself in an integrated, cohesive way to the simultaneous and more or less schismatic or conflicting tasks of social survival and treatment of schizophrenia. The primitiveness to which I refer involves an absence of internal integration and cohesion, beyond the superficial cohesion implicit in the term "hospital." The hospital contains a heterogeneity of professions and occupations, with an almost equal diversity of understandings and treatment philosophies about mental illness, to say nothing of the variety of views toward the practical survival considerations already alluded to. The tensions between different views of mental illness embodied by different personnel—the naive psychological view of the therapist, the naive organicism of the psychopharmacologist, and a perspective born of pressures toward symptom relief and rapid discharge that is generated by insurance companies and an externally responsive hospital administration—all foster at best (if there is a strong, treatment-dedicated leadership) a state of overt conflict and at worst a state of symptomatic nonintegration.

Moreover, hospital staff inevitably use the work setting as the arena in which to struggle with issues of career goals and satisfactions, to say nothing of more personal loves, hates, rivalries, and problems. Differences of departmental affiliation and geographical location of office or work setting within the hospital make communication difficult and enhance splitting. Often, the therapist does not work on the ward where his patient resides, which makes therapist and other staff ready reciprocal targets for splits and projections. Conflicts related to professional rank and status or, in some instances, to more personal hostilities are as frequent in the mental hospital as in any other arena of work. Matters are further confused by the fact that the hospital is not an organization committed to a tangible external task of work, like producing automobiles, but is one that focuses on personal problems and relationships.

Pressures on the hospital as an organizational system come not only from external sources and from the variety of agendas and orientations of its personnel but from, of course, the disintegrated and undifferentiated schizophrenic patient and his family as well. Ward staff, who may have very limited training to understand the nature of schizophrenic thinking and who must spend long hours in unmitigated contact with patients, are particularly susceptible to these pressures. Permeable boundaries and susceptibility to confusion based on projective–introjective modes of relating characterize all poorly integrated systems, and the mental hospital is no exception. The disintegrated elements of patient and family and their fluid differentiation boundaries provide fertile soil for the projection by staff of personal hostilities, dissatisfactions, and differences at the same time that the lack of integration and weak boundaries within the staff itself make its members susceptible to introjecting and enacting latent but undifferentiated and unintegrated tensions and differences projected from within both the patient and his family.

In the course of successful treatment, mobilization of destructively internalized and delusionally bound affect, particularly rage and despair, may lead patients unconsciously to create wedges between therapist and family and between therapist and staff, and to incite all these individuals to vicarious enactments that threaten the integrity and cohesiveness of the staff and the continuity of the therapy. The nonintegrated patient may confide one emotion-laden set of ideas and may choose one empathic staff member and may share the contradictory set with another, leading each to believe that he represents an unconflicted totality and in this manner setting staff at odds with one another. As family integrity has depended on denial and suppression of many of these feelings and attitudes, other family members may become disturbed as well and may direct hostility and blame toward the hospital in general or toward particular members of the staff. In short, rationalizations concerning therapy to the contrary, the welfare and growth of the patient is but one element in a system comprising poorly integrated and differentiated elements and driven by external sociocultural and internal patient and familial rein-forcement of primitive processes.

How problems play themselves out when primitive systems collide, as the hospital attempts to treat patient and family, will be illustrated in the re-mainder of this chapter. No matter how consciously and sincerely hospital staff intend to undertake the substantive modification of schizophrenia, the hospital as a representative of society and culture will tend, in the guise of treatment, to enact and to pathologically compensate for the elements of schi-zophrenia in patient and family, and will tend toward disorganization or en-tropy in response to specific and poorly contained and integrated pressures from patient and family, on the one hand, and from those who wish to objectify the entire process and institute a treatment based on understanding and work-ing through, on the other.

What happens in practice when a hospital consciously attempting in-tensive treatment in fact enacts the social view of schizophrenia outlined in Chapter 11? The patient is most likely to be covertly devalued and treated as a disabled person whose thinking and ideas are not to be taken seriously and from whom relatively little responsibility can be expected. Because the schizo-phrenic tends to be averse to people, stimulation and the affective contents of his mind, the hospital is likely to protect him from emotional stimulation and to avoid contact with him other than what is required for caretaking. The staff is likely to accept the unintegrated viewpoint of patient and family that neither has personal responsibility for the illness and that it is not related to uncon-scious family conflicts, to resonate with their tendency to interpret the pa-tient's disturbed thinking and upset feelings as a toxic epiphenomenon of an organic illness rather than an integral aspect of his personality, and to project blame and responsibility onto other people and things. A commonplace re-sponse of staff is to blame the therapist for stirring up problems and conflicts, to see these as a regressive consequence of the psychotherapy, and to attempt to eradicate them through the use of medication.

Perhaps the most common way in which the hospital tends to enact social and familial views of schizophrenia, ironically, is by encouraging regression (disability) in the guise of treatment, by emphasizing a combination of psycho-tropic medication and behavior training, producing patients who are superficially quiescent but as chronically adapted to the institution as to the primary parent. Working productively with schizophrenia involves the containment and channeling of rage, as Searles, Winnicott, and numerous others have noted. But if ward staff encourage the patient to express himself rather than to turn rage inward and become docile, thus deadening his capacities for thinking, feeling, and constructive living, they are, with full awareness of their limited resources to help, exposing themselves without insulation and for 8-hour shifts to a suffering and disabled human being. And they may evoke the wrath of family members who want to know why their loved one seems worse. The therapist, after all, has only to sit with the patient for an hour at a time, during which he can take defensive refuge in his theories ("He doesn't really hate me; it's just transference") after which he can turn to other activities.

So staff have an understandable stake in maintaining patients in the compliant, affectless, zombie-like (tranquilized) state that ensues when the adaptation related to the psychotic core becomes chronic, rather than allowing them to become actively affectively aroused and troublesome, as occurs during the effort at analytic therapy. Such a regression may be iatrogenically enhanced or prolonged by overtranquilizing patients with medication and subtly infantilizing and devaluing them as "pets." Hospital staff are very susceptible to the seductiveness of such approaches and by the nature of their roles perhaps even primed to enact a primary object countertransference with the schizophrenic patient which is qualitatively similar to the collusive countertransference of the therapist during the pathological symbiosis phase (outlined in the previous chapter). Staff need much help to learn to bear the disturbing emotions they experience in response to schizophrenic affect.

In other words, efforts at psychologically focused treatment in the mental hospital setting inevitably lead to institutional tensions between familial-social forces of infantilization, suppression, denial, undifferentiation, unintegration and projection, forces that are unconsciously enacted in various ways by all parties—patient, family, staff, and therapist—and lead to angry, divisive attacks on the more constructive efforts to raise the psychological and intrafamilial issues of schizophrenia to a level of awareness and expression at which they might be worked with more constructively. The effort to treat is inevitably and more or less unconsciously undermined by the very process of unintegration and undifferentiation that characterizes the illness at the personal, familial, and social levels. And while I have focused in this chapter on pathological elements contributed by the hospital and its personnel as a representative of society, the reader may recall from the previous chapter that during the stage of pathological symbiotic collusion it may be the therapist who subtly infantilizes his patient and encourages him to avoid personal responsibility while the two bask in a tranquil state of regression masquerading as therapy and share projections of transference anger onto staff (and at times even family), who may express their disquiet over the patient's real lack of progress and may point out certain realities of the patient's disability and disturbance that the therapeutic duo do not seem to be dealing with.

The Matrix of Hospital Treatment

When the powerful homeostatic familial, social, and patient personality forces collide with the forces of change embodied in the hospital, which is a primitive, unstable organization, the result is a maelstrom of mounting disturbance, characterized by a sense of loss of control and incipient disruption within the treatment team. Accusations of poor treatment and iatrogenic regression often emerge. Searles would perhaps say that the therapist and the rest of the treatment team must all deal with the unconscious efforts of patient and family to drive them crazy, and with the efforts of society and culture to make them accept the process and rationalize it. I would put it that hospital staff and therapist must recognize ways in which they, as representatives of society and culture, tend blindly to enact rather than reflect and communicate about the schizophrenic process. They must find ways to resist these disorganizing pressures and strive to become a more mature and cohesive organization, capable of containing the fragmentation, regulating the rage, and establishing appropriate boundaries. If they fail they merely replicate schizophrenic forces of disintegration and undifferentiation, but if they succeed they may foster reorganization of social and familial pathology at a higher level, one characterized by conscious conflict and mature forces of conflict resolution. I believe it is the handling of crises of this nature, with their potential for regression or for growth, that routinely characterizes the hospital analytic treatment of schizophrenia and that determines the fate of the treatment. In order to successfully treat the schizophrenic the hospital staff must strive to treat itself, doing so through a process of information gathering involving communication between members of the treatment team, institutional self-reflection, conflict resolution, and self-modification. In other words, the hospital must simultaneously attempt to treat the primitiveness in itself at the same time that it strives to treat the schizophrenia in patient and family. Wards on which analysis of group process and enactment is not practiced usually become hotbeds for destructive repetition and reenactment of problems, as various authors, for example, Main (1957) and Stanton and Schwartz (1954), have pointed out.

Chapter 17

Crises in Hospital Treatment and Family Treatment Considerations

T he success of psychologically focused therapy of schizophrenia depends on the efficacy of treatment interventions at other system levels, including the hospital system (Chapter 16), the somatic or organismic system (Chapter 18), and—possibly the most important—the family system. In my psychotherapeutic efforts, with but few exceptions, I have had to become personally involved in family therapy, adjunctive to my role as individual therapist, for some period of time. Even in the case of Celia, the only one where no formal work with family members occurred, I was called upon to meet with family members on several occasions when crucial decisions about the patient's treatment were being considered, for which their support was needed. In some instances, as in the case of Joanna, family work was occasional and sporadic, not systematic. In others, as in the case of Emily, Edward, and Rachel, it accompanied individual work for the better part of a year.

The exceptions to the need to work concurrently with family, in my experience, are those cases in which the primary family constellation that "nurtured" the pathology has been disrupted (for example, by the death of one or more members or by divorce) and has thereby lost some of its contemporary clout. For example, Celia had been functionally (though not psychologically) independent of her family for many years, despite her psychosis; her father was dead and her mother had remarried and moved to a distant city. In each of the cases in this book in which I worked with families, even the two that failed, various family members, who were often initially quite threatened by the mere prospect of such meetings and who were defensive and hostile in response to the issues raised early in their course, ultimately came to be very grateful and commented on how much they benefited personally and as a family from the freedom from pathological bonding with the patient that the work helped them to achieve. As a bridge to further consideration of such work I would like to present some illustrative examples of crises in hospital treatment, all of which involved work that needed to be done with the family system.

Illustrations of Crises in Hospital Treatment

Regression: Intrinsic and Iatrogenic

The case of Edward illustrates both the basic regression that characterizes schizophrenia and the noisy and silent kinds which may arise as a result of flaws or inadequacies in the hospital treament regimen. Edward's functioning appeared to have been primitive and marginal for years prior to his hospitalization, but this was unnoticed by his family and by the university he had attended, which was accustomed to overlooking eccentricity in its students— or perhaps it looked upon it, with bemused resignation, as an aspect of their special brilliance. After the bizarre behavior and delusional thinking that led to Edward's admission, the hospital staff, like his family, seemed more invested in tranquilizing him, normalizing his behavior, and getting him back to the community than in getting to know him. Because he created little disturbance on the ward in the early stages of his hospitalization, Edward was more or less neglected; staff members were preoccupied with more tangibly disturbed patients and were probably just as happy not to have another demand for their attention. When Edward was less floridly disturbed and more tractable and amenable to interpersonal influence, staff perceived him as better (in the sense of having no further hospital-related needs), discontinued his medication (when, in retrospect, he needed it), and encouraged him to make plans toward discharge. Although I continued to tell his administrator that he was underestimating the severity of Edward's illness and his need for restriction and containment, and overestimating his capacity to live outside the hospital, I also failed Edward by neglecting to underscore his need to continue on antipsychotic medication.

Edward began to talk about how he felt his parents had denied his needs and had assumed he could take care of himself during his growing years; he also began to convey the message that he needed ward staff to perceive and respond to his distress and thus differentiate themselves from his perceptions of his family and from his projections or undifferentiations of his own omnipotent, sadistic and rejecting behavior, but the staff continued to provide him with little attention. He remained aloof and bizarre with me until just prior to my vacations when he became vocal about his need for me. During each vacation separation he regressed markedly. In other words, his expression of need was reciprocally related to the real possibility of obtaining a response.

Not until Edward developed the second form of regression, which was more noisy and overtly destructive, later in the treatment, did the hospital staff belatedly recognize their mistake and begin to institute a more active program to contain him and involve him in therapeutic relationships and activities. At that time Edward's psychotic grandiosity, aloofness, and demonstration of sadistic rage proved to be powerful, adaptive interpersonal tools, behaviors that were more effective in getting attention from the ward staff than being sane and direct about needs would have been. Edward acted toward staff and me much as he must have experienced his mother's behavior toward him, and we experienced him as inaccessible to our efforts just as he must have felt incapable of reaching her. He must gradually have learned that, in the hospital, as in his family, disturbed and destructive behavior was the best way of mobilizing and controlling others in his environment and getting attention. In response to our renewed efforts Edward became increasingly destructive, proving his contention that hospital treatment was indeed harmful to him and challenging us to still greater efforts. Family therapy revealed that this was part of a larger pattern where one member at a time would become more open, receptive, and interested in the others who would characteristically respond with rejection, withdrawal, and destructive behavior.

For those who might think that Edward's regression proves how harmful the effort at intensive psychotherapy and prolonged hospitalization can be, it is important to note that the gamut of somatic therapies, including a variety of medications in considerable doses and a course of electroconvulsive therapy, was no more effective in controlling Edward's behavior and thinking. All forms of treatment, alone and in combination, failed. What finally happened was that Edward was eventually transferred to another hospital where he was simply contained, medicated, and treated as disabled, and no efforts were made to actively engage him and work with him. At that time Edward again became quiescent insofar as overt symptomatology is concerned, as he had been at home.

Progress Misinterpreted as Iatrogenic Regression

The issue of iatrogenic regression arose in one way or another in each of the other cases. Emily's mother confused her destructiveness in the hospital during the early stages of therapy with regression, even though Emily had behaved similarly prior to hospitalization. Mother had no idea how much and in what ways she herself contributed to the disabled aspect of her daughter's behavior until she participated in family therapy and began to learn about her inaccessibility to Emily's more mature efforts to communicate affectively with her, and her readiness to infantilize Emily and to respond with undifferentiated distress of her own to Emily's regressed state, which Emily was then able to deny. Different staff members were at various times openly antagonistic toward Emily's psychotherapy because of its association with her increased ownership and more open expression of some of her chaotic emotions, and they argued vigorously that I was promoting her regression.

When Joanna was quietly psychotic, passive, and superficially compliant, showing what she later described as her "Colgate smile" and her "china doll" facade, few people were seriously concerned. But when I began to experience success mobilizing the affect and ideas she had been avoiding, some of the psychiatrists in offices surrounding mine found her screams during therapy sessions disconcerting and expressed their concern that I was fostering her regression.

Confusions of Psychosis and Normalcy

Because Rachel's father was only interested in cosmetic repairs, no matter what lip service he paid to other goals, he manifested little concern when she was quietly psychotic. Ward staff likewise tended to leave Rachel alone and were relatively inattentive, choosing to direct their interest to more overtly disturbed patients. When Rachel began to speak up more and express feelings, as well as views of her own about family life that differed from those of her father, he not only became upset with her but equated her newfound expressiveness with craziness (regression), even though to most people she appeared much more normal. Father then suggested that Rachel be hospitalized nearer home ostensibly because she was not improving.

The False Self

Celia exemplifies the most extreme form of a false self: the maintenance of a semblance of normalcy as a key constituent of psychosis, a posture that induces confusion in those who attempt to work with such a person about what constitutes progress and regress. The most disturbed, psychotic elements of Celia's personality were manifested by a denial of her needs and problems, and involved, in essence, a destructive attack on her cognition and affect awareness; this quiet but global self-abnegation made her appear to lack the needs or problems that attract the attention of others. This false self was fervently invested in and believed to be normal by Celia herself, and while it employed her significant capabilities, from the standpoint of her total personality organization, her broader ability to adapt, and particularly her emotional needs, it had no constructive element. Any expression of distress or admission of a need for help of any kind was antithetical to maintenance of this position. Celia intuited the image or false self that would make her blend in and seem normal or unremarkable in whatever culture she happened to live. She sought relationships modeled after the self-destructive non-nutritious feeding and caretaking experiences which had comprised her early experiences with her mother, in which she was required to deny and attack her basic needs in order to enhance her mother's narcissism and, by reducing demands on her mother, to maintain the semblance of her sanity. On a mental hospital ward Celia's maintenance of a false self led her to act like a junior staff member, and in a most convincing manner, except on occasions when her psychosis burst through. The hospital staff mistook her psychotic facade for normalcy and interpreted as psychotic her subsequent healthier efforts, as a result of her therapy, to articulate her distress in a superficially more disturbed manner. The fact that Celia and her family perceived matters in the same way and confused facade with normalcy did not help matters. At times I was just as confused as they. When Celia's facade was most effective, when in fact she was most delusional and subtly destructive, staff tended to let her go rather than contain and hold her. When she showed more chaotic affect and admitted that she was confused and troubled, that is, when she was in fact better and more self-aware, they tended to get upset about her, pronounce her more disturbed, restrict and try to control her, and they would begin to question to value of her therapy.

Confusion of Treatment with Regression

Betty, a woman in her late twenties, of whose treatment I offer but a vignette, had tried to jump out of a window and had nearly bitten off her tongue in a delusional state while in another hospital. Shortly after her admission to the hospital where I began to work with her, she nearly succeeded in killing herself. In the hospital she appealed to staff in a childish way, like an ideal if at times somewhat insatiable patient, eager for their help and idolatrous of them. She spilled her mental contents indiscriminately to anyone who would listen, caretake, and advise her with rules and programs. She figuratively devoured slogans. Her typical day consisted of one therapeutic group or staff talk after another, in which she would obtain advice, often contradictory, would write it down in the form of sayings or rules, and would try to comply, without contributing any thoughts of her own. Her life became an anxiety-ridden combination of pleas for advice and constant scheduled activities. The staff quite naturally assumed that the more anxious, confused, scattered, and upset Betty was, the more of this kind of advice and scheduling, which they perceived as therapeutic support, she needed, but paradoxically she seemed to feel increasingly empty, frantic, out of control, and suicidal in proportion to their efforts. Eventually, after substantial doses of antipsychotic medication did not seem to alter matters, electroshock treatment was contemplated.

When I met her Betty was a vacuous walking container of slogans and lists. As I got to know her in depth I came to realize that her anxious, scatterbrained, seductive appeal to others to care for her and their consequent zealous therapeutic and empathic efforts to help her represented the successful enactment of a powerful magical wish Betty maintained to be free of responsibility for her thoughts, feelings, and life, to be a kind of princess who would be so completely taken care of that she would never have to do any cognitive or emotional work at all. She consumed what others had to offer insatiably and was unable to set limits in any area of her life, leading to an eating disorder and sexual promiscuity with narcissistic men who were to magically impregnate her with their imagined wonderful identities.

After Betty managed to get just about as many different kinds of advice and programs as there were helping professions and groups in this therapeutically eclectic hospital environment, I came to realize that the hospital, with all good intentions and some well-rationalized but substantively empty beliefs about caring, holding, and empathy, was literally encouraging my patient to lose her mind and to disintegrate. It was very difficult to convince hospital personnel of this, however; they were all flattered by Betty's sycophantic interest in them, and each thought himself unique and indispensable to her mental health. My repeated efforts to suggest that they limit their contacts with her, try to dis-illusion her, make things more conditional on her personal responsibility tak-ing, and encourage her to think for herself not only seemed fruitless but evoked staff hostility. Such advice was interpreted as the result of my failure to under-stand the extent of the patient's fragility and vulnerability, as suggesting that personnel cruelly deprive her of what she needed, as evidence of my not valuing other members of the treatment team and their professional roles, and reciprocally, as a kind of therapeutic conceit of my own stemming from a wish to render the patient totally dependent on me.

At the same time, Betty subtly fomented discontent and antagonism among her family, staff, and me by encouraging us to articulate those aspects of her hostility she could not own and express herself and to compete over who could offer her the most. She selectively flattered her immediate caretaker, appeared to comply with that caretaker's agenda, and then proceeded to com-plain about him and his agenda to the person she chose next, subtly distorting matters so that it seemed his efforts had been hurtful to her rather than helpful, thereby inflaming the anger of the new helper against his predecessor. In the countertransference I experienced some of the anger at her family for in-fantilizing and devaluing her that Betty was unable to face; they, in turn, enacted her anger at me for expecting her to bear feelings and to take more responsibility for her life and for refusing to infantilize her. Soon the family stopped paying my bills and began raising questions with my patient and the social worker about her relationship with me; when I requested payment, family members depicted me to the social worker as greedy and unreasonable, cited alleged transgressions of manners on my part in relation to them, and began to complain that my abrasive and insensitive manner was responsible for the patient's "upset" behavior and their equally upset response. Other staff, who were invested in their roles as Betty's advisers and caretakers and who felt that I expected too much of her, also came to believe I was needlessly upsetting the patient and offending the family. Family members denied problems and conflicts among themselves, and when I pointed out to ward staff some of their latent conflicts and hostilities, and encouraged Betty and the social worker to face and explore these, the ward administrative psychiatrist accepted at face value the social worker's articulation of family assurances that they loved the patient and were doing everything in their power to help her and concluded that I was acting as a disruptive influence. He announced to everyone in a staff conference that my problems were interfering with the therapy and that I was trying to destroy the patient's essential loving relationship with her family. He proceeded to call other conferences and consultations to deal with *my* splitting and to ascertain whether the patient ought to have a new therapist. Meanwhile, in this bizarre setting the cost-conscious and insurance-dominated peer review arm of the institution was encouraging the use of more and more supportive and symptom-relieving forms of treatment, which I felt simply reinforced the chronicity of the illness. Of course, by that time I was in fact feeling angry at everyone—family, ward staff, hospital administration and my patient.

Betty was eventually discharged. She continued in treatment with me, and five years later she was doing better than ever in her life. She was more or less self-supporting for the first time and more accepting of the need to bear her own painful thoughts and feelings. She was more aware of some of the intrafamilial hostility and of the tendency to create splits and scapegoats. In turn, family members and others in her life who would previously have infantilized her felt a bit freer to confront her with some of the things about her they were unhappy with. One of the more interesting developments involved Betty's awareness of enormous shame, an emotion that others would previously have tried to tell her was unreasonable and unnecessary, but one that seemed to be meaningfully linked to her increasing awareness of her own past responsibility for her disabled and irresponsible state. With the wisdom of hindsight, it appears that getting Betty out of the so-called therapeutic hospital setting and teaching her that she needed to become more responsible for herself was one of the most difficult but useful steps in her treatment.

The Family System

One inescapable conclusion from this analysis of the processes, thickets and pitfalls of hospital treatment is that successful psychological treatment of schizophrenia must take into account the homeostatic forces favoring an organization based upon varying degrees of individual disability within the family system. Lidz (1973) doubts that "effective therapy with any youthful schizophrenic patient can be carried out without paying considerable attention to the family in actuality as well as in the patient's psyche. Neglect of the family has been a major cause of therapeutic failure" (p. 118).

The core problems of the schizophrenic (which are described in detail in Chapters 7 and 9) are both sustained and compensated for by the activity and caretaking of his family (described in Chapter 10). He is deficient in the processes of integrating a cohesive sense of self, or identity, and differentiating elements of the self from the environment and other persons. This leaves him with a severely impaired and unreliable reality sense. By projection and introjection across fluid boundaries his family provides him with a mode of thinking—sensorimotor–affective enactment—and relating. They project into him an archaic unintegrated narcissistic sense of identity, by encouraging his grandiose thinking and by infantilizing, hence implicity devaluing him, and they define his reality sense using a combination of denial and inversion of ordinary meanings, such as right and wrong, good and bad, existent and nonexistent. The schizophrenic has great difficulty with internal and external stimuli and related self-regulation, both external (sensation and perception) and internal (drive and affect, particularly rage and aggression). The family supplies the missing regulation and control in the form of avoidance and overprotection in relation to external stimulation and in the form of avoidance, invalidation, and hostile suppression in relation to internal stimuli. They respond to the schizophrenic's people aversion by providing an isolated and overprotected environment, and to his aversion to his mental contents by denying their existence and validity, encouraging their suppression, and by not providing him with the attention that might raise these mental contents to conscious awareness.

Response of the Family System to Hospitalization

Following the initial hospitalization it is not uncommon for the family to reinstate their briefly shaken belief that they and the patient are relatively normal. As family equilibrium depends on avoidance of latent hostility and conflict, the family cannot be expected to view with equanimity initial therapeutic success in mobilizing affect and conflict, particularly in the earlier chaotic phases when its significance is not readily apparent, and in their threatened state they tend to respond to any disturbing thoughts and feelings emanating from the hospitalized member as though these were regressive abnormalities induced in an otherwise more or less normal person by the hospital, and particularly by whatever representative of the hospital, usually the therapist, the patient seems to have become most involved with. When the therapist supports efforts of his patient to recognize and express his feelings and to resume (or in some instances initiate) conflictual family relationships, family members may respond with covert or overt fear and hostility. As I noted in Chapter 15 on psychotherapy, dealing with the rage of the schizophrenic is one of the most important and neglected or misunderstood aspects of the treatment; however, the average therapist is even less prepared and knowledgeable about dealing with the hostility of his patient's family, and when his well-intentioned efforts at treatment of their member are not responded to with their immediate gratitude he may become enmeshed in hostile interaction with them and feelings of devaluation, which he may rationalize with theoretical beliefs about schizophrenogenic parenting.

Therapeutic Intervention in The Family

Since the source of much of what passes for good feeling in families of schizophrenics in fact consists of a combination of denial, infantilization, inversion of meaning, and totalitarian suppression, the task of the social worker, who is most often assigned to work with family members in an analytic treatment setting, is not the one often naively assumed, namely, to assist the family to cope with the external tragedy inflicted upon them and to help family members feel better about themselves. While such work is entirely appropriate and necessary in situations where treatment has a supportive, rehabilitative goal, it has no place in psychological forms of treatment, where it is, however well-meaning, little more than a combination of complicity in denial and neglect both of family and patient. While earnestly beseeching the social worker to expedite efforts of other members of the treatment team to alleviate the symptomatic distress of their schizophrenic member, the family is likely to present convincingly its view that any alteration in the direction of identifying problems, conflicts, painful feelings, and the like is creating problems where heretofore none existed, and to recruit the participation of the social worker in finding the cause or the culprit and restoring the status quo. If the social worker is not psychoanalytically trained to look beyond the obvious, and if he functions in a setting in which ongoing dynamic institutional self-analysis of the kind I suggested in Chapter 16 does not occur, he is likely to unknowingly enter into a kind of symbiotic transference or collusion with the family (which has some parallels with the narcissistic collusion of patient and therapist I described in Chapter 15 and with the familial–social transference enactment by hospital staff described in Chapter 16). For example, Emily's mother took an initial dislike to me because Emily continued to be upset and particularly because of efforts Emily made to initiate discussion of areas of conflict with her. She thought I was upsetting Emily, and the social worker agreed with her and supported her belief that it would be too upsetting for Emily to attend family therapy sessions. (The treatment of Betty, just summarized, provides another example of this problem.)

Who should be involved in the family work? As many members of the primary family as possible, but at least both parents and the patient. In some cases not all siblings need be present, and not all members need attend simultaneously. Emily's siblings did not attend, and her therapy progressed well; in contrast, the presence of Rachel's sister was essential to understanding and working with the dynamics of the family, and Edward's younger sisters, even the youngest who was barely into her adolescence, brought a crucial element of reality to his treatment that was lacking in both parents. In the course of our work together Joanna brought in each of her parents separately when she felt the need to work on a particular relationship. Often the family does not wish to participate as a unit, and it takes time to understand the meanings associated with the presence and absence of various parties and to determine whose presence is actually crucial and whose is not. What about the patient's individual therapist and the social worker? I do not think it is intrinsically required that either party be present for family therapy sessions, but in family units characterized by disintegration and undifferentiation the pressures on therapist and social worker are so extreme and often so subtle that the presence of all parties in the same room simultaneously may be necessary to clarify them. In my cases each of the social workers tended initially to be so enmeshed in the enactment of familial attitudes of denial, inversion of meaning and projection comparable to the unconscious symbiotic collusion of patient and therapist (which I described in Chapter 15), that he was unable to achieve effective working clarity until we all sat down together. No doubt I too brought some of that collusive blindness into family meetings and was also able to use the settings as a corrective in which to acquire a larger, better integrated and differentiated view of each of the family members. I have concluded that it is more important for the family therapist(s) to be highly trained in identifying and understanding the implications of primitive thinking, including disintegration, undifferentiation, and projective–introjective and enactive modes of relating than it is that he represent a particular profession or simultaneously be the patient's individual therapist.

What is involved in family therapy work? Since detailed discussion of this subject would duplicate much of what has already been outlined elsewhere in this book, I will but cursorily review a few of the salient issues. To begin with, the work is predicated on the propositions that it is the active, albeit authoritarian, combination of infantilizing, attribution, and neglect on the part of other family members that enables the schizophrenic member to continue in his dysfunctional state, and that their "success" in this achievement is at the expense of each member's capacity to fully identify his own thoughts and feelings and experience the freedom to act autonomously. In other words, all family members, knowingly or not, experience a degree of personal disability, a loss of freedom, and the imposition of obligatory, oppressive, coercive bonding with other family members. It is the purpose of family therapy that is conducted to facilitate psychological treatment to elucidate how the family system functions in a manner that is interpersonally undifferentiated and lacking in boundaries, a manner that is based on projective identification and introjection and that makes the family look more like the parts of a single organism than like an affiliated group of separate, autonomous individuals. The therapist or cotherapists of a family must attend to and help validate the thoughts and feelings of each family member, without prejudice as to whether that member is patient, parent, or sibling, and must intervene when efforts are made at suppression, invalidation, and inversion of meaning. The systems view just outlined, psychologically equidistant from each family member, is critical if the therapist is to avoid participation in a system of victimizing and scapegoating, either of patient or of parents.

Since assisting the individual treatment of the schizophrenic member is the immediate stimulus for undertaking family treatment, the latter will naturally focus on the infantilization and overprotection of the schizophrenic member, including attribution of the unowned thoughts and feelings of other members to him in lieu of a mind of his own, suppression and invalidation of his actual thoughts and feelings, and overprotection of him from the responsibility for his mind and actions and their consequences, and on the irresponsible, grandiose (but covertly devalued) state in which he is able to live as a result. But the broader goal of treatment is to assist all family members to become more psychically differentiated from one another and for each to become a more internally integrated person. One result of the increasing individuation and autonomy of each member, including clearer recognition of the extent to which he has been bonded to the others not so much by love as by hitherto destructively internalized, enacted, projected and denied hostility and conflict, may be overt disintegration of the family unit and formation by the members of other, hopefully more mature, units. More frequently, in my experience, members realize more personal freedom from the painful, obligatory ties to one another, accompanied in many instances by physical separation, and the basic family unit remains intact, if not so exclusively vital to the interests of its individual members. Latent capacities for true mutual respect and friendship, if not always love, may emerge, as the case of Emily illustrates, or the family may simply become a much less significant element in the life of each member.

When should such treatment be undertaken? It is probably not possible for a schizophrenic to benefit significantly from family therapy until at least some of the fantasies and illusions characteristic of pathological symbiosis have been uncovered, and the patient has made some choice or commitment to try to work on them and bear and assimilate the resultant feelings of disillusionment, conditionality, and rage. Ideally but not necessarily, family members ought to have expressed some real curiosity or interest in getting to better understand the sick member and the dynamisms of family functioning. It may take a year or more of individual psychotherapy with the schizophrenic and preparatory work with his family before it seems useful to commence family treatment.

As with individual therapy, the personal assets, liabilities, and motivation of each of the family members (apart from their various collective pathologies) will determine success or failure of the family therapy undertaking. There was little flexibility or support for change in Rachel's family, even when some of the pathological dynamics and their generally deleterious effects could be more or less agreed upon by all members. In the case of Edward it did prove possible to engage the family and promote significant changes, but by that time either the presence and attentions of his family no longer seemed to matter to Edward, or they provided him with a long-awaited opportunity for revenge, or the changes in members of his family were so threatening to his psychotically based identity that they had the paradoxical effect of exacerbating elements of his psychotic withdrawal. Perhaps the work with Emily's family was most successful, consistent with the generally positive outcome of the case. Initially the family social worker was quite convinced that it would be too upsetting to mother if I were to participate in family therapy. However, since family therapy was something Emily seemed to want and I supported, the social worker and mother eventually acquiesced to a trial. Before and during our early sessions Emily had dreams graphically portraying the disruption the family work threatened to her family unit and to her psyche. But years later, when all was said and done and our work was coming to an end, she not only felt that the work had been crucial to her achievement of functional separation from mother but noted various ways in which her mother had flourished because of it as well.

Chapter 18

Treatment of the Organism Under Stress: Pharmacologic and Somatic Modalities

A n understanding of the hierarchical systems model (proposed in Chapter 2 and elaborated in Part III) will have prepared the reader for the otherwise curious statement that all known treatments of schizophrenia are organic. So the task in a chapter devoted to organic treatment is not to delineate a class of biological or somatic therapies from a class of therapies that are social or psychological but to compare and contrast some of the unique features of all treatments as viewed from the perspective of the organic level. Among other things, this requires us to reconceptualize in physical-organic terms what we are ordinarily accustomed to think of as psychological, interpersonal, familial, and social elements, both pathological and therapeutic, as they impinge upon the patient and as his nervous system responds to them. Whether they do so knowingly or not, this is what occurs when psychiatrists and neuroscientists speak of stress and stress reduction and employ a stress-diathesis model for schizophrenia. This way of looking will help us to be aware of the unique contributions and limitations of models and treatments of schizophrenia at each hierarchical level. At the conclusion of Chapter 15 psychological therapy is conceptualized in organic terms, utilizing concepts such as neural plasticity, critical periods, and development of compensatory function.

Stress

The concept of stress in physiology and medicine is generally attributed to Walter B. Cannon and Hans Selye. Cannon (1935) defined stress as physical stressors or stimuli that are disruptive of internal homeostasis and productive of an organismic strain. His emphasis on stress as a stimulus corresponds to the casual use of the term today. Selye (1950, 1956) was less concerned with delineating external causality and more interested in delineating a configuration of organismic response, which he referred to as stress. So it is useful to be aware that when we speak of stress we may sometimes be referring to the stimulus and other times to the organismic response. In any case, schizophrenia may be conceptualized as a stress-related impairment, due to a combination of constitutional and experientially elaborated alterations in the nervous system.

Stress Reduction Treatments in a Hierarchical Systems Context

In each of the preceding chapters in which I delineated one level of treatment I also noted how a hierarchical systems perspective requires us to reconsider our traditional distinctions between what constitutes disease and what constitutes treatment. The same requirement applies to understanding stress and its treatment. Stress is not a variable to be viewed on a single dimension, simply as undesirable. It is an inescapable aspect of life, and maturation may be described as enhancement of an organism's adaptive capacity to handle it. Therefore, the question of whether treatment should aim to reduce stress or to enhance the schizophrenic's ability to cope with it is a critical one. Reduction of organismic stress by means of psychological and social interventions, which are conceptualized as concrete physical forces, and by medication, is unquestionably an appropriate therapeutic enterprise when somatic therapies constitute the sole form of intervention, and when for whatever reason, a goal of therapeutic enhancement of whatever latent psychological capacity the patient may possess to become more socially responsible for his thoughts, feelings, and actions and their consequences does not appear to be feasible. On the other hand, stress reduction therapies applied with the unexamined assumption that the patient is too disabled to be expected to function like others are little more than higher-level reflections and reenactments of the basic pathology of schizophrenia at the individual, familial, and social levels.

A more useful way to consider the issue of stress is to ascertain the optimal level an organism is capable of coping with adaptively, and to gear treatment toward to maintaining this level or, if possible, expanding it. Turning more specifically to pharmacotherapy, the use of medication, we must carefully consider whether the intent is to titrate and maintain an organic level of stress consistent with maximal motivation and capacity to work on problems psychologically, with the objective of progressively enhancing the capacity to handle stress, or whether it is to reduce the manifest level of disturbance and produce a more tractable and "tranquil" patient who is less troublesome to his family and to society by reinforcing and compensating for the essential elements of the schizophrenic process, including denial, avoidance, disintegration, and suppression of unruly thoughts and feelings. In other words, a hierarchical systems model sharpens our awareness of what is involved when we utilize organic treatments alone or in concert with modalities from other levels, most notably hospitalization and psychotherapy, and requires us to examine whether the treatment goal is to fundamentally alter the schizophrenic pathology and attempt to enhance the capacity to handle stress or whether it is to restore and enhance the status quo, a goal based on the view that the disability is an immutable fact but that suitable intervention may assist the patient to achieve an adaptation that is more benign and humanitarian.

Realistically, many (and perhaps even the majority of) schizophrenic patients are not candidates for major personality and social overhaul, whether owing to the extent of their constitutional vulnerability, their other individual assets (intelligence, ability), their family structure, or economics and the availability of therapeutic resources. There will always be an important place for efforts to restore the pathological status quo humanely, and although from the perspective of individual autonomy such a measure may be viewed as reinforcing pathology, from the perspective of society such minimizing of disruption may be viewed as a normalizing process. In other words, as with all treatment, stress reduction therapies of all kinds, whether interpersonal, environmental, or pharmacologic, should be done in the context of a sophisticated systems perspective.

A second difficulty of an organic stress reduction model is that, without a complementary psychological model, we cannot know for certain what is stressful to a particular person (that is, what meanings particular configurations of the environment and of experience have for him) and what is not. Within a broad range we all respond idiosyncratically to events and interactions, and what is stressful to one person is not necessarily so to another (Lazarus, 1966). Without a complementary psychological theory we are restricted to the most simplistic physicalistic conceptions of stress, for example, extremes of sensory-perceptual experience.

Principles of Pharmacotherapy

However medication is to be used, in order to be as clear as possible about the boundary between therapeutic assistance of optimal, albeit perhaps turbulent, functioning with the goal either of maintaining homeostasis or of expanding the capacity to handle stress, on the one hand, and "therapeutic" tranquilization in order to make existing pathological elements less apparent and disturbing, on the other, it is necessary to understand how medications affect the organic substrate of such dysfunctional elements as passivity, denial, disintegration of psyche, and alienation from self and other.

The major classes of antipsychotic medication—phenothiazines, thioxanthenes, butyrophenones, and dibenzoxazepines—are clearly capable of mitigating such constitutional vulnerabilities as disorganization or fragmentation of thinking, disturbance of attention and concentration, stimulus flooding, and rage. As yet there has been little effort to try to refine our understanding of these vulnerabilities and, by using measures such as magnetic resonance imaging (MRI), positron emission tomography (PET), psychophysics, neuropsychological testing, and simple interviewing, to attempt to ascertain which medications prove more or less effective, ameliorating which particular areas of vulnerability.

In the four decades since the discovery of antipsychotic medication (Delay, Deniker & Harl, 1952; Delay & Deniker, 1952) little has been learned about their mode of operation except that they appear to be dopamine antagonists (Snyder, Banerjee, Yamamura, & Greenberg, 1974). With a single exception there is no significant evidence that they work selectively on particular regions or pathways in the brain. That exception is clozapine, which appears to specifically inhibit the mesolimbic dopaminergic system (Gardner, 1992). It lacks the neuroleptic side effects (extrapyramidal reactions, tardive dyskinesia, and neuroendocrine disturbances) of the other antipsychotics, which seem to be attributable to their action on the nigrostriatal dopaminergic system. Furthermore, the question of whether the tranquilizing effect of a medication is achieved by mitigating or by reinforcing the pathological processes typical of schizophrenia may be decided not only by the nature of the medication itself but by such things as dosage and the psychological and interpersonal context in which it is used.

Pharmacologic treatment that makes the manifest effects of impairment less apparent while in some instances enhancing the impairment itself may be viewed variously as undesirable from the standpoint of individual autonomy, as desirable if no other options are available, as undesirable in terms of the social critique of schizophrenia as suppression of individual differences, or as desirable from the socio-cultural level standpoint of restoring social order.

Before examining the differences between medication used as the principal treatment modality and medication as an adjunct to psychotherapy, I would like to enumerate some general principles of drug treatment. As I am not a psychopharmacologist I will not attempt to discuss in detail the complex issues related to choice and dosage of neuroleptic or psychotropic medication.

First, we must remain vigilant to the potential for lasting damage from neuroleptics, either the damage we know for certain, such as tardive dyskinesia, or that which we do not know for certain, such as the loss of brain substance among chronic patients, most of whom have histories of heavy medication.

Perhaps more alarming is the tendency toward polypharmacy, which characterizes too much of contemporary psychopharmacology. Drugs from all major categories are often administered simultaneously; it is not uncommon to encounter patients receiving five or six different psychoactive drugs simultaneously. While the era of psychopharmacology has been touted by many as the advent of science and reason into a situation hitherto dominated by magic and witchcraft, the so-called reasoning process behind the selection of medication often differs but little from that of the chef who tries first a little of this and then a little of that until the recipe seems to suit his taste. One need spend only a short time on an average psychiatric ward to observe such a multiplicity of side effects from drugs—often administered in bewildering combinations with a "let's try this!" attitude—that it is sometimes difficult to distinguish "pharmacophrenia," the iatrogenic illness comprising the side effects, and even toxicities of multiple powerful medications on psyche and soma from the intrinsic manifestations of the basic disease process of schizophrenia itself. When asked to consult on patients drugged in these complex ways, usually because they remain disturbed or have developed new disturbances, I often find myself unable to differentiate elements of basic personality from responses induced by treating the brain like a machine and using drugs like the buttons or levers.

The administration of medication—like the introduction of any other variable into treatment, even a psychological interpretation of what things might mean—should be looked upon as an experiment. Insofar as possible it should be done in a controlled setting in which the effect of other variables is minimized. This is done by introducing new elements or modifying existing variables one at a time, if possible. Unfortunately, new drugs are often introduced into the patient's system before thorough trials on existing ones have been completed, or before existing ones that might interact with the new ones in strange ways are discontinued or their effects eliminated from the body. In shortsighted economic terms such actions are understandable, for it may take weeks or even longer to thoroughly eliminate the effects of some of the psychotropic drugs from the nervous system and nowadays it is difficult to get insurance companies to agree on hospital stays of longer than a single week.

Another important principle of drug prescription is that the effects of all the major psychotropic medications are significantly dose-related, and the dose that is ineffectual or that produces side effects for one patient may be just right or too much for another. If it is deemed important to try a particular drug, then it is important to gradually push the dosage to the recommended limit or to the point of side effects before concluding that it is not effective and trying another one. While we are probably more familiar with the effects of overdosing patients, it is by no means uncommon in my experience that patients are treated homeopathically.

In an era in which patients go in relative personal anonymity from one treatment resource or set of therapeutic personnel to another, a patient's specific drug dossier looms large as vital identification, achieving a place of importance rivaling the social security number, and each medication is treated with a degree of reverence it may not merit. If the patient appears to be disturbed, therapeutic personnel often hypothesize not that perhaps he is over-medicated or mismedicated, but that there must be a good reason for the particular combination and dosage of drugs he is receiving, that they should not be discontinued lest the patient's condition worsen, and that perhaps it is best to add something new to the brew. The fear of removing patients from a drug regimen that oftimes was arrived at in a haphazard and inadequately validated manner to begin with, lest greater disturbance result, is probably one determinant of schizophrenic chronicity as well as a potent cause of some of the long term neurological consequences of medication. In this respect the psychopharmacology era unwittingly duplicates the worst features both of the post–World War II psychoanalytic era and the asylum era—indiscriminate overdosing and chronic inflexible treatment with a single modality.

When the psychiatrist prescribes medication it is important that he be sensitive to its psychological meaning to the patient, whether or not the patient is concurrently in psychotherapy. If medication is the exclusive treatment, the psychological issues are narrow ones related to compliance. In the case of psychological treatment more complex configurations of meaning will be encountered at the time the drug is introduced and again, if all goes well, when the patient is finally weaned from it. Giving medication is an enactment and primitive thinking is enactive (Chapter 9), and to the extent that there is accompanying meaningful discussion, the introduction of medication may also be part of a psychological interpretation.

When Joanna was seriously decompensating during our second year of treatment and progressively less able to sleep at night, her thoughts full of associations concerning maternal deprivation, oral longing, despair, and rage, I prescribed chloral hydrate for her, which helped her to sleep. When she read the *M* in my name and in the *M.D.* on the label, she associated to the word *mother*. She needed the medication; it helped her to sleep, to reorganize herself, and probably to avoid rehospitalization. My effort, embodied in the action itself and what discussion we were able to have at the time, was not to be a mother to her but to demonstrate that I was a reliable holding person and that, whatever the actual and psychological reality of her earlier experiences, it was possible at critical times to depend on others for help.

I prescribed a small dose of trifluoperazine at bedtime to help another patient quiet an internal dysphoric and disruptive state whose effect on her ability to sleep was profound. We worked with considerable success to help her understand the infantile origins and meaning of her tendency to generate and repeat a state familiar to her from childhood, one that was characterized by barely comprehended feelings of diffuse internalized rage and hurt, and to help her substitute feelings of caring and pleasure and associated behaviors, first developed in her relationship with me, which were frightening but clearly more adaptive and satisfying. These behaviors were associated with copious salivation, which the patient at first disparagingly labeled "drooling" but which she gradually came to realize was a mouth-watering, appetitive feeling. Many associations to disrupted and completed infantile feeding experiences emerged in concert with this development. When it came time to renew her prescription she came to the conclusion although she was feeling better than ever before in her life, that while she might no longer need them for purely pharmacologic reasons, the two tablets taken at bedtime represented a good breast-feeding and it would be premature and disruptive to be weaned from them just then. Yet a year later, when she again initiated the discussion of weaning, it emerged that trifluoperazine (brand name Stelazine), represented "Stella," a generic name for her mother, who had infantilized her and led her to believe, and to function as though, she were not required to experience and bear any intense emotion in her life.

Noncompliance

The phenomenon of noncompliance with a prescribed regimen of medication is most difficult to account for from a purely organismic perspective, from which the patient would be at least as invested as his caretakers in any treatment that would reduce stress and render his subjective state of mind and affect more normal. After all, who would not want to feel better? Yet a significant proportion of psychotic patients refuse to follow a prescribed drug regimen even when it would objectively seem to be making them better. Some even go so far as to secretly discard medication while trying to fool the doctor into believing they have taken it. While some noncompliance may relate to autonomic and extrapyramidal side-effects, understanding requires psychological level considerations of meaning and of the sense of self and, in particular, recognition that medication threatens to disrupt the chronic psychotic identity.

Celia had numerous trials on antipsychotic drugs before and after I made her acquaintance, and invariably they were stopped because she claimed that not only were they of no help but they interfered with her "clear thinking" and made her feel "worse." This was the case even in instances where she seemed unequivocally better. She was so convincing in her clamor that medication made her feel worse that I considered at times that she might not be schizophrenic, despite overwhelming evidence to the contrary. In fact, her problems of denial of illness and a reversal of a her sense of what constitutes sickness and what constitutes normalcy had to be worked out in exquisite and time-consuming detail in her therapy before she could accept the effects of medication and correctly define the feelings they induced as "better" feelings rather than as something harmful to her identity and a cause of "bad" feeling and "craziness." When after nearly 7 years of treatment Celia was finally able to accept medication from me and report that it ameliorated some of her psychotic distress and made her feel calmer, more focused, more able to contemplate her inner life, and even able to sleep for more than brief, disrupted intervals of time, I came to realize that what she had previously meant when she insisted medication interfered with her "clear thinking" was that it helped her to be more integrated so that she was less able to erect a facade of normalcy and utterly deny her problems, her feelings, and her needs. What she meant when she told me medication made her feel worse was that it helped her to be more in touch with her painful feelings, which were otherwise externalized in the form of delusions and hallucinations. Even then she was so heavily invested in maintaining a psychotic identity based on such things as denying anything was the matter or that she had any needs, and on attacking her own caring and positive feelings, that she remained threatened by the drug effect and ultimately had to stop medication. Even in the face of palpably clearer thinking and better functioning, Celia intermittently tried to convince herself and me that medication was driving her crazy and that she could not tolerate it.

Pharmacotherapy as Primary Treatment Modality

From the standpoint of the humanist, in even the most optimistic of scenarios, Voltaire's "best of all possible worlds," probably the majority of schizophrenic patients will be too impaired or chronic to be candidates for intensive psychotherapy, and even among those who might otherwise seem amenable, family attitudes, economic factors, and scarcity of therapeutic resources will make it impossible to use this modality. For perhaps the majority of schizophrenics the most realistic and hopeful prospect that can be envisioned involves the judicious use of medication as the principal treatment modality.

It is extremely unlikely that medication alone can bring about permanent organic structural change, or that somatic treatment of any sort can alter pathological paths of development and adaptation with their associated neurological substrates that were learned over the course of many years and that are not simply transient products of reversible regression. But, as already noted, medication may target and ameliorate some of the core and presumptively constitutional elements in schizophrenia such as disintegration, defective stimulus handling and rage processing, and problems with focus, attention, and concentration, and thus support the highest level of adaptation of which a patient is currently capable. Unfortunately there is a thin line between medication used in this truly therapeutic manner and medication used to reinforce familial and social attitudes and beliefs, including denial and suppression, and to promote a compliant and uncomplaining "adjustment" to the very limited circumstances in which the schizophrenic may find himself, and that line is frequently and unknowingly transgressed.

Perhaps the medical-reductionistic model of disease and treatment is the major reason for such transgressions. To the extent that medication is used to further alienate the patient from awareness of his feelings and to relieve him of the responsibility of facing and being responsible for his life, such "treatment" might better be conceptualized, from the individual psychological if not from the broad socio-cultural standpoint, as part of the illness itself. Of course, we can no more expect the average psychopharmacologist to acknowledge such an attitude than we can expect the psychotherapist I described in Chapter 15 to be aware of his narcissistic symbiotic collusion to keep his patient disabled. But because the schizophrenic who is encouraged and expected as part of his treatment to try to cope with himself and his life as others do with theirs can be a terribly disturbing influence on his environment, to say nothing of being a danger to himself, it may be assumed that when medication is used alone as a primary treatment modality, even with the best of intentions, it is likely to be administered in such a dosage and with such accompanying environmental attitudes and expectations as to go at least somewhat beyond the bounds of simply counteracting constitutional vulnerabilities, into the area of reinforcing existing psychopathology. I do not say this critically, for it may be that such a situation is the best we have to offer most patients. In that case our efforts should be directed to effect compromise between the needs of the patient and the needs of society in the most enlightened, humane, benign way possible, so that we do not unwittingly replicate destructive family attitudes and produce a crop of bland, passive, tranquilized human vegetables.

Particularly with newly admitted acute schizophrenic patients heavy medication is often used to relieve their apparent suffering, ameliorate symptoms, and normalize behavior. This use of medication during the period of evaluation resembles giving analgesics to patients in pain from medical problems; it is not specific treatment and it may remove motivation at the same time it produces a more tractable patient. In this regard it is of interest that in the old asylum days narcotics were sometimes used to sedate psychotic patients.

Pharmacotherapy and Psychotherapy

In all but the mildest cases use of medication at some point may be indispensable to maintaining the minimum level of cognitive and adaptive functioning necessary to participate in psychotherapy in a way that will ultimately enhance the patient's capacity to bear stress. I doubt that I could have engaged most of the patients I have worked with without the assistance of medication, and I marvel at reports in the literature of successful treatments in the era prior to the introduction of phenothiazines following World War II. When medication is employed adjunctively to exploratory psychotherapy the purpose is not to remove awareness of feelings and suffering, but to facilitate the patient's capacity to join with the therapist in doing the work of treatment in the face of overwhelming anxieties and pressures that would otherwise lead to fragmentation and withdrawal into an unrelated and self-destructive state. When I was in psychiatric training I acted as psychiatric administrator for a patient in the Massachusetts Mental Health Center longitudinal study (Grinspoon, Ewalt, & Shader, 1972) who was being treated by Elvin Semrad, my mentor. Semrad often accurately guessed when I had raised his patient's dose of chlorpromazine, and would wryly remark to me that I had made his patient "drunk." The dosage of medication must be titrated in close conjunction with the progress of the psychotherapeutic work; if it is being administered by a separate psychopharmacologist (and I do not think it interferes with treatment for the therapist to administer the medication if he is comfortable with the use of drugs, for doing so is simply an enactive form of intervention, such as I outlined in Chapter 11), he needs to understand that the drug is not the primary treatment modality, and his goal is not symptom eradication and relief of suffering but facilitation of therapeutic work. Psychotherapist and psychopharmacologist must remain in frequent communication.

While no discussion of psychotherapy is considered complete without examination of issues related to termination, when medication is prescribed for a schizophrenic patient, with the possible exception of the early stages of the first psychotic "break," it is almost always with the conscious or unconscious assumption on the part of the psychopharmacologist, based on a neo-Kraepelinian conception of schizophrenia, that such treatment will probably be required for the remainder of the patient's life, as insulin is for a diabetic. This may well be true when, for practical considerations or because of the results of evaluation at the psychological level, the goal is one of restoration of the social status quo, perhaps accompanied by ameliorative, educative, or rehabilitative efforts. I have indicated that this use of the concept of the organic component of schizophrenia is unnecessarily limited, and have cited evidence that psychotherapy, conceptualized as physical force, may facilitate the development of compensatory processes based on structural modifications of the central nervous system. In such instances it may eventually be possible for the patient to relinquish medication. This was possible in two of the three successful cases in this book, those of Emily and Joanna. In the third, Celia's repudiation of medication because she was subjectively disturbed by its normalizing effects on her psyche made the initial stages of treatment more difficult than they might otherwise have been, but spared us the subsequent work of weaning her.

In commenting on my published discussion of the subject of removal of medication (Robbins, 1992), one reviewer wondered why I assumed my patient should dispense with medication first and psychotherapy subsequently. The answer, aside from the physical hazards of prolonged medication, resides in the humanistic bias that informs this book, in this case couched in a neuroscientific model: It is important, wherever possible, to develop to the fullest each patient's autonomous maturational capacities to deal with stress. Termination of psychotherapy before weaning the patient from medication, except when one is compelled to do so by practical considerations, makes no more sense than placing an obese and sedentary patient with mild hypertension on a long-term medication regimen designed to lower blood pressure, cholesterol, and maximize cardiac function, without first and thoroughly exploring the therapeutic effects of a program of exercise, diet, and stress reduction.

Part V

Cases:
The Middle Range
of Outcomes

Chapter 19

Joanna:
A Positive Outcome

History

Joanna was 20 years old when she was admitted to the hospital at the end of the summer preceding her senior year of college. She had become progressively disabled, incoherent, and delusional in the preceding months.

Joanna was the third of six children. Her mother, a concert pianist and music teacher, was an overcompliant woman who had been dominated by her own father. Joanna's father was an antisocial, intellectual curmudgeon, a man who had abandoned his engineering career to start his own business in the area of environmental preservation. He had episodic rage reactions and often engaged in sadistic teasing of other family members.

Joanna was named after her maternal grandmother, Joanna, and her maternal uncle, John, a chronic schizophrenic. Within Joanna's first 2 weeks of life her mother developed a breast abscess, which made it necessary for her to wean Joanna, and was hospitalized. In the early months of her life her father developed a serious eye problem, was hospitalized, and lost the sight of one eye.

Some of the parental breach was filled by Joanna's namesake, her schizophrenic Uncle John, who lived with the family for long periods of time, and by a family maid. Uncle John believed Joanna was destined to be like him, an empty person with a social facade, and he urged mother to prevent this by not smiling at her, a bizarre idea that turned out to have a grain of truth when we discovered the mechanical smiles that were a trademark of both Joanna and her mother. The maid who cared for Joanna convulsed and went into labor when Joanna was alone in her care at age 2; she never returned to the family.

Joanna sucked her thumb until puberty. There were chronic toilet training battles with her parents, and she suffered from constipation and encopresis.

She developed a sickly sweet facade, for which she was teased by her older siblings. She had recurrent nightmares, in which she made unsuccessful efforts to hold on to a precipice to avoid being devoured by a monster, had her fingers fused together so that she could not grasp, and had her hands run over by a train. She had a variety of phobias (including a school phobia) and terrors, and suffered from recurrent stomachaches.

When Joanna was 5 a sibling was born. In response to her question about mother's sudden absence father joked that she had left and was not coming back. Before she was 10 Joanna acted as father's helper and enjoyed considerable physical contact with him. Around age 10 a brother was born, and after that time father drank increasingly and was much less available to Joanna. When she was 11 her uncle John committed suicide. Her menarche occurred at age 12.

As an adolescent Joanna seemed intelligent, talented, and popular. However, she could not make sense of the world and concretely perceived that it was composed of unintegrated fragments or pieces. Tangible signs of Joanna's illness coincided with the beginning of college. Father had a recurrence of his eye problem, which threatened his vision and required him to undergo repeated surgery. Joanna felt inwardly chaotic and unable to communicate. Although she could not feel emotion she often felt physically cold and in need of physical attention. Although she feared men she began to seek out relationships with self-centered, domineering, erratic, angry men who were concurrently involved with close women friends of hers. These men included another patient of the psychiatrist whom she had begun to see and the brother of a friend; often they were from other racial or cultural backgrounds. Joanna became sexually promiscuous. She felt she was being controlled by external forces, and began to experience auditory hallucinations; she felt intense anxiety associated with the belief that her face was dissolving or fragmenting.

Following her sophomore year of college Joanna developed a protracted, ostensibly physical illness and had to spend much of that summer in bed. By the start of her junior year of college she was marginally functional and utterly dependent on her boyfriend Deeg, a black man from a very different cultural background. When he went home for the summer, and Joanna correctly suspected that he wanted to end their relationship, she became unable to leave her house, was confused, agitated, and disorganized, and was convinced she was pregnant. Finally, when she became incoherent and bizarre, she was hospitalized.

On admission Joanna was disoriented, hyperactive, and unable to sleep. She compulsively rearranged the furniture in her room. Her emotional flatness was punctuated by outbursts of inappropriate laughter, rage, and weeping. Her speech was pressured and often incoherent, a flood of loose, idiosyncratic associations. Reasoning was concrete. Some of the time she confused her identity with that of her dead Uncle John, believing he was inside her body and had cast a spell on her. She said that both of them had an "unnatural" love for her mother. She expressed confusion about the water she splashed on her face when she washed, thinking it might be her own tears. When she became angry she feared this meant she was becoming a man. She thought that she might be pregnant by her father, that she had just had a baby, that she had been given a large fortune, and that a book had been written about her.

One week after admission Joanna had psychological testing, which revealed an acute schizophrenic reaction with a strong affective component. The tester commented on sexual identity confusion, fluid ego boundaries, affective lability, primary process thinking, hallucinations and delusions, much introjected rage, strong symbiotic ties to mother, chronic depression, and a compliant, overachieving style.

During the 6-week interval before I began working with her, Joanna gradually recompensated with the assistance of modest doses of thioridazine. She remained physically wooden and emotionally flat, and, although she developed a brittle social smile and became somewhat more functional, she continued to harbor delusions that she was a machine or that other people were machines controlling her.

Treatment

Year One

Joanna and I began therapy relatively early in my own professional career, more than 25 years ago, and we continued for 7 years, until she was 27. At first we met three times a week, later four times, and toward the end we cut back once again to three. Joanna presented a "good-girl" facade so extreme it was like a caricature. At our first meeting her speech was pressured, she was very anxious, and her thinking readily became disorganized. She expressed fears of being hurt if she became dependent on me, and she actually felt the hurt as a pain in her stomach.

In ensuing meetings Joanna was affectless and robotic in her expression and movements. She was naive and confused, not nearly so bright as her college background suggested. She had perceptual distortions and a terror of disintegrating, being abandoned, or being attacked. Her self and object boundaries were very fluid and there was much projection. In lieu of feelings she experienced varying degrees of anxiety, nausea, and body sensations; for example, she would feel cold and believe that she was ice or a stone. Sometimes she thought that I was calling her names or that I might attack her. Much later I learned about her numerous delusions; all she told me at the time was that the longer the intervals between our meetings, the more I came to seem like a monster or a machine to her. At times she admitted she believed that I was Hal, the robot from the movie *2001*, an idea not entirely so preposterous as it might seem, since I tend to smile infrequently. In fact, as I learned later, her belief became something of a joke among the other patients on her ward, who would observe me when I came to see her.

After about 2 months Joanna hinted that she was experiencing dependent and sexual feelings about me, although she remained flat and distant in manner. Awareness of this attachment frightened her and was regularly followed by episodes of perceptual distortion of my face, disorganization, inappropriate laughter, and exacerbation of her belief that I was a machine. She cried and told me how hopeless and entrapped she felt; at times her body felt as though she were stooped over under a counter and could not get up.

In the second 3 months of our work I began to direct Joanna's attention to her generalized and extreme inhibition of feeling, which made our sessions not only uneventful but soporifically boring for me. I pointed out how she walked around like a zombie, stiff and without feeling, and Joanna was able to relate this behavior to her inhibition of feelings that she believed would be destructive and to her belief in the possibility of retaliation or abandonment should she express them. I observed that she was the robot. Although she claimed she did not like the constricted feeling, and although she worried that she was emotionally frigid, as she imagined her mother to be, she seemed untroubled by my comments.

She then tried to talk about how angry and hopeless she felt, but her account had a distant and unreal quality. Then she became silent and uncommunicative; she said she felt empty, as though she had lost her limbs, and just wanted to lie in bed and keep warm. She believed her reaction had some relation to the loss of her boyfriend Deeg, who had been like a part of her body. I felt sleepy and could not entirely conceal the fact from her. Joanna realized she was putting me to sleep. She tried to express her anger by shouting but it had a forced, nongenuine quality, and when I questioned why she was doing it she responded that she was trying to win my approval. Negating her inner life, she added, was part of an effort to attain the kind of perfection that would bring her closer to father, a scientist who looked upon emotion as a flaw in the system. Rage was stuffed in her stomach, she said, where it was boiling.

Joanna dreamed that there were many birthday cakes, and I went into a meeting with the ward staff but she was not allowed. She dreamed she was in a car driven by a man. They crashed into a pond and she was suffocating, trying to come up from the bottom. This account led to a discussion of the part of her that was choked off and swallowed. She recalled being constipated as a child, and she felt urges to defecate as well as nausea. She recalled toilet battles with her parents and enemas from the family doctor. She seemed to want me to act like her father, whom she experienced as punitive and censorious about emotional expression; when I did not comply she concocted her own justifications for censoring her productions. Her emotionless ruminations continued to make me feel bored and sleepy. Despite my own struggle to be a "perfect therapist," to be attentive in the face of her boring lifelessness, I became increasingly unable to hide my drowsiness. Joanna, in turn, tried her best not to notice. Despite the relative success of our collusion I eventually thought it best to begin to call her attention to my behavior. In response she began to articulate her own wishes to be asleep, even to be dead, and to put me to sleep because of her fear of me and of her feelings. As we focused on what she was trying to put to sleep in herself, there was some evidence that it had to do with her genitals and sexual feelings about me. She commented that she had missed her most recent menstrual period. She imagined, and at times seemed to believe, that she was a machine, Sleeping Beauty, or a china doll.

In the fifth month Joanna and I agreed to meet four times a week in the hope that the new schedule would be useful in dealing with her extraordinary inhibition. Joanna began to express envy of other patients, who she believed were able to be more genuine, but at the same time she maintained that she had to try to be a "good girl" or a china doll, since what made her innately evil were her feelings.

There was increasing evidence of Joanna's wish to make a fuss and to express herself as angry, needy, and jealous. Now there were occasional eruptions of rage, in the form of real shouting, and expressions of sadness. At first her rage was expressed as great incoherent sounds which appeared to combine explosion and inhibition, and did not seem particularly human. Her shouting gradually attained more of a ring of conviction and less of a squelched and compliant quality. She described her experience in physical terms: broken intestines, an enormous sore or blister. She discovered that she hallucinated female voices that prohibited her from having feelings. There were rage at her parents for not letting her be a person, envy of others who were more expressive, and anger at people who had left her or disappointed her, particularly her boyfriend Deeg. Joanna imagined getting attention from her mother and revenge by committing suicide, as her schizophrenic Uncle John had done. I commented that she seemed much more real when she expressed her feelings, and she responded that her abdominal pain and constipation had ceased. She recognized a growing attachment to me and to her therapy, for it was the only situation in which she felt she was alive.

At this time I informed Joanna that I was being unexpectedly called away and would be absent for 2 weeks. Her ward administrator felt that she was suicidal, moved her to a locked ward, and increased her daily dose of thioridazine to 200 mg. My plans changed and my trip never took place. Joanna dreamed a black mother-substitute was trying to have intercourse with her using a foam penis substitute; although she was excited Joanna felt something was wrong and she awoke. She resumed acting and talking like a china doll, stiff and affectless, and she complained of feeling unreal. Our sessions again became soporific. I heard from father about his dissatisfaction with Joanna's progress. After I had been seeing her for more than 6 months, I gave Joanna something of an ultimatum, informing her that it was unlikely she could get better and have a life of her own unless she became more accepting of her inner life of feelings and thoughts.

My recollection is that I struggled with sleepy, detached feelings in response to Joanna's extreme emotional deadness for a seemingly interminable period, until I worried not only whether I could continue to remain alive and wakeful in my sessions with her, but also whether she might be a chronic schizophrenic who would be unwilling or unable to involve herself with her emotions and with me. According to my notes, however, the soporific stage of treatment could not have lasted more than 8 or 9 months. I now view my relative impatience and the associated ultimatum as a countertransference replication of Joanna's hopeless infantile depression, which will shortly become more evident to the reader, and as my protest against experiencing it and being driven crazy, as she had been.

Joanna was then able to tell me that her emotional deadness was in part a form of retaliation against me because she did not feel as special as she wished to be. She had a very pleasant dream in which she was first my secretary and then her father's, in which she took an hour lunch break to take a bath. She associated the bath in the dream to bathing before intercourse. It turned out that some of her father's restlessness about her hospitalization was because she was presenting to him the "normal" (that is, affectless) facade to which he was accustomed, which made him think she was ready to leave the hospital. She took issue with this idea, and he revealed to her the extent of his anger at the hospital. After this Joanna realized she had provoked her father to enact her anger at me for not making her special. A disruptive crisis was averted through a family meeting which turned out to be more amicable than I had anticipated. Father behaved like a curious little child who also wanted attention, but both parents agreed that Joanna had become a more three-dimensional person since her hospitalization, and they seemed pleased.

Joanna remained on a locked ward because of her suicidal preoccupation. Once again she shut down emotionally, acted detached, felt unreal and empty, and experienced pain in her stomach, and I had to struggle with drowsiness and wishes to sleep during her appointments. Yet her menstrual functioning returned for the first time since hospitalization, and she dreamed that she had found two interesting blue balls and had sent them to a man to be refined, and that she was swimming with me. She felt I was encouraging her to become a woman. She reverted to her wish to be special, and told me that her emotional detachment was her solution to intolerable frustration over her wishes to have an all-consuming sexualized union with me. She recalled that she would get herself to eat by imagining Deeg eating, and told me of her wish that I would literally speak for her, as I had done, in a sense, in the family meeting. She dreamed of being held by an older man and wanting to have a climax, then woke with menstrual bleeding for the third time in a month.

Gradually Joanna's depression lifted, and after 8 months of therapy she was able to get a part-time hospital job. As my summer vacation approached she was more aware of the frustration of her passive wishes to merge with me, and she began to scream in my office with rage and frustration, hour after hour, in a way that I now found as frightening as I had found the preceding deadness boring. Psychiatrists in offices adjacent to mine began to complain about the noise and offer polite expressions of their disquietude and skepticism about what they thought I was doing with Joanna to make her regress, which made me uneasy because of my relatively junior status. Joanna's rage was associated with cannibalistic wishes to cut me in little pieces and devour me, penis first, or with a wish to get inside me and somehow possess me and my idealized attributes, which would make her strong. When she ate she sometimes became convinced she was eating me, which made her nauseated. She recalled wishes to eat previous boyfriends, especially during separations. We learned that her promiscuity had been an effort to actualize these fantasies, and that when she lost a relationship, such as the one with Deeg, in which her wishes seemed potentially attainable, the longed for state of fusion would occur through psychosis, through, for example, the belief that she was becoming a man. She needed help with boundaries, reality testing, and limit setting (once I had to remove from her hand an ashtray she was about to throw at me).

As stormy as our relationship had become, Joanna now seemed better to others; as the anniversary of Deeg's departure loomed—the event that seemed to have precipitated the acute psychosis, her discharge was also planned. Joanna cried about the loss of Deeg and expressed fears that she might not be real and concerns about the summer separation from me. Without a man and a penis she felt empty and inadequate. Her speech was again full of eating metaphors. She wanted to devour me or Deeg to obtain qualities she felt were missing in her. She wanted to go to medical school and become a doctor, like me, but wasn't sure she could "hack it." At times she felt full, sometimes even nauseated. Then she would feel no need to talk to me, mention wishes to terminate therapy, and even act as though I were not there; at such times it turned out she had transient delusions she had indeed devoured me. When she saw me after brief separations and realized she had not in fact succeeded in consuming me, she felt both relief and rage. She acted very inhibited when she reported a dream in which she smeared feces and was then told by her doctor that she had to bury them or to shove them back into the sink and up the drain again, which she could not do; then her father came and marinated meat in the sink that the feces had been in, and they ate it. In a subsequent hour she recalled a childhood memory of soiling herself, and she realized that she equated feelings and feces.

It began to dawn on Joanna that I would not be around to help her if she were to kill and devour me. Our now tumultuous relationship included shouting rages, wishes to beat me into submission as an act of control and revenge, and wishes to possess my attributes. She insisted that she would become a doctor and someday I would marry her. This led to plans to return to school as a premed in the fall. Her feelings and behavior as she negotiated interviews with the dean and the university psychiatrist who had once treated her and now had to approve her return to school all seemed very appropriate and assertive. At the anniversary of her separation from Deeg Joanna recalled her psychosis after his departure, and she feared this would happen again during my summer absence. She had an urge to get involved with another student from Deeg's country who reminded her of him.

Thioridazine was reduced to 25 mg and soon thereafter discontinued. After 9 months of hospitalization Joanna was discharged from the hospital to an apartment which she shared with other formerly hospitalized patients. She slept at the hospital five nights a week and continued her part-time hospital job, which she seemed to enjoy. Withdrawal from thioridazine left Joanna quite shaky. She reported the following dream: She was coming to a strange city to see me and didn't know how she would make the connections; suddenly, without knowing how she got there, she found herself in my office. I had just finished seeing her sister, and I was laughing and eating clams. I told her she was jealous and refused to see her, saying that I was leaving; she burst out crying.

In fact, Joanna did spend many of her therapy hours crying and expressing fears I would leave her because she was not interesting enough; she also expressed rage at her sister, who she felt was more interesting, and at father, who paid attention to sister and mother and not to her. For the first time she realized that the heavy feeling she had experienced when Deeg left was rage. When I had to cancel an appointment, she tried unsuccessfully to make a date with a countryman of Deeg's and then canceled her next appointment. Next hour she reported the following dream: She had played the leading role in *A Doll's House*, a play, which she attributed to Tennessee Williams, about a married woman who was separating from her husband because she had been nothing but an extension of him. There were two schoolteachers, one with very low self-esteem and the other rather manic and inappropriate. In a final scene some students were angrily rebelling against the university and trying to overthrow it. Joanna's associations were to her efforts to become an individual rather than a china doll, to my forthcoming vacation and her previous summer separation from Deeg, and to her fears of an anniversary repetition of her psychosis. She was particularly afraid that when she saw her previous psychiatrist as part of the screening for her readmission to the university, she might express her anger at him for having been unavailable to her when she needed him, and that he would think she was crazy and not allow her to return to school.

Joanna seemed more vivacious and spontaneous, and her work was going well. As my vacation approached she felt a wrenching sadness, but her tears were strangulated as she recalled how much her parents disliked crying. With a week remaining she called to cancel an appointment, saying she had burned her hand and was sick to her stomach as a result of having caused an explosion when lighting her gas oven. I urged her to keep the appointment, and she had an enormous affective explosion in the office, including rage, tears, and feelings of helplessness about my vacation. She said the light, warmth, and security were going out of her life, and she just wanted to stay inside me. It turned out that she had realized a split second before lighting the stove that there might be an explosion, but had sensed that she wanted such an external distraction. I worried to myself, and to her expressed my hope that she would keep future explosions for her therapy sessions.

Year Two

Joanna did well while I was gone, and when I returned we began our second year of work. She had rejected opportunities to enact sexualized mergers with men, including one with her old boyfriend Deeg. She had been able to express some of her anger at him for leaving her. She was able to review her illness, and although she had entered therapy involuntarily, she now chose to continue it and was able to define some broader goals for herself. She concluded that it was best to postpone her return to college. She seemed more vivacious, warm and alive, and a degree of intelligence more consistent with her previous record of accomplishment, which I had not hitherto seen, was much more evident.

The initial flurry of constructiveness was quickly superseded by Joanna's feelings of hurt and anger about my vacation and my involvement with my own family, and by her wishes not to reinvolve herself with me. She dreamed of conflicting allegiances to two male patients, one of whom was compliant and cooperative with the hospital and one who had to be restrained because of violent rages. She wondered whether my influence over her had been good or evil. A dream of a patient who cut off the top half of her torso was associated to her war against her feelings. Nonetheless, she cautiously began to feel warmly toward me again.

In the course of discussing her strong attraction to a young man Joanna began to be more aware of her search for a particular configuration of charisma, controlling, selfishness, and rejection which resembled her descriptions of her father. These men tended to be involved with other women, and the triangle represented her father and her more successful sisters. Her aim was to merge with such a man in order that she might become what he idealistically represented male strength to be: a person without the flaw of emotionality. She wanted to become a doctor like me and thought of pleasing her father by going into his scientific field; perhaps she might obtain a penis. Joanna had recurrent dreams of going crazy, exploding, trying to call me but being unable to reach me or speak. She dreamed I would not see her because I was "specialing" another patient. She experienced churning in her stomach, nausea, and muscular tension in her arms; these represented her inhibited longings to be more involved with me and her wishes to hit me. She dreamed of being on trial for shooting a man in church; she was about to be acquitted because of mental illness, but she told the jury she was responsible for what she had done.

As Joanna began to enact her search for a father substitute I became aware that in recent weeks I had been finding her particularly appealing. In anticipation of her menstrual period it occurred to Joanna to tell me that she had recently had her first sexual encounter since leaving the hospital and might have gotten herself pregnant, as she had not used a contraceptive. She had picked a repressive man in order to help her inhibit sexual feelings. I pointed out the seeming contradiction between the qualities she sought in a man and her belief that such a relationship would provide her with security and self-esteem. Joanna then dreamed that mother had distracted her for 40 minutes from tuning her violin, and that she had to move out of a house with a garden and kill all the plants, which were twins, with a syringe. She dreamed she had a baby boy who went crazy and tried to rape her, and that she was pregnant but was able, with father's help, to obtain an abortion.

I pointed out the fact that sex in her dreams was never consummated. Joanna realized that she had felt enormously inhibited sexually in her home and that she had gone to great lengths to avoid being seen in her bedroom. She talked about "letting her hair down" in ways simultaneously concrete and metaphorical: by coloring her hair for the first time and wishing to be less inhibited. She bought a diaphragm. After a visit home in which a sister brought up the issue of Joanna's behavior with men (Joanna told her it was none of her business) she dreamed of being in a room with a door which opened suddenly into an adjoining apartment; she entered with curiosity, only to be attacked by a man.

Joanna was accepted back to school for the following year, and she had the feeling she was getting well. Then she overslept and was late for work, having had a dream that she had a severe heart condition and the doctor prescribed complete bed rest. She realized the need to see herself as sick had to do with wishes not to see father's problems, for to do so left her feeling very insecure. Her associations became chaotic and bizarre. Her perception of father had been of a creature all head and brain who waxed eloquent about science; now he seemed smaller and more fragile. If she were sick and crazy then she could avoid perceiving and responding to father's sickness, and she could continue to see me forever.

It seemed that Joanna selected unsuitable men in order to externalize and avoid her own difficulties sustaining close and sexual feelings, and to avoid the aggressiveness she feared she might show with a more accepting man. Men of other races were safest because she perceived deep commitment with one to be impossible. She began to talk of her enormous mistrust of men and of their dark, angry, crazy, rejecting side. She literally felt she could not trust me unless she saw the whites of my eyes. She felt like a helpless victim in a world of gigantic attacking cockroaches. These images shifted between metaphor and concrete delusion and hallucination. She called me between sessions, distraught and frightened, but came into the next therapy hour bearing a container of milk and feeling like a more trusting little girl. After a weekend separation Joanna acted distant from me and reported a dream in which a boy had attacked her and bitten her throat and she had swung from tree to tree like a gorilla in order to escape. She dreamed she was trying to protect an angelfish from a large predatory catfish, which turned into a man; she associated to the sexually impulsive and angel-priggish sides of herself. As Joanna became more aware of the problematic nature of her relationships with men and of the fact that she had turned to them for mothering because of a failure in her relationship with her own mother, she began to seek out more closeness with women.

As the time to return to school approached Joanna terminated the relatively undemanding job she had held since her discharge from the hospital, and with it some important close relationships she had formed with older women. She made demands for a more personal relationship with me, and then dreamed that a former college friend became psychotic because her father had slept with her. She feared she would search for a sexual father-mother to assuage her loneliness and replace the relationships she was losing at her work, and she recognized some of the secure attraction of being a hospital patient again, along with fears that she might become psychotic. She called me in a state of panic following a dream in which she lived with a foster family with whom she could not communicate (because they spoke only Italian). Just before resuming school she dreamed the episode of Deeg leaving was happening again, but in her dream she was aware of and expressed all the anger and sadness she had previously inhibited. But she also dreamed she was being attacked by a man, and was paralyzed and helpless.

When she commenced school Joanna was surprised to discover in herself a new sense of capability and aggressiveness, a new ability to express her needs, and a sense of freedom from internal disruption. There were many memories of rejection by her mother, who seemed to prefer Joanna's schizophrenic Uncle John, and she recounted that mother had been required to stop breast-feeding her because of an abscess. She wished for a warm, secure mother and experienced a strong pull toward the hospital to meet this need. Her language became almost completely oral. She woke in the mornings nauseated and starved. She was compelled to eat sugar cereals for comfort when she felt needy and disappointed; they were safe, she could control them, and they stayed inside her. She longed to be fed and to get "feedback" from me. She experienced feelings of rage and rejection associated with nausea, and urges to vomit and rid herself of what was bad and untrustworthy—at times her mother, but often me. She was never sure I would be the same person from one hour to the next; she continually felt our relationship to be endangered, and at times she again perceived me as a machine.

Under the stress of her first examinations at school Joanna could not eat or sleep. She began to dream while she was awake, which we recognized as a prepsychotic symptom. When she again wished for me to feed her I prescribed some chloral hydrate and offered to accompany her to the hospital cafeteria while she ate. Instead, she took the chloral hydrate at bedtime with milk and noted that the *M* in my name on the prescription also stood for *mother.* She was able to sleep and eat and get through her first examination. A former hospital patient she befriended stole half her medication, and she dreamed I told her I could not treat her because I was paralyzed, for I had a mother who was bad. She was hungry to fill the cold emptiness inside; at the same time she felt angry and wanted to vomit. Joanna sobbed in a desperate, pathetic manner, like an abandoned child, and wanted to cling to me and to be my Siamese twin. She wanted to kill me, dissect me, and find out what made me tick, wanted to make me into a mummy or doll she could carry around. After seeing Deeg again and spending the night with him, at which time each acknowledged that the other had changed and that they had no future together, Joanna remembered playing on the floor next to father's desk, wanting to be near him but very invested in the sight, smell, and texture of her dolls. Suddenly, she remembered her favorite doll was black, like Deeg!

Now Joanna began to spend more time visiting the hospital, having involved herself with Dean, a patient. Joanna was remarkably unable to perceive his blatant psychosis, which included delusions and hallucinations, and was furious at ward staff for restricting his freedom. She kept secret his plans to escape from the hospital, and he was found in an extremely disturbed condition and returned. When I questioned her judgment, Joanna experienced a hateful rage at me. She told me that Dean dressed and looked like Christ, and she added that she believed the mentally ill were special, chosen people, whereas the rest of us were either ordinary or a part of the world of machines. As she relinquished her identification with Dean's grandiose paranoid attitude and her conviction that he was normal, she alternately raged at me and cried with sadness, and her own deep suspiciousness of others became more apparent. After 19 months of therapy Joanna suddenly and without warning announced that she was not going to see me for a week; on her return she admitted she had been so angry she could not face me. She began to relate her recent preoccupation with Dean to an unrecognized attachment to her Uncle John, who died when she was 11.

Joanna seemed more disorganized. There were loosened associations, hallucinations of mother's voice, and buzzing in her ears. I began to provide more reality and structure in her sessions, and started her on trifluoperazine, 6 mg, which she took erratically because of her suspiciousness. She could not feel skin sensation and cut herself without knowing it. Joanna wished to devour me and possess my good qualities but also feared that I was poisoning her. She was convinced that she literally possessed the worst qualities of her psychotic uncle, her facade mother, and her partially blind father.

Once again Joanna became less suspicious, more trusting and more obviously sad. She felt more vulnerable and human, and acknowledged that she no longer aspired to be a machine-perfect student. She recalled positive memories of being fed by her dead maternal grandmother, Joanna. Dean turned out to represent not only maternal Uncle John but, more fundamentally, a suspicious, inhibited, hostile part of herself. Recognizing that mother had been attached to crazy Uncle John much as she herself was attached to Dean, Joanna concluded that Uncle John had similarly represented and enacted this role for mother. While Joanna and mother acted normal, with their smiling facades, holding on to Uncle John or his proxy was a way of holding on to other parts of themselves, and to one another. Then Joanna realized she had also enacted this angry suspicious part for mother. This made her first enraged, then absentminded and disorganized. She punned, felt pressure in her head, and was convinced that her eyes were unusually bright.

Again Joanna became less suspicious and more depressed as she struggled over relinquishing her role of being special to her mother by virtue of her insanity, but this change frightened her since she felt more vulnerable and dependent on others. She began to form a relationship with Bob, a fellow student who seemed more gentle than her typical boyfriend, but when she wanted to be physical and he wanted to study she felt rebuffed and became first enraged and then concrete and confused. Joanna began to act flirtatious toward men without realizing it, and got upset when they responded to her. She hallucinated a comforting voice calling her name. During weekend separations she tried to keep me in mind, but her rage did not permit it. She hallucinated men making overtures to her and in fact allowed herself to be picked up by and have sex with a stranger. During an ensuing therapy hour she became panicked that I might rape her, until she realized she had lost her stable image of me. As we talked she made a retching noise, then felt she wanted to chew gum or eat, and finally, she was able to own up to some of the affectionate and sexual feelings and wishes she had toward me, as well as rage that I did not gratify her.

At the 20th month of therapy Joanna's efforts to internalize a stable good object intensified as we prepared for a week I would be away. She struggled to hold on to close positive feelings about me, and experienced sadness. There was much orally centered conflict, with ambivalent caring and depression alternating with rage, vomiting, and ridding herself of my visual image, which left her with a world experienced as mechanical and monstrous. While I was gone Joanna employed writing and picture drawing (she drew stiff, childlike portraits of me sitting in my chair) to attempt to maintain object constancy and stave off rage. She was all right when she could think about missing me and talk about it with others, but when Bob left one morning she posed for nude pictures for a photographer, then felt flat and zombie-like.

As she told me about this after I returned Joanna had the urge to tear my eyes out. I increased her trifluoperazine to 8 mg. She transiently believed she was a man and did not have to feel. Her rage was so intense it made her go limp and clutch the arm of her chair during her therapy hour, and at night she needed to get out of the bed she shared with Bob and put the light on to reassure herself she had not killed him.

In the latter part of our second year of work there was evidence of Joanna's renewed vigor and intelligence and of a capacity to more efficiently concentrate on her studies, despite the periods of psychosis. She passed all her courses in the spring term, managed to maintain a job, and began to make new friends. Once again men became the subject of interest, and we realized she only related to them in terms of wishes, fantasies, and delusions of merger. In contrast, she could sustain positive thoughts, feelings, and fantasies about me only as long as we were at a physical distance; if she approached me with caring feelings and shook my hand, for example, terror of merger, self-loss, or her own death led her to commit psychic murder on me by obliterating her perceptions of my physical characteristics until I appeared flattened and lifeless.

Dean called from the hospital and Joanna had the urge to visit him. When

I questioned her assumption that because she had been psychotic she knew how he felt whereas I did not, she launched another rageful, screaming attack on me and claimed I was untrustworthy. Eventually she became calmer, and in subsequent hours was able to discuss how she picked psychotic men in order to deny her own psychosis, and how she maintained the hermaphroditic delusion that she was a man-woman, or perhaps a woman with a man inside her, in order to feel totally self-sufficient and to protect herself against the threat of having feelings about people. A paranoid man such as her Uncle John or Dean was looked upon as particularly powerful, as a kind of Promethean figure. Without the conviction there was a man inside her Joanna was terrified that she could not handle her angry and sexual feelings. She went ahead and visited Dean, perceived his psychotic thinking, and then informed me his problem was that he was terrified of feelings. Having done so, she was able to experience warm, close body feelings about me.

As she relinquished more of her omnipotent beliefs Joanna gave up the idea of going to medical school and becoming me. She began to ask my advice more, and we worked to help her establish more realistic sources of power and control. She talked with her parents more openly about Uncle John, hitherto a taboo subject, and about her concerns that she was like father, and father was able to point out to her ways in which she was different. Uncle John turned out to be a kind of transitional object; Joanna had given his name to her teddy bear and her violin. When father would reject the family or when Joanna felt rejected by a man, she would gain strength by imagining Uncle John sitting cold and aloof.

For the first time Joanna felt vulnerable, soft, and feminine, in need of and attracted to men as separate beings. She dreamed she was with a man, felt sexual, and asked him to touch her vagina; his hand came away with blood on it. She talked about the feeling that she was losing her penis. Her image of the men she had to depend on, however, was a frightening amalgam of father and Uncle John, men who were unreliable, distant, and paranoid. But now she also had some awareness that this image was colored by her own rage, and that her need to attach herself to such a man had to do with an attempt to deny it. She then turned to the conviction that other people carried knives and that she needed to also. She felt her body disintegrating, felt her head separating from it. Wishes to be close and to be accepting of her feelings alternated with wishes to withdraw, harden herself, get her uncle back inside her through sex, and play psychotic duets with Dean. She dreamed she met a wonderful boy named Joanna.

Year Three

After 2 years of treatment Joanna made a 10-day trip to see Bob, who was away for the summer. Prior to her departure she wished to be in my stomach, like baby Roo with Kanga in the A. A. Milne story, or, if this were not possible, to become a psychiatrist. But she remarked that the work necessary to become a psychiatrist would kill her, by which she meant that she would lose her identity. She was angry to be confronted with the impossibility of her wishes, felt nauseated, and wanted to spit me out and turn off her feelings. During the interruption, nonetheless, she was able to keep me in her emotional awareness, and she was only tempted to merge with Bob once, when she heard him playing the piano and impulsively rushed to get her violin.

In the fall I moved my office to a new location, outside the hospital setting in which Joanna had heretofore seen me. She became disoriented, experienced perceptual distortions in which the new office and objects in it were flying around and falling apart, felt depersonalized and suspicious, and wished literally to see things through my eyes. We realized the extent to which her identity was merged with her surround rather than based on her emotions. To make matters worse, Joanna somehow guessed that I was going to get married, and I thought it best to confirm this as well as my plan to take some time off afterward. At first Joanna felt sad and fearful of loss, but soon she experienced rage, the wish to kill me off, and "puke" me out. Although she wanted to close herself off from the world of feelings and people, Joanna now began to realize that by so doing and by erecting what she called her "Colgate shield" (a reference to her fake toothy smile) she avoided the feelings and involvement necessary to form a relationship of her own like the one she imagined I had. Then she had an urge to have oral sex which was associated with the belief that she was an omnipotent boy-girl. In response to these insights she felt cold, covered herself with clothing, dressed like a man, clutched her hands together, and would not speak in order to avoid acknowledging she needed me.

Joanna felt increasingly disintegrated, panicky, and impelled to withdraw and sleep. Although she was enraged at Bob, when he returned she insisted on living with him. After I pointed out how her wish to merge and feel invulnerable through sex led to various of her symptoms, she experienced a terror of identity loss when she began to experience loving or caring feelings for Bob and for me. I suggested that it was not the loving feelings that led her to identity-destroying efforts to be merged. Joanna realized that she wanted to plunge into her relationship with Bob in order to avoid her feelings about me, and by imagining herself merged with a man who was actively working on his career, to avoid facing decisions about her own career after she completed her remaining year of college. She tried to set limits to their physical intimacy, but experienced rageful wishes associated with actual stomachache, to consume me and acquire my supposedly superhuman powers.

Joanna began to talk more about her career choices, and as she faced new situations, such as auditioning for a string quartet, she experienced anxiety. As my wedding approached she felt a literal hunger to incorporate strength, which alternated with murderous rage, the wish to vomit out the world, and paranoia. These forces were counteracted by her realization that she needed to preserve our relationship in order to use it as a practice ground for other relationships. She dreamed she came to an appointment and my office was in a state of flux, with books and furniture all around. There she met my wife, a warm, friendly woman. They had a cordial conversation during which Joanna acknowledged, "You've won, hands down!"

In preparation for my absence we reviewed what we came to call Joanna's rules for becoming schizophrenic, which she eventually wrote down and determined she would struggle with during my absence. These included (1) calling her feelings "crazy" and repudiating them in favor of the belief that she was a machine; (2) somatizing her rage and vomiting me out, with the result that her inner world was devoid of people and the external world became peopled with frightening monsters and robots; and (3) withdrawing to bed and seeking a dreamlike oblivion.

At the 26-month point of therapy I got married and left for a 3-week honeymoon. On my return Joanna told me of a recurrent dream the first few nights of our separation, in which I hugged her and said I was leaving to get married; it had been very satisfying but equally painful to waken to reality. After an initially positive response to my return Joanna began to dress like a man again and express rage and wishes to leave me. It seemed that she had shut me out of her life until she suddenly realized one morning that her stability depended on her awareness and acceptance of her feelings. She dreamed of having to cross a river where a drawbridge was open; a black man made futile efforts to close the bridge by striking the water, but then a stereotypic young Anglo-Saxon man came along and was more successful helping her across. This led to thoughts about Deeg's problems and her own breakdown and her efforts to "bridge" the two of them by merger.

During a visit home Joanna's mother shared with her her own goal in life—to be superefficient—and revealed that she had a recurrent dream about a large machine with a defect! And her father and sister expressed their convictions that people were not to be trusted and that the world was headed toward doom. Joanna made subtle efforts to trick me into revealing whether I was in fact human or machine. Gradually, we concluded that my marriage had shattered her conviction that she would merge with me and had led her to attempt to rid herself of me and substitute machine delusions. Although this awareness first made Joanna depressed and angry, she soon experienced feelings of liberation and greater closeness to Bob, and she was able to talk about her career choices and make the decision to go to graduate school.

When Joanna felt less than perfect she believed that her body was disintegrating and that she was about to be attacked with a knife. When I acknowledged to her during the course of a discussion about her music that I could not read music she felt disorganized and vulnerable, and believed that I might be imminently rent into shreds, or that I had a knife with which I was about to attack her, and she tried to manipulate me into admitting it was true. After this hour she had a repetition of a dream she had before my marriage in which she affirmed that she could still love me and we could have an affectionate relationship even though I was married.

We began to construct Joanna's somatic model of her mind and of her disintegration experience. Her body image was all stomach and mouth. She felt as though her body were porous and in imminent danger of disintegrating, with gaps or interstices where another person such as myself, or a knife might get in. She could connect the occurrence of these fears with the presence of oral wishes to merge with me. She dreamed she bought some seductive clothing, but it was from the men's department. She realized that the disintegration feeling was related to her female body image and that, to protect against it, she wished to be a male; men have no holes, and have the weapon that pierces holes. I remarked that the problem had much more to do with control of her oral and oral-genital rage-fueled longings to obliterate identity.

As we were able to put words to her disintegration experience and talk about her wish to armor herself by believing she was a machine Joanna began to feel better. Her college grades were excellent and she scored very high on the Graduate Record Examination. When we had to meet in my hospital office for logistical reasons, Joanna felt sad and tearful as she recalled how needy, lost, and confused she had been when acutely ill. She felt smaller and less omnipotent and the hospital seemed smaller to her and not so interesting. But she realized that in getting better she was inexorably separating from me, and she imagined that remaining crazy might be a way of preserving a place for herself in my family.

As Joanna became more aware that her intense mothering needs had never been satisfied, she wanted to discuss this with mother. However, she feared that she might learn that mother hated her, or that mother's brittle facade might crack and she would disintegrate; she associated to the surprise birth of her sister when she was 5 and recalled how when she asked father where mother was, he had joked that she would never return. Joanna invited her mother to come to therapy in order to discuss their relationship, but mother declined to come for fear of being blamed, or of crying. Joanna felt a familiar rebuff, which made her realize how she had turned to men for the mothering her own mother had failed to provide. She recalled going to father's workshop as a child, where she would suppress her tears and rage and surround herself with the whine and buzz of his machines. Again she approached mother; this time they had a good talk in that she learned more about the problems in her infancy which had not been her mother's fault, including mother's breast abscess and hospitalization. They talked about the maid who had cared for Joanna, and how she had suffered a toxemic convulsion and miscarriage in Joanna's presence when she was 2. Joanna realized that (though she consciously recalled nothing of this experience), she had acted out the convulsion in the very spot it had occurred when she was becoming psychotic. More material emerged involving her intense orality and rage, her jealousy of her younger sibs when mother fed them, her efforts to curl into a ball and transform herself into mother's breast, her fear of harming mother's breast, and the relation of her fear of expressing her emotional hunger and anger to her delusions of bodily disintegration.

Mother reconsidered her decision not to come to therapy, and 2 years and 7 months into Joanna's treatment we began a series of conjoint meetings. At first mother was impenetrable, acted as if she knew everything and monopolized the conversation, paying little attention to Joanna. But eventually the two cried together and mother was able to assure Joanna that she cared about her. The meetings provided historical clarification and included a discussion of the powerful influence Uncle John and his delusions actually had on mother's child-rearing practices; for example he had convinced her to inhibit her caring responses, insisting that if she smiled at Joanna, the child would turn out psychotic like him. Joanna, in turn, was able in these meetings to express her rage at Uncle John and her envy of his psychotic state which she felt had preempted mother's attentions. And Joanna and I were able to see the grain of truth in Uncle John's beliefs: since mother's false "Colgate smile" was a repudiation of her individual identity, Joanna's emulation of mother's smile was indeed a step on the road to being psychotic.

As Joanna and mother worked out some of their issues, Joanna began to struggle more with her caring and sexual feelings toward me. She dreamed she was in a mental hospital but was dissatisfied with its restrictiveness; in response to her wish I held her hand and kissed her, but this interfered with her thinking. She had another dream of lovemaking with me, from which she awoke before consummation. In this context Joanna recalled father's intense jealousy of the involvement of any of the women in his family with another man (Uncle John in the past and currently, myself). Joanna dreamed she had come to our session wanting to seduce me, but had avoided it by talking about caring for a sick person who was trying to cure himself by vomiting up his badness and then selectively re-eating it. In this dream I had informed her there were three people out to kill me. She hid, and father appeared, threw her a gun to defend herself, and then shot at me. Joanna shot her father in the eye, but this did not hurt him. As she thought about the dream Joanna realized how difficult it was for her to be herself, and how great her tendency was to take on mother's problems, or to live totally in the world of one man. She was much more aware of father's blindness, which she now interpreted more abstractly in terms of his suspicious, anti-feeling, anti-relationship, man-against-the-world ideology. She felt rage and wishes to separate herself from him, but realized that whoever failed to adopt father's ideology seemed to become his mortal enemy. She also recognized that this separation would mean relinquishing a crazy part of herself. She and her father had shared a kind of paranoid isolationist religion in protection against a shared though unspoken sense of vulnerability and weakness.

Joanna now initiated a good talk with father, in which he acknowledged some of his problem areas and supported her treatment, and she began to feel more separate, but also flat and structureless and in need of an ideology, a strong man, an MD degree, or some equivalent. She said she felt like an unsteady toddler. Themes of burial and mourning pervaded her thinking. In a dream she said goodbye to Deeg because she was about to graduate; he responded that when she left him he had fallen apart, and now he was feeling like two people, with a baby inside him. Associations were to separation from merger, and to relinquishing her psychosis and regretfully leaving it with him, a somewhat angry reversal of the way things had actually happened. She dreamed that I told her not to try to remake herself in the image of the deity but to try to paint herself in her own colors.

Joanna began to question her tentative choice of a career, one which might involve relating to people who were ill. She dreamed I had written two books: one about a schizophrenic girl's experience in a mental hospital and the other a perfect treatise on violin playing in which I had named and described the dynamic range of tones. It sounded like she was talking about her conflict between wishes to regress, merge with a man, and return to the hospital and wishes to grow, do her own thing, and tolerate the range of her feelings, as well as about her conflicts over who would write the script or score for her life and who would play it. For the first time and with some difficulty she began to reject advances from men. Joanna showed much assertiveness, decision-making capability, and emotion. She got the highest grades she had yet achieved at college. At times I felt superfluous to her functioning.

The time of graduation from college approached, as did the anniversary of the birth of her sister, and Joanna became convinced I was about to leave her. She recalled the experience at age 5 when sister was born, and father had teased her that mother was never coming back. She had turned to her father for something perfect to solve everything and had merged with his belief system in her grief. Now she felt I had given psychological birth to her. On her sister's birthday she told me of a dream in which she was riding in a car with a friend named Moe with whom she was trying without success to communicate. A dog turned into a bear and attacked her; someone gave her a gun and she shot it. Then she hungrily cut open its belly looking for meat, but there was none on its bones. It turned out that the dog was Moe, and she visited him in the hospital where they sewed him together, and she apologized. Associations were that Moe was shorthand for mother, that she had been starved both for food and affection as a child but had been unable to communicate, and that she had feared her anger had sent mother to the hospital. She recalled how her mother had her pet dog killed when her younger brother was born for fear it would harm him. She recognized in the dream her tendency to regress to an oral incorporative mode of thinking under stress.

At this time Joanna noticed that my eyes were very red, and that there was medication on my desk, and asked why. I responded that I had glaucoma (which had just been diagnosed) and was taking medication. This reminded her of her father's chronic eye problems and of her concrete condensation of his difficulty seeing and his withdrawal and unresponsiveness to members of the family. She thought about her own overreliance on vision and her tendency to experience visual distortions and two dimensional flatness when she was anxious.

Joanna was increasingly aware of her sexuality, a swollen feeling in her vagina, and of needs for her boyfriend Bob; simultaneously she was more aware of his constriction, including his relative lack of interest in sex. She realized she had chosen him because he made few demands on her. She then dreamed of a fat female medical student who was asked to leave school after the third year and who had swollen legs. Joanna felt that her experiences must be trivial in my eyes, and that if she didn't entertain me I wouldn't look at her. She felt alone and vulnerable, literally tiny, without a charismatic man to merge with or a protective delusional system. She contrasted this with how, in the hospital, she had felt big with the beliefs that she had just had a baby, had just been given a million dollars, and had just had an article written about her.

    We were in fact approaching the end of our third year of work together, and Joanna graduated from college with honors and was accepted into graduate school. She made significant progress in her music and reveled in new friendships. She found herself longing for a more satisfying male relationship than the one she had with Bob. She told me that she was experiencing breast sensations for the first time in her entire life, and that her breasts were actually growing in size! In a dream she told one of her instructors, a man who had some eye problems, that emotional communication and vision were different things, but with me she was afraid to dress more seductively and be more demonstrative of her love for fear I might fail to see her and respond to her.

    For the first time Joanna found herself interested in men who were actively sexual and interested in her. She dreamed she gave a man dinner, and was shaken to realize that what heretofore she had taken for sexuality was really displaced orality. She became increasingly aware of bodies and of her extremely limited capacity to fantasize about sexual relationships. We had long since realized that she never had a dream of consumated lovemaking, and that she never imagined a man undressed; in fact her intimate fantasies consisted of isolated fragments. Joanna realized she was threatened by acknowledging my masculinity, and she needed instead to perceive me as mother. She realized that her relationship with Bob was fraternal or maternal. When Bob had to be away for a night, she took a dart and a can of Mace to bed with her. When she tried to explore fantasies about hugging me she became anxious and felt that she had no body, that she was just a collection of atoms with space between them, and that if she actually tried to hug me she would faint.

    Joanna began to spend some nights alone so she could work on these issues, and this occasioned sadness as well as a sense of growth. Without Bob to comfort her at night she was more aware of having nightmares; he would have awakened her at the first sign of distress. She dreamed about a deformed boy who was thrown from an airplane by his mother; at first he appeared to be dead but was not, and she decided to care for him. Associations were to the feeling that mother had rejected her because something was wrong with her and to the belief that she could now care for herself and could relinquish fantasies of being a male. Bob turned white and acted dead, she told me, when she informed him she wanted a man who would treat her like a woman. She then dreamed she had killed me and had been taken by my wife, along with other patients, to a house where they were to remain, as they would get sick again without me. She rebelled, saying I would not have wanted them to do this; took my body and put it in her white car, along with some "sinful things"; and drove off, feeling frightened by the challenge. She realized she believed that she had a meat grinder inside her vagina, and that she killed and incorporated the men with whom she had sex, turning them white and cold, and realized that one of the explanations she had given herself for why others carried knives was to protect themselves from her.

Joanna became interested in men as sexual beings in situations where previously she would have become paranoid and felt threatened by a knife, and this led to acquaintance with Tom, a man who seemed delighted by her wishes to be affectionate and sexual. But she continued to dream that the men in her life died or became crippled. She realized that she was still crippled by her tendency to entomb her strong feelings, particularly angry possessive ones.

Before my summer vacation Joanna feared that if I could not see her she would not exist for me and life would stop, and she experienced retaliatory wishes not to care about me. During our single appointment halfway through my vacation break she experienced powerful wishes to hug me associated with fond memories of her grandmother and regrets that she had not demonstrated such feelings before grandmother died. She wanted to prove to herself that she could hug me without merging, and she came over to my chair, hugged me and was overcome with feelings of derealization, depersonalization, and fragmentation. But she rapidly calmed herself and we were able to talk about her feeling that her skull had come off and her brains were unprotected, as well as about her sadomasochistic fantasies that she would be mutilated or I would die. She subsequently wrote me a letter saying that she had not forgotten about me and could recall my face and some of the pleasures of our relationship. She described some of her summer experiences playing in quartets with her friends, experiences she had found "closer to pure joy than any psychotic merger could be."

Year Four

My return after my summer vacation marked the beginning of the fourth year of our work. Joanna experienced an exuberant sense of herself. But it was also the time of her birthday, and she reenacted events of her early infancy in an uncanny way: at first she experienced rage at men, particularly her father, some of her more dogmatic professors, and then me. Next she felt bitter and skeptical about me and experienced me as a "bad mother," one whose breasts were flat and nipples were not good; I could not nurse her. Joanna wanted to go off by herself and "have visions in the wilderness" or eat a great deal and roll up in a blanket, activities reminiscent of some of her childhood efforts to soothe herself. Finally, she enacted what we concluded was a sour grapes or "sour milk" attitude, withdrawing into an emotionally and physically retentive posture in which she ate little and was constipated. Joanna realized that she reexperienced these same issues every fall, around the time of her birthday and the start of school, and concluded that in infancy she had moved from a position of active frustration and protest to one of hopeless, bitter withdrawal.

Joanna dreamed she came to see me in a new office. She asked if I had been away, and when I said I had not she allowed herself to have warm feelings about me and to kiss me. When it was time to go she noticed my right hand was just skin, stretched over a mannequin mold. In her associations she remarked how flatness/roundness (or emptiness/fullness) were her basic perceptual parameters about herself and others. The alternation of perception depended on whether the other person seemed real to her. She experienced the limits in our relationship in terms of flatness, emptiness, and sickness. I told her that all relationships are limited, and we reviewed the reasons for the limits in therapy. In a dream she filled her own nursing bottle because no one else would.

Joanna began graduate school. She continued to experience periods of despair, and paranoia, feelings of disintegration, and perceptual distortions; at these times she was concrete, her associations were loose, and she tended to pun uncontrollably. Through a dream of a man who had features both of me and of her father she realized she required a depressed, angry, unhappy man as a kind of "security blanket" and externalization of a part of herself she had not yet been able to face. She became more aware of the hopeless rageful depression she felt over the mothering she had received, and she realized that it was this sense of utter futility that had led her to withdraw early in our relationship, which in turn tended to make me sleepy during her therapy hours. Then she began to be aware of a more rageful, demanding, infantile, "Lizzie Borden" part of herself, as well as of a more adult belief that she now had the eyes (the capacity to perceive) and the voice and words (the capacity to act) to solve problems in her life and meet her own needs. Joanna experienced a new hunger for learning and for therapy, a sense of wanting things "right now," along with concerns lest she devour the object of her appetite. She feared that intimacy was inherently destructive to one or the other party and that if she were not psychotically crippled the other would be destroyed by her rage and neediness. She wondered, did she want to devour people or could she be satisfied simply getting something from them?

We were preoccupied with Joanna's conviction that satisfaction was unattainable, a conviction associated with memories and images of an unapproachable mother. Joanna experienced hunger pangs whenever she would see a nursing mother and baby. We began to piece together a portrait of a helpless infant with enormous wants and anger who was unable to make any gesture toward mother without feeling that she alienated her. Joanna allowed herself to speak of her needs to her mother. At the conclusion of their visit and for the first time in her memory, mother spontaneously kissed her goodbye. Their interchanges made Joanna aware of how controlling mother tried to be of the distance and all the activities in their relationship. For the first time Joanna began to contemplate the possibility of birth and motherhood for herself. In repeated dreams she attempted to give birth to and nurture a whole baby in the face of myriad complications.

Meanwhile, Joanna continued to experience a busy and increasingly productive life as graduate student and now part-time music teacher, along with more gratifying peer relationships. In one hour when she was utterly negative and depressed about the potential of a human relationship, feeling that she would rather remain as she was than take a risk, I told her my response was to experience a wish to reach out and comfort her. This made her feel much better, and helped her to realize that she needed to correct her belief that others were like mother. Increasingly it seemed to me that Joanna concretely experienced the classical psychoanalytic mirror position as identical to the maternal emotional barrier that had crippled her activity and initiative, so I began to share a bit more of myself with her in response to questions she had always asked but that hitherto, in my efforts to be orthodox (I was finishing my own training at the time), I had not answered. We talked about music and I shared with her the fact that I was also interested in music but had never learned to play a musical instrument. She began to encourage me to try to make more active efforts to learn to do so!

By 3 years and 3 months into her treatment Joanna was doing so well maintaining a positive sense of self that she began talking about the possibility of cutting down the frequency of her therapy. In retrospect I think this was the first of a series of efforts to leave before she was entirely ready. She struggled to keep in mind her "good objects" and used a treasured old shawl to hold on to positive memories of her grandmother. She reported the following dream: She had to steal food, but there was garbage in it. A little blonde girl came and told her they would have to leave because the Nazis were coming. She tried to call a male friend but first an answering machine tried to block the conversation; then he told her he didn't want to talk with her, so she put her shawl around herself and went off alone. Joanna was increasingly able to objectify and reflect on her whining complaining sense of pessimism and "sour milk" futility, and she was more consistently able to feel security and sustenance from her relationship with me.

At Christmas Joanna took a 2-week vacation in order to visit her sisters. Rage at me during our last hour threatened her sense of stability and well-being, but she recouped by writing me a loving letter in which she cited a disagreement she had had with her father when she mentioned a mutual friend's problem and father had criticized her for being judgmental:

"I was reminded of how I hollered at you for being 'psychoanalytic' before I left . . . as if to say that to cite problems in me was to call me evil. I have been feeling sad that I became so angry with you on a day when I would like to have been friendly. I am relying on you to take what I said with a grain of salt as big as a boulder, which you usually do. Still, I am very sorry I said so many things I don't mean, even if I was angry."

Despite her efforts Joanna returned feeling not only angry at me but skeptical that I thought about her when she was gone; she felt "taken in" by our relationship. Her affect was flat, I looked flat to her, and she was detached; she had to make a conscious effort to restrain an urge to pun. I, in turn, felt detached. Joanna dreamed she was in my office looking at a picture of my children. In the background was the portion of Picasso's *Guernica* that depicts a grieving mother holding her dead and dismembered child. Her parents came in and Joanna told them to leave, but then she did not know what to do with me and got down on the floor like a child and played with another child who was there. This dream seemed to mark a new awareness of her symbiosis with mother and to herald a struggle to separate. Joanna told me her holiday visit had made her aware that she could no longer turn to her sisters for mothering. She worried that mother might die or become schizophrenic, and she realized that in her childhood such concerns had led her to act like a human sacrifice and try to take care of her mother, an activity she came to think of as being mother's "blood clotting factor." She attempted to discuss with mother what might have caused her to become ill and mother suggested that it was a vitamin deficiency. For the first time Joanna not only vigorously disagreed but set limits to the conversation. She realized that her "love affair" with mother had kept them both from being intimate with men. As she discovered that she had been the vehicle for enacting her mother's anger at father, some of his lifelong bitterness became more comprehensible to her and in response she moved closer to him.

Joanna realized that her deadening merger with mother, including ritualistic inhibitions, had been a form of security like being in a coffin. When I was absent for a week, Joanna experienced fears of disintegration and hopeless depression and referred to me as her "clotting factor." In turn, I wondered to myself, as I reviewed her generally charming, cheerful manner—which may not be so apparent to the reader of all this hostile, destructive material—and all the positive feedback about myself I received and perhaps had come to depend on from her, how attached I had become to her and even whether she had made herself indispensable to me and had somehow become *my* "clotting factor." I selectively shared some of these concerns with her, and she responded quite readily by citing situations where she inhibited anger at me, put what she believed to be my interest before her own, and did not allow herself as much freedom to be late or miss appointments as she might wish.

Joanna realized she was generally more sensitized to others' needs than to her own. When she observed Tom or a woman friend unhappy, her own body felt depressed, heavy, and blob-like and she would think about what she could do for them; but she had little awareness of her own needs. She was strikingly unable to conceptualize her own infantile needs for love in interpersonal ways so that she might satisfy some of them; she was only able to think of them in autistic and impersonal terms. In the office she rubbed herself against the arm of the chair; at home she took a warm bath. Cautiously, she began to articulate some of these needs to her father and to Tom and was able to get some comfort from them. She invited father to dinner, and they commiserated that they had both been isolated and lonely and had been angry at one another when they should have been trying to be closer. She put her head on Tom's shoulder and cried when she was upset. Concurrently she experienced wishes to confront her mother, which in turn elicited the familiar disintegration feeling, a terror of abandonment and rejection, and fears that she might kill mother or make her ill.

Joanna dreamed she was caring for a little baby who was near death and stiff with rigor mortis; she was unable to feed it, and it did not respond when she gave it a warm bath. Then the scene shifted and she was sitting at home, between her parents. She grasped and pinched mother in anger, and felt joyful that for the first time she was able to do such a thing and still feel whole. Father got angry at her for what she had done, but she confidently disarmed him by walking up to him and telling him she loved him. In her associations she realized she had always felt the need part of herself pinched off when she got close to mother. In reality, when Joanna approached and talked more with mother about her needs, she was struck by the fact that mother's response, which served to "pinch off" further attention to Joanna, was to cry, feel sorry for herself, and quickly change the subject to her own needs and problems.

With me Joanna felt guilty after being 10 minutes late because she had indulged a wish that seemed more interesting and had gotten into an interesting conversation; she was unable to sit in a chair near me because she perceived me as dangerous. She was fearful that she and I had made a Faustian bargain, and that if she were to get closer to me she would discover it was now my turn and I would devour her or reclaim her in turn for having given Pygmalion-like birth to her.

At the 3½-year mark Joanna began to talk about separation and termination, and after 3 years and 7 months of therapy we agreed to reduce the frequency of our meetings from four to three times per week. As I review the material now, I wonder why I was almost invariably so ready to acquiesce to her various suggestions to meet less frequently, and eventually to her desire to terminate. Because this treatment occurred almost 25 years ago, before I had completed psychoanalytic training, I cannot say for certain. I suspect it was a combination of factors, including a self-esteem problem that did not enable me to fully appreciate just how important I was to Joanna; a certain rigidity in my personality; a related idealization and misunderstanding of independence and autonomy which included an overvaluation of termination; and a belief that prolonged analytic treatments were somehow wrong. These attitudes were mostly reinforced by the psychoanalytic culture of the time and by my status as a trainee.

At the same time that she talked about termination with me Joanna began to realize that in Tom she had chosen yet another passive, unassertive, relatively uncommunicative man who was himself in search of a mother. Their relationship became more stormy as she raised these issues, and perhaps I should have attended more to their transference implications. Nonetheless, Joanna felt a firmer sense of personal identity and greater self-esteem and was able to purchase more feminine clothing and to be more assertive.

I told Joanna that in 2 weeks I would need to interrupt our work to have eye surgery for my glaucoma. At first she tried to deny this, but then depressive memories of father's preoccupation with his eye problems and their estrangement began to surface. She then began to consider for the first time what loss of vision must have meant to father, and how she had distanced herself from him when he must have been in need. She was flooded with awareness of positive, tender, maternal, and sexual feelings toward me and toward her father, and she was able to be much closer to him. She wanted to hug me, but no sooner did she acknowledge the wish than she experienced perceptual fragmentation, body fragmentation, a panicky sense of impending annihilation, and the overwhelming urge to pun. As she reconstituted herself she was aware of a need to inhibit her depressive and angry feelings out of a fear of burdening me excessively.

After 3 years and 9 months of Joanna's therapy I had surgery on one eye and a month later on the other, interrupting our work for about 10 days on each occasion. Joanna brought me some flowers prior to the first surgery, and afterward she expressed a kind of whiny anger which she associated with the cold, annihilating part of her mother, and a wish to eliminate a man who cannot be controlled and essentially made a part of her. She struggled to maintain contact with father and with me.

After my second eye surgery we began to attend more to the question of closeness in relationships, literal and emotional. It became apparent that Joanna avoided emotion—particularly intense feelings about closeness and separation, both of which seemed to connote death—by maintaining a fixed physical distance from me in the office, including an invariant seat position. She imagined we were two boxes connected by a steel rod. In situations where she had to be physically closer than was comfortable for her, she would imagine that she or the other person was someone else. At her instigation we began to experiment with different seating arrangements to help her face and explore these feelings. We learned that she was unable to sit closer than 6 feet from me without experiencing depersonalization, derealization, and bizarre fragmentation, including the belief that she had no skin or skull.

As Joanna became more involved with her father, she learned, to her surprise, that both of them had shared an idealization of mother. She realized mother had depreciated femininity, had taught her to scapegoat father, and had made it seem taboo to be wholeheartedly involved with me; for his part, father had participated by self-devaluation, conveying the belief that he wasn't worth caring about. Joanna brought father into one of her sessions with me. Although he was a bit gruff and suspicious about Joanna's treatment, what was most impressive was the extent to which he devalued himself and his importance to Joanna. After this visit Joanna had a dream in which she cuddled up to me and enjoyed it; the feelings and associated imagery uncharacteristically persisted for the ensuing weekend, giving her an unaccustomed sense of well-being.

My summer vacation and the end of our fourth year approached. After efforts to deny and withhold, Joanna became more depressed and angry; then she began to experience a kind of hopeless, frantic, infantile depression along with the twin convictions that she was about to be poisoned and that I would not return. She was unable to evoke positive sustaining fantasies. In this context it came as a surprise to both of us that, during the separation itself and without conscious volition, she began to experience positive fantasies and dreams of closeness to me, which served to sustain her.

Year Five

As our fifth year commenced, the war between Joanna's demanding, uncompromising body and her self-critical rationalizing mind became more conscious. She withdrew from me and then recognized it was part of her self-abnegating response with mother. One had to be "perfect," that is, without needs and with a willingness to be used and consumed by others, in order to be allowed to play in mother's chamber group, so to speak. Joanna briefly experienced nausea in the morning, and recurrent delusions that she was a machine; she realized that these were related to rage that she had allowed herself to play "second fiddle" to her mother. She felt hunger in all parts of her body, accompanied by wishes for hugging, feeding, and physical contact, and a rageful feeling that she was like a starving person in the middle of a smorgasbord. Nothing anyone could give her seemed as though it would be enough. There was a wish to grind her mother up and eat her. She dreamed that she was going downhill in a car and that a policewoman told her to stop; she could not, so somehow she ended up in a mental hospital. When mother made a characteristic call requesting some favors, Joanna uncharacteristically said no.

Joanna struggled over her inability to make any demands of me, such as requesting that I adjust the time of one of her hours a few minutes to accommodate a difficult schedule conflict. She felt that nothing short of total mothering would meet her needs; much of her refusal to get closer to me had been motivated by an unwillingness to experience her rage and disillusionment. As she began to realize that our relationship was limited, she began to temper her previous idealization of me and to experience us as more separate. When she began to be aware of her closeness to me she would angrily reject her body sensations and then experience both of our bodies fragmenting into threatening parts, of uncertain ownership; after weekend separations she perceived herself as disintegrated, with holes in her body. She recalled the incident when she had posed for nude photos while I was on vacation and realized it had represented her effort to retain a sense of bodily integrity. A satisfying dream of hugging me was followed by paranoid feelings and rage at the limitations of what I had to offer her. In the ensuing hour she felt cold and experienced her face as numb and disconnected from the rest of her, but after recognition that her anger had made her reject her bodily needs she rapidly regained touch with her body sense. It dawned on Joanna that for some time she had almost literally been thinking of me as her functional mother (not the mother of deprivation), and that when she was lonely she would repeat to herself, "Michael will mother me."

Joanna's fantasy life became more vigorous, her sex life with Tom improved, and she gave evidence of being better able to negotiate in her own behalf in school, where she seemed to be doing quite well. However, after a visit home in which she experienced mother as controlling and using of other family members, she vomited and became mildly paranoid. She dreamed she was late to see me because she was in a museum; when she finally reached my office I was gone and in my stead there was a black woman who was my wife. Joanna liked this woman, but the two of them were arrested by police for being whores and were taken to a mental hospital. The museum represented her own sense of deadness and related to her willingness to sacrifice some parts of herself in hopes mother might change. Since mother's perception was that expressive women are whores, Joanna thought that perhaps mother was the black whore, a person who manipulates others for supplies. Joanna realized that her first effort to separate from mother had involved enacting an identification with this aspect of mother by becoming promiscuous and crazy and by choosing a black partner.

Joanna's efforts to feel close to me and sustain positive fantasies were regularly followed by feelings of loss, desolation, rejection, and anger, all of which she associated to her mother. I suggested that what she wanted when she expressed positive feelings toward another person was a response, but that her very sense of identity and stability was predicated on believing that there was none and on not allowing one. In this context I offered to hug her or hold her hand if she wished.

I interrupt the narrative to anticipate the concerns of the reader, for in certain respects the culture of today is quite different from the one almost 25 years ago in which this treatment was conducted. There is a heightened awareness of and concern about issues of incest and abuse, and related questions about physical contact between patient and therapist. At the time of Joanna's treatment not only was there less social consciousness about such things, but we were not far removed from the belief in therapeutic re-mothering (elaborated in Chapter 15), which led such respected therapists of schizophrenia as Sechehaye, Schwing, Rosen, Winnicott, and even Fromm-Reichmann in the earlier stages of her career to become very involved with the care of their patients in ways that not infrequently became physical. From my perspective at the time, the hugging seemed compellingly necessary because of the concreteness and fixity of Joanna's belief that her basic needs would not be responded to by another human being, her utter lack of a sense of personal instrumentality in obtaining need satisfaction, and the organization of much of her pathology around distance modes of perception and nonaffective modes of cognition. There seemed an unfortunate congruence between the physical distancing, exclusive reliance on words, and associated rules of classical analytic technique, on the one hand, and Joanna's beliefs, on the other. My offer was an enactive way of highlighting and interpreting a fixed pattern of thinking that did not seem susceptible to verbal intervention, probably because words spoken at a distance were too similar to the perceptual and auditory distance which characterized the early contact between this patient and her mother to have any mutative value, or perhaps because they did not have the meaning to Joanna that they might have had to another person who had had different early nurturing experiences.

I would like to emphasize that I was aware of my attraction to Joanna, and was in some conflict over whether I ought to engage in an action that would be wish gratifying to me. My conscious intent, at least, was not to provide wish gratification to either of us (or nurturance or good mothering) but to challenge the veracity of a belief that lay at the core of Joanna's pathology. In fact, I probably gratified Joanna's wishes (as contrasted with her needs) more when I remained distant from her. Would I have encouraged hugging had the patient been male? I doubt it. Would I do the same thing today? I cannot say, for an encounter between Joanna and the me of today might well be different in many respects. The reader will have to judge whether my actions complicated the remainder of her treatment, particularly the termination phase. It is also possible that, had I not allowed hugging and hand holding during this period, Joanna might not have been able to engage with me in her treatment as fully as she did. Certainly this is what Joanna subsequently believed. This dilemma illustrates a basic problem in the study and evaluation of therapeutic technique: It is not possible to arrange a controlled experiment by splitting the patient in two and trying one method (or one therapist) with one part, and another with the other.

Finally, I would like to place my action in a larger context: probably in every successful treatment of a schizophrenic person some therapeutic laying on of hands occurs. To be sure, this is most often done by hospital staff rather than by the therapist, and most often involves the control of destructive behavior, but it is just not possible to deal with a schizophrenic exclusively in the realm of words (an observation I elaborate in Chapters 15 and 17).

To return to the story, with some difficulty Joanna instigated a period of experimentation with distance and touch. The experience was disequilibrating (she had to reassure herself that the office was not moving), but she felt that the disruptive feeling was related to growth and not disintegration. We began to see more clearly the dichotomy between her proximal and distal senses; the former were more emotional and destabilizing, the latter more cognitive and stabilizing, albeit inextricably linked with depression and pessimism. That is, Joanna gained stability by having people at a predictable, isolated, unavailable distance, where good feeling and closeness were not possible. From this I inferred that her infancy must have been a period in which stability had been gained not through maternal recognition of bodily and emotional need, and satisfaction through the proximal senses, but by precocious dependency on vision and audition (recall that her mother played the piano). Joanna realized she could not be physically close to Tom for long without having to back off and look at him. She began to perceive me as a more controllable source of gratification and began to struggle more with her own ambivalence and to develop, slowly, a new physically and emotionally based sense of identity related to closeness with me. It disturbed her to realize that she didn't need to think all the time, that a stable sense of herself might come from simply responding to her feelings in the present rather than anticipating the future. As her emotional life expanded her sense of boundaries became more stable. She had a very satisfying dream of nursing a baby, including good feelings about her breasts, which she had always disliked.

Joanna began to see herself as a passionate woman, with vitality in relation to both sexuality and anger, in spite of bouts of depressive feelings of hopelessness and rage which we related to her infancy, moralistic prohibitions related to her mother, and fears of identity loss and helplessness. Her relationship with Tom deepened, and they decided to be married at Christmas, 9 months hence. Tom surprised Joanna by telling her that the only reason he had equivocated was that in the past her urges to marry had always come at times of separation from or dissatisfaction with me. Joanna dreamed of dining at a Greek restaurant with Tom, paying an exorbitant bill, and then being chased by killers. This led to her awareness that she equated marriage with loss of identity and annihilation by mother, and she decided that she had better postpone the marriage until she was in better control of her response.

In the process of decision making during this period of therapy Joanna adjusted her physical distance from me, keeping further away when she wanted cognitive help to solve problems and moving closer when issues of warmth and affection predominated. A key variable in determining her distance seemed to be the anger she felt toward me when she was confused and in turmoil, that is, she believed that she was protecting me from it by keeping her distance. Joanna worked hard to try to integrate close feelings with her rage, using her ability to control the physical distance between us, and therefore the possibility of hugging me, as a way to counteract her depressive and rageful fantasies. Feelings of helplessness, depression, and rage related to satisfying her needs in our relationship were now countered by an entirely novel and satisfying sense of active control over her need satisfaction.

After 4½ years of therapy Joanna earned her master's degree. I was away for 2 weeks, around the time of the important anniversary of her younger sister's birth. On my return Joanna had a delayed reaction of rage and hatred of me and of people in general, and was able to tell me about a variety of previously withheld ideas about people that she now realized were "crazy." These provided some discouraging evidence that her psychosis, characterized by paranoid attitudes in which I was the master and she was the slave, body feelings of coldness and nausea, deep pessimism about the possibility of need satisfaction in a human relationship, and inability to maintain positive object constancy, had not been resolved as completely as I had wanted to believe. A combination of being able to touch me and to stay a while after the scheduled end of the therapy hour (it was the last of my day) served to shake some of her psychotic convictions; in turn the freedom to enact her wish made her conscious of wishes to enslave me.

Joanna began a new job. We soon realized she had chosen a dictatorial boss and was acting like a slave. She wished for the simple security of identity-less enslavement, to be like the selfless tool that was carried in her father's toolbox so that she could avoid dealing with the unfamiliar turmoil associated with closeness, which stirred pains in her stomach. She dreamed that she beat me up because I said she had no effect on me. When I was away for a long weekend, she dreamed she came to my home looking for a place to sleep and I allowed her to stay in a guest bedroom. It turned into her parents' living room. Someone else was there, they were both crippled, and in 2 minutes one of them would have to die. In a panic she jumped from a second story window, landed unharmed, and fled, with a pursuer close behind throwing grenades with lit fuses. Associations were to her own short fuse and her difficulty being close to me because of her rage. After realizing enslavement was a way of blocking out her awareness of parts of herself and her intimate partner she decided to quit the new job, and she was able to have sex without concurrent depersonalization and fragmentation for the first time in her life.

These events led me to focus on the slave master or killer part of Joanna's own personality: a self-mutilating conscience, which had been largely projected (for example, as the knives she had once been convinced others carried). She exacted ritualistic punishments of herself each time she allowed herself to be close to someone. With me she was literally paralyzed; each time she allowed herself the wish to move closer she experienced a physical kick in the stomach and heard a voice calling her a "shit." She dreamed of asking me to sleep with her, but we found ourselves trapped in her family's house. In contemplating her dream Joanna realized she was not supposed to have insides (organs, feelings) of her own or seek pleasure but was expected to remain a prisoner in her family. Joanna planned a vacation and then experienced escalating attacks of sadistic conscience. She came to her hour hardly able to lift a finger, sobbing convulsively and feeling that her insides had been kicked out, and reported having spent the preceding several hours calling herself names. At this time I adopted an "open door" policy. In response to her belief that she was a "little shit" and could expect nothing, that there was never enough time for her, I left my door open for her at the end of the hour so that she could come back if she wished. We discovered that in order to do so she had to give up power, control, and a feeling of pride, which she associated to the biblical injunction "The meek shall inherit the earth." Interestingly enough, these were three attitudes her conscience hitherto had not required that she sacrifice.

I noted that her sadistic conscience never seemed to be active when Joanna was with me; it was always in hiding. So I suggested that she move from one chair to another in the room as the different parts of her spoke in order to define and delineate more clearly the "conscience," the identityless slave or "little shit," and the growing woman with pear-shaped feelings inside who wanted to touch, be touched, and discover the pleasure centers within herself. I sat in the fourth chair except when the nascent pleasure self wanted me to sit next to her on the couch. The results of this combination of enactment and discussion were fascinating. As the conscience became articulate and subject to commentary from other parts of herself and from me it lost respect and then power, for it was palpably dictatorial and sadistic, unable to think or reason clearly, and lacking in a sense of social tact or diplomacy. But at the same time Joanna noticed that selected elements of this conscience might be useful to her if modified. For instance, the threat of kicking out her sexual insides, which led her to wonder if her mother's history of miscarriages might have represented somatic hostility toward the kicking fetus, became an admonition not to have affairs since doing so might jeopardize her relationship with Tom. The "little shit" part of her was gradually redefined as the thinking, tactful, diplomatic part and became more valued. For the first time Joanna realized that her conscience, not her feelings, had been the part of her that had run wild, acting out of control and entitled, and that it had something to learn from the rest of her, rather than vice versa.

Joanna began to seem more integrated; the reports emanating from the various chairs began to sound increasingly similar. Name-calling of herself ceased and her moral admonitions to herself seemed to take more cognizance of her needs and of reality. Her sexual and affectionate needs and behaviors now seemed more connected. Her moral sense began to focus on family issues involving the use of money; in particular, Joanna felt a growing outrage that her parents would not give her information about monies held in trust for her, and instead made her feel guilty that she did not earn more money and fearful that they would withdraw their support if she failed to conform. In the hour preceding the vacation she had planned she initially sat in the conscience chair and expressed anger, helplessness, and feelings of impending annihilation. This led her to associate her rageful conscience, with its overblown threats, to an infantile tantrum which she had turned against her own needy, infantile self.

Year Six

Joanna took a 3-week vacation and we commenced our sixth year of work. She began a new job. She was more comfortable sexually and had a more reasonable conscience, better diplomatic skills, and a greater capacity to hold on to a positive sense of herself and to experience ambivalence in the face of frustrating situations, such as her continuing disappointment that our love relationship seemed to her so one-sided. This led her to decide that she really needed me as a doctor and that she should begin to set limits on the closeness she had enjoyed with me, both the physical and psychological closeness. She defined some of her remaining goals in therapy in the areas of relationship and work. In the process, however, Joanna realized that she tended to split off anger at Tom and project it onto other men, and she wondered if she might prematurely have committed herself to him. She was terrified by a new awareness of just how attracted she was to men who seemed to share more of her basic interests than he did, and she realized that she tended to reject her sexuality rather than experience fantasies of being annihilated or risk the possibility of actual rejection, which was still associated with the now-familiar hopeless infantile state of depression. In her fantasies sperm were parasitic and became babies that would devour her. Joanna recalled her own parasitic behavior when she was ill. She decided that, by settling for less than what she wished for with men, she was perpetuating her depressive conviction that satisfaction was unattainable. Joanna began to take note of mother-infant situations that seemed to work out well. She dreamed of two mothers with babies; I enjoyed holding the babies and then she tried and found it gratifying. Though she was still susceptible to periods of terrible depression and paranoia, it appeared that Joanna now had some basic hope and trust to sustain her.

At the end of a therapy hour Joanna felt her arm aching. Then she dreamed her right arm was accidentally cut off. Although she complained, nobody noticed; finally, someone told her to put insulin on it and she did. Then a doctor she liked came along and propositioned her. They slept together but he too, failed to notice the absence of her arm. Then I came and she realized the arm had been there all along. In her next therapy hour Joanna realized she had been angry at me at the end of the hour when her arm ached. She recognized how angry she was at father and at men, and she became aware of the unsatisfactory choice she felt she had to make in relationships, that is, between losing the man on the one hand, or relinquishing feeling parts of herself on the other. (The purpose of the insulin in her dream was to lower her feeling level.) The arm dysfunction, which continued to dominate her symbolism for some time, denoted her paralysis in expressing anger and her tendency toward masochistic submission to charismatic but narcissistic men, who symbolized her own individuality, and who tended to use her. She became more aware of her rage at being used and her sense of entitlement. She dreamed she had left her baby in order to go to work; when she returned, the baby was angry and inconsolable, and although she apologized profusely, hugged the baby (in ways that she had hugged me, in fact), and promised it that she would be better, the baby would not forgive her. Joanna then questioned me, as she had lately begun to do, about some of the emotional satisfaction she was convinced I derived from being a therapist in general and from being her therapist in particular. In the past she had asked if I ever had sexual feelings about her; now she focused on my gratification from the idealization and dependency of someone as bright and attractive as she, a gratification I readily acknowledged. This raised in her mind the question of whether, if we both got pleasure out of the relationship, did that make the relationship bad?

Again Joanna and Tom began to plan marriage, and again she felt threatened and depressed and made some flirtatious and clearly inappropriate efforts to involve herself with other men, including her father and an older music teacher. As we identified the pattern, memories emerged of how little help she had received from either parent during adolescence to enable her to emerge from the role of neuter companion or helper into a more sexual identity; Joanna understood that father, in particular, must have been threatened by her developing sexuality and, consequently, tended to avoid her.

At the 5 years and 3 months point of treatment I noted that Joanna was not bringing sexual issues into therapy. One of the reasons turned out to be her confusion of feelings with actions, related in part to the hugs that had characterized the previous stage of her treatment. We agreed that in order to work on this there should be no more physical touching. This enraged her but it apparently permitted her to feel an increased body awareness. Joanna characterized the status of her sexuality in musical terms; she could state the theme, but she managed to disrupt things so that the "development" section and the "climax" would never occur. After attempting to break our new physical contact rule (and my reminding her of the necessity for it), Joanna was able, for the first time ever, to describe a consummated sexual fantasy. Then she seemed concrete and somewhat fragmented and reported two dreams: In the first she went on a trip with a 10-year-old rather than pursue Tom; in the second she was searching for me, and though she found many traces, she could not locate me and ended up getting raped. These seemed to represent the solutions to frustration and disappointment she had attempted in her adolescence.

Before our last appointment of the year, and my absence for 2 weeks, Joanna had a very satisfying dream of aggressively making love to me, in which she felt all her feelings. In reporting it she said that she wished it had actually happened and, at the same time, that she knew it would be unwise to ever have a sexual relationship with me. In a second dream, the same night, she was trying to reach me at the hospital through a series of mazes and frustrations but could not; she awoke shaking. She realized this dream represented her relationship with her father, and was the harbinger of loss of body feelings. She asked to hug me when she left, saying that her capacity for positive memory and anticipation were very much related to her body contact experiences with me, and adding that she realized a hug would now also leave her feeling sexually frustrated. We hugged at the end of the hour.

During the 2-week separation, though she dreamed of depression and body loss, Joanna was able to maintain a warm sense of her body, a close relationship with Tom, and a separation of fantasy from action. Though there was a typical delayed whiny, depressive, depleted, angry reaction after I returned, along with some loss of judgment and urges toward a sexualized clinging dependency on me, it was brief and attenuated. Joanna was more aware than she had ever been of her need to challenge her passive, depressive, hopeless, autistic view of life, in which one person loses and becomes the "blood clotting factor" for the other. She realized how insecure and threatened by her conscience she felt whenever she perceived herself as a sexual woman with freedom of choice and multiple possibilities for satisfaction in fantasy and in action.

Joanna attempted further financial separation from her family, and she tried to challenge Tom's passivity and lack of responsibility in the face of her own regressive inclinations to act out sexually and to use illness to get attention. Her primitive conscience attacked her new autonomy and she experienced herself as a depressive nonentity attacked by a man. To her surprise, Tom told her he was relieved that she now stood up for herself more in the face of frustration, for it meant he no longer had to take care of her. She also got feedback that her musical skills were improving rapidly. And she realized that in music, as in love, she picked partners who were more bland and less skilled for reasons of safety. In a dream she told me to spend my efforts helping her rather than trying to mold her sister from a dish into a three-dimensional object. Then she had reached down and touched my penis. I had been disconcerted and had responded that my penis was not the most important part of me, but she said that to her it was.

Now Joanna began to think about decreasing the frequency of her therapy from three to two times per week, and about changing her job, which involved trying to help an essentially unpromising, perhaps even hopeless, group of people. She concluded that her decision to marry Tom was prompted more than anything else by her conviction that she should sacrifice herself for someone else. She realized that sex was so threatening to her because she had used it to achieve a deadening, identityless security and that this need for security had prevented her from finding a man with whom she had intellectual, physical, and spiritual rapport. She decided not to marry Tom. Then she reported a dream in which she came to see me, but was frozen like an iceberg. I hugged her and she began to warm up. As she did so she became aware both of sexual feelings and of anger at father. The she found herself at her parent's home, in bed with her married music teacher.

Although Joanna felt more alive and acted like a more vibrant person, there were periods when she lost touch with her sexual feelings during the night, while sleeping, and had to make a conscious effort to get herself "together" again after waking. She dreamed she was involved with a man who owned a restaurant; he offered her tea and toast as a prelude to sex, but she told him she would just take the food.

Joanna raged at me for all the sacrifices I "demanded" of her in order to come to therapy three times a week, and for the way I had used threats of illness (presumably, my eye problems) to keep her dependent. She insisted she wanted to come less often, but when I said I would agree to whatever she thought best she became sad and panicky, and felt that she could not survive if she saw me less often. She dreamed that she aggressively initiated sex with me in the office and took great pleasure from it, particularly oral aspects, but we were discovered by a colleague of mine; at first she took it upon herself to protect my reputation by denying that she was my therapy patient, but then she decided this was my problem to handle. Subsequently, in the same night, she dreamed she was trying to get to her parents' castle but was submerged in an ice avalanche. On another night she dreamed she was with father and had the option of allowing herself to feel sexual about him; she decided not to because of his unresponsiveness and the incest taboo, but she was punished by being caught in a a Gothic torture device, called a sex machine, that dismembered people and transformed them into machines.

After 5½ years of therapy Joanna had a dream in which she was compelled by circumstance to make love to her mother, who was bisexual and had a small penis; they had to try three times before mother could have an orgasm. In the dream Joanna became very angry and had to masturbate to climax. In another dream she struggled with regression once again: She was in church near her parents' home, afraid she would fall off the pew into an abyss; as part of the service she swallowed a vital fluid, then saw several women undress and realized they were like her. She associated to her belief that I "had the stuff" and that I was a kind of prostitute she required. Joanna realized she thought of herself as asexual for fear she might otherwise seduce her unhappy father away from her frigid mother. Instead she had engaged herself in the lost cause of being a prostitute who attempted to animate a "dead" mother. She expressed some concerns about homosexuality as she became more aware of her interest in women, but she realized that the dream intercourse with mother had not primarily involved sex, but had involved relinquishment of her sense of self in an effort to replenish her mother's narcissism. She concluded that in her life she had relinquished her sexuality so as to avoid competing with mother for the affections of her father.

Joanna struggled with renewed attacks from her conscience, both internal and projected onto moralistic male supervisors at work, as she began to dress and act more seductively, and she developed an unshakable conviction that she should die, or that she should not have lived at all. She struggled with feelings of disintegration and bodily dissolution, concrete thinking, and difficulty generating positive fantasies about her future. She recalled how her sisters had fought vigorously for her father's attentions, whereas she had been unable to compete. Nevertheless, she was able to be more aggressively self-interested. She played successfully in a chamber group at a public concert. She dreamed she was a 12- or 13-year-old who had let a stallion out of a barn in the face of admonishments she should not, and then became involved in an exciting interaction with a grown man.

Joanna began to realize, with sadness, that she and I could now live without one another, and she began to contemplate termination. Because I simply sat and listened she felt I was giving her permission to go, rather than taking advantage of her loving and needy feelings and her conscience, thereby assuming the role of cripple myself, and forcing her to repay a debt. Although she was grateful to me, at the same time she was angry at me that I would let her go and not seem to be upset about it. Issues of growth, separation, and intimacy dominated her associations; these included the separation feelings of dying people and their families, wishes to infantilize her own music pupils into perpetual dependent lovers versus pleasure in helping them to become more independent, and many thoughts of having a family of her own. A sense of internal stability was accompanied by a grieving for infantile linkages: Joanna realized that she could play passionate music without necessarily having to read the score and that while she had a new power in relationship to her father, she would never have a nurturing father.

At the 5¾-years point in therapy I took a week's holiday, and Joanna realized she no longer needed to know where I would be. In reaction, she told me that being her own person was driving her crazy. She went on to describe an interaction with Wendy, an old friend from her hospital days who was still psychotic and believed Joanna was trying to control her. Feeling the pull to linkage, Joanna got angry and told Wendy that she cared about her but that Wendy needed to see her psychiatrist and get rid of her crazy thoughts. In an important committee meeting at work Joanna spoke up and disagreed with others. She was less idealizing of others and she recognized the edge of aggression in being her own person and keeping others at a certain distance. Her married violin teacher tried to seduce her; as she coped with the situation she recognized his personality limitations, and how much she contributed to the ongoing stability of their relationship. When I remarked that this was true in therapy also, that is, that she herself introduced the material and organized the sessions, she was pleased and more able to own her activity and, at the same time, depressed by a concomitant deflation of my image.

Joanna next took a week's vacation, during which regression to feelings of ineptitude and envious wishes to be me alternated with evidence of a more mature assumption of various of the functions I performed for her, as well as of some of the constructive coping mechanisms of her parents. She reported a dream about a male violinist she had idealized from her youth. He propositioned her sexually, and she was very turned on but said no. He wanted to play her violin, which would make her second fiddle, but to this too she said no; she wanted to take her own sexuality and her musical ability and use them for her own agenda and to relate to all the people in the orchestra. Joanna seemed to have a better sense of her own boundaries and her own abilities to handle things, and after a weekend in which she did particularly well she realized again that she could do without me.

Joanna planned to move in with Tom, with whom she was again involved. She feared falling asleep lest she have nightmares about her family, and she was aware of a wish to kill off her own body awareness and feelings and merge with a powerful mother. As she prepared to move she realized how much her identity was still diffused in her surroundings. She became nauseated while packing her things and from this she realized that her identity was not body-based. She never admired her nude body in a mirror. Instead her warm feelings were associated with her kitchen, her humor and poetry were located in her books, and her music in her instrument, all external to herself. As she reviewed this familiar and primitive mode of self-experience, Joanna realized there had never been any place for her anger and sexuality, two feelings she now felt had a secure place within herself. She recalled the period of her therapy that she described as "presexual," when she hugged me and sat next to me, and realized this was the first time she had really felt as though she possessed someone else, and she remembered the time when she began to feel an integrated, warm sense of self.

The move back with Tom and our talk of termination seemed to stir a kind of identity crisis in Joanna. On the one hand there was a proliferation of ambition, self-interest, feelings of entitlement, and fantasies of sexual, professional, and musical satisfaction, along with a more spontaneous expression of sexuality and agression both in and out of therapy; these functions seemed to be integrated in relation to Joanna's wishes to be "grabby," which literally made her arm ache. On the other hand, she briefly experienced nocturnal hypnopompic visual hallucinations or illusions of spiders. She felt she could not keep track of her identity without my regular mirroring. She ridiculed her feelings and at times believed that I was ridiculing her. She recalled how during her hospitalization she had wishes to rip out the bad parts of herself with a knife. As she became sexually excited about me she attributed her feelings to "this person in me." She became preoccupied with the fact that there was only one penis between us; since one of us had to have it, how could both our needs be met? From these preoccupations we realized that her intimate feelings were still depressively bound up with the dyadic hopelessness related to her mother.

Joanna's regression intensified. She anticipated my summer vacation with disintegration of a sense of self, a despairing, panicked belief that she was losing the only person in the world, and wishes to obliterate me and to curl up in a womb and sleep arose. In a dream she could not find any of the men in her life to make love to, and tried to make love to a black woman who she felt represented her mother instead. The regression was leavened by recurrent dreams of her house, which had more rooms than in the past but was empty of furniture. In one such dream she resisted blandishments of an older woman who was moving and who wanted to sell Joanna all her old furniture at a very high price.

Year Seven

During our ensuing summer vacation separation Joanna was able to fantasize a soothing cheek-to-cheek relationship with me and to maintain a gratifying physical and conversational relationship with Tom, one which she knew was quite different from her relationship with me. But her image of me was "all good," and when we resumed she had to deal with disappointment and rage. When we began our seventh and final year she reported a dream: She was heading for a concert which was to be held in a church in her hometown, but found herself instead in an old room with her mother and sister. She made love to both of them, having orgasms and the unique experience that she got more pleasure than she gave, yet not enough to make her want to stay. She continued to the concert and found Tom. She wanted to make love immediately, but he reassured her that there would be enough time afterward. She was offered some food, which she declined, convinced that there was a tapeworm in it. Joanna associated the food to her parents' home, the nonnourishing quality of the family interactions, and her belief that there had not been enough supplies for both herself and her mother. She struggled with a reemergence of passive, whiny, angry depressive feelings associated with the idea that she had to act grown-up before she was ready. She dreamed of lying close to me at night in a satisfying way after a hard day, and was able to come into her therapy hour in a mood that was positive but also feisty and combative, as she realized that this dream could never come true. She avoided Tom out of mistrust and a belief that she had to protect him from the annihilating intensity of her needs, for she still held her fundamental belief that only one member of a dyad could survive.

These separation and reunion developments helped us to define our therapeutic task: to consolidate and internalize an image of mother, who seemed to be pervasively diffused in the environment. Mother bought Joanna a birthday gift that reflected what she, mother, would have liked to receive, rather than anything Joanna wanted. Joanna accepted it uncomplainingly, and then dreamed that Tom was turning into mother and that there was a growing unbridgeable gulf between them. After we discussed the dream Joanna called mother and told her of a number of specific areas where mother had not considered her feelings and needs. When the conversation ended she felt curiously separate, aware perhaps for the first time that mother could not satisfy all her needs. She realized that in her dreams the recurrent image of going home really meant regressing to a walled-off, self-pitying state of passive depression. Joanna began to invest more of herself in fantasizing, planning, and obtaining current satisfaction, particularly from Tom. Once again she realized she had picked a man who was not very emotional, in preference to men whom she found simultaneously more exciting and more threatening.

As Joanna was reminded of her difficulty tolerating emotional excitement we began to talk about her repressive use of relationships, her equation of love with inhibition of emotional aliveness that would "rock the boat," and her efforts to be a china doll with Tom as she had been with mother. I reminded her that she had long since made clear that she believed I loved her, yet I was constantly saying things to her that upset her in a way she found constructive, and that she increasingly experienced pleasure from our intense, emotional give-and-take exchanges. She feared that a fuller expression of her emotions would lead her to become promiscuous—or play music all the time! It was again clear that her cognitive organization was based on infantile deprivation. She began to challenge Tom more, and her challenges elicited some of his passivity and fundamental avoidance of intensity in relationships. She dreamed she was going to marry Tom's sister, but at the last minute she halted the ceremony and disrupted social convention by asking, "Who has the penis?" and remarking that since she did not, she needed a partner who did! As her sexual relationship with Tom was one of the few things she found satisfactory, she realized the penis in her dream signified the climax of a whole relationship with another active person.

It seemed that something basic was changing within her. Joanna reported a greater capacity to concentrate, to appreciate subtle nuances, to obtain satisfaction from a variety of activities, both solitary and with others, and to delay gratification when necessary. Joanna had the novel feeling that she was entirely on her own side. As she tried to work problems out in this new way with Tom, it became apparent how expert she was in taking on problems internally and "killing herself" to work them out; this quality was at once her basic problem and, in many situations, an adaptive strength. I neglected to inform her of a change in therapy hour. When I realized my error I called her, and by considerable mutual accommodation we were still able to meet. With minimal prompting from me (but also in her usual friendly, diplomatic manner) she was able to admonish me slightly about my problem, and to suggest that she would like an apology, which I tendered her.

Joanna experienced what seemed to be an almost overpowering self-interest, including wishes to have her own place, play music, dress elegantly, and be courted. She felt very angry with Tom and wanted to move out again and look for a more satisfying relationship. She began to take steps to separate from him, and experienced all the familiar feelings: self-castigation, abandonment anxiety, and depression, as well as a limited sense of disintegration. Her conflict was accompanied by great difficulty sleeping, with its attendant passivity and helplessness, which seemed to enhance the regressive propensity. She recalled earlier efforts to separate herself from her mother, which involved interest in her father and his tools. She would spend long periods of time in his workshop, with fantasies of making boxes and putting things in them, an activity she now associated to wishes to make a baby. Eventually, she only felt coldness, that is, cut off from her feelings, and ceased her visits.

As Joanna felt less of a pull to use sex to merge with another, and a more healthy sense of personal ambition, she elected to stop sexual activity with Tom. For the first time in her life she began to get satisfaction from masturbation, although she felt that it was not as satisfying as having a man. She consolidated her plans to separate from Tom but she feared and confused "breaking out" with "breaking down." There was a burst of new appetites and interests. Joanna became aware of wishes to be the greatest in what she undertook, to be admired and mirrored, and she experienced greed, rage, and envy related not only to her awareness of the limitations imposed by her abilities, which were considerable but not extraordinary, but also to her awareness of her lifelong tendency to become the satellite of a narcissistic male. Halfway through the seventh year of her treatment Joanna separated from Tom and for the first time since I had known her, commenced living alone. She dreamed she was going up and down uncontrollably in an elevator but somehow managed to say no, get out, meet a man, and have an experience of progressive closeness culminating in her declining to have sex because she was "unprotected." She experienced the old feeling of her skull peeling away.

Joanna began to experience rage and envy at me for not giving her something. This led us to examine her tendency to choose self-centered men, and to try to enhance their narcissism, that is, to make them feel good, all the while feeling hidden rage and envy that they possessed what she lacked and that all she had was the illusion of the strength and normalcy she was unable to provide for herself. Because of her own discomfort with her emotions, she continued to discourage overtures from more attentive men who might have had more to offer her. Efforts to relate to me with sexual feelings and fantasies turned into wishes for me to narcissistically exhibit my sexual appeal, accompanied by almost delusional somatic self-denigration, including ideas that she had sores in her mouth or cancer and was disintegrating. She could feed my narcissism but was unable to feed herself. She was tempted to get some "fast food" (sex). In fact, she was not eating well in Tom's absence. She was unable to perceive her own insides as interesting. As we worked on these issues I became increasingly aware of my own narcissistic investment in her, that is, of her ability to interest me in her in a way that enhanced my own feelings of importance, at the same time that she could not feel self-important. She had a very positive experience with an interesting man, but its limits were so apparent to her that it led to rage at men and to an impulsive episode of unprotected intercourse in mid-cycle with a shallow, self-centered man. When she told me about this I felt angry at her for not valuing herself more, and decided to tell her about it. She experienced my reaction as caring, and felt both moved and angry at herself for not having cared more. She realized there was a grandiose aspect of herself that believed she could circumvent process and expect instant and total gratification; the mirror image of the devalued part that looked for "fast food" through enslavement to a narcissist. She was impatient with the time and the frustration involved in forming a substantial relationship, and reluctant to expose her areas of vulnerability. When she attempted to be patient and get to know a man she found exciting and desirable, she had difficulty differentiating patience from mindless compliance, and negotiation and compromise from taking on his problems as her own.

Joanna reminisced about our relationship and told me how astonished she had been in the early hospital days that I had addressed myself to what might be her interests. She recalled that she had literally believed I was the heat generator in the hospital, a delusion she now looked upon as her earliest efforts to make sense of these positive feelings. Then she began to talk about termination in the context of her difficulties holding on to the image of a loving relationship and generating her own heat. She dreamed that she made and drove a rickety car. We both noted the contrast with her recurrent dream of being in cars that lacked steering mechanisms and were out of control. She began to do what she called "shutting the door," that is, having a more appropriate sense of privacy and limits in her relationships with men, even in the face of frustration and wishes for "fast food." She reported several dreams in which she angrily held her own with men who did not treat her well, including her father. After nearly succumbing to temptation to sexually use and be used by a self-centered man but at the last moment "shutting the door," Joanna dreamed first that she was in a house teetering on the edge of a cliff, but managed to get out in time, and then that she was in a car being submerged in floodwaters but was able to roll up the windows.

I was both distressed when Joanna informed me that she had smoked some marijuana and pleased that she experienced nothing more than lassitude and a sense of time slowing. For the first time she began to experience what seemed like ordinary depression. At first she mistook it for fatigue, as it was so mild in comparison with the more familiar hopeless infantile despair. She related it to her work, which brought her into contact with people who were dying, and she contemplated changing to an area where she might be able to experience more optimism.

Six and one-half years of therapy had now elapsed. Joanna realized how she had overidealized her father and had taken on his self-devaluation problem as though it were her own in her efforts to achieve his grandiose expectations. She recalled how they would walk in the woods together when she was a child and how he would make no effort to adjust his rapid pace to hers, so that she would exhaust herself running to keep up. This memory, she realized, was a metaphor for how she had conducted her relationship with her father. Joanna felt calmer and more able to be alone and to soothe herself once she realized she could go at her own pace and not her father's. She was able to confront father appropriately when she felt he had not treated her well. Her body felt more integrated, particularly her genital area. In her new single life Joanna was flooded with requests for dates, and she was confronted with the need to discriminate and to decide whom she liked, and whom she did not, and let them know. For the first time she began to be able to detect significant problems in the men she met, which previously would have been covered over by her denial and introjection of those problems. She could now "shut the door" before becoming entangled with such men. In this more mature context Joanna met and began to date Robert, her future husband. The theme of our sessions became "opening the door a little and then drawing back to look out the window." This meant expressing herself, evaluating the consequences, and then taking selective and appropriate action.

Joanna began to work actively on termination issues, and hours were filled with separation dreams and feelings. She could do this without evidence of psychosis or hopeless, infantile depression, and she felt that she could live without me because she now had resources within herself. Moreover, she now believed that if she should need help there would be other people from whom she could obtain it. At the same time she wondered how she would deal with what she now called her basic death wish, that is, the wish not to have to continue to deal with her feelings. She dreamed that I was too tired to give her therapy, and wanted to play the piano instead. She assented, then heard me playing a duet with a violinist and became angry. In another dream we met at the top of a tall building, where I talked with her about infantile prevention of mental illness, a subject that bored her as she felt she knew it already. In yet another dream she was on a hospital ward as a patient at the same time that she was also out of the hospital on her own, and she felt angry that she was being displaced from her sick place. Associations led to rage at me and wishes to retaliate by seeking "fast food" from inappropriate men. She told me that if she had the choice she would never again invest herself emotionally in a relationship whose possibilities were as limited as ours. Finally, she dreamed we had an appointment in her bed and I hugged her. We were both turned on sexually, and then I said goodbye and left. Her association was that goodbye might be a human experience of gratification and frustration for both of us. She anticipated a termination 3 to 4 months hence, which would bring us to my summer vacation and the end of our seventh year.

Joanna felt mounting rage toward me, along with a sense of having invested in lost causes and having been used and betrayed, and a recrudescence of the infantile feelings of hopelessness, but these ideas and feelings were self-limited. As she realized again the sense of love and trust she felt toward me, the feelings evolved in the direction of healthy skepticism about where and with whom to invest her affections in the future. A sense of excitement and optimism about her life was accompanied by crying and grieving over our termination, which left her feeling better afterward. She predicted she would be depressed for about 9 months following our termination and realized she would like to see me after several months to check on her success in differentiating normal loss feelings from her sense of infantile hopelessness, for she realized the latter feeling might lead her to compromise herself in fundamental ways. The fate of this wish to check back with me was to have longstanding consequences in her life. We reviewed what Joanna had internalized, and she felt she had her own "watchdog," namely, the capacity for anger in her own behalf if she were to "open the door" and get a hurtful response from the world. She menstruated and felt like a fetus longing for mothering; simultaneously she had fears that what was coming out of her—hopeless depression—might contaminate others. Joanna revealed that 2 weeks earlier she had had her first gynecologic exam in several years and that it had evoked familiar thoughts about holes and knives but also newer concerns about coping with her own sexual feelings. She had a succession of dreams indicative of her struggle to remain integrated: In one of these a woman offered to remove the painful part of conflictual feelings and Joanna repeatedly said no; she felt her abdomen splitting apart under the pressure but pushed the halves together and felt better. She realized that the lure of psychosis was great, because of the freedom it offered from the experience of conflict. In another dream a formerly idealized male violin teacher offered to fix her instrument; each time he returned it, however, there was something basic wrong with it, which she was able to identify and object to.

We had a 2-week separation and Joanna experienced some fragmentation and mistrust, as well as depression, but she remained able to experience her attachment to me, to feel competence and pleasure in her work and her music, and to maintain a positive sense of herself. There had been two bad days when she felt her skull peeling off and her body fragmenting into parts and into the corners of the room, but she had been able to understand this reaction as a product of continuing infantile mistrust of me and to control it. In anticipation of a concert she elected not to talk about her feelings about me, which she felt might prove disorganizing and interfere with her performance. After the concert, which was very successful, she explored her powerful wishes to maintain a crippled relationship with me, including fantasies of being back in the hospital for "fast food" pleasure. Her rage and frustration led to reciprocal wishes not to allow me to be separate, that is, to wishes that I not take with me the narcissistic pleasure of curing a schizophrenic. In this way we would remain pathologically interdependent.

In the face of the regressive pull Joanna set a termination date 2 months hence. We were both somewhat surprised when she experienced an actual enhancement of her sense of self-esteem. She dreamed she was taking a trip but she wasn't sure what the temperature would be and how best to dress; at first she wore an old raccoon coat with holes, but she realized this was inappropriate and would hamper her mobility. Associations were to her old mode of coping by isolating and insulating herself and destroying her body awareness. In another dream she was in father's car with the rest of her family but realized that in order to have a man of her own she would have to get out and find someone else; she wanted the car stopped but said nothing. In this she recognized her old tendency to stop loving herself under conditions of stress and pain, such as our termination, and to seek a narcissistic male (whom she now generically and disparagingly referred to as "pukeface") to use her and give her attention.

Joanna realized she was avoiding full disclosure of her termination feelings and then movingly expressed love, grief, and anger toward me in ways that seemed very appropriate. Then she struggled with her old belief that I was an indispensable part of her, with feelings of confusion, and transient thoughts that her scalp was peeling and she was dead. We discovered this kind of regression occurred when she was unable to recollect a "clear" dream from the previous night and would waken with a depressive sense of need and a vague sense of mother. She realized that the problem was her inability to sustain a "maternal" image of her relationship with me so that she could be optimistic about her self-worth and the possibility of a loving relationship. On awakening in the morning she would think about our separation, experience first anger and then her maternally introjected prohibition of such feeling, and then try to evoke an image of me, which was at first one-dimensional and like mother. She would experience internal conflict similar to dialogues we had had about being accepting of one's feelings and would gradually feel calmer and be able to recall loving images of herself and of our relationship. Joanna dreamed she had taken on two jobs at once and was unable to function; she could not remember who she was until someone told her that her past was burned and gone. Then she felt relieved, realized it would take time to feel better, and felt she ought to take the day off from work to rest. For the first time in her life she was able to say to herself, "I love you."

Joanna dreamed about trips and obstacles. The theme was choosing the unknown, the trip, the future, over the security of the known, which was symbolized in one of the dreams by an immobile, tearful, Christlike figure protected by "mother church." This messianic image represented herself and one of her former self-centered male friends.

During our final month Joanna and I worked more on her psychotic rage and pessimism, and the problem of maintaining positive internal images in the face of her sense of a world of abandonment and hopelessness where only one person survives. First she felt that all life resided in me and termination meant death, and she experienced rage accompanied by cramps and diarrhea and wishes to destroy her image of me. Then she experienced real grieving and surprising optimism about the future. She was distressed by the lack of manifest response from her parents over her growth and impending termination, but she had the sense that her beloved grandmother was in heaven watching over her. About 3 weeks prior to termination Joanna had the following two dreams: In the first of these she was caring for a woman who bled to death through holes while laboring under the illusion that she was simply menstruating; the woman manifested great emotional integrity while dying. Associations were to the fact that her period was due around our termination date, to her fear that she would die without me, and to her wish to have a baby boy and name him after me. In another dream she dealt with her morning waking difficulty by having someone hand her a baby she could hold. This was accompanied by an upsurge of loving and maternal feelings toward herself.

Joanna nostalgically reviewed our work together, remembering some of her psychotic ideas when I had first met her in the hospital, and made it clear that she was managing her outside life well. She felt full of herself in a positive way and told her parents proudly about our impending termination. But although she told me she was crying over our termination outside her sessions, she was afraid to cry with me lest it revive more regressive feelings. At the same time she was upset with me for being unaware of the intensity of her termination feelings. In the next to last hour she reported a dream in which she came to see me, found me in bed, and got into the bed and tried to prod me into having a session with her, only to find that I had terminal liver cancer, a circumstance that did not deter her from her efforts. She associated to how she had learned to say goodbye through experiences with people who were dying, and to her realization that love could persist in the face of bodily assaults and other traumatic circumstances. She also realized she was accepting the death of her wishes for a physical relationship with me.

Joanna was surprisingly regressed during our last meeting, after almost 7 years of therapy. She brought me a pot of flowers, but her gift-giving was overshadowed by a feeling of loss of love, a tearful rage accompanied by nausea. Her distraught state reminded me of the spasmodic hiccuping of an infant who has cried to the point of exhaustion. She herself associated her reaction to a wish to get rid of my internal image in order to survive. I was distressed and perplexed: Should I act to alter the termination plan at the very last minute? I tried with little success to engage her in a constructive discussion about this. I expressed my concern and perplexity to her and reminded her of her earlier wish to see me again after a period of time had elapsed; at my suggestion we agreed that she would call me in 3 months to schedule a follow-up appointment.

I have often wondered about our termination. Might I have anticipated her regression in the final hour? What does one do when the patient does not actively collaborate in reviewing and perhaps modifying the decision to terminate? How many of us have had enough experience terminating successfully with such disturbed patients to answer such questions? Certainly I did not, so early in my own career. I felt I was steering a treacherous course between the Scylla of encouraging a chronic symbiotic merger based on invalidism and deadness and the Charybdis of allowing her to leave with what she, at least in part, experienced as a repetition of the emotional rejection that characterized her infancy; in other words, both options contained elements of her symbiotic dilemma with mother. In retrospect I think that in those days I was still learning the sense of timeless patience and ad hoc flexibility it takes to work with schizophrenics, and just as I may have been too coercive in my zeal to initially involve Joanna in the treatment, perhaps I was too rigid in failing to recognize that she might have benefited from another year or so of work. I suspect that I should not have assented so readily to her various wishes to cut down her frequency of appointments long before the actual termination. My relative inflexibility and paralysis in the final hour may have been a counter-transference repetition of Joanna's infantile feelings of passivity, despair, and rigid distance, and my allowing our grand plan of termination to override my feelings of the moment may have mirrored similar unresolved tendencies within her.

Joanna did not call for an appointment, as we had agreed. After a year had elapsed I wrote to inquire how she was and to remind her of our agreement, and she came in to see me. She and Robert had married, she had a new job, and she seemed to be doing well, but we had no substantial discussion about the termination hour.

Years passed and I heard nothing further from Joanna. Perhaps 15 years later, in the course of writing this book, I made inquiries of her mother of her whereabouts and well-being. Mother replied promptly, enclosing a picture of Joanna with her children in a letter saying that Joanna was happily married. Mother concluded with the following words: "We were glad to have a chance to thank you for your successful work with her. It was miraculous." Soon I received a letter from Joanna. She reported that her life was very full with family, work, and her music. She said, "There were many aspects of our work which have helped me to lead a very full life. I attribute some of my family happiness to my ability to recognize and express my feelings and accept those of others. You functioned as an emotional mother and father to me, and I have persisted with many of your characteristics." She commented on my "durability, unflinching regard for the truth, and wish to see me free to be myself" as having been very important to her. However, she said that, in retrospect, she had been unready for termination, which she experienced as "unbearably painful." She said she had left with the belief that I did not want to see her again, and that our separation was "inflexible." Some 3 years later she had consulted another analyst because she was depressed, and was referred to a woman therapist with whom she worked intermittently and occasionally for several years on separation issues. As she did not volunteer this person's name, I was unable to obtain any further information.

Chapter 20

Rachel: The Choice to Remain III

Rachel was hospitalized shortly after she completed her sophomore year of college. She had hallucinated voices instructing her to jump out the window, to take an overdose of pills, and to hurt other people. She became confused and frightened, could not sleep, and wandered around the campus at night in her nightgown.

Rachel was the younger of two daughters in a wealthy family. Her father, a successful businessman, had a genial demeanor and seemed eager to please. He was full of banal slogans and precepts. Family therapy revealed that his political facility thinly veiled a sense of grandiosity and contempt for any point of view different from his own. While family members tended to be mutually supportive in superficial and material ways, they tended to negate in one another manifestations of separate identity and feelings. Father took the lead in this regard, and established a variety of material bribes and sanctions that seemed designed to keep the others subservient to his will.

Mother also had a successful career. Her independence and leadership skills in her work belied her ideational compliance within the family, where she seemed to be in charge of the material aspect of the members' lives. Although mother showed no evidence of a mind of her own in discussions with her husband, he repeatedly indicated that in their marital relationship she was frustrating and withholding toward him sexually, a subject she refused to discuss.

The family valued action, achievement, success, and even stardom. They had but scanty vocabulary for feelings and relationships, and tended toward mechanical imagery. For example, father talked about "reprogramming" Rachel, and in stating his ideas about her treatment he said, "Rachel doesn't have time for people." Family members shared an idealized image of the family unit and a somewhat paranoid view of outsiders.

Rachel was described as a restless child with a short attention span. Because of unspecified behavior problems, referred to by her father as "outlaw" tendencies, she was taken to a therapist at one point in her childhood and was briefly placed on tranquilizers. She described her childhood as happy and full of friends and activities until the age of 8, when her upwardly mobile family moved from a middle class neighborhood to very affluent surroundings and she was separated from her friends. Rachel engaged in sports from the time she was very young, and rapidly gained recognition for her unusual skills. By the time she was 10 or 11 she was a "track machine" with grandiose fantasies about her future. Father became her coach and manager, and the family organized much of its leisure time around travel to and from her meets. Rachel's menarche was delayed until age 16, a phenomenon mother volunteered was common among serious athletes. Beneath her superficial charm and intelligence Rachel remained extremely naive about social mores and relationships, and she grew up without friends, spending much of her noncompetitive time alone in her room. She claimed she was not even aware that her high school classmates dated. In retrospect, she described this period as living in a "bell jar."

When she was 15, in tenth grade, her sister left home to attend college, and Rachel began to experience commanding auditory hallucinations. Her parents observed her lip movements and were aware of some of the content of these experiences but did not seem particularly concerned. When questioned about this subsequent to her hospitalization father said it did not seem unusual, and he added, "I do the same thing." Gradually, Rachel became convinced nothing was real and all the world was a game.

After high school Rachel had cosmetic facial surgery and her striking appearance made her the object of much male attention. Compliantly and passively she went through the motions of dating. Father took it on himself to write her college admission application, including her entrance essay. Rachel spent the summer preceding college at a private summer school distant from home, where she formed a relationship with an understanding woman faculty member, who, she recalled, was the first person to convince her that she might be human and have feelings.

Rachel attended the same college as her older sister. There her superficial social compliance led her to respond readily to male overtures and to become sexually promiscuous even though she was aware of no particular interest in or enjoyment of either the sex or the young men with whom she became involved. During the summer following her freshman year she began to experience an active interest in one of the young men with whom she had been intimate, and it was then, for the first time, that she became overtly psychotic. She wandered aimlessly, spoke rapidly, became abusive, drove her auto at outrageous speeds, spent huge sums of money, called people in the middle of the night, engaged in shoplifting, had ideas of reference, and hallucinated. She was hospitalized for 2 months and treated with loxapine, 40 mg.

Rachel returned to college midway through the following school year. No definitive arrangements were made for follow-up care, and since she resumed her compliant behavior and her grades seemed adequate, school authorities paid little further attention. Rachel stopped taking her medication, however, and during the summer following her sophomore year she became psychotic again, at which time she was rehospitalized at the institution where I met her.

Treatment

Year One

On admission to the hospital Rachel was disheveled. She believed the admitting doctor wanted to "screw" her. Her affect was flat, her speech was blocked, and she hallucinated voices admonishing her to jump out of the window. Her manner subsequently became stiff and robotic. She paced the floor repetitively, with an enigmatic smile on her face. She believed that there was a conspiracy against her involving the Mafia and major stars of the track and field world, and she was convinced she had cancer. She was placed on 30 mg of haloperidol and I was asked if I would become her therapist. At that time ward staff informed me that Rachel was the most reclusive patient on the ward. We met three times a week for 1½ years.

Rachel was a tall, slightly overweight, attractive young woman. When I first saw her she was scantily clad in a manner that seemed more heedless than provocative. In my office she looked drugged, showed little facial expression or emotion, and claimed to have little energy. She preferred to lie on the floor with her eyes closed. Occasionally she postured bizarrely, and looked almost catatonic. Although Rachel had a large vocabulary, a good memory, and some intermittent capacity for self-observation, and although she made some perfunctory efforts to find out what I wanted and to comply in a mechanical manner, she was mostly silent. She claimed unconvincingly that she trusted me, and told me she was frightened of other patients and of staff. But when I would attempt to rephrase something she said in order to see if I had understood, she would typically retort, "That's not what I mean; you're putting words in my mouth!" Nonetheless, during our first four exploratory sessions she mentioned feelings of fear, anger, and guilt, as well as a belief that her parents were persecuting her; said she was not sufficiently self-assertive; and finally asked if I might be able to help her with this and if I would agree to be her therapist.

During the first 3 months of our work Rachel's demeanor was little changed. When she was not with me she made no personal contact with anyone and spent as much time as possible in bed. She so thoroughly stuffed herself with food that she gained 25 pounds. She seemed helpless, puzzled and naive about the world around her and waiting to be told what to do. For the most part Rachel acted as though she were alone when we met for therapy. Constant lip movement and subvocal speech, along with occasional gestures and facial expressions, suggested hallucinations and a lively inner dialogue.

This apparent internal animation was in marked contrast with her interpersonal deadness and withdrawal. Her infrequent coherent comments suggested delusions and auditory hallucinations about such subjects as cancer, hysterectomy, conspiracies against her, and her special place in the world of sports. She continued to respond to my attempts to articulate what she seemed to be saying or doing by telling me not to put words in her mouth. After the first month haloperidol was replaced by thioridazine in doses as high as 1,000 mg; after another month this was replaced by mesoridazine, 500 mg.

A recurrent theme was Rachel's conviction that there would be a magic cure and she would be released from the hospital to go home, a place she described in womblike imagery. She spoke as though this event were to transpire after she had served a sentence of some sort, or perhaps as a kind of childlike reward for her superficial efforts to comply, which seemed to constitute her idea of recovery. Her attitude was not inconsistent with the stance of the ward staff, who tended to believe she was better when she was compliant and who rewarded her with privileges, much to my dismay. Otherwise, they tended to leave her alone in her isolated state because she did not create a gross disturbance like so many of the other patients and because contact with her tended to be so unrewarding. I often struggled with my own tendency to withdraw and feel drowsy in response to her, and I began to be aware of countertransference wishes to be somewhere more satisfying, which strikingly paralleled her own wishes. During one hour I pointed out the contradiction between her assertions that she had faith in doctors and was in the hospital because the doctors told her she should be, on the one hand, and her lack of involvement with me and rejection of my comments on the other. She rapidly changed the subject.

Things were not totally bleak, however. From time to time Rachel acknowledged that she knew she was ill. Occasionally, she displayed a sense of humor. And she reiterated that she did want to continue meeting with me, though she responded to any attempt I might make to encourage her to focus on an issue or a contradiction, or even to own the content of her remarks, by withdrawing, forgetting, or changing the subject. I tried to mobilize some activity on her part by not automatically scheduling appointments before inquiring about her own interest in doing so.

After 2½ months a staff conference was held. The social worker presented new information from Rachel's parents that she had been hallucinating at least since her mid-teens; hitherto, despite questioning, they had not considered this fact sufficiently remarkable to mention. Psychological tests reported at the conference revealed "a classical pattern of longstanding schizophrenia," an acute disorganizing disturbance superimposed on a chronic deteriorating process. Intelligence was low normal, with verbal scores higher than performance scores. Signs suggestive of catatonia led the tester to observe that the prognosis was poor. A consensus was reached that Rachel was a chronic, deteriorated schizophrenic with a private inner life she was unwilling to share with anyone. It was agreed that more vigorous treatment efforts were advisable. Medication was switched to loxapine, 200 mg, staff began to give her more feedback and to pressure her to relate to them, and I began to challenge Rachel's desire to go home by asking her why she didn't do something about it rather than waiting so passively.

Although her preoccupation with food and sleep persisted, after about 3 months Rachel began to look more alert and to sit in a chair and do needlepoint. When she stopped to express guilt that she should be paying attention to me instead, I responded that it was not necessary for her to try to please me; she then resumed her needlepoint with evident relief, simultaneously chattering away like a little child about nothing of consequence, as though she were trying to make me feel good by being companionable. She took more interest in grooming herself and began to diet. She realized that she had been in a kind of daze, playing "mind games" having to do with special patterns and meanings in the way she walked and in the things she touched. She realized she had been very withdrawn—not hallucinating, she assured me, but "talking to myself." However, she was certain that those behaviors were all gone now and were not, therefore, a problem we need concern ourselves about.

Next Rachel decided that she wanted another therapist. She reasoned that therapy had not been a serious matter up until now, and that this must mean that I was not a serious person. In fact, she said that I looked like a clown to her and thought that perhaps I had been laughing at her and not taking her seriously. I need not have been concerned that she might act on this idea, however, for, like most thoughts, the wish to get rid of me did not last long and was soon replaced by a more characteristic stance of trying, in a naive, childlike way, to get me to tell her what she should do. Her affect remained flat, and her presence rather mechanical and staring.

Rachel began to talk about her lack of self-confidence, confusion about what she wanted, inability to assert herself, and tendency to comply with others. She was overwhelmed with the realization of what a "pushover" she was and with feelings of helplessness and hopelessness about altering this characteristic. She told me that she and her older sister, Nina, were both "mice," bossed by their parents. Father had "programmed" her to be an athletic machine and kept her "on a leash." She realized that since the fifth grade, when the family had moved, she had been a withdrawn and isolated person who had no fun and had no idea how to relate to other children and that her parents had not seemed to notice.

Rachel informed me that whereas once she had been convinced I wanted to hurt her, now she was reluctant to leave her appointments. She recognized that she had "no mind of [her] own" and that in the past her parents had made all her decisions for her. Her imagined solution was to get me to tell her what to do, and thereby replace a "bad" master with a "good" one. After 3½ months her parents visited for a holiday. In anticipation Rachel felt depressed and impotent to deal with them, and wanted to do what she had done so often as an adolescent, namely go to her room, shut the door, get under the covers, and go to sleep. She was surprised and gratified by my suggestion that she might ask a ward staff member to be present in case she needed help. After the meeting she was more stylishly dressed. Initially she was pleased that she had been able to tell her parents not to overpower her, but as she reflected on their ready acquiescence she realized they had only been placating and indulging her.

Rachel was sad that her life had turned out as it had, and wished she had another chance; she thought that perhaps things would be fine if she could leave the hospital and try again. I said perhaps she would have a better chance outside the hospital if she could first use her treatment to work out some of the problems that had led to her difficulties. I questioned her about her relationships with other patients and staff, and she realized, to her amazement and dismay, that she was not able to relate to anyone in the hospital.

Rachel and I began to establish consensus that she was preoccupied with avoidance, distraction, and immediate pleasure seeking. She immersed herself in external activity, or paid endless attention to her clothing. She had an almost literal sense of having no insides and not being human, expressed in its extreme form by her intermittent delusion of having been hysterectomized. Since I realized she was quite unaware of having an inner life, I encouraged her to attend to her dreams, fantasies, and feelings, and she began to tell me about suicidal preoccupations. Gradually we identified a variety of other fantasies, subsumed under the phrase "marking time," which she originally coined when I asked her about her characteristic shuffling-in-place body movements. "Marking time" fantasies included pleasurably reliving a time at around age 8 when she had lived on a lake, imagining herself back at college, looking forward to the next opportunity to sleep or eat, or imagining she was on a South Seas island. She much preferred these to anything real. She realized that people frightened her and she wanted to withdraw into a "bell jar." She reported her first dream: A former roommate was riding in a balloon with her parents but fell out; Rachel ran to her in a state of distress. In the ensuing days she told me two others: In the first she was touring the track-and-field circuit with a famous woman athlete, and in the other she was covered with red nodules of skin cancer. The first dream involved her belief that women athletes are like herself, not human beings, therefore, were she with them she would be more comfortable. The second dream led her to recall that at puberty she had been convinced that she had breast cancer and during a previous hospitalization she believed she had a brain tumor; now, she admitted, she believed she had undergone a hysterectomy. I questioned her about her sexual functioning and learned that her menses had been late in onset and were sporadic. I remarked on her rich fantasy life and her longstanding belief she was different from others, physically and emotionally; she was surprised and saddened, and talked about the the need she and her family had to pretend it was not so.

In the next hour her associations indicated a fear of her feelings, and a sense of security she got from father who protected her from having to deal with them, as well as of her tendency to comply superficially with others while not really letting herself be involved. She returned to the subject of marking time in her head, wishing she were somewhere else. I wondered if she was doing this now, and she reluctantly talked about anticipating dinner. I remarked on her misleading compliance and asked if there was anything she truly enjoyed. She responded, "eating and sleeping," and when I asked if anything else in life was pleasurable for her she admitted with much embarrassment that sex was. I remarked this must mean she had sex organs, and I asked if she ever had sexual feelings when she was with me. With more embarrassment she responded that she had but that this was not appropriate because she knew I was married. It was clear that she had trouble distinguishing thoughts from things and from actions. With disconcerting directness and great naïveté she asked if I ever had any sexual feelings for her. I responded straightforwardly that I had not because she had been so withdrawn that she had hardly been a presence in our relationship. As the conversation progressed she began to blush and she realized that for the first time in a long while she was not "marking time" and had lost the preoccupation with impending dinner, but she felt overwhelmingly excited and guilty, and on the verge of physically shaking!

In subsequent hours Rachel rapidly returned to a state of passive depression, "marking time" until she could sleep or eat. She said she looked forward to seeing her father, for he made her feel secure. When I asked what had happened to her feelings about me she remarked, with some asperity, that they were gone, that if it was impossible to have a physical relationship with me, there was no point in having thoughts and feelings. In subsequent hours we both felt a sense of emptiness and purposelessness. My pursuit of inadvertent remarks about suicide led to the uncovering of extensive fantasies about suicide and also about killing someone else, and in return getting put out of her misery. When I remarked on the paradox between her belief that she had no thoughts and her rich fantasy life, she responded that there was no reason for us to pay any attention to these ideas or take them seriously, as she was not about to act on them. I then tried to explore the reason for her most recent withdrawal, and she was able to acknowledge that it was fear of the feelings she had begun to have.

Although Rachel continued to be withdrawn, she was intermittently able to talk about sex. She said that she had hated herself and her sexuality since the promiscuity of her freshman year. She apologized for her withdrawal, and said it was because human relationships were so unsatisfying, and that I shouldn't take it personally. She expressed some anger at her father for training her and her sister to be "performing robots" and not allowing them to have fun or friends.

By 6 months Rachel's loxapine had been reduced to 100 mg. She said she was feeling good and planned to return to college, but her affect was flat, she yawned repeatedly, and she talked exclusively about what the future would be like. When I commented on her withdrawal and avoidance of her immediate experience she acknowledged boredom and lack of pleasure, and verbalized then a variety of fantasies, ranging from bloody suicide to pleasure in her tropical island paradise. She said she was "marking time" and told me how moved she had been by the inscription on Martin Luther King's tomb: "FREE AT LAST!" When loxapine was reduced to 50 mg, Rachel acknowledged some fears of becoming overtly crazy again. I suggested one way to prevent this might be to try to understand what had caused her psychosis to begin with. She expressed surprise at this seemingly novel idea and returned to her wish to deny her sexuality. She talked about how she had lived in a "bell jar" at home. When she left for college she had never even kissed a boy, and was both naive and terrified of others. She had compliantly engaged in sex, like an automaton, because that was what she thought a college girl was supposed to do. It was not so bad until she met a boy she started to care about, and he jilted her. At that time, she said, she gave up on boys and on sex.

The social worker and I speculated that Rachel's mindless state was related to family issues, but since the social worker's efforts with the family to identify any problems had elicited nothing but the insistence that everything was quite normal, we decided conjoint family therapy might be a useful adjunct to individual therapy and separate meetings with the parents. After about 6 months, as the first meeting approached, Rachel dreamed she was secretary to a once respected public official who had been found guilty of a crime. She then realized that her father was coming to the meeting from the city where the crime had been committed and that, in fact, he was involved in business dealings with a "firm of ill repute" in that city.

Father dominated our first meeting. He had explanations for everything. He denied Rachel's claim that he had pushed her into athletics, and he insisted that he understood her completely because she was so much like him. Calling attention to her bizarre thinking did not sway him in this conviction; he merely insisted that her behavior and thinking were a normal response to being in "a place like this." No one in the family but father seemed to have a mind. Rachel and her sister literally changed their minds as he talked; to my amazement and consternation I heard Rachel grossly contradict things she had told me. When father disagreed with Rachel's claim that he had pushed her into athletics she retracted it; he, in turn, denied that they had ever had a disagreement to begin with. Mother said she did not agree with father, but she was unwilling to elaborate.

After this meeting Rachel talked with me about lacking a mind of her own, and depending on others for an identity. She realized that she behaved like a chameleon, enacting whatever people wanted her to be at the moment, and that for her the real problem came when the music stopped, so to speak, and she felt depressed and jellylike. When her Loxapine was reduced to 25 mg, she became more active on the ward and at a job she had taken, but she expressed fears of being mangled.

For some time the family meetings centered around Rachel, who was designated by everyone as the family problem and was quizzed by other family members, who seemed to present themselves as her therapists. At first Rachel compliantly responded to her family's questions and concerns. Father con-

tinued to be the dominant force, and the meetings had the flavor of a doc-
trinaire party meeting in a totalitarian state. Father could be quite perceptive
about others at times, but he generally tended to be pontifical and full of
slogans, long-winded and obscure, and was utterly blind to the possible
significance of his own behavior. Though he claimed to value learning highly,
and defined it as listening and taking in what others have to say, it was a case
of "do as I say, not as I do," for his convictions of the moment, however
self-contradictory, illogical, and changeable, were unshakable. With scarcely
a ruffled feather he invalidated the perceptions others had of him, even when
they were unanimous. Father was troubled that Rachel no longer seemed the
vibrant daughter and famous athlete he had known and obviously gotten much
gratification from, but when she attempted to disagree with him he would
become directly upset with her and began to question her sanity. The women
in the family rapidly withdrew from any confrontation with him, in this manner proving their contention that it was impossible to have a dialogue with
him. In this quite subtle way, father, like Rachel, was a scapegoat.

There was a curious reciprocity between father's unreachability in the
family meetings and what he reported was mother's disengagement in the
concurrent couple therapy they had commenced in the city where they lived.
While father seemed willing and even eager to talk about some of their marital
problems (and claimed that his wife was not sympathetic to his feelings or
needs), mother declined to discuss these matters in front of the children and
reported flare-ups of her colitis whenever the subject was broached.

After 9 months of hospitalization Rachel was taken off all antipsychotic
medication. I had seemingly inexhaustible opportunities to point out her lack
of "a mind of my own" since she would repeatedly, grossly, and blithely contradict herself in her individual work with me and in the family meetings. Rachel
began to express determination to leave the hospital "prison" and return to
college, where she was convinced she would somehow find a mind of her own
and everything would be fine. In this fantasy scenario I was readily replace-
able; she would just get another therapist. I discovered that no one was unique
and special to her; Rachel secretly devalued everyone. She referred to the other
patients contemptuously as "born losers." As we talked about these things
Rachel became more aware that she was a cold, aloof, and judgmental person,
and this depressed her. In our concurrent family meetings, Rachel shared her
new insight, and in an uncharacteristic family interchange other members
responded with awareness that each of them was in one way or another, more
or less consciously, withdrawn and aloof from the others.

Rachel formed her first ward relationship, a distant idolization of a bright
male patient who clearly devalued her. She daydreamed about him and about
being back at college. I pointed out to Rachel that she used these fantasies to
fill the void where feelings, attachments, and commitments might otherwise
be. When her plans to leave the hospital began to be more concrete, her ward
administrator recommended that she remain. After a surprisingly brief and
minimal reaction of disappointment, Rachel began to become more involved,

and I began to hear feelings of sadness about her life, anger at her administrator, a hunger for relationships, and even an awareness of sexual feelings, which she continued to consider too private to share with me. She was most distressed by her sexual feelings, and made it clear that she had to keep them separate from the people she cared about.

In our family meetings Rachel now became more active and curious about the other members. It became clearer that father was not exclusively responsible for the family impasse, for when he would point out in a seemingly realistic way issues he had with Rachel's sister and with his wife, they refused to discuss them. Rachel began to be aware that she was generally angry, and at times she got angry at me. She began to intimate that she had a mind of her own, had something valuable to say, and would like to differ with father. She wanted to challenge his prohibition against speaking with her paternal grandmother about a contradiction she perceived between grandmother's professed love for her and her shame that Rachel was in a mental hospital. Rachel realized that she devalued herself and that she shared her father's devaluing attitude toward feelings and human relationships. In fact, it emerged that she literally thought of father as God and turned to him to guide her.

The process of self-discovery and the prospect of living on her own were very exciting to Rachel. She became much more appropriate in her relationships, work plans, and plans for discharge. She shared feelings of depression and fearfulness about recurrence of her psychosis, and realized that she needed to talk about her hitherto unspeakable sexual concerns. After about 10½ months of hospitalization Rachel was discharged to a halfway house, with a job in the community (which she seemed to enjoy though it was not intellectually demanding), a partial hospitalization program, and tentative plans to attend a local college in the fall, about 4 months hence.

Following her discharge, to her surprise and mine, Rachel was full of feelings and eager for communication and relationships with others. It was like watching a starving person discover a steak. She became very involved emotionally in her work with me and was reluctant to end her therapy hours. I was amazed to note that, except for a certain naive, "born yesterday" quality, she often seemed quite normal. Rachel felt herself separating from her family and was filled with self-doubt and the need for guidance. She was quite excited about living on her own but remarkably unsophisticated about the simplest matters of self-care and self-regulation. She had great difficulty making decisions and setting limits on her impulses, for she literally did not seem to know how to integrate her wishes with her values and with reality or how to reach decisions and judgments that were her own. She was unable to budget her expenditures and commented that her parents had always encouraged her to buy anything she wanted. As I worked with her over control and decision making, she literally got a headache, recalled father's "perfect" advice, and longed to take the easy way out by asking her parents to take over. She looked upon me as an umpire or referee. If her judgment was not ratified she became terrified, felt out of control, began to be actively self-devaluing, and expected retaliation for her "bad" ideas. She pressed to see me more frequently. As she became more excited about her life and active in her own behalf she became increasingly uneasy, and tried to define the changes as crazy and to appeal to me for medication and restraint.

As she became more aware of her need for people and her specific dependency on me, Rachel was shocked to realize that I was an autonomous person who was capable of leaving her at any time. She became sad about the departure of a young medical student she had gotten to know in the hospital, and she said she felt angry much of the time but did not know why. People were no longer just objects to Rachel, for she seemed genuinely curious and empathic about others and was able to sustain her investment during periods of separation. But she realized she was confused about her dependencies. How was she to decide which were good and which were not? Though she appeared to be thinking things through, she wondered if she was assimilating what I told her and following me as mindlessly as she had followed her father—and, in my silent reflection, so did I.

There was a striking shift in the family balance as we approached our summer vacation interruption and the anniversary of Rachel's hospitalization. Rachel had become more open with her opinions and feelings. She expressed concern for her older sister, Nina, who had begun to act more withdrawn and to manifest a set of feelings and behaviors, including devaluation and idealization, inhibition, accompanied by escapism fantasizing that the "grass will be greener," that Rachel recognized all too well. Mother was also withholding and would not talk about her issues; she argued that she was talking about them in couple therapy, but father disagreed. Father, in turn, was concerned about each of the others, although he would not talk about himself. He complimented Rachel on her maturity but expressed his concern lest she become ill again. He and Rachel expressed interest in continuing family meetings in the fall, but mother and Nina did not want to; we decided to have more meetings in the fall to try to resolve the stalemate.

Rachel seemed to be growing by leaps and bounds in work, friendships, and self-care. It clearly made her uneasy that she was so happy, and her conviction that there was something the matter with her escalated proportionately. As she checked out the various situations in her life in which she was exercising initiative and on reflection found each unexceptionable, she turned her focus of worry toward her body, particularly moles and amenorrhea, and began to obsess about cancer and to have escalating fears of going crazy.

Although Rachel felt that her relationship with me was secure and productive, she began to ruminate that perhaps it was a crutch, perhaps the sense of security was an illusion. She ruminated that she was bad, wrong, and defective, and her search to identify the defect accelerated, darting frantically from one thing to another despite my efforts to continue a more abstract dialogue with her about her relationship with her father, her fears of separateness and of her feelings, and her issues about personal goodness and validity. I wondered to myself if she should have more medication but felt conflicted;

she might interpret such a suggestion as my confirmation of her equation of autonomy with craziness.

In anticipation of a date with an eligible graduate student Rachel realized how important men were to her, and how her fear of losing them clashed with her need to set limits. She began to think about a boy from home she had once had a crush on but had not seen for several years. Her date went surprisingly well, and Rachel sounded calm and reflective afterward; she and the graduate student had enjoyed one another as separate people and Rachel had experienced no pressure.

Near the first anniversary of her hospitalization there was a long holiday weekend. Rachel did not realize we would miss the Monday hour on which the holiday fell until our final appointment of the week, which was on Thursday. The following day she came to my office unannounced. She demanded I return letters from her old boyfriend from home (which, in fact, she had not given me) and talked rather impulsively about the urge to visit him immediately. I heard her out but did not act. Over the ensuing weekend she made several phone calls to me, sounding increasingly panicked and somewhat hostile but not clearly psychotic. In the middle of one night she called the police and asked them to bring her to the hospital. There she paced the floor, delusional and giggling. She had multiple somatic delusions about her vagina, her teeth, and her eyes, and hallucinated a female voice informing her about a Nazi conspiracy to exterminate her. When I saw her after the weekend she was withdrawn and seemed afraid of me. She walked out of the office in the middle of our first appointment.

Year Two

Rachel was floridly psychotic for the next 2½ months. Her posture was wooden and her affect was flat or inappropriate. She was indifferent to the people around her. Her lips moved and she seemed consumed with an inner dialogue. She hallucinated swastikas, believed the Nazis were plotting to kill her, and that her food and medications were poisoned. Possibly these beliefs accounted for the periods during which she refused to eat, to take medication, and to see me. She believed she had cancer, was becoming bald, was losing her teeth, and had undergone a hysterectomy.

Rachel acted as though I were not there. When she was not more obviously immersed in her psychotic world she would do needlepoint or make the most superficial efforts to relate to me by introducing trivial topics of conversation, or expressing a kind of Pollyannish belief that everything was fine. During our meetings her mood and thought content fluctuated rapidly and bizarrely. At times she would smile blandly and vacuously, and at other times laugh for no apparent reason. There were episodes of paranoid terror associated with tears, total body tremor, and the conviction that I was about to kill her, followed abruptly by laughter and the declaration that she loved me and wanted to sleep with me. Numerous antipsychotic medications were tried without success.

Loxapine, which had been effective in the past, was discontinued despite my doubts, because her administrator believed it was inducing parkinsonism and was responsible for her wooden posture.

I realized that I felt shocked, dismayed, and angry at Rachel, as though she had somehow betrayed an agreement with me by becoming psychotic again. When I discovered that the young woman who had seemed to be so invested in life and so involved with me was replaced by one who grinned vacuously, uttered facile yeses, seemed indifferent to her surroundings and preoccupied with an inner world, I expressed my feeling of sadness to her and wondered aloud if she would regain her interest and begin relating to me again. As though in response she called me at home and asked me urgently to come to the hospital before her next appointment for she had something important to tell me. With sudden hopefulness I did so, only to hear that she had decided to marry her old boyfriend from home. I felt disappointment and anger and told her so. She refused to attend our next several meetings.

Now, in striking contrast to her previous levels of energy and interest, Rachel would not deal with the most elemental issues in her life, including seeing her family and the arrangements she had made prior to her decompensation to attend a local college in the fall. To further complicate matters, I had to introduce another issue, namely, that my wife would be giving birth in about a month, and I would be interrupting our work for a week or so at that time. When I tried to call her attention to an issue she would ignore me entirely or remark, "I can't be bothered about that." Sometimes she would withdraw into a state of muttered cursing.

Shortly before my wife's due date Rachel apparently had a menstrual period, a relatively unusual event for her. She became preoccupied with her vagina, complained of itching and pathological bleeding, and repeated her belief that she had had a hysterectomy. When I reminded her about the impending birth of my baby she became preoccupied with its name, and wanted me to call it Rachel. When I returned a week after the birth, the ward staff shared with me their impression that Rachel had been suspended in a state of waiting for me.

My countertransference feelings of helpless dismay led me to forget one of her appointments. When I remembered and rushed to the ward half an hour late, it seemed that Rachel had not even noticed. On another occasion she said she did not want to see me again, then smiled, paced back and forth in front of me, and invited me to make more appointments. I had the feeling she was trying to involve me in some childlike game and I had to struggle with the urge to laugh inappropriately.

After 2½ months of regression and about 15 months of therapy I urged Rachel's administrator to discontinue the current antipsychotic medication and resume loxapine. He agreed to do so, despite his reservations. In the week or so following resumption of a 50 mg dose there was a significant improvement. Rachel's thought disorder was less apparent and she was gradually more able to concentrate, to show appropriate affect, and to be realistic. It began to dawn on her that she had "dismissed" everyone, given up all her activities, and gone into a state of withdrawal. She showed what appeared to be appropriate signs of depression and loneliness. She began to think about people again, initially in terms that were black and white, concrete, and utilitarian. First she talked about her dismissal of mother, which she justified by saying that mother was a bad person who yelled at her. It took another month for her to decide to initiate a rapprochement with mother; by that time the ostensible reason for banishing her had been forgotten. Then, in the context of wishing for someone to run errands and bring her things, she recalled the existence of her sister, but she realized that she didn't even know where Nina lived or how to reach her. Finally, she began to show interest in me again. First she called me at home to express her fear that she would die in her sleep. In our next meeting, when I expressed surprise that she had turned to me, Rachel laughed ruefully and acknowledged a reawakening of interest in our relationship, adding that I should consider myself privileged to be one of her "chosen few." She concluded this hour by matter-of-factly requesting me to fetch her a pencil!

Rachel's awareness that she once again had been quite ill was at first naive and superficial; "I worked too hard," she explained. As she thought more about her illness and her rehospitalization she cried. Gradually, with my help, she was able to conceptualize her recurrent psychosis, to talk with some measure of perspective about her paranoid ideation, and to show some interest in working to keep the problem from recurring yet again. Now her idea was that her decompensation related to her date with the graduate student, specifically, to the fact that sex and men frightened her, and that she had an all-or-nothing way of dealing with these things. She began to show interest in a job, school, therapy, and in resuming visits with her family, and she was able to come to my office for her sessions. Once again she had a compelling and initially mindless urge toward activity. I pointed out the alternation between her active, excited states and the periods of passivity, withdrawal, and indifference, both historically and as these trends fluctuated in her day-to-day living, both relatively mindless, and I suggested that there was an intermediate state of self-awareness that she wanted to avoid. It was apparent to me that she required regular contact with me to maintain any kind of serious, organized introspective effort; even a weekend separation usually led to disruption.

Her psychotic regression had more or less spanned the planned interruption in family meetings, and as our planned fall family reunion, with its agenda of deciding whether there should be further meetings approached, Rachel became more passive and lethargic, her affect flattened, and she was preoccupied with wishes to live in the past or in a home with her family, envisioned as a warm, hedonic retreat. The most striking development in the meeting was the emergence of Nina (who at the time of the interruption had shown personality characteristics similar to those of Rachel and who had wanted to discontinue family therapy) as a thoughtful, questioning, therapeutic ally. Since other members were unable to make a commitment to family therapy it was Nina who articulated how all family members tended to avoid commitment, and persevered in activities and relationships only as long as they seemed gratifying and did not require any soul-searching and self-modification. Family members gave Rachel considerable feedback about her psychotic withdrawal and she was appropriately upset, but evasive. Father complained that family members were keeping secrets from him; at the same time, he dropped broad hints, which he declined to elaborate, that he and Rachel were engaging in secret conversations about the possibility of her leaving the hospital and returning home. Increasingly father played the part of therapist, exhorting Rachel with slogans such as "Go jogging," "Read the *Wall Street Journal*," and "Go into computers," and she in turn acted like a cult follower.

Rachel expressed to me growing unhappiness that she was so passive and interested not in people or reality but only in hedonic pursuits such as eating, sleeping, or her escapist fantasies. I suggested that she perceived herself as a princess from whom nothing is expected, who banishes summarily people who have in any way offended her, even by encouraging her to think or feel about painful matters. She realized that she had enacted this regal role in her adolescence as the family athletic star.

After about 16 months of therapy and 1½ months back on loxapine, Rachel decided she had to have a job immediately. She reported feelings of being controlled and "bugged" when her willfulness was in any way challenged. When she presented herself one hour with racing thoughts, mounting panic, and restlessness, I escorted her from my office back to the ward, where she was restricted, and the dosage of loxapine was increased to 75 mg. Rachel experienced the ward as a prison. I talked with her about her impulsivity and grandiosity, and suggested that she was unable to stay still anywhere for long without feeling persecuted by all the painful feelings she was unable to own. She experienced me as unsympathetic and said that when I did not agree with her I was dismissing her as a person. I maintained that matters were quite the opposite, that she was dismissing me and herself as a person, acting like the queen who only wanted a mirror in which to admire her image, and that she expected me to take no issue with her and to be as crazy and inconsistent in my beliefs and states of mind as she was in hers. My interpretation made her angry, and with thinly disguised rage she joked that perhaps she would pronounce the verdict on me "Off with your head!"

Rachel next became determined to have sexual intercourse, heedless of my reminders of how stressful she found sexual issues, and quite convinced that she could not get pregnant even though she did not use a contraceptive. She pressed to leave the hospital and get a job, convinced that identity and direction would flow into her from it. She admired a very hostile psychotic woman patient and believed that by emulating this woman's behavior she would acquire a mind of her own. Over my objections her hospital administrator permitted her to get a store-clerk job. After two weeks she found the job boring, and quit, with fantasies of becoming a sports superstar.

By contrast, in family meetings Rachel seemed to be waiting, spongelike and passive, for others to decide her future. It was inadvertently revealed that father and Rachel had again been talking secretly about her going home, and a seemingly irreconcilable split emerged between father, on the one hand, and mother, Nina, the social worker and I, who confronted him with our shared concern about the destructive nature of what he was doing. Nina was especially vehement. Of all the family members she seemed to have derived the most benefit from our sessions; her life had improved dramatically as a result of insights about the family. But father was unshakable and his response was openly devaluing to the point of calling all of us "crazy." Rachel subsequently cried in her meeting with me and told me that I was the only nonfamily friend she had; at the same time she refused to listen to anything I might say that seemed to differ from what her father told her. She viewed herself as ready to return to school and unjustly imprisoned in the hospital. When I wondered if she had been upset by the recent family meetings she could not recall that there had been anything controversial about them until I really pressed her. Then she was able to agree that she was externalizing her own conflicts, that her world consisted of a deity and a jailer, and that she was now looking for the deity to rescue her from the prison of having to deal with anything she found distressing. After this discussion she called her father and with much difficulty expressed to him her concern about his devaluation of me and the family members, but she promptly lapsed again into superficiality.

In the next therapy meeting each of us, I discovered, was wishing to be elsewhere (my fantasy was to be with a more gratifying and productive patient). Finally we were able to share some of our mutual frustration. Rachel told me, "You read me like a book," and I countered that she was not interested in reading any part of herself that was disturbing, such as her dreams, fantasies, feelings, and family relationships. Although she claimed not to understand what I was saying, she suddenly realized that about a week before (probably around the time of the distressing family meetings in which she and father were aligned in opposition to the rest of us) she had dreamed that she was being devoured by the shark in the movie *Jaws*. She told me of her belief that others often capture her thoughts, and then recalled another dream, in which she repeated to me, over and over, "I don't understand what you think my problem is!"

Loxapine was increased gradually to 150 mg. Around the weekend of her 21st birthday Rachel's push to go home ("where it's warm") and get away from the hospital, which she found a cold place, and perhaps from a coldness she had begun to observe in herself, hardened. She rationalized her demand so that it did not seem like an act of opposition to her therapy and to me by means of a kind of sloganized perversion of the discussions we had had about her need to have a mind of her own. She was superficially compliant with me, with other patients, and with staff, but I was aware that she had altogether stopped listening to the content of my comments and knew from what she told me that she consciously lied about her mental state to the ward staff in her efforts to get more privileges. She preferred to sleep and to daydream, and she imagined that she would marry her old boyfriend and live happily ever after. I expressed mild skepticism but felt that it was unwise to actively oppose her. When I would interject some aspect of reality that ought to have given her pause she simply brushed aside my concern. Finally, I said that she seemed to be saying goodbye to me. Her response was to ask casually if I would refer her to a therapist near her home.

What turned out to be the final 2-month portion of Rachel's hospital stay was ushered in by a conference reviewing her treatment. She had been re-tested by a psychologist, and there were surprising signs of improvement: Rachel had gained over 30 IQ points, but subtest scatter was still evident. Her concentration and memory were especially improved, but her social judgment and ability to draw logical conclusions in interpersonal situations were both very impaired. She was less rigid. Her relationship with mother seemed more "humane," and her problems centered much more around relationships with men, especially father, and her sexual identity. On the Rorschach she identified herself as a butterfly trampled by two hippopotami. I noted the cyclothymic nature of Rachel's illness, with 4-month cycles of catatonic-like behavior fol-lowed first by psychotic depression and then by a reconstitution, during which she was at first more active and constructive, albeit with compliant and gran-diose undercurrents. As a result it was decided to taper her off loxapine and place her on lithium, a decision which, perhaps unfortunately, was not im-mediately implemented because once again things seemed to improve.

Rachel told me that her sister had "lit a spark" under her by expressing anger at Rachel's willingness to give up, go home, and let their parents take over her life. We were able to discuss her conflict between her uncritical worship of her father and his thinking, and her awareness of his unwillingness to face his own problems. When members of the family told father they were depressed about their inability to communicate with him Rachel could see how he would deny any part in the matter and focus solicitously on their depres-sion. She was also impressed by my suggestion that her somatic delusion that something was wrong with her insides might reflect a partial awareness of her inability to control her own life.

At subsequent family meetings Nina pointed out that neither father nor Rachel would acknowledge that they gave contradictory messages. Father said he was eager to participate in therapy; simultaneously he made it clear that he felt I was "nuts." Rachel pretended interest but remained passive and in-different. This led to an open family discussion about my competence, in which mother and Nina made it clear that this was not an issue for them and father allowed that his opinion that I was insane might be his way of dealing with his inability to understand what I was saying. We talked about the difficulty all family members had in dealing with differing points of view. This led to an expression of how mother inhibited her chronic anger at and sense of differ-ence with father, with the result that everyone thought she was an angry person but no one knew why. Rachel and her sister, in turn, pointed out how difficult it was to disagree with mother, and how she always had to have her way in a dispute. Father agreed, and said his only choice was to withdraw from her. We concluded that family members experienced relationships in terms of the polarities of engulfment and withdrawal. After this discussion the family all concluded that they wanted to commit themselves to family therapy. But father added that Rachel would have to show progress in the next 3 months or the family would consider a less expensive treatment program.

These changes turned out to be more apparent than substantive. Rachel vacillated between periods of seeming involvement and motivation and periods of a more superficial compliance covering a painless world of delusions. One of these delusions involved the conviction that she would marry her old boyfriend (despite the fact that he had recently indicated, in response to a letter Rachel had sent him following a discussion in therapy, that he had no special interest in her). Another delusion involved the belief that she might indeed be the suicided poetess Sylvia Plath, and in yet another she ruminated about an elaborate scheme in which she had somehow bested and killed a famous male track star, so that his continued appearances were impostures.

Loxapine was raised to 175 mg. Rachel complained that the medication made it difficult for her to talk, but did not comply when I suggested she speak with the administrator about lowering the dosage. She dreamed that she was taking a lethal medication that was putting her to sleep; in this dream the nurses asked if she was certain she wanted to take it, and she insisted that she did. In another dream she was talking with me but I had a hangover. This related to her accurate perception that she was exhausting me. I remarked on her willingness to destroy her life and thought to myself, sadly, that others such as myself were expending much more effort in her behalf than she was. She, in turn, reluctantly shared with me more of the details of her delusional system and her confusion about its reality, and we were able to agree that the delusions were a passive way of feeling important. She agreed to struggle with them more, and we decided that a way to do this would be for her to share these beliefs with others. When Rachel encountered a young male patient who seemed genuinely interested in her she became terrified, and talked with me about how much easier it would be to be a shapeless amoeba, and be kicked around. She told this patient some of her delusions and was impressed that he seemed more upset that she should believe such things than she was. It made her realize how little she cared, and she shared with me some of her beliefs that nothing was the matter and that she had no need to worry. Meanwhile, her administrator finally agreed with my request that he lower the dose of her medication; a month after the conference and a month prior to Rachel's discharge loxapine was reduced to 50 mg and treatment with lithium commenced.*

---

*At the time of this treatment, about 15 years ago, many of the current antipsychotic drugs such as clozapine, were not available and psychiatrists were not as ready to prescribe lithium as they are today.

In the next series of family meetings the issue was how family members try to act for other family members who are perceived as having problems, rather than for themselves. Then they talked about a ski trip they had made the previous weekend. Father blandly reported how pleased he was with himself that he had pressured Rachel to ski "for therapeutic reasons," quite oblivious to the relationship between his remarks and our preceding discussion, and to the fact that her skiing had been a superficial act of compliance.

Rachel seemed preoccupied with the wish to go on more skiing trips with the family rather than remain "imprisoned" in the hospital. She parroted her father's definition of what would be best for her, regardless of her own acknowledged hatred of some of these things. After the meeting she began an eating binge and wanted only to sleep and daydream. She reported a dream in which she was lying in bed with her eyes closed, feigning sleep, while others came into her room, talked, and were active. During one therapy hour she lacked feeling but talked about what everyone else thought she should be doing, elaborated her own wishes to leave the hospital and therapy, and then voiced some of her delusional beliefs—that she might be Sylvia Plath and that she had dated a male sports celebrity; afterward, I found myself feeling exhausted, faint, and "spaced out."

In the face of Rachel's commitment to delusion, and the boundaryless, self-contradictory thinking she engaged in without apparent distress, I made what turned out to be my final interpretive efforts. Rachel talked about the insecurity of experiencing feelings and conflicts in relation to a male patient she had some interest in. She said her method of feeling secure was to believe that he had been sent to her by a friend in order to take care of her, and to construct a fantasy about their special relationship, rather than to think about her real feelings and the problems and uncertainties she and the other patient had in relating to each other. I talked with Rachel about security, real and illusory, and tried to explain to her how her system in fact left her about as vulnerable as a person could be. She said she wished she could do her life over again and be more related to others, and then went on, blandly, to tell me how she wished she were home where it was warm, for a vacation.

A family visit impended and Rachel decided to ask her family to take her home. She was sad and embarrassed to end her relationship with me, and she joked that perhaps I might move to her home state so that we could continue. She told me that she was not really ill, and that when she got home she would have friends and a job and would go to school. In our final family meetings it emerged that more secret negotiations had been occurring between Rachel and her father for some time. Father had decided to remove Rachel from the hospital for what he purported were financial reasons. When I suggested that he might instead request of the hospital a reduction in rate, he responded, quite oblivious to the significance of his remark, that he wouldn't think of doing so because he knew he was too wealthy to be eligible. With similar disregard for consistency he said that he had learned that Rachel's problem was an overdependence on her family. Mother made no objection even though Nina noted that several days earlier, when Rachel had claimed she was capable of leading a normal life and had pushed the family to take her home, mother had responded, "If you are so well, show us you can do it here first." Nina added that at that time she had predicted to mother that, by the time of the family meeting, mother would allow herself to be talked out of her opinion. In our last meeting, about 5 weeks after the commencement of lithium treatment, Rachel had trouble understanding that, while I would be interested to hear from her again, the door would not be unconditionally open for her to return to therapy. Even during our very last meeting she tried to discuss some of her thinking problems with me as though we were not saying goodbye. Finally she thanked me, gave me a hug, and left, feeling sad.

Over the next several years I had several letters from Rachel of a progressively more delusional nature. After a month and a half she wrote that she missed me and was having second thoughts about her decision, and had even talked with her parents about returning. They had said she should live with the decision she had made. She said that she had seen her old boyfriend but there was "nothing there." and that she often thought of how happy she had been a year ago, when she was seeing me and was out of the hospital. She concluded, "Basically I'm just working and going home to the TV. Mom and Dad are pleased with how I'm doing. I feel like I'm making decisions for myself, but you'd probably say I was passive and I guess you'd be right." Five months after leaving the hospital she wrote that she had quit her job because it was boring, and that she needed a "change of scenery." She was planning a vacation trip and added, "I miss you and feel you were really very dedicated to me." A year after her discharge Rachel wrote that she had been rehospitalized near home, and for the next several years during which I heard from her intermittently, she remained there. In these letters she told me that she missed me and that I represented the part of her that wanted to make attachments to others. She said, "I carry a part of you with me," and added that she wished she had never left and hoped she would see me again. The content of subsequent letters became increasingly disorganized and delusional, and she began to use me as a kind of postal delivery service for bizarre notes and messages written to a variety of people in the area, most of whom I had never heard of.

About a decade later, in the course of writing this book, I wrote to the family requesting a follow-up, and Rachel responded. Her writing was more coherent, but quite scrawled and messy, and there were peculiar references to such things as crushes on unavailable men. She told me that she had been hospitalized for a total of 10 years after terminating with me, and that she had been out of the hospital now for about 6 months and was taking antipsychotic medication. Her parents had divorced, and she lived with her father and held a menial job in a firm run by a relative. She seemed reasonably satisfied with this dependent, semidisabled state of affairs. Of her therapy with me she wrote the following:

I have thought about you often. At the time that we worked together I was just too sick to take advantage of ... the opportunity. ... Much of the immaturity and selfishness is gone ... you are one of the nicest doctors I have worked with. ... I think gratefully of your kindness and understanding when I was unaware of so much going on around me including my problems. ... I hope I have learned from your example how to treat people and maybe because of what was started in our relationship I have been able to polish some of my rough edges. I regret that at my sickest and worst I have been offensive at times and selfish ...

Chapter 21

Celia: Treatment of a Chronic Schizophrenic

History

Celia was 28 when she consulted me. She had recently been asked to leave graduate school in the midst of her first year, and at the time of our initial meetings she was hospitalized in a small private institution in a city near where I practice. She had obtained my name from a former therapist in a distant city, but a friend took responsibility for making the initial contact with me since Celia was too frightened and suspicious to call.

Celia was the second of four children and the oldest of two girls in a wealthy and status-conscious upper-class family that valued achievement, particularly in its male members, and devalued women, whose purpose it was to serve the men. The family treated any open manifestation of feelings, needs, problems, or dependency in family members as "weakness" or abnormality.

When I initially asked her to describe her mother and father, Celia responded that they "would seem perfect to anyone who has restrictive parents. They let you do anything you want." By this she meant that they just did not seem to care. What little time remained after his work, which was his consuming passion, father spent with his sons; he would take them on trips and leave his daughters behind. The only attention from him Celia could recall was in the form of reprimands about her schoolwork or spankings for infractions. He divorced Celia's mother and gained custody of the children while mother was in a mental hospital (Celia was about 10), and when Celia was 12 he remarried. When Celia was 14 he died after a brief illness.

Information about Celia's mother was obtained from Celia, from the hospital social worker, and from records of mother's 2-year mental hospitalization. In my brief telephone contacts with mother after Celia's hospitalization she was angry, demanding, and accusatory. The relatively brief marriage of Celia's parents was full of crises. Mother seemed unable to accept her assigned

372

role as subservient appurtenance to father's career, and seemed to lack maternal feelings as well. She repeatedly enacted scenarios in which it appeared that she was trying to get rid of her children. For example, she habitually failed to make enough food or to set enough places at the table for all of them. When her children were very young she took them sailing and threw them all into the ocean, reasoning that she was attempting to demonstrate that she could rescue them from drowning. When Celia was about 7 her mother became depressed and anorexic and took to bed. She had always been thin but at this time she became emaciated. After a brief hospitalization and what, in retrospect appeared to be two suicide attempts, mother entered a psychoanalytically oriented mental hospital for what turned out to be a 2-year stay that involved the permanent rupture of the nuclear family. Celia was 9 at the time. The children were told only that mother had arthritis. During this hospitalization Celia's father divorced her and gained custody of the children, but these matters, as well as mother's fate, were never explained to them directly. Psychological test results from mother's hospitalization are compatible with a very severe borderline personality organization, although that term was not in use at the time. According to hospital records she was an extremely difficult woman—passive, insatiably demanding, hostile and blaming. She managed to defeat the efforts of everyone to relate to her and to blame them for it. According to hospital records she manifested little or no concern over the welfare of her children during the prolonged separation from them.

Celia's early childhood appears to have been characterized by a combination of neglect and terror. Father was effectively absent from the family, and Celia's memories of mother were of a terrifying, bizarre individual who was prone to incomprehensible fits of rage or to strange ritualistic behaviors possibly governed by hallucinations and delusions. Celia learned to be as unobtrusive as possible, even to freeze and play dead, especially when she was in need, for if she called attention to herself, mother might attack her, certainly verbally and at times physically as well. In this way Celia felt that she was controlling mother and keeping her sane. For example, around age 8 Celia broke a milk bottle and cut herself; rather than call to her mother for help she shut her eyes, walked through the broken glass, then picked the pieces out of her bare feet and cleaned up the mess so no one would know.

Celia never had a favorite possession, such as a teddy bear. She was isolated from other children, and spent much time in the basement of their home with her brothers, often engaged in hazardous activities such as using adult tools in peculiar ways without supervision. In contrast to her paralytic docility with mother, she sometimes provoked one of her brothers, who had a hot temper, until he would attack her viciously. She stayed close to the basement furnace as though it were home, even though she got severe burns from touching it. In the winter she spent long periods of time in snow tunnels, where she felt "at home," oblivious of the cold.

Celia developed strange obsessional thoughts and ritualistic behaviors, many of which centered around the number 8, which must have been her approximate age when mother became clinically disturbed, and which she eventually informed me symbolized breasts and therefore a generic mother. In school she had just one friend; she was a good student but spent her time in ritualistic activities, such as shredding paper and stuffing it through the ink hole. At that time, she recalled the world looked strange to her. Her teachers were apparently concerned about her poor work habits, not her emotional disturbance, but neither of Celia's parents responded to their requests for conferences.

Mother was hospitalized without warning when Celia was 9 and never returned home. Celia was not told where mother had gone or whether she would return. She learned about both her mother's mental illness and her parents' divorce from school peers, who presumably had learned from their parents. Father simply acted like mother no longer existed; he hired a succession of caretakers for the children and paid little attention to what they did. Some were apparently disturbed and mean or neglectful to the children; none stayed for long, perhaps because the children, particularly the boys, were quite difficult. Celia was dressed and treated more or less like a boy. Her occasional visits to mother were a source of puzzlement and resentment, for she could not comprehend why mother was living in a pleasant environment with many recreational facilities rather than at home. Father remarried when Celia was 12, to a neighbor with whom he had been having a longstanding affair.

When Celia was 14 her father developed a rapidly fatal illness. He sent her siblings to stay in a foreign country with relatives and sent Celia to stay with a business associate whom she did not know. It was only when she saw the shocked and disturbed reaction of members of this family to the letter informing her that her father was dying that Celia grasped something serious was the matter. She was summoned home for father's funeral, and when she began to cry she was admonished not to. Her stepmother was awarded custody. The only positive element in the seemingly unmitigated horror of this family story, as we discovered well along in Celia's therapy, was her occasional contact with her paternal grandmother, a woman who seemed to genuinely care for her, however much she was also imbued with some of the basic family traits of denial and rejection.

Around this time Celia lost the last vestiges of trust or desire to relate to others. During the years between her mother's hospitalization and her father's death she began to hallucinate. She had always accepted her teachers' description of her as one who annoyed them by talking aloud to herself, but in the course of treatment she realized that she must have been hallucinating even then. After her father's death Celia began a pattern of running away from home to distant cities and slum areas, where she would blend in with a marginal, often criminal subculture and become involved with men who used her sexually, and often abused her physically, in exchange for food and a place to sleep. Her stepmother and extended family seemed relatively unconcerned. Finally, at age 15 Celia was arrested, apparently in a psychotic state, and placed in a youth detention center, where she was allowed to remain for a time until, despite the affluence of her extended family, she was committed to a public mental hospital that at that time specialized in psychotherapy. There she remained for more than half a year, the recipient of antipsychotic medication and unsuccessful efforts to engage her in psychotherapy. She was calmed by the routine and the limits and was not shocked by the presence of psychotic adults; evidently it was like a more controlled version of home to her. She blended into the destructive adolescent subculture so well that eventually she was expelled from the hospital because she was abusing drugs.

Celia then went to live with her mother, who had remarried and regained custody. Mother was still subject to hysterical and paranoid outbursts; for example, she became convinced that Celia was about to throw her from the window. Again Celia tried to be as selfless as possible and to soothe and tranquilize her mother. As a "reward" for her help with renovation of her mother's new house, mother and stepfather surprised Celia with an airplane ticket to a distant city where she knew no one and had no place to stay. In this unfamiliar place Celia once again allowed herself to be used and abused sexually and physically in exchange for food and a place to stay.

Despite these hardships Celia somehow managed to complete high school with some distinction—another manifestation of her extraordinary ability to blend into and appear a normal member of whatever relationship or subculture she was in. She went on to complete college over a period of years, punctuated by many leaves of absence and prolonged stays on a skid row in a city distant both from the university and from her home. The pattern was similar: Celia would apprentice herself in a kind of slave role to a sadistic, abusive man. At the surface level she would act and feel as if she had no will of her own, but at a deeper level she felt she was superior to and controlling of both the man and the experience of pain; in particular, she would take a kind of satisfaction, as though she were watching a movie, in being able to absorb near-lethal beatings without showing any upset. She maintained an active hallucinatory and delusional life filled with imaginary threats and terrors, and elaborate rituals for avoiding danger or expiating badness, in order to remain "safe" and to obtain permission to satisfy basic survival needs for food and rest. On a number of occasions she had a brief hospitalization, including treatment with antipsychotic medications; she was secretly contemptuous of her psychiatrists and convinced she was manipulating and controlling them.

Celia was accepted by a graduate school in a city near her home, and it was about half a year after enrolling that she became floridly psychotic again; she was hospitalized and sought me out, having been given my name by a former therapist in another city. She was on antipsychotic medication when she came to my office from the hospital for her first appointments, and while she denied any unusual behavior and expressed contempt for the acumen of her administrative psychiatrist, he informed me that she spent long periods of time huddled in corners, mute and in catatonic-like postures or making bizarre, stereotypic facial expressions.

When we first met, Celia was a rather nondescript overweight woman in sexually neutral, body-concealing attire. I was impressed by a vacant quality about her gaze; she had a whispery voice, flatness of affect, no eye contact, and vague speech. Although she claimed to be nervous, almost panicked, she was outwardly composed. When I inquired why she had come to see me, in a characteristically ambiguous and affectless manner Celia described "spacing out," that is, an inability to concentrate and to study. She claimed that she lacked a sense of self, though it was not until well along in her treatment that it became evident what she meant by that. As we talked she reported a sensation of the top of her head lifting off and said she was hearing voices instructing, admonishing, harassing, and frightening her. She claimed she knew these were not real voices, but as I got to know her better I realized that she did not believe they were a part of her and that their effect on her was more compelling than the voice of any real person. She said it was difficult to think clearly since thoughts would "short-circuit" in her head, making strange new connections so that she could neither understand the ideas of others nor express herself sequentially. While I concluded that she was probably schizophrenic, I was impressed by the vigor with which she seemed to fight for her life, however maladaptively, and I found about her a certain wry, feisty, likable quality.

We did not reach an immediate agreement about whether to work together, and over a period of 4 hours Celia told me something about her life, including, since her early teens, numerous prior unsatisfactory encounters with psychiatrists, each characterized by her contempt for them both because of what she perceived as their fear of her strangeness and the ease with which she felt able to deceive and manipulate them. What I found most impressive, even frightening, was her seemingly syntonic self-destructive attitudes and behaviors, that is, her predilection for placing herself in alien and dangerous situations and for abusing herself or unconcernedly acquiescing while others abused her, all of which were rationalized by a delusional and hallucinatory system. It appeared to me that she was trying to get herself killed, while disowning responsibility, and much later she confirmed that this had been so.

After four meetings Celia expressed a wish to work with me and I agreed. She was then discharged from the hospital, whereupon she promptly discontinued the antipsychotic medication she had been given. We met three times a week for a total of 49 hours in the approximately 5-month period prior to my 5-week summer vacation, and then for another 30 hours, for a total of 79 hours or approximately 8 months, until I found it necessary to hospitalize her. In order to explain some of the problems that arose in the course of her treatment it is important to reiterate that Celia sought my help for her sense of detachment and lack of identity, and that not only were her self-destructive attitudes and behaviors of no concern to her, but she was thoroughly convinced that she knew how to care for herself better than anyone else could.

At the outset I will note several repetitive features of Celia's behavior which need to be kept in mind as background by the reader, since they cannot be repeated with anything like the frequency with which they occurred. For example, on entering the office Celia would not look at me but would regularly glance out the windows. Whereas another patient might make a greeting, she would characteristically and inappropriately laugh or issue a burst of *sotto voce* cursing. Then she would sit near the door with her head averted, often with her coat on or her purse clutched to her lap, so that it appeared that she was always poised to leave. She could hardly wait for her therapy hours to end, and often bolted out the door a few minutes early. She manifested a general air of passivity and detachment, including flat affect, absence of eye contact, a fixed posture with rather rigid automatic movements, and little indication that she cared about anyone or anything other than her delusional ideas and hallucinatory voices. Speech was sparse in quantity almost to the point of muteness and vague in meaning. Although my impression was that Celia was unusually intelligent, and possessed a large vocabulary, she did not seem able or willing to think in depth, express herself with clarity, or share any details of her inner life. For some time I found her hours very boring. From her reports, outside our sessions her flight took physical as well as psychological form and included nocturnal roaming in response to delusional commands and impulsive, delusionally based trips to distant cities, which at times interrupted the early years of our work.

Celia perceived herself as a kind of actress or chameleon in the world, whose job was to give others what they wanted and to fool them into believing it was genuine. She perceived herself as stronger than others and above having feelings and needs of her own. In her previous and rather extensive contacts with psychiatrists she believed she had acted crazy because that was what was expected of her, although as time went on I wondered if it was really the act she claimed it to be. She prided herself on being able to survive on an emotional and physical starvation diet, without even adequate sleep.

Out of graduate school and the hospital Celia soon procured a menial night job that was much beneath her evident capabilities. She was frustrated because she felt I gave her little clue about what I might want from her, but most of her attention seemed directed to what "they," her voices, wanted, which was usually in opposition to relating to me at all. Underneath all this, and muffled by flatness and detachment, Celia gradually revealed a generalized hatred and mistrust of others, centering around her belief that they had no real interest in her but simply wished to use her for their own purposes. Ironically, she seemed to reserve her most bitter thoughts for those who claimed to care in one way or another, such as family or psychiatrists, and to experience less hatred toward those who were quite open about using her, such as the pimps on skid row; perhaps she saw that they, at least, were not hypocrites.

Celia was generally suspicious and at times floridly paranoid. She felt that people were out to kill her, that I had poison in the office, that bombs were planted in the walls, or that the building would fall down around her. She anticipated that I would throw her out the window or strangle her, and was relieved to hear a cough from the waiting room, for it meant there was a witness and I was unlikely to act. Helicopters and sirens outside meant that "they" were coming, perhaps through the window, to "get" her or to put her in a hospital, and she would begin to panic and want to flee from the room.

After a time there appeared transient indications of a wish to relate to me. At times, particularly when she made eye contact with me, Celia showed brief and tantalizing flashes of feeling, which she struggled internally over whether to express or suppress. The feelings consisted of a deep sadness, heralded by incipient tears, wishes to share some of her deep hurt, and a rage including wishes to "scream bloody murder" and to kill everyone. As these feelings and associated wishes surfaced, Celia cut off her thoughts, talked about "short circuits" in her head, and sometimes even bolted from the office before the hour had ended. The content of her hallucinations and delusions reflected the war over these wishes. "They," a Greek chorus of female voices that at times she could localize (and perhaps at times visualize), seemed to control her life, requiring that she deprive herself of food, sleep, and contact with me, or else she would be made to suffer terror and disorientation and would have to be punished and make restitution. Our sessions consisted of a curious triadic relation among Celia, myself, and "them." But only she could talk with "them" and "they" had ultimate authority. It soon became clear that "they" disliked, mistrusted, and ridiculed me.

I could not help but be appalled by Celia's self-destructiveness, and even though I did not really have her permission to take issue with her about it I attempted to point out to her the striking contradiction between how she deprived herself and constantly put herself in harm's way, usually at the behest of her hallucinated voices or delusional thinking, and her conviction that she was an expert at taking care of herself and surviving in a world of perceived hostility. But I felt helpless and frustrated, defeated by "them," unable to talk to "them," and without an ally in my endeavor.

Prior to the 12th therapy hour Celia felt depressed and frightened to see me, but once that hour began she claimed everything was fine and experienced herself in a kind of Olympian position from which she found everything "comical" and ridiculous. When I suggested that she might be trying to distance herself from depressive feelings she became frightened of me and imagined I was about to throw her out of a window. In the 14th hour she recounted her first dream: It involved a cylindrical eight-story building, open inside and resembling a great family dining room, with tables and chairs floating around. One false move and one could take a dangerous fall. Her sister was dining there, unaware of the danger, which only Celia could see. A clown began to entertain everyone but pushed her sister, who began to fall.

In subsequent hours Celia talked about her need–fear dilemma: mistrust of others so great that at one time she had made herself live all alone in a forest for 2 weeks, and a paranoid terror when she was alone of such intensity that she felt forced to approach people again. At times her psychosis was impressive: She mumbled gibberish about shapes and patterns, fearfully misconstrued noises from the street, and experienced hallucinatory retaliation from her Greek chorus of voices in the form of disruption of her concentration and threats of terrifying consequences, especially each time she confided more in me. Within a single hour she could shift fluidly from nascent tears and depression to a paranoid hallucinating position, glancing furtively about the office, and, for instance, becoming convinced that my telephone answering machine contained a bomb. "They" admonished her not to talk to me and to stop coming to see me. In our 21st hour Celia told me of a dream in which she could not reach her sister because of a gunman who accompanied her and was killing people; afterward she said she felt some connection to me, but then she perceived changes in my countenance and my eyes became so frightening that she feared I would try to kill her. Her "test" for whether she liked someone was whether she thought she could kill them with a gun; she acknowledged she would have much trouble shooting me. When she violated "their" rule that she was not to sleep more than 4 hours a night, "they" terrified her all the following night with the belief that she had jumped from an airplane and her parachute would not open.

As psychotic elements became more apparent, and there was increasing blocking of speech, I began to talk with Celia about taking medication. She had taken many antipsychotic medications in the past and had experienced little subjective benefit, so it was not at all clear to either of us that she would take anything I prescribed, much less that it would help. Nonetheless, Celia reluctantly agreed with my suggestion of medication, and after our 28th hour she began a 6 mg dose of trifluoperazine. I prescribed gradual increases to 30 mg by the 49th hour, just prior to my summer vacation.

Celia and I began to talk about the resemblance between her voices, with their admonitions not to sleep or eat and not to confide in others, including me, whom "they" perceived as dangerous, and attitudes and memories she ascribed to members of her family. Her awareness was heightened when she attended a family dinner mother had just prepared for sister's birthday, and she realized that mother, characteristically, had made insufficient food for all the guests.

After the 30th hour one of Celia's friends phoned to inform me that Celia had fled to a gambling establishment in a distant city, where, as Celia later informed me, she had flirted with dangerous involvements with undesirable people and had placed herself in situations that might have provoked assaults. Her stay was brief, and when she returned it was clear that, while in one sense she had been panicked while gone, suffering delusional terrors, in another sense she had felt more comfortable in a setting where no one knew or cared about her. She showed me a list of instructions she had written to herself while there, including the following: "Don't leave the room, even though you think it isn't safe; it is less safe in the middle of the night on the street; eat something tomorrow—only 2 cups of coffee; sleep, you will get more crazy if you don't." It turned out that one factor precipitating her departure had been her interpretation of some of my comments to mean that I did not care about her, and she acknowledged having been angry with me. She told me about how she had been a repeated runaway in adolescence, and about her belief, which seemed consistent with the facts as she reported them, that her family was never very concerned about her absences, and never made much effort to find her. The remainder of her explanation of her journey, which was based on her hallucinations, was incomprehensible to me. Some 10 hours later, after describing her often delusional and hallucinatory preoccupation with incipient disasters, and then telling me of her fear that I might die, she said that if I were to die it would be a relief, for she could then go to a gambling establishment, lose all her savings, purchase a gun, and kill herself.

I could often tell when Celia was hallucinating because her lips would move. "They" were sitting on the couch, she informed me (it was not clear if she could see them), and it became apparent that she made Faustian bargains with "them" in which certain things were allowed her in return for self-punishments. Things that might be need-gratifying were interpreted to her by "them" as hostile and dangerous, and because "they" gave her such information, and even threatened her if she were to pursue such things, "they" were experienced as helpful and caring—even, in a way, as parental. Celia told me that if she tried to defy hallucinatory injunctions, "they" would punish her by confusing and terrifying her. For example, they might convince her that she was driving the wrong way on a one way street (when in fact she was not) and that she was about to be smashed by an oncoming car. "They" regularly arranged punishments for her after any occasion in which she might have been more open and communicative with me. The bargain that became particularly important in the ensuing months of our relationship, to which we both often referred, had to do with a building under construction that she could see from the window of my office. Once it was completed, she said, "they" would no longer allow her to continue to see me! Her description of "them" and their role in her life led to her telling me more about how she had been abused at times by her brothers, and how she had been beaten up and raped in various skid row communities in which she had lived. But she continued to stoutly maintain that she had no difficulty taking care of herself.

During our 33rd hour Celia told me I was "shaking [her] contraption," that is, challenging her belief that she needed and could trust no one; she said that she wanted to share some sad feelings with me, but she was convinced I would die. "They" kept telling her that I was dangerous to her and might kill her or poison her and that I was a "fool" and a "joker." We were both taking a risk, for I became increasingly concerned about the harm she was capable of doing to herself.

By the 43rd hour Celia was, I assumed, taking 25 mg of trifluoperazine, but there seemed to be little change except that "they" were letting her sleep somewhat longer than her customary 4 hours. About a week before my summer vacation Celia began to express the conviction that I would not return and our relationship was coming to an end. I felt somewhat alarmed, since I interpreted her certainty to be a veiled statement of her own intention not to return in the fall. I therefore suggested that she at least return in the fall to check out the accuracy of her belief, and she agreed. Occasionally she admitted she would miss me, and was near to tears, only to suppress them and talk about the rain clouds outside the window. She admitted being angry and wanting to kill me, because I had gotten her to like me and to rely on our appointments. She had the wish to poison an elaborate cake she had agreed to make for a family wedding. I gave her a number where I could be reached during the interruption, even though she did not ask for it. After 4½ months (49 therapy hours) we interrupted our work for 5 weeks.

Celia did return on the date we were scheduled to resume our sessions, and we were each surprised and I think visibly pleased to see one another. Celia had stopped taking trifluoperazine after I left because of her conviction that our relationship was over; since it was not clear to me that she had benefited from taking it, I did not prescribe it again. In her customary flat tone she expressed wishes to shoot and kill everyone in the world with a machine gun; at the end of the hour she told me that she had not decided whether she was going to "have anything to do with feelings and people or go completely crazy."

In ensuing hours Celia was clearly engaged in an inner struggle over whether to talk to me; sometimes she acknowledged that her voices were cutting into our conversation. Much of the time she claimed she had nothing to say and wished to leave, but felt obligated to talk in order to please me. I said that she did not need to talk unless she wished to, that I would read the newspaper and she could let me know if she wished to converse. When I started to read, however, she became agitated and tried to leave the office. I urged her to stay long enough to tell me why, and she burst into tears and informed me that she was very "pissed off" at me, that my behavior (reading the paper) made me just like everyone else in her life, and that she felt lost and alone.

In our 55th hour, about 2 weeks after we had resumed meeting, Celia dropped a bombshell: She very convincingly confided that the symptoms of psychosis she had been regaling me with were all part of an elaborate act she had learned during her initial psychiatric hospitalization at age 15 and that, in fact, she had never really hallucinated. She talked of her ability to give people what they want, and described how in the past she had played the roles of a heroin addict in withdrawal, a tough street person, a good girl, and a scholar. She revealed her contempt for all "shrinks" because we were so readily fooled and manipulated. She seemed sincere, and in fact she acted more integrated as we talked. She said her real problems were absence of a stable sense of identity and feelings of superiority or inferiority to others. She said it was a relief to tell me this though she feared I would be angry with her for deceiving me. After a few sessions in which she was able to talk more directly about her struggle against feelings and dependency and there was no sign that she was hallucinating, I felt both pleased and fundamentally unsettled, as though the rug had been pulled out from under me. I wondered how I could have been so gullible and thought that perhaps I could not trust my own perceptions and reality sense. I actually consulted informally with two colleagues in an effort to make some sense of what was happening.

This seemingly healthier state was short-lived; soon Celia once again became much more detached, silent, and affectively dead, spoke in a monotone or not at all, and did not look at me. I felt drowsy in response, and comprehended that I was struggling with her ambivalence; that is, when she noted "her" detachment in me she felt hurt and angry and wanted me to be more involved; when I was attentive she withdrew.

After the 71st hour Celia began to appear more obviously psychotic. She had seen her mother and realized that she was jealous of the attentions mother gave to her dog, but added that her mother was planning to have the dog put to sleep. Her mother had also casually inquired whether Celia had stopped her therapy yet, thus expressing her assumption that, as in the past, Celia would find it valueless. Although her speech was halting and affectively deadened, Celia reported that her thoughts were racing. She said that when she attempted to communicate it served to destroy her thoughts but that she did not need to communicate with me for I knew her thoughts without her telling me. She fantasized kidnapping a famous female chef and forcing her to cook lunch, and went so far as to call the woman but hung up when she answered.

Celia's face began to acquire a hunted look. The room had a sinister appearance to her, and she wondered if the wiring was connected to explosives, if I had a gun in my drawer, and if I was about to strangle her. Between therapy hours she went to a bar, got drunk, and invited seduction and attack from the owners, although she managed to escape unharmed. In the following hour paranoid suspicions that I was going to hurt her alternated with sadness and a longing to tell me about her suffering. She described in a detached manner, as though watching a movie, some of the instances in which she had gotten herself attacked and nearly killed. After the hour she became more paranoid and wandered the streets for much of the night.

In our 78th hour, after 8 months of therapy, Celia wished she could communicate with me better, and then became frightened that LSD would enter her mouth while she was smoking. In the 79th hour she became very agitated and suspicious and lost contact with me almost totally. She clutched her coat, mumbled to herself, occasionally expressing bizarre fragments of ideas, (for example, that people and thoughts were perpendicular) and darted furtive glances around the room. Her facial expressions changed frequently and strikingly, without reference to external events. Gradually I gleaned that she thought people were trying to kill her, and that she would have to flee to a distant city. She finally became convinced that "they" were about to come in through the window for her, became acutely panicked, and paced the room, preparing to flee or fight. I took control, called two of her friends, and arranged for her admission to the hospital, where she remained for the next 1½ years.

Celia immediately barricaded herself in her hospital room. For the first several days of her stay she required seclusion, and at times restraints as well because of her paranoid terror that people were trying to kill her and the assaults her belief led her to make on staff when they approached her. In her meetings with me she showed both more feeling and more evidence of her visual and auditory hallucinations. She said she was having waking dreams and saw acrobats performing on the walls.

Our 86th hour was spent together in the seclusion room. Celia was confused and suspicious, uncertain who I was, disbelieving that her mother had tried to visit her, and preoccupied with her hallucinations. Toward the end of the hour she began to talk with me about how abandoned and uncared about she felt. Our discussion led us to wonder whether her hospitalization was an effort to convey a message about her needs to me and to her family, and that she was in the midst of a struggle between being more aware of her feelings and being unfeeling and superior to it all. This vague acknowledgment of need was followed in the 89th hour by the belief that someone was going to strangle her, which was accompanied by strange bodily feelings, including deadness and levitation.

Celia told me of a recent telephone conversation in which she had tried to tell mother how disturbed she was; mother had responded that it was nonsense, that she herself had experienced all the symptoms Celia reported and that they were of no consequence. Mother had suggested that Celia go to another hospital and had then ended the conversation by telling Celia she loved her and wanted to help. Celia had not let mother know she was upset by her comments, for doing so would have proved she was not psychotic and didn't need help! Mother had expressed her opinion that Celia had always been manipulative, and had threatened to hang up the phone if Celia implied she was in any way to blame for all this. Celia had the urge to slash her wrists. Some of my natural tendency to doubt the veracity of Celia's account was tempered by the social worker's account of a session with mother in which mother had virtually succeeded in convincing her that Celia was only pretending to be ill.

It was a relief to Celia when she learned that it was the consensus of the initial staff conference about her that she was quite disturbed and in need of help. I suggested, and she consented, that we increase the frequency of our meetings to four per week. Some tearful feelings of insecurity and longings to confide alternated with deadness, distancing, isolation, and increasing paranoia. She felt that the office was being sealed shut and that we were about to be dumped into the ocean, where we would drown. I wondered if she was threatened by the prospect of being involved with and dependent on me, but she seemed to have forgotten that she had ever acknowledged any needs in the first place.

Celia continued to be very disturbed and to spend much of her time in seclusion. She told me she had pleaded with the staff to move her out of the quiet room because screaming patients in adjoining quiet rooms had been terrorizing her, but staff had confused her emotional pleas with psychotic loss of control. I offered to intercede and help her with the room issue, but she spurned the offer. I said that I felt she was trying to be more genuine about her needs and that I would intervene anyway. Celia was moved to another room, and she subsequently admitted that she had had a good night's sleep. She then talked to me about "getting it on the sly"; as a child she would feign sleep when in the car with father at night so that he would pick her up and carry her, for she believed he would refuse to do so if she asked him directly. As an adult she would drive off in her car in the middle of the night and follow big trucks, often for hundreds of miles, so as not to feel lonely!

Celia expressed anger at the social worker, who questioned the accuracy of her perceptions of her family. She feared that if she gave up trying to take care of others, mother would go crazy and that if mother was nice to her, she, Celia, might have to feel good. As a meeting with mother and the social worker impended, Celia became frightened, convinced that the social worker was her stepmother and that I was someone else. Afterward she had little to say about the meeting but she complained about people who invalidate her perceptions and deny her needs. At the end of the 111th hour, in a transient moment of contact, she remarked that she was "getting a few crumbs."

Over the weekend she wrote me a remarkable letter, the first of many in which she seemed much better put together than she appeared to be during our meetings. In it she said:

"I rarely think I am alive, and if I think about it, like I am thinking about it right now, I get so sad because it has been pretty lousy and I get really angry. . . . When I sit in the room with you and I let myself believe you are there I feel so safe I just want to sit there forever. But I can't, and I can't seem to be able to believe it for very long afterwards. . . . I had no idea what I was getting into [by entering therapy] and I'm scared and I do hate you, but I also wish I could be with you every minute."

Over the ensuing weekend Celia attempted to escape from the ward in near zero temperature, without a coat. In the following hour (the 115th) she began to talk about how she took care of others in order to survive, and she wondered if there was another system, and what it might be based on. I suggested that it was learning to take care of herself, and that it was based on knowing more about her needs. In response she became more aware of her passive magical longings: I was supposed to see through her and take care of her so that she would not have to think about what her needs might be. She said she wanted to be "carried" by me so that she would not have to assert herself. Nonetheless, she began to experiment on the ward by asking for things, although it stirred her anger to have to do so. When we could not find a room on the ward in which to have therapy, she saw me question the staff about reserving a room in advance, and felt taken care of, but after telling me this she began to hallucinate more.

In the 118th hour I announced my vacation. Although Celia tried to minimize its importance to her, she told me, angrily, "You have screwed up my system," by which she meant her self-sufficient form of adaptation. As she began to show more anger and depression to ward staff she elicited a mixture of gratifying responses and alarm. I realized that most ward staff had bought into her "everything is fine" facade and had interpreted her show of feelings as an indication that she was getting sicker.

A similar problem became apparent with regard to her brother when, in the 119th hour, she showed me another of her precocious letters, this in response to his expressed concern that she was becoming "institutionalized." Celia was angry at being perceived as being much "better" than she believed she was:

"I am furious that would even come up, I am in no way, shape or form institutionalized, the thought is rather ironic. But my fury at you isn't really justified as I haven't told you what the hell I'm doing in here . . . I am not dependent on [the hospital], in fact I have trouble even asking the staff for a towel or for change. . . . I have been operating under the delusion that I am very competent in taking care of myself. And I have been very concerned with maintaining this illusion and persuading everyone as well as me that this is the case, but it is not. Hanging out on skid row, getting beat up, putting myself in very dangerous situations wandering around the streets of [a big city] at 2 or 3 A.M. totally paranoid, in my apartment all day in what Robbins calls psychotic terror, alone and pretty nuts. . . . My ability to come off 'rational,' function in jobs, school, talk to people, etc., is an integral part of the craziness. When I sit in a room with another person I focus on them entirely, try to figure them out and organize my own self around information I can pick up. It could be described as human Saran wrap, weak ego boundaries. . . . I get the majority of my definition from outside. The process avoids feelings. . . . The day I arrived I thought the staff was going to kill me. I ended up in 4 points, restraints, flat on a mattress with my arms and legs strapped down. . . . I am struggling for my life here, because I have gotten crazier as the years go by. I am fighting myself, the part that hates the whole goddamn world and doesn't want anything to do with anyone, that part is supported by Ma saying shit to me like 'I hate Dr. Robbins,' or when I hear that you think I'm becoming institutionalized. I react by saying to myself to get the hell out of [the hospital], stop seeing Robbins, avoid dependence at all costs. . . . Part of [the treatment] is being dependent on Robbins, forming a real human relationship with him, telling him I hate him for exposing me to all the rage, sadness, feelings; that I like him. . . . I have to practice asking for things, saying no to people. . . . I need a safe place to take risks. . . . It feels good to tell people how I feel. It also gets me absolutely terrified. What puts me into seclusion is when I get so far away from people, paranoid, isolated. But you see I always have thought it was the other way around. . . . One last thing. It might appear that I have worked everything out. But I can intellectualize til the cows come home."

I could not have described it better, but I was left with my own confusion, to which I was becoming more accustomed, about whether this eloquent letter was a manifestation of insight or of denial.

Celia alternated between being more involved and being "a million miles away" as a separation of a week and a half approached. In hour 128 I suggested that she was trying to leave before I did, and she responded to this with increasing body awareness of her "feet on the floor and [her] butt on the chair."

In the next hour her voice and manner were softer and she said, sadly, that she felt less tough, but that night she escaped from the hospital into a cold, rainy night. At our final meeting before my absence I pointed out that she was creating a world of rejection, misery, and abuse and proving she could control it by not acknowledging how much it disturbed her. She then tried to end our final hour before I could do so.

On my return Celia continued to oscillate between attachment feelings and distancing maneuvers accompanied by more florid psychosis; moreover, it was apparent to me that at times she was trying to deceive me into believing that she was not hallucinating. When I took this up with her there were brief tears and angry memories of how her father had always overlooked her obvious problems, even when the school tried to alert him, and of how he had sent her to a foreign country where she knew no one and did not speak the language when he was dying. After a brief attempt to leave the hospital against advice Celia admitted apprehension about an impending conference to review her treatment; she worried that she would be let go. In our 135th hour, after some of her concerns had been clarified, she remarked to me sheepishly, "I'm addicted to you; a Robbins addict." On the cold and wintry day of her 139th hour, shortly after telling me of her wish that I would "surround" her, Celia remarked, without awareness of any connection, about her powerful wish to go out into the woods and lie in the snow, where she was virtually convinced it would feel warm and secure.

Year Two

The second year of treatment commenced. We had to meet in a basement office for the 141st hour, and Celia recalled how she had spent much of her childhood in the basement of her home, snuggling next to the furnace for warmth and using dangerous power tools without supervision. In her adult life she maintained a belief (with some truth to it) that she was an expert in a variety of building and repair trades; however, her belief transcended her actual knowledge and on more than one occasion she had come close to electrocuting herself. After telling me this she remarked that she had informed the supervisor in the hospital shop, where she had used some power tools, that she was frightened and that she had been stunned when he responded that he was glad to hear it, that if she weren't afraid he wouldn't want her to use the tools. A distasteful sexual encounter during a weekend pass led to a discussion of how much effort she spent in her life attempting active mastery of childhood trauma by recreating experiences of hurt and abandonment and proving to herself by emotional deadening and grandiosity that they did not bother her. As we discussed these things some of her hurt and rage at her mother surfaced.

For the first time since her hospitalization Celia attempted to leave the hospital and return to my private office for her appointments. At first she felt both excitement and shock as she recalled how she had believed that my telephone answering machine was a bomb, but soon she became more silent and detached, and I noted that her lips were moving and her eyes were darting about the room. In the course of the eight appointments she had in my office her functioning deteriorated. Finally in hour 153 it seemed as though she were angrily withholding in response to feelings of being deprived. She felt "drugged" and I felt sleepy. When I inquired more actively about her state of mind, she said that her hallucinations had stopped but that she was experiencing murderous feelings and fantasies about everyone, including ideas of cleaving my skull with an axe. She felt better having told me this, but in our next hour she was vague and muddled until, in response to my active questioning she talked of her wish for a womblike world where she could believe everything and its opposite and it would not matter because I would take care of everything. I decided it would be better if we resumed meeting at the hospital.

Back on the ward for our 157th hour Celia was nearly catatonic in posture, silent, and affectively frozen, but she was able to acknowledge, in response to my questions, racing thoughts and active hallucinations, which derogated her sense of reality and attacked her relationship with me. Gradually, we reestablished some contact and Celia told me how leaving her "home" at the hospital to come to my office in the city had required her to deny her feelings of sadness, anger, and terror and to act normal, lest I think her out of control and psychotic. She remembered the years after mother had left, when father was totally absorbed in his work and an affair and had no time for the children, when she lost her only friend and there was a succession of caretakers, several of them abusive, and no one even told her what was happening so that she could use her mind constructively to comprehend matters. She conveyed to me rather poignantly the pathetic, hopeless quality of a resourceless child who had no choice but to turn against feelings and attachments in order to survive.

During our 163rd hour Celia gave me a picture she had made (Figure 5). She told me it was a self-portrait. There is a large empty space in the middle, surrounded by busy, angular webs and plots. She then proceeded, it seemed, to enact what she had drawn: She was withdrawn and obfuscated meaning for the remainder of the hour, all the while claiming she wanted to make contact before our weekend separation. Later she said she was "all wired up" over some impending family visits. When I saw her staring at some electrical wiring on the wall and questioned her about this, she admitted she was becoming paranoid and then recounted a nightmare of being crazy in a place that resembled both a dungeon torture-chamber and a mental hospital. She began to recall her first hospitalization at age 15 and mother's disparagement of psychiatry and of the hospital (when Celia would run away from the hospital, mother would act proud of her "accomplishment"). After telling me this, Celia abruptly denied there was anything the matter with her and ridiculed the possibility that she might have become attached to a departing member of the hospital staff who had spent much time working with her.

By hour 172 Celia was paranoid and hallucinated prohibitions and

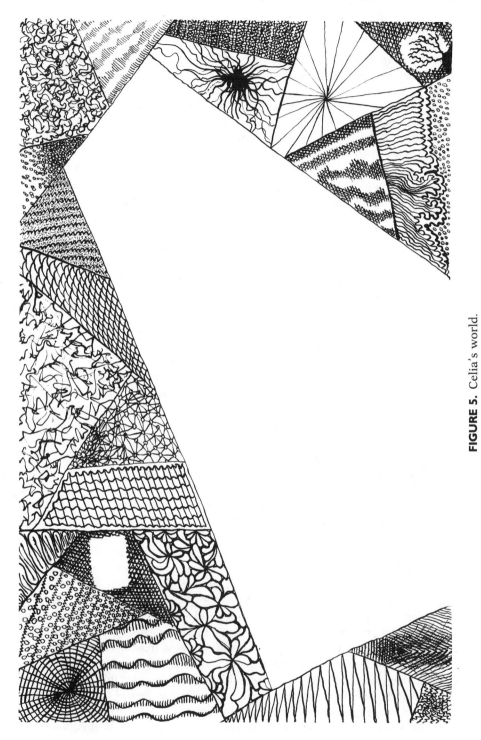

FIGURE 5. Celia's world.

threats; however, unlike her reaction in the past, she was now able to volunteer that these phenomena were occurring. More florid psychosis continued for the next 10 to 15 sessions over several weeks. Awareness of her needs for me and the hospital alternated with her customary withdrawal and with voices telling her that she must not trust me or talk with me, that I was going to kill her.

During this time Celia told me more details about her sexual experiences, about how she would attach herself to men who were abusive and had poor impulse control, and how she would be utterly compliant while they enacted their at times violent scenarios on her body. She viewed these abusive men as actually or potentially crazy and out of control, and saw herself as supplying the missing control. Her task was to endure and to show that she was invulnerable. In so doing she had the grandiose feeling that she was controlling the situation and tranquilizing the man. Celia felt no pleasure from the sex—in fact, she made it a point to have nothing to do with anyone who "threatened" to give her any pleasure.

In our 179th hour Celia was more aware that her delusions and hallucinations were reflections of her own fear and hatred. She said that it made her feel more confused and crazy to realize this, that it was much more normal and comfortable for her to experience herself as being on the ceiling (the analytical self, as revealed in the letter to her brother) observing the war between herself and "them." It made her hate and fear me to be so shaken up in her way of thinking, and she wondered if I was driving her crazy. In our 181st hour she was convinced that I had yelled at her the previous day. But she also realized that I was providing her with a kind of care and attention she had never experienced before. For the next 5 or so hours she alternated between a florid paranoid psychosis and suicidal depression. My impending vacation enhanced her distress. She was particularly frightened of the violence of some of her wishes about me. She received high doses of chlorpromazine and trifluoperazine, and much of the time was in restraints or seclusion; she was even temporarily boarded on another ward, one designed for the most disturbed high-risk patients.

After one episode of seclusion Celia was convinced the staff had gone berserk and had attacked her. Because she was totally unable to tell me what part she had had in all this, I suggested, and Celia agreed, that a staff nurse come into our session as a source of information. Celia was confused when told that her disturbed behavior could evoke powerful responses from others. This was so different from the "normal" neglect of her family that it seemed to her that the staff must be crazy. By our 184th and 185th hours Celia was more aware of and disturbed by her confusion and her fluctuations in orientation and memory. She wondered if some of the illusions or perceptual distortions and hallucinations she had been having, including floating furniture and faces, were experiences she had been having regularly in her life but had not acknowledged, and she thought that the vision of things floating represented her disorientation and the sense that everything was "up in the air." She was struck by the enormity of her family's denial—of mother's illness and treatment, of father's illness and dying, of a serious and chronic medical condition of her sister, and, of course, of all that was going on with her. She felt rage at her family for their failure to appreciate her needs, and she began to raise objections when mother and brother seemed to ridicule and devalue psychiatrists and mental hospitals and brought pressure to bear on her to leave the hospital. At the same time her hallucinated voices admonished her not to talk to me, and when I pointed out that they represented her own thoughts she expressed rage at "this place" and at me for not leaving her alone and for making her face reality.

After our 188th hour there was a hospital conference reviewing her treatment. The staff response to Celia was remarkably polarized; many of the staff, led by the nurse in charge, expressed their disbelief that she was very ill and their doubt that hospitalization was necessary and psychotherapy was of any benefit. I remarked that Celia had a dissociated, contradictory set of responses to almost everything of importance; that, while she might appear to staff to be sicker than before, this was due at least in part to inroads in her own denial and covering over; and that her ability to convince herself and others that she was normal was perhaps the most malignant aspect of her illness. The consultants recommended prolonged hospitalization and continuation of intensive treatment.

In our 192nd hour Celia told me that she was very sad ("When I think about it," she said) about just how much of her life had been spent in a state of terror and isolation, living on the fringes of the civilized world, being used and abused, and trying to drown out and otherwise avoid knowledge of her thoughts and feelings. She realized that she had hitherto lacked a sense of herself as an entity traversing a lifespan marked by the calendar and by her accomplishments, both because there had been so few emotionally satisfying events and relationships to measure by and because her anger led her to obliterate memory. She remarked that she was beginning to note the passage of time in relation to the rhythm of our appointments. Celia said she was sad about our impending brief vacation separation. In subsequent appointments she was detached, flat, and distant, with inappropriate laughter. Just prior to our separation I preceded her to the office where we were to meet, a sequence we had long ago agreed upon to avoid the paranoia she experienced when I followed her, but when I got there she was not behind me. I found her sitting back on the ward, convinced that I had gone elsewhere. When she looked at me she felt good, but gradually my face acquired a malevolent cast and she felt frightened of being attacked and killed. She realized that this had to do with terror, sadness, and rage about our forthcoming separation. She was particularly terrified because she saw me as her only source of reality. As we talked, the striking similarity between those attitudes of her mother that enraged her and her own denial, confusion, hallucinations and ridiculing laughter was apparent to both of us. She recalled that mother and stepfather had removed her very sick sister from a hospital when she was young because they claimed that she was too upset to be hospitalized. Celia struggled with the part of herself which wanted to leave the hospital before I left for my vacation and to run away from her distress. After observing the similarity of her attitude to that of her family, I pointed out that she was viewing our separation once again as a final ending, rather than seeing her caring feelings as signifying the beginning of a meaningful relationship.

When I returned tears came to Celia's eyes but she quickly laughed and avoided the subject. In the hours that followed (the 198th and 199th) she showed a more emotional commitment to our relationship, along with fears that having a needy and demanding self would inevitably cause it to end. Now her central concern seemed to be my forthcoming summer vacation, and an impending visit from the relative who was helping manage the trust funds that were paying for her hospitalization. Celia was now more able to acknowledge that her hallucinations represented her hatred, associated with memories of father's repeated rejections of her, which culminated in his sending her abroad as he was dying, and her wishes to be strong and harden herself so she would need no one. She lamented the loss of what she considered to be a strength, namely her "ability" not to care, and admitted that she intermittently felt contempt for me and viewed me as weak because I continued to care and did not give up on her. She admitted having feelings of caring about me; when I asked her where they were, she pointed mutely to her heart.

The visit of her trustee-relative went better than Celia had anticipated, and she was able to acknowledge that the hospital was her home for now, and to make positive plans for the coming months, during which she would begin to admit to having needs and would for the first time show awareness of a sense of time and future. These plans included the idea of bridging our separation with a series of letters to me, which she would show me on my return. In the last hours before my vacation Celia acted detached, but she was able to tell me how angry and tearful she had been in a ward meeting in which she had taken issue with a group of adolescent patients who were negative about the hospital and who devalued staff. In our final meeting she alternated between aloof disengagement, in enactment of an acknowledged wish to kill me and destroy our relationship, and fears that I might die.

The following are sequential quotes from Celia's diary notations during our 5-week separation. At first she sustained images of me:

"I miss you. . . . I think of sitting in those crummy little offices, and I think about you when you get bored and close your eyes, and I get hysterical inside that you are going to leave and tell me to go to hell if I can't do more to keep you at least awake. And when I think about it I get really sad, and I want to scream and yell at everyone, and then I feel like a stupid fool for getting so upset about you going on vacation, like what the hell is the big deal."

Celia felt fearful when she walked through the wooded path from the hospital toward town:

"I would never have been scared like that before. When I get paranoid I am not really scared of something happening to me, it is just a vague, intense fear of some cataclysmic end of me, death. This is different."

Then I seemed to her to be gone:

"Here comes the depression like a ten ton truck with no breaks. I just want to be dead . . . I want to blow my brains out, die, implode . . . You're dead, gone . . . why the hell were you so important to begin with, because I don't give a damn now . . . I want to . . . take off for [the foreign country where she was sent in adolescence] . . . I hated it, so why do I want to go back? I want to get drunk, stoned, wasted . . . if I did I know I would kill myself, quick. . . . And what is frightening is that I'm not frightened about it at all . . . the thought is reassuring."

On a pass out of the hospital Celia went so far as to buy a plane ticket to a distant city, but after a prolonged internal debate, and a conviction that the plane would crash, she returned to the hospital. After another week and a half Celia missed me again:

"You don't put up with a lot of bullshit . . . I guess I like being taken seriously, and I like you, I like being with you. You are really reliable, and I do trust you. I know you are coming back. I don't really understand why you put up with me, but I am really glad you do. I miss you. It makes me cry."

About halfway through the separation Celia involved herself with a male patient with a history of dangerous, violent behavior, and with a combination of rage and insight she imagined returning to old familiar activities:

"I am really lost. GONZO. I am a million miles away and I don't know where that is. I have all these fantasies (this is rare to begin with) about taking off with him, staying stoned, drunk, getting pimped out, beat up."

She concluded with rage and sadness at her parents:

"I want to cry and scream and hit people and I am so angry. You know, I am really smart, I am really creative, imaginative, I could have done a hell of a lot with myself, and here I am coming up on 30 and I am sitting in a nuthouse kissing a fucking psychopath."

Then she wrote that she still had things under control, but that it was difficult for her. It made her angry that she was struggling to do better, and she wished she could get drunk and escape self-care responsibilities:

"I am so angry at you . . . I want to scream, I want to tear the room apart, I can't handle anything anymore. I wish I was dead."

As the time for our reunion approached, she began to talk about what she had gotten out of the hospital, namely, safety, structure, support, and a sense of the future—"something [she] never thought about before" and associated with missing me. But because of her murderous rage Celia feared seeing me again.

Over the weekend preceding my return from my summer vacation Celia became floridly psychotic, and that fall she was intermittently destructive, enacting delusional or hallucinated scenarios and requiring restraint. In our 210th hour, after expressing gladness to see me, Celia said in detached tones that she was enraged that I had left her but that it had not been safe for her to leave me until I had returned. When I came to the ward for our 211th hour she huddled in a corner, preoccupied; she laughed or giggled at everything and reported racing thoughts and hallucinations of voices whose content I interpreted as hostile. Associations suggested she both felt unsafe and was being maliciously destructive. My feeling was that she was trying not only to let me know how difficult it had been for her when I was gone but to make me feel responsible, and when I suggested this, her laughter confirmed it. Her voices told her not to look at me lest she be tempted to feel good. As she put it (in the 216th hour), her rage was "bouncing all around," sometimes manifested as a fear of being attacked or assaulted, and sometimes as a hostile hallucination. In our 220th hour I noted to myself that Celia was making me feel some of the hopelessness she felt about reaching and being related to another, a feeling she did not want to deal with.

Celia's administrative psychiatrist expressed doubt to her and to me that psychotherapy was helping her, and wondered if perhaps her treatment program should be changed. He informed me that he was experiencing pressure from his staff to justify the continuation of Celia's psychotherapy with me, and he increased her dose of chlorpromazine. Celia was shaken, and she surmised that somehow she was setting others up to enact her hatred and her belief that I was driving her crazy; the part of herself she now associated with family attitudes and with her hallucinations. Now she complained that staff did not understand her. I empathized with her feeling like a little child with no dependable adults to meet her needs, but pointed out that she was giving contradictory messages and could not expect to get her needs met until she could be clearer within herself and more consistent with others about what they were. She guessed what bothered her most was seeing more clearly when people cared about her. It seemed strange and it confused and angered her.

Celia hallucinated voices calling her by a childhood pet name and voiced fears of imminent earthquakes and airplane crashes. She made a half-hearted effort to escape from the hospital, and subsequently was found banging her head against the wall. Staff returned her to the quiet room, where she giggled and hallucinated. I commented on her efforts to avoid thinking and facing her feelings of caring, sadness, and rage and remarked on how "dumb" she was about taking care of herself.

Celia seemed to assimilate what I said, for she began to talk about feelings, and signs of psychosis diminished. Again I suggested to her that the feelings she was encouraging staff to enact represented an uncaring part of herself and her family. One of her brothers offered to bring in some beer when he came to visit; mother sent a banal postcard that seemed to imply that she and Celia were vacationing from one another, and then wanted to bring her dog (which Celia had never met) when she came to visit. Celia remarked that her family equated facing and talking about real problems as being sadistic, uncaring, and trying to drive the other crazy, whereas denying problems was believed to be caring and considerate. Celia was furious with me for forgetting the time of her (233rd) therapy hour and coming late, but it turned out that she had confused the time as part of her dread over an impending visit from her mother. She subsequently told me that she had tried to talk to mother about some of her feelings of having been neglected, and in response mother became enraged, called Celia a bitch, threw an ashtray against the wall, and resisted efforts of staff to calm her. Not long thereafter, mother suggested that she and Celia might spend some time together looking at flowers. I wondered about the veracity of Celia's strange story, but it was subsequently confirmed in all respects by a staff member who had been present. This commenced a series of visits between Celia and mother, most of which occurred in the presence of the social worker.

To Celia, a trip away from the hospital in a van with a number of other patients she referred to as "crazy" and a single ineffectual staff member seemed like a metaphor for her childhood. We talked of her terror of "crazy" people and her characteristic placatory behavior around the other patients, which simulated maturity and insight and was part of the reason staff tended not to consider her ill. She recalled a time when her mother had been convinced Celia wanted to throw her out of the window and another time in childhood when mother, in a rage, had literally thrown the children around the room. Celia vacillated in her ability to identify "craziness" in herself and others. After subsequent visits with mother she fully expected the social worker to conclude that mother was normal, but it turned out that the social worker was impressed by mother's caged pacing around the room during their interview and her threats to leave, behaviors Celia found unremarkable.

Celia had a resurgence of hallucinations, which she could acknowledge was her way of trying to believe I was driving her crazy. In response to my observation of her inappropriate laughter (during the 239th hour), she claimed she was dead, then got angry at me for "getting on [her] case," and finally began to hallucinate commands that she should leave. She experienced herself in parts, sitting in several different areas of the room, one part running from me, another feeling attached to me and sitting near me as protection against mother. She found this fragmented location of herself very disturbing.

In subsequent hours (the 246th to the 248th) I began to take up with Celia her increasingly apparent pattern of avoidance of contact with me until the end of the hour, when she characteristically made brief eye and emotional contact with me. This seemed to be Celia's way of proving to herself that there was no point in caring, as one always gets left, but she admitted to being perplexed by the fact that she felt better each time she allowed such contact to occur. It was also her way of avoiding feelings, particularly rage; the wish to kill me; and awareness of the sexual difference between us. In our 250th hour, immediately preceding another hospital review conference, she was more aware of her rage and worried that her success in sabotaging our relationship might lead to the loss of her relationship with me. This led to the novel thought that in some respects she was not the victim she had believed herself to be and that perhaps she could be an active agent in her own life.

At the review conference I commented on Celia's impressive aversion for thinking and feeling, and on her skill at denying her problems. In my note for the conference I wrote, "The craziest part of her is her capacity to deny she is crazy and to fool others into thinking she is well, competent, and understands herself when in fact none of these things are true." I commented on her deep hatred of people, on her pattern of living within herself while placating the world and keeping it at bay, and on how, at the same time, she continued to harbor a fantasy that somehow others would magically divine her needs and take care of her. I noted that, despite her periodic protestations about how important our relationship was to her, she still made minimal affective contact with me. Once again the nursing staff voiced their near unanimous belief that therapy was not working; they were responding not only to statements Celia made to them about therapy but also to painfully accurate perceptions and comments she often made about them and their various failures. Once again the consultant held things together, asserting that progress was being made in Celia's treatment and supporting continued hospitalization.

The recommendation of the conference for prolonged hospitalization raised financial issues that necessitated contact with the male family members responsible for administering Celia's trust funds. Celia reported conversations with them in which they allegedly implied that she was wasteful of money and unappreciative and said that they had her best interests in mind but had doubts about the hospital and her doctors and wanted to consider other alternatives. This stirred feelings of rage at her dead father and memories of how he had sent her away to camp with protestations that he had her best interests at heart and had then, unbeknownst to her, taken her brothers on a special trip to a distant resort. She recalled numerous other instances of discriminatory treatment against the women in her family, and commented wryly that at least mother had gotten two years of hospitalization out of the family patriarchs.

Following our 256th hour Celia escaped from the hospital. I was not notified by the staff, though it was customary hospital procedure for them to inform the patient's therapist, and first learned about it more than a day later when I found a message from Celia on my answering machine assuring me she was safe and would return to the hospital. My subsequent investigation of the reason for staff failure to contact me revealed that the nurse who acted as Celia's treatment coordinator in the hospital did not believe in long-term psychotherapy. Celia had "found" some ward keys and had gone to a distant city noted for gambling, where she became paranoid but resisted the prompting of her hallucinations to walk the streets late at night. She remarked that she had not called me sooner because she feared it would make her have feelings and hence "fall apart," and no help would be near. She perceived the gambling city's environment as one in which people are out of control and do not care about one another but try to use and exploit one another, an environment from which there is no escape (because of its isolated location, nocturnal egress from the city is actually very difficult). I suggested that in such a "normal" environment her external situation matched her inner life so well that she had no feelings whereas in the hospital environment she could not readily ignore efforts to care for her, and these stirred awareness of her neediness, rage, and sadness. Following this therapy hour she called me at home at night, in conflict over whether to "split" again. Talking calmed her, and we realized that "splitting" really meant cutting herself off from her feelings. She admitted she was frightened of her caring feelings for me, of how out of control and harmful to herself she was, and of how changeable her thinking was. When she observed herself hallucinating she asked staff to keep her in the quiet room, where she felt safer.

We began to talk about whether the chlorpromazine Celia had been taking since her most recent stay in the quiet room was helping her, and I learned that Celia unequivocally believed that no neuroleptic medication was beneficial; if she sensed that a medicine that another person gave her was affecting her, she was profoundly frightened, would conclude that she was being driven crazy, and would then do everything she could to fight its effects. She then informed me that she had taken very little of the trifluoperazine I had prescribed for her soon after making her acquaintance. Now she was genuinely confused about what was sane and what was crazy and was unable to tell whether the chlorpromazine was making her crazy or making her better. She was also aware of a constant undercurrent of thinking that her food was being poisoned. I found myself sharing her confusion about the significance of the changes she reported when she took neuroleptic medication.

Around the 270th hour Celia began to manifest a generalized, rage-related "stop the world, I want to get off" reaction, in which she both articulated and enacted a refusal to think and to allow any meaningful contact with anyone. In response I found myself coming late for her appointments. I talked with her about her attitude, and it turned out that she was withholding much information concerning her preoccupation with me and my importance to her, including how she typically looked out the window for my car before her hours, felt secretly solicitous and guilty about the trip I made to the hospital to see her, and, more recently, was upset with my lateness. To her further chagrin she realized, entirely on her own (I had not been aware of it), that she tended to mimic my gestures. In the 274th hour, following these revelations, Celia was withdrawn again; she decided to leave a few minutes early, which, she realized, represented her wish to destroy our work. As this became clearer she expressed her rage at me more directly, at the same time maintaining her litany of complaints about how family and others did not understand her needs. After an hour in which I remarked on her passive complaining, and her refusal to clarify and be consistent about just what her needs were, she planned to "split" from the hospital, but this time she experienced an uncharacteristic sadness and awareness of what was important to her and what she would lose in doing so. Again she complained about uncaring family attitudes, but I pointed out to her, being aware of some feelings of anger at her as I did so, that the "the hell with you" attitude that she so vividly described and decried in family members was in fact her own attitude in much of our relationship.

In our 283rd hour, at Celia's request, we once again attempted therapy in my private office, off hospital grounds. Celia recovered a series of memories dating back as early as age 7 or 8 in which she associated needing and seeking help with being mistreated. She became paranoid about me and began to obsess about leaving the hospital. When questioned about her avoidance of feeling she said to me repeatedly, in a way that was more offhand than defensive, that she felt very depressed and angry "if [she] stopped to think about it." When I pointed this out she made a conscious effort not to play her car radio on the way to therapy so that she might think, and in the 287th and 288th hours she told me some of her rules of functioning: to not talk to a nurse she liked because her appearance reminded her of mother; to not look around when entering my office so that it would not be real and she would not feel; to make meaningless pseudo-responses to people (she often tended to speak in cliché or jargon) so that they might be fooled into believing she was involved and communicating. When I pointed out that her refusal to know how she felt left her without a constructive way to orient herself and make decisions, and therefore very much at risk, Celia became frightened. I responded that I also found her conscious rejection of self-care signals frightening. Next hour she feared seeing me, as though I were a monster. She told me she was much more comfortable relating to Mike, a frightening patient on the ward who disliked people and assaulted them; she was convinced she could "handle" him. Once again she had the urge to escape and to disappear; she did leave the hospital but soon returned and was flooded with feelings, first of being an unloved orphan or waif and then of anger at me for being "hard" on her and not giving her positive "feedback." I remarked that while she wished that I would love her the only treatment she seemed able to tolerate was a reflection of her own uncaring attitudes.

Sadness, anger, and related childhood memories began to surface more regularly. Celia recalled running away from home and how she had sought out people who wanted to use and abuse her and had allowed them to structure her life, as though she was trying to prove that she could endure anything, even death. She looked forward to her hours with me more openly, and said (in our 293rd hour) that she felt safe and secure with me, a feeling she claimed was entirely novel in her life. It also seemed she had stopped hallucinating.

Spurred by financial considerations Celia seriously began to contemplate hospital discharge. For the first time since I had known her she seemed to care enough to try to plan constructively for her future. She became preoccupied with an adolescent female patient who repeatedly ran away from the hospital and got herself into destructive predicaments, and she began to adopt a motherly role with her. She began to be more aware of her lack of attention to and care of herself. She told me that she avoided looking in the mirror or buying clothing, and that she often bruised herself because she bumped into things.

Then she said she was beginning to feel secure, warm, and comfortable in her hospital bed; once she even elected to remain in bed and miss a therapy meeting. This was in marked contrast to her former nocturnal paranoia and restless wanderings.

When a staff member Celia wanted to talk to was busy, at a time when I was away for a few days, Celia hallucinated and became convinced people were not who they seemed to be. She imagined there was a missile silo in the yard behind the ward, panicked, began to run, banged her head against the wall, and fought off efforts to help her; finally, she required restraint. Once in seclusion diffuse rage began to surface, with fantasies of literally ripping herself apart and bombing the hospital, blowing it and me up. She felt her head swelling and occupying all corners of the room. Then she began to talk and puzzle about who it was that tortured her, finally concluding that it was herself, and that when she was kept in seclusion she was forced to face that fact. In our 300th hour she told me about her frightening awareness of how incapable she was of taking care of herself. She reread some old diaries and was horrified to see how paranoid and self-destructive she had been. It was even more frightening for her to contemplate wishes to be held like a baby and cared for by Mike, a ward nurse, and it filled her with rage that her wish could not come true. Sharing of her insight was punctuated by active self-ridicule.

These out-of-control psychotic episodes led to increasing ward restrictions, which in turn began to jeopardize our regular meetings because of difficulties I had in arranging my schedule to visit her. They also effectively halted discharge planning. At the same time Celia told me how alone and depressed she felt, and how angry with me she was for not understanding and appreciating all the efforts she was making. She stared out the window, remained detached from the affect, and vague in her speech. There were some affectless associations to father not caring and leaving her with hired help (presumably the ward staff), and Celia learning to "tough it out." The more I pointed out the connection between her childhood memories and what she was telling me of her current wishes, the more impressed I became by how she did not seem to be attending to or absorbing anything I said, and how she always seemed to change the subject. When I took this up with her and suggested the presence of an active and destructive element in her, Celia laughed and tried to convince me that my perceptions were not accurate. In response, now that I had become more confident of my own sanity in our relationship, I suggested she might tape-record her sessions to help her determine who was accurate, and she began to bring a tape recorder to her therapy sessions.

In our 308th hour Celia began to insist that she wanted to leave the hospital in 2 months. When I pointed out the incongruity of her wish with the way she had been acting and the things she had been telling me, she fought with me and bitterly accused me of not understanding. However, in the next hour she said she had learned from the tape recording how little she actually listened to me, and she began to talk more than she had ever done before about her attachment to me, and its meaning; this was the first experience in her life of a caring relationship with another person in which her needs were satisfied! She said this realization stirred incredible depression and rage in her and made her think that her caring was a chink in her armor and a threat to her "independence." At the end of the hour she looked at me and acknowledged that she felt good, but then she became detached, laughed bizarrely, and recalled how mother had recently told her (with the conviction that she was sharing a memory that proved how much she had cared for Celia) that when Celia and her siblings were all under age 5, mother had taken them sailing in the ocean and had thrown them overboard so she could teach them not to be frightened and prove to herself that she could rescue them.

In subsequent hours Celia giggled and was detached. She went to a bar, got drunk, and had casual sex with a man who picked her up. I expressed my concern and she first said she was suicidal, wanted to shoot herself, and didn't care about anything and then said she was avoiding me so as not to have feelings. She submitted notice of intent to leave the hospital, and then left a tearful phone message for me saying that I was all she cared about, and that she was trying to cut herself off from me but could not. In the 311th hour we reviewed the sequence of her feelings and behaviors: Caring stirred depression and hatred, and these led to attacks on our relationship, including withdrawal, forgetting, not knowing anything, and a chilling, sadistic triumphant laughter. I was impressed when, in discussing the power of her rage in our relationship, Celia told me, "You can only destroy what you have," adding that her relationship with me was all she had ever had.

When Celia described how her mother seemed to be trying to manipulate the social worker into doing her bidding while simultaneouly denying she was angry or had problems I remarked on the similarity of this description of mother to what we had been seeing in Celia herself. Celia initially became enraged and shook her fist at me, but then she began to speculate that perhaps both she and mother were trying to drive others crazy, and to consider how disturbing it must have been to her as a child to have mother act crazy and pretend she was normal. Then Celia proceeded to foul up the tape recording process, which had been responsible for some of our recent constructive conversations. Her hallucinations were clearly hostile and ridiculing. As I persisted she began to talk about her rage at people who claim to care, but really don't; her wishes to destroy were so intense that she actually used one arm to restrain the other.

Year Three

As we commenced our third year of work Celia was again confined to the quiet room, where she had been placed when she began to pick at the skin on her face in what she told me was an effort to tear her face off. When staff restrained her she became paranoid and thought they were trying to kill her. In her sessions with me there was much laughter, which we agreed was mocking and sadistic, along with much hostility toward me, expressed by her hallucinated voices. Celia admitted to being in distress, but said that "they" were keeping her from me. I shared with her my feelings of helplessness and dashed hopes, and pointed out to her how she was destroying resources—money, time, staff patience, my caring—and we both marveled at the power of her hatred. In subsequent hours (the 315th to the 320th) she regained self-control and was allowed out of the quiet room, and after listening to the tapes of our sessions she became very sad as she realized her need to destroy what was important to her; specifically, she realized that she seemed to be trying to drive me crazy. In an evanescent way she seemed more positive and caring, and more able to focus her rage on her parents, but this was followed by fears that mother would kill her, and rageful wishes, which she actually shouted at ward staff, to smash the ward and blow up the world. Celia baked muffins for everyone on the ward and then hallucinated that she had poisoned them. She became confused about the time of our hour and then thought perhaps I was sick. Then, in the 320th hour, she recalled from her childhood an instance of her mother's psychotic behavior: She had thrown Celia, her brothers, and Celia's friend into a corner and was terrorizing them. Her friend called her mother and was rescued, but Celia had no recourse but to train herself not to fight back.

Celia became more detached and flat in affect as she planned a visit with mother. She felt isolated and alone, frozen like ice, and I did not seem to exist in her mind. But she could associate some of her feelings about the impending visit to her childhood experiences, and she was also better able to turn to staff and ask for help. She recalled her efforts at age 9 (the year mother was hospitalized) to keep her gerbil calm and quiet after she gave birth, for she knew that mother gerbils are hypersensitive at such a time; the housekeeper disrupted the cage during her cleaning, and the gerbil ate its babies. Another memory that surfaced involved the death of her gerbil: Celia became so upset that she denied it had happened and covered the cage; only after a month, when the stench became unavoidable, did the death come to the attention of anyone in the family. Celia recalled the time after her mother regained custody: She had spent many months literally helping mother renovate her house, and as a "reward" mother sent her to a distant state where she knew no one. I told Celia that I was reminded of her original pact with her voices—that when the building across from my office was finished she would have to stop seeing me.

In her meeting with mother Celia vented some of her feelings of sadness, deprivation, and anger, and mother soliloquized (probably accurately) that she wanted to hold Celia, but would not attempt to do so because she knew Celia would not wish her to. After the meeting with mother Celia again became paranoid and hallucinated; she gave notice of her intent to leave the hospital, and left a message for me that she did not want to see me again. I responded that I would respect her choice, and she called back to say she had been foolish and wished to change her mind. I became ill and had to cancel her next hour, and she left another message on my answering machine, punctuated by tears, saying how much she cared and how upset she was; it was painful for me to listen to.

Again serious discharge planning commenced, but now Celia was more realistically worried about herself and her future. She struggled over whether this state of heightened awareness of the distress and confusion within her meant that she was becoming more disturbed and abnormal. She was amazed to discover that she had not noticed that my face had been grossly swollen from a dental infection for several days. She told me she had closed a door on her own arm, something that happened to her with regularity. As we articulated her state of being "lost" and confused, we began to wonder about whether this was a chronic and "normal" state of mind for her. Intermittently, and possibly for the first time, she began to view herself as human.

Celia was now driving to her therapy appointments at my office off the hospital grounds. When her car would not start after a therapy appointment, Celia frantically pushed it away from my house and down the hill—almost pushing it onto a main street and into rush hour traffic in the process—so that her need for help would go unnoticed by both of us. When I pointed out that she was trying to get lost, she became aware of a powerful longing to be taken care of, which reminded her of countless instances of being alone and in need, the contemplation of which filled her with depression and rage. She realized it felt secure and orienting, albeit frightening, to be closer to me. This state alternated with her usual detachment, sadistic giggling, and denial of need, as well as with an inner fight against urges she experienced to imitate my mannerisms.

The time of discharge from the hospital grew near, and Celia became increasingly sad and apprehensive about whether she could take care of herself. She began to realize how much many of the hospital staff meant to her, how secure the hospital felt to her, and what a good home it had become. She did not know how to say goodbye. She felt more positive about me, as well, though this was accompanied by thoughts that I might harm her, which were frightening even though she knew them to be irrational. She literally plotted escape routes out of my office. When she looked at the skyline she had the feeling the earth was falling out of orbit. She volunteered that she felt "affectionate" toward one of the staff; how to express such feelings genuinely perplexed her. As she planned to enter the halfway house where she would be living, she made the following remarkable statement "I never realized when you leave someplace you can have some other place you want to go to!" After 26 months and 355 hours of therapy (and 1½ years of hospitalization), Celia was discharged. After several hours of being rather affectless and detached, she revealed her fear that, if she faced how confused, frightened, homeless, alone, and sad she felt about leaving the hospital, she would be unable to function. Gradually, however, she began to relate to people in her new setting, and to feel somewhat better. She was particularly relieved to visit the ward and discover that she really did not want to be back there.

In one respect Celia felt a novel sense of freedom, but we began to realize that she also felt oppressed by the omnipresent experience of her mother—in the person of a psychotic older woman at the halfway house, in her fearful anticipation of me at the commencement of each therapy hour, in her fear during the hour that her mother was sneaking up behind her or was hiding behind my office plants, and in her belief that a lion was outside her room at night. She was overwhelmed with the realization of how terrible her life had been. As she anticipated my summer vacation with terror, and articulated her fear that I was abandoning her to the clutches of a crazy woman, we both realized that the woman was no longer her mother but herself. In the 364th hour Celia began to feel that the world was literally disintegrating. She feared that the ceiling was about to fall, that trees would fall on her, that her car would split apart, that big trucks would smash into her room at night. She began to avoid looking, thinking, and feeling, and then realized how little attention she paid to herself, and how unaware she tended to be of injury, illness, fatigue, hunger, and sexual feelings. She said she felt entitled to a vacation, as well, and by this she seemed to mean the freedom to go crazy, and not to think or feel. The halfway house was near a children's zoo, and the patients often spent time there as volunteers. Celia identified with the small and orphaned animals, and experienced horror when a raccoon killed a baby chick. She became increasingly detached; nonetheless, as we struggled over whether she would allow herself to feel, she informed me that she no longer had a choice.

In anticipation of my forthcoming summer vacation Celia realized the difficulty she experienced taking over from the hospital important self-care functions. She lacked a normal danger response to certain signals, such as the pain of handling a burning pot (instead, her reflexive response tended to stem from a belief that nothing could bother her). For the first time Celia realized with alarm that her self-protective instincts were deficient and that the things that upset most people did not bother her. I added that the things most people felt at home with, such as intimacy, terrified her. She was detached and continued to hallucinate and be delusional, and we wondered if she ought to return to the hospital while I was away. She imagined a nest for herself in the corner of my office but was quite late for our appointment. In our remaining hours (the 380th through the 383rd) Celia struggled with wishes to beat me up, tie me up, and put me in a dark place, as though this would make me feel as she did. These wishes terrified her, and she deadened herself, and kept needing to reassure me that she would not do such a thing. Arriving at our 384th meeting she was relieved to find me intact, but she was so detached and numbed that I did not seem quite real to her. She recalled episodes of running away and being physically assaulted while feeling numb and frozen.

Finally, Celia concluded that she needed to return to the hospital while I was gone, and immediately she felt better. She said she loved me and she gave me a gift, a lovely ceramic car she had made, which she called her "getaway car," but sadness, hurt, and rageful sadistic feelings followed. She wanted either to be crazy to avoid these, or to drive me crazy in a vengeful effort to bind me to her. Her wish to deprive me of hope, activity, and sanity alternated with a wish to preserve my autonomy. Her affects remained quite muted, but there were poignant memories, including one of swimming much too far out in the ocean, until she was no longer certain she could get back, only to realize that the prospect of returning was so terrifying she did not know if she wanted to try. We could understand her embrace of death and craziness in preference to what others might consider security, and comprehend the sense of no place to go but out of her mind. Celia experienced me as torturing her. Turning off her feelings was a form of triumph; it meant no one could hurt her. She imagined torturing me in return, imagined beating and terrifying me to the point where I realized that there was no longer hope, that whatever I did or did not do would only provoke her more, so I would finally remove myself from body and feelings and go crazy. These ideas alternated with memories of having such things done to her—first by mother, then brother, and ultimately by some of the sadistic men she apprenticed herself to in her adolescence.

We separated for my month's vacation, and though Celia reentered the hospital as planned, she quickly realized she no longer knew anyone there. She escaped, eventually going to London, where she knew no one; she called to reassure me that she was well and taking care of herself and sent me a card from Freud's house.

When I returned for our 387th hour Celia was pleased to see me; she seemed quite clear about the importance of our relationship, her problem with self-care, and the emotional distance she maintained from me. Characteristically, the following hour she felt "awful," laughed inappropriately, acted distant, and told me she wasn't certain I was really back. She hallucinated opposition to relating to me, and she felt like running away. In response I soon felt bored and detached. Toward the end of the hour she began to talk about wishes to make me feel alone, terrified, and trapped, and to drive me crazy, but near the very end she was able to realize that her involvement with me enabled her to remember childhood feelings that would otherwise be intolerable.

Amidst an ensuing hour marked more or less by silence and fragmentation Celia told me her thoughts were exploding in midsentence; she perceived me as strange and dangerous and felt stuck, all alone, with no one there. I said that she made me feel alone, as well. It seemed we were both immobilized, isolated, and in the throes of a pull to lose our minds. In our 392nd hour Celia literally sat on her hands as she told me of her global hatred, her wishes to beat me up, and her terror that I would think the person who had recently committed murder near where she lived was, in fact, she. I remarked that what impressed me was her inability to be actively and directly angry and aggressive. When a destructive act was committed at the halfway house, and although the perpetrator was known, Celia worried that she might have done it or that she might be accused of it. She became very frightened, believing that I was not me, that the real me had been kidnapped, and that someone was about to attack her from behind. At night she believed her house was being burned. She had urges to scald herself so someone could see her suffering.

At the end of our 394th hour I expressed to Celia my concern that we were reaching limits beyond which we might have to rehospitalize her. To my surprise she cried, felt closer to me, and in subsequent hours felt better. She construed my setting limits on her as the actions of a good father, but this made her feel a total body numbness, and a wish to leave. At the same time she recalled a single incident, in her teens, when mother had stroked her hair, and it had felt so good she wanted it never to end. She felt pleasure when a policeman stopped her for speeding, and she contemplated not leaving the office when the hour ended and hitting me playfully, both of which seemed to express her wish to be physically contained and held. In the next hour she reported having had the startling urge to ask a good-looking man she had spied while eating to marry her. She phoned me at home one evening to see if I was really there.

Starting in the 399th hour, and continuing for the next ten or so sessions, Celia began to experience and to remember, in a form at times global, enactive, and paranoid, and at other times more reflective, her terror of her mother and her need to hide from her, particularly to hide feelings of caring and need. After experiencing the wish to share with me sadness and rage, she experienced herself as a small terrified child with a huge and menacing mother standing over her. She called me the next night, in near panic, wanting to run from the halfway house because she was in a rage and wanted to smash everything. I spoke with a staff member and arranged for the two of them to talk. Celia dreamed chickens had escaped the coop and the raccoon was about to kill them. She recalled how, as a child, she had spent much of her time hiding in the closet of her room with the door closed. Once she had tried unsuccessfully to conceal from her mother the fact that she had cut her finger rather badly; when they got to the hospital and the doctor wished to suture it, mother fought with him and would not permit it.

Now Celia began to feel secure and to enjoy life and people more. She took some courses. When she had the urge to run from the waiting room at the sound of my approach at the start of a therapy hour she guessed that she was frightened of confronting her sad and angry feelings; she left the hour furious with me for "making" her feel, and crying hysterically—very unusual behavior. When she observed an infant throw its toy on the floor she was convinced its mother, who was near by, would attack it; there were suggestions that ideas like this veiled memories. On the road a truck driver waved to her and winked, and she felt good. She recalled being forced by her mother to eat things she did not want, and responding with efforts to be invisible and to swallow whatever mother fed her. These memories, in turn, stirred others of having to perform endless fellatio on some of the men who had abused her and of thinking that in so doing she was controlling them. She hallucinated the command to bolt from my office befor I "clobbered" her, but soon admitted that she was very angry at me and wanted to clobber me and throw me into the corner as mother had done with her. In our 410th hour I commented that her tendency to act as she had as a child in her mother's presence brought about the very destructiveness she had sought to protect herself from.

In hours 411 through 418 Celia showed signs of caring about her life, having hope, making plans, asserting herself, and expressing needs in situations where hitherto she would have been passive and compliant. She was able to concentrate and read, enjoyed her classes, and talked of moving to more normal surroundings. When she lamented how totally compliant she had been in the past, I remarked, "Not entirely," and commented on how stubbornly defiant she was when it came to suggestions that she think, feel, pay attention, and take better care of herself.

During a weekend separation Celia called me because she was terrified of imminent attack, and felt the need to run, and in the ensuing 412th hour she sat in a corner, virtually unable to look at me, focus, talk, feel, and remember. In sparse, affectless phrases she told me that the room was floating and about to explode and that my face had changed and become sinister; at the end of what was for me an incredibly boring hour she became obsessed with the possibility that she might even cease breathing! The following hour she was much more lively—in a quiet rage about irresponsible people at her halfway house, a description that was consistent with the facts of her living situation as it was described to me by staff—and expressing entitlement to normal comfort and cooperation. But when I pointed out that the problem had less to do with how she was treated by others and more to do with her inability to take good care of herself, she denied that it was she I was talking about.

In our next hour (415th) Celia confided that she had been feeling suicidal and estranged from me for several weeks; the reason, she said, was that she had not been able to tell me that she really didn't hallucinate, and that the stories of abuse in skid rows were fabrications; she concluded by saying that if I believed such things I was unreal to her. She added that when she was in London during my holiday and had wanted attention and sympathy, she had gone to a restaurant and convinced the waiter that she was a bereaved widow revisiting the scene of her marriage. I felt shocked and a bit sick to my stomach, and wondered aloud what to believe and how I could tell when she was being truthful. Celia tried to convince me that she was telling me these things because our relationship was so important to her, but she could not assuage my suspiciousness. She said she felt suicidal for she had ruined our relationship when in fact she loved me and needed to feel close to me, but she was sitting in the far corner of the room as she said this and her affect was flat. I pointed out her detachment and she talked about her fear; the whole room began to change to her, things became animated in sinister and threatening ways as she attempted to tell me she cared, and she feared I would change, go crazy, and attack her. I could only comment to her that she was the un-predictable and changeable party in our relationship, and that at times it was next to impossible for me to know what was real and true about her because she herself apparently did not want to know. Celia could see what I meant, but said such behavior had become so natural to her that she was no longer upset about it.

Once again Celia allowed herself to be used sexually by a man she did not care about; she told me that she had to obliterate self-awareness in order to do it. Our discussion led to the realization she was staying "in training," that is, testing out whether she could still "get away" if she had to. My attentions made

her realize she wished to be invisible, and she imagined attacking me physically and making me hide, freeze, or become invisible so that I could not
attend to her. At the same time she realized she enjoyed my attention, particularly a kind of bantering or playful interchange we had gradually developed
where she would "give me trouble" and I would "get on her case." But this was
almost impossible for her to talk about, since she had almost no vocabulary
with which to express positive body sensations, feelings, and wishes. In language muffled by vagueness and obfuscation she began to tell me that life was
becoming meaningful to her, that she was taking better care of herself and was
grateful to me. Now she felt immediately when she had jabbed her hand on a
nail head, though she might still do nothing about it. And she was making her
room more comfortable. She marveled that I seemed to keep her focused and
to know just what she could deal with; for example, the last time she threatened
to run away I had said, knowing that she now had the capacity to make a
choice, that if she did she should not call me; this had made her angry and yet
she had liked it. She also liked it when I smiled and laughed. At this point in
the hour she became petrified of impending attack and said she couldn't
breathe; indeed, she looked as though she felt she was being strangled. When
I shared this observation she agreed and said that when that happened she
couldn't let herself feel, for that made it worse.

   I wondered about related childhood memories, and in our subsequent
hours (the 424th to the 426th) the issue of childhood abuse arose again; this
time Celia had an urge to talk with her stepmother, various family members,
and mother's former therapist, or to view court and hospital records in order
to find out more about what had actually happened. She found the prospect of
asking her mother directly so terrifying that her conscious thinking literally
stopped. She recalled a recent family gathering in which mother had egre-
giously flunked a child-care quiz in a woman's magazine and then had caus-
tically attacked the makers of the quiz for knowing nothing about parenting.
She had proceeded to label her infant grandchild hysterical when it fell down-
stairs, and she referred to its mother, her daughter-in-law, as overprotective
for comforting it. As this hour concluded Celia became paranoid; she perceived
that my voice changed and that I became distant and ridiculing. She retained
some capacity to differentiate this state of mind from me and was aware that
she imagined mother about to attack her from behind. I wondered why she
continued to sit in the most distant chair, near where she imagined mother
was, and with a look of surprise Celia moved nearer to me, looked at me and
said she felt much calmer, and added that the idea of turning to me for help had
not occurred to her.

   After this hour Celia was in a rage and had a powerful urge to get drunk
and go to a bar, but she made herself return to the halfway house, where she
took the initiative to involve herself sexually with a very passive, "spaced out"
adolescent male; much to her surprise, she enjoyed the affectionate contact.
Self-consciously, and for the first time in her life, she took a stuffed animal to
bed with her. After much avoidance, vagueness, and denial, interspersed with

paranoid panic that she would be killed, Celia discussed her plan to ask mother's permission to speak to mother's former therapist. In our 430th hour Celia reported that mother had not only given verbal permission for Celia to see her hospital records but had expressed solicitude that I should be with her when she read them!

Celia began to anticipate her wishes and needs over the forthcoming holiday season, which were accompanied by the usual counterpoint of rage, detachment, and struggle against acknowledging them. She felt locked up in her head, with the urge to explode, and wanted to cry out to people about how upset she was but felt she could not. She did not look at me, her thoughts were disorganized, and she was speechless about her inner experience. She wanted to rip me up and tear my head off, and I noted that this was what she was doing to her own thinking. She was paranoid that there were snipers outside her room, and her attention was totally devoted to protecting herself. At times she could sense her extreme disintegration, which she likened to "trying to drive two cars going 200 miles per hour at once."

At this time she wrote me a series of letters from which the following are excerpts:

"I thought I had something to say but I am in a muddle now. . . . I hate the whole fucking world. . . . Not only does my head get splintered up but the room does too and words get blasted into meaningless letters. So the four walls of the room no longer join and I don't feel safe here. Everything gets unglued. . . . Life really does suck. I start thinking about it and I get so angry I just want to blow up the world. . . . Where the hell are you? I don't know. I haven't been able to see you hardly at all lately, everything is drifting away. . . ."

She was flooded with memories of being abused by men in various ways, including being forced to perform fellatio for long periods of time. She experienced nausea and wishes to vomit, which alternated with massive rage and wishes to hit and kill and blow out brains in revenge. She imagined asking someone to knock some sense into her. With me her wishes fluctuated rapidly, from wanting to cry and share sadness, to wanting to beat me to a pulp, to wanting to hug me and be close, to secretly laughing at me, to wishing to have nothing to do with me at all. I found the effort to follow and make sense of her extreme and rapid fluctuations exhausting. She told me angrily that she had originally come to see me in order to perfect her psychosis, that is, to prove she could defeat the efforts of yet another "shrink," but that I had confused her.

Celia began to focus anger on mother, who, had done nothing to follow through on her promise to ask her former therapist to talk with me and/or with Celia, and to request the mental hospital to release her records to me. She remembered the many times when mother had failed her, times of need when mother would become hysterical, preempt attention, and get Celia to take care of her instead. She realized, with much rage, that she had been mother's "tool," which involved disconnecting from her own feelings and needs, and repudiating caring, in order to do what mother seemed to want. For Christmas she bought her mother a hand vacuum, but mother appeared to have the last word, serving grossly undercooked meat at a holiday meal and giving Celia a gift of a season ticket for one to a local theatre (which turned out to be in the very last row, at that!). Celia felt hurt, sad, and in need of a home, along with her usual wishes to rid herself of the feelings.

During our 450th hour, following a brief holiday interruption, Celia told me of a holiday family get-together in which her brother's young children were punished and called manipulative for head-banging and for expressing fearfulness. Afterward Celia dreamed she was in a world of seductive vampires, and had to decide whether to swallow a concoction and become like them. When she came for her 451st hour she felt stunned by reorientation to her feelings of sadness and rage, which she had lost contact with, and she wanted to hit me just hard enough to stun me. She had virtually simultaneous wishes to be involved with me, to hit me, and to run away and have nothing to do with me, and Celia realized she was of two minds about everything, and therefore of no consistent mind at all.

Once again Celia urged her mother to request that her former therapist talk with her or with me, and this time her mother responded with anger, hysteria, and suspiciousness, contradicting some of the things she had told Celia about the past, and accusing Celia and me of attempts to persecute her. In the following hour Celia said she didn't want to be with me, laughed in her ridiculing manner about herself and her feelings, and told me she was becoming more paranoid. After some encouragement she began to talk fearfully about her rage at mother and her wish to kill or terrorize her into insanity. She was convinced that one of them would kill or drive the other crazy. The talk was punctuated by disruptions, laughter at herself, and the sensation of being unable to breathe. She seemed more aware than usual of how thoroughly identified she was with some of mother's attitudes, and of how unreliable and inconsistent both of them were.

Celia began to plan a teaching career with adolescents. In a confused way she began to articulate a wish to be closer to people, but in the next breath she informed me that it had not even occurred to her to tell me she had a bad stomachache. She felt things coming together in her mind in a positive way. When she answered the phone at the halfway house and the caller mistook her for another resident and referred to her as "honey" it made her feel sad that she had not been anyone's honey, and she realized she wished to be. She began a new job which was much more constructive than previous ones, if not really challenging of what I was increasingly aware were her unusual skills and abilities.

Once again, around the 463rd hour, Celia became frenzied and confused, even as to the date, and reported hallucinating. She told me she had been awake and paranoid for two nights and that she needed to shift seats in the office because she was convinced an attacker was behind her. She felt choked into silence, unable to breathe, and she hallucinated negative remarks about me. Perhaps I was unreal, or perhaps I was crazy too. She realized her hatred of people was directed mostly at me, but she also had urges to cut up her teddy bear.

In the following hour Celia informed me that mother had written to her former therapist and then to the hospital about releasing information to me. As the possibility of getting data about mother and her illness became more real it turned out that Celia did not believe mother had been in a mental hospital or had been mentally ill at all, and that she subscribed to the family myth that mother had been absent because of a physical infirmity. We realized that no one in the family really knew the dates of mother's hospitalization or any facts about it, and Celia did not want to disrupt this tacit understanding. I told Celia we would need to have mother's input about how whatever information I might get was to be shared, but it turned out that Celia did not believe anything would be sent me and was convinced mother felt the same.

When I received mother's hospital records she told Celia she did not wish to be involved in the sharing of them and gave me permission to use them in any way I chose. I asked Celia what she wished to know, and in response to her specific questions I gave her a few simple facts about dates, nature of illness, and response to treatment. As I read the lengthy and biographically detailed record to myself, one of the most striking elements was the complete lack of interest and concern Celia's mother seemed to have had about both her marriage and her children. When I shared this with Celia, explaining how pre-occupied mother must have been with her inner experience, just as she herself was, Celia had great difficulty dealing with the discrepancy between her unimportance in mother's mind and how terrorized mother had made her feel. Celia's attention then turned to the memory of her father, who had perceived her only as someone with something wrong with her, and had attended to her in a sporadic, cursory, and moralistic way. Celia had difficulty experiencing me as real. Inwardly she mocked reality, truncated her thoughts in the middle of an idea, and literally felt she was choking back massive rage. She thought she was keeping a distance from me for fear she might kill me.

Illusions of a terrifying woman in the doorway of her room at night made Celia wonder if mother had acted bizarre and threatening. As we now had the hospital records to refer to, I read her a nursing report that mentioned mother's abusiveness and overt destructiveness; threats of violence and suicide; running away; periods of disorientation and of immobility, lasting for hours; and terrifying hallucinations of a persecutory old woman. Celia realized that when she experienced strong feelings she would freeze, not breathe or make a sound, and draw herself inward, and that this behavior must have originated as a protective effort to avoid drawing attention to herself and to make mother go away. She recalled seeking out relationships with bizarre and destructive men and selflessly catering to their whims in order to keep them tranquil, and she speculated about her unusual capacity to deal with disturbed people at the hospital, which had made her a kind of auxiliary staff member and had led most staff to grossly underestimate her own level of disturbance. Again we returned to Celia's feelings of loneliness and pain, and her belief, which seemed all too true, that, except for me, no one in the world seemed to care what her needs might be. She cried plaintively.

Suddenly and without warning Celia told me with satisfaction that she had stopped her three-pack-a-day cigarette habit, and although she could not say why, she was convinced she would not resume it. She said she was feeling good, and was more aware and self-protective when people mistreated her. After a week she resumed smoking just as abruptly as she had stopped, and seemingly without real concern. She would not take seriously the issues of credibility and consistency that I pointed out to her. Finally, after commenting without success about my growing drowsiness in response to a vague, amorphous, affectless quality about her, I picked up a journal and read. When Celia got upset I explained how she repeatedly set me up with hopes and expectations and then proved that her presentation of reality and her intentions were not real or were not to be taken seriously. Again Celia began to realize how self-contradictory and out of control she was, and it frightened her with something like the intensity she imagined she must have felt frightened of her mother as a little girl. She realized how negative, oppositional parts of herself existed without her even knowing about them, so that she could stop smoking (or start again) seemingly without conflict. She observed herself laughing at things she thought were serious, and realized that when she was angry at me it was as though she were sitting and watching someone else. This led to a more basic awareness of the two sides of her: her wish to experience contempt and superiority by proving that nothing affected her, which she now realized was not triumph over another but a bad joke on herself, and the wish to care and be involved. She said, "You confuse me; I used to have only one idea about all this." She realized that she didn't like dealing with crazy people as much as she thought, that it was too much of a challenge, but I responded that it was not nearly so challenging for her as was dealing with normal people. She confirmed my comment by recalling the utter confusion and discomposure she experienced following a positive experience with a friend.

Year Four

The 489th hour heralded the fourth year of our work. Celia visited her old university and felt confused and disturbed when she realized she had gone through college without any awareness of feeling, but it was not clear whether she considered the past or the present situation to be the abnormal one. On the trip she spent some time with the family of a friend and felt herself included in their lives, becoming aware in the process that she had so thoroughly and reflexively absorbed her mother's attitudes of mockery toward family life that, in the past, she would not have allowed herself to be aware of caring feelings. We began to contrast some of her destructive attitudes and behaviors with me with her attitudes toward others at the halfway house, where she had acquired a reputation for being caring and constructive. Through her usual screen of laughing and calling what was crazy normal and vice versa she described for the first time since I had known her some fantasies of having a home and a husband of her own. Following this she told me that she was crazy and that there was a bomb bursting in her head, and she enacted fragmentation of her thinking and noncommunication. But again she returned to the topic of change. Now it was the discovery of ambivalent feelings; she continued to care about people even though in some respects they frustrated her. Even though she felt in a rage at me and wanted to hit me and prevent me from influencing her in any way, nonetheless she said she loved me.

Celia began to notice hitherto denied discomfort in her body: for example, a splinter or symptoms of the flu. We talked of how she wore form-disguising garments and tried to avoid looking at or thinking about her body or even knowing of its existence. As was characteristic at such times she felt more vulnerable and appeared more disturbed. She said she feared her food was poisoned, and her solution was to avoid eating. I commented on how she habitually engaged in potentially lethal behavior toward herself in the illusionary belief that she was being self-protective.

Celia's birthday approached. She could not recall any instance of family celebration of this occasion, and she recalled how as a teenager she and a friend had run a successful business making birthday parties for children of parents who were too busy to do it themselves. She felt alone and homeless, with no family to care for her and treat her as special. She wanted to cry but feared if she did she might never stop. She giggled and thought I looked crazy and then told me she had been paranoid and hallucinating. She rhymed and punned but also said that she thought she seemed more crazy because she was less successful dissimulating and putting on a facade. Now she struggled to remain in contact with me, and recognized that the root of her difficulty in doing so was her fear and rage at mother. After telling me this she began to chop up her thoughts, and there was a stream of self-ridiculing hallucinations accompanied by bizarre laughter and a sense of terror. On her birthday, before our 501st hour, Celia had the urge to get in her car, speed, get picked up by police, attack the policeman, and get killed, and she recognized this would be her way of demonstrating to mother what mother had done to her. She recalled ill treatment by police, the staff of mental hospitals, and others who ought to have cared. But she made her needs clearer to the people around her, and as a result friends and even her sister gave her some very gratifying attention on her birthday, Celia realized that although the hate feeling was still strongest it was now, for better or worse, accompanied by caring.

Once again Celia became so frightened by her hallucinations and delusions that she was unable to sleep, and after she sought the help of the staff at the halfway house, she had a brief and constructive rehospitalization. When I first saw her at the hospital she was overwhelmed with feelings—gratitude, wishes to hug me, sadness, loneliness, and massive rage. She could barely deal with these and her wish to run was enacted in the form of changing the subject and retreating into hallucinations. The end of this 502nd hour was most impressive: Celia asked to shake my hand, to which I agreed, and she then remarked with obvious relief, followed by crying, that I was human and that it felt good. In the hospital terrifying convictions that mother would come and kill her alternated with murderous feelings about mother, and these were accompanied by a new awareness of all she had missed in terms of human closeness and by wishes to hug me. On the ward she was much more direct in making her needs known and getting responded to; she said to me, "If I'm going to feel all this stuff, then I want to have people around all the time to share it." She even initiated a successful phone call with mother, in which mother poignantly indicated how threatened she now felt by Celia, and how hard she had tried to pick a birthday gift for her that Celia would not interpret as a rejection. Celia came away from this call with a more balanced view of a mother who, despite her obvious limitations, was making an effort. Celia was able to articulate to me wishes to be my little child and to crawl into my lap. She realized she had become increasingly committed to a world of feelings, although she admitted that, at times, she tried to fool herself and tell herself that it was just another one of her tricks, her acts, and that it was not real.

Celia was discharged from the hospital after about 2 weeks, and initially felt suspicious that I was crazy, a creature from Mars, someone who was tricking her into caring in a world where no one else really did. She told me she had gone to a family gathering at her mother's house determined to confront one of her brothers who had for some time been avoiding her. She was direct with him about his importance and her need for him as well as about her anger, but she reported a response of anger and withdrawal on his part, along with a mocking laugh she was very familiar with. This had touched off a remarkable and atypical emotional family scene in which mother empathized with Celia and made episodic efforts to stop the quarrel, and her sister was also supportive. Celia felt good about this. Afterward she had very much wanted to talk to me about it, and she dreamed she was baby-sitting in my family.

Beginning in our 512th hour, in a manner that combined remembering, repeating, and somatizing, Celia began to talk about her experiences being abused by men. She spoke of her terror and about her belief that she was placating the insane (that is, sexually aroused) man by sucking on his penis. She felt nauseated, along with a terrifying sense of helplessness, but felt she had no choice but to go out of her mind (that is, not think or feel). This sequence was repeated numerous times in the ensuing weeks as she recalled various instances of allowing herself to be abused, and we talked about their significance in relation to her mother and to the men in her family. Once, during this portion of her therapy, Celia came close to enacting the scenario in a bar to which she had been attracted by the warm, dark, drunken, convivial feeling, which she associated with family. I emphasized that she had enacted more than enough of these experiences for a lifetime, and that the issue was remembering them and working on their meaning, not putting herself in renewed jeopardy by her actions. I told her I wanted her to agree not to go into a bar again, and she did so reluctantly. The following hour she volunteered that she was angry at me and wanted to "slug" me, but she said it with a warm smile. She said that she felt trapped and deprived by our agreement, and had been longing to go to a bar since, but she had made her promise and I could rely on her to keep it. It became clear that the bar represented the home of deadness, the raucous music drowning out thought and feeling, the darkness preventing perception, the booze confusing her thoughts. I said that I suspected she was feeling more than she had told me, and she replied with a combination of passion and anger that she was putting herself in this box or trap because she loved me and that it felt good. She went on to elaborate a fantasy of getting married, like her sister, but said the idea made her angry because she realized all the work she would have to do if she were to have any chance of success. The theme of being enclosed or boxed in continued in subsequent hours; the box she was accustomed to (abuse) had not seemed abnormal but was often accompanied by paranoid fears of danger and snipers. She told me that as a child she had often made her bed in a closet. There were more realizations of male chauvinism and sadism in her family, both historical and contemporary (for example, such birthday "gifts" from her brother as a ripsaw and a picture of his crotch). As she told me these things she hunched over self-protectively and experienced a combination of sadness and anger. Then she had a nightmare of a man who was awaiting a verdict in an execution apparatus that would decapitate him, but who cut off his own head first. This made her think of her father, who had died before she had an opportunity to deal with her feelings about him. Such awareness alternated with disorganization and paranoia, with beliefs that snipers were after her, and the alternation seemed to relate to how well she was able to face a plethora of childhood memories of having been abandoned or left with sadistic caretakers in dangerous situations that she had hitherto viewed as normal and expectable. She began to have more wishes to be a teacher.

Celia was overwhelmed with feelings of homelessness and rage, further stimulated by her beginning search for a housing arrangement of her own that would allow her to leave the halfway house, and by anticipation of my forthcoming summer vacation. She was more aware of the strangeness of her previous behavior when she was homeless, when she would search out and submit herself to brutal men in bars; now she felt the terror and rage related to those times, but frequently these feelings were directed toward me because she experienced me as assaulting her with these ideas and memories. At other times the anger was in response to having just 4 hours a week of my "home" or attentions. When she talked about her fear of the potential insanity of the man, and about how she would retreat to an inner space where no one could get her, fooling the man into believing that she cared and that he was affecting her, we realized the similarity to the many times she had fooled me. I commented that while she might have fooled men, thought them insane, and believed she was in control, in fact the loss of control and sanity in these situations had been her own.

Celia arranged to move into a house jointly rented by several women. She felt that she was changing, becoming committed to a world of feelings and relationships. People were important to her: mother, who was planning to move; her paternal grandmother, the only family member who had shown her any caring and whose death she feared; a male staff member at the halfway house, whom she admitted having a "crush" on and who would be leaving; and of course I, who would soon be leaving for a vacation. Celia could now imagine work, marriage, and family whereas before she did not think of herself as being a person and having roots in time and space. She told me she no longer hallucinated. At night when she was terrified and at times paranoid, she now hugged her stuffed animal. But as she became more aware of how she had lived in a nonhuman world where no one had needs and people were stereotyped with epithets and used by one another, she worried that, in my absence, she might not be able to sustain feeling real and wondered if she could bear all the feelings involved. She felt the urge to ridicule caring and return to her previous condition of not thinking and feeling. She said at the end of the 537th hour that she loved me, wanted to hug me, and would miss me terribly when I was gone, but this enraged her and she felt that I had "set her up" and that the rug would be pulled out from under her and she would be made a fool of. She felt weak and trapped; previously, she had been a "rock" and could "get away" when she needed to.

Around our 539th hour Celia moved out of the mental health system and into a house she shared with several women. She felt fearful and insecure. After her characteristic prelude, "If I let myself think," she remembered that the house in which she grew up had not felt like home because terror of her mother had led her to try not to be visible and to avoid calling attention to herself, and because father's rules made most areas of the house, save the basement, literally out of bounds to the children. There ensued some withdrawal, inner ridicule of others, and cutting apart of her own thoughts, followed by diffuse rage with wishes to bomb and destroy the entire east coast. I pointed out how identified she was with the uncaring attitudes of her family that deprived her of a home, and how she kept oscillating between her angry belief that other people did not care and a rageful uncaring attitude of her own. Her response was a kind of rageful withdrawal from me and a perception that I was critical and blaming of her and about to leave her. As we struggled with this she acknowledged that she had never cared about anyone before or accepted that she needed anyone, or considered thinking and feeling to be natural, and that she had to force herself to do it now. She would not let herself recall the beginnings of our relationship because it would involve acknowledging that she had been helpless and dependent on me, and this would violate her conviction of self-sufficiency.

I was away for a week. When I returned, Celia's mocking laughter and puzzling ambiguous comments soon led to articulation of her hatred of thinking, feeling, expressing herself clearly, and of course caring, and of her need to feel invulnerable, and then to a more subtle feeling of sadistic revenge that she experienced from having once again "fooled" me into believing we were getting closer, only to frustrate me. By the end of the next hour I found myself struggling with boredom and drowsiness while she talked of rejection and mistreatment from father and brothers. Finally and critically she noted my reaction. When I wondered aloud why it was happening, she responded vehemently that it was because she didn't want me near her.

In subsequent hours, as my longer summer vacation approached, Celia remained cold and aloof. Seemingly oblivious to what she was doing, she tracked mud over my office rug with dirty sneakers. We talked about her rage, some directed at mother for moving ("Mothers aren't supposed to do that! She set me up!"), and her own wish to retaliate by going to a foreign country where there could be no communication because Celia didn't speak the language. I commented that that country was called the land of back-ward schizophrenia. Once again Celia began hallucinating ridiculing voices and expressing paranoid fears of imminent attack. This time she was able to talk about some caring efforts she had made to plant and cultivate seeds in the halfway-house garden, which had met with failure owing to the indifference and lack of cooperation from others, and as we traced her growing sense of futility about expressing her feelings, to the point of wanting to give up and become psychotic, her hallucinations abruptly ceased. Identifying herself with the ill-fated seeds, Celia began to recall how mother would come into her room when she was a child and commence an escalating verbal attack on her while messing about with her things and telling her it was not her room at all; in defense, Celia relinquished her sense that anything was important.

As chance would have it, Celia learned at this time that her mother was seriously ill and would require immediate surgery. This heralded a period of emotional disengagement on Celia's part which extended throughout my summer vacation and well into the ensuing fall. Celia was affectlessly and obsessively preoccupied with mother's illness, and with the fact that mother was acting as though nothing were the matter. I suggested that the present situation might be like her childhood, where she could not live her own life but had to devote all her energies to avoid presenting mother with any needs or demands and to maintaining mother's sanity. She recalled how mother had seemed to capitalize on the sick role to get attention.

Despite her state of mind, Celia survived my monthlong vacation without obvious psychosis or destructive activity, as she informed me on my return (in our 562nd hour). She obtained her first job since leaving the hospital, as a teacher's aide to small children, and she promptly informed me of how ridiculous her mother had found her description of how these children's mothers doted on them. Celia now seemed of two minds, all enjoyment and all pain, about everything. On the one hand, she seemed quite invested in her life and enjoyed her new job and some course work she had undertaken; simultaneously she reported despair, constant suicidal preoccupation, and chillingly graphic images of how she might kill herself. Since she was mostly detached in our sessions, I struggled much of the time to master my sleepiness and boredom, responses that seemed to inflame Celia's fury at me and to remind her of (or to be confused with) the neglect by her family, although at times she recognized that my reaction was a reflection of her own detachment. It was becoming increasingly worrisome to Celia that she kept claiming she wanted one thing while enacting the opposite.

Our 569th hour was a poignant one. Upset because she had not slept and worried that she was becoming crazy, Celia forced herself to look at me and make contact. She talked about her school job, and particularly about separation, infants crying for their mothers and mothers coming for them—and her overwhelming sadness and rage that no mother was coming for her. Wondering how she had managed when she finally realized her mother would never again return home led her to feelings of rage and sadness about my recent vacation, and some confusion about whether or not she was a small child and I had in fact done something unforgivable.

During the next hour she remembered how she had dealt with mother's presence by suppressing her feelings and trying to be inanimate. She recalled mother's rageful injunction to "get lost" so mother would not have to see her face again, and the implied threat that if she did not mother would do something terrible to her. After this hour she visited her mother and realized that she was in a state of terror for fear she would act on her wish to tell mother what we had talked about. Instead, she went to a bar and got drunk. As she told me about this (in our 571st hour) she mentioned another wish she had not acted on: At the end of the previous hour she had stood outside the office door, wanting to knock and to tell me she needed a hug, for security, before she could leave.

The theme of motherless child continued. Celia experienced intense empathy for the separation feelings of her nursery school children. She told me of a dream in which she was to teach a group of underprivileged minority slum children while the other children all went somewhere else with the "real" teacher. She realized that in her own school days she had had no sense of orientation except survival, and had felt she needed to learn a set of rules that made no sense to her in order to do so. As she continued to talk about these painful themes she felt at times that I was torturing her. The crux of her thinking seemed to be that an abandoned child feels so overwhelmed with pain that eventually she no longer wants anyone to come back and make her aware of it; nonetheless, she acknowledged that when she could allow herself to make contact with me the pain did seem to be bearable.

Celia needed to ask to change an appointment time, something she rarely did, and at the prospect she became frozen with terror of impending attack. We talked about how she did not wish to be hurt but refused to bear the feelings which would serve as signals. I acknowledged that I too would hate people if I felt so helpless to deal with them as she did. Despite her denial I could tell from her darting glances and moving lips that she was becoming more psychotic, and she finally acknowledged paranoid thoughts (her coffee was poisoned, troops were mobilized against her in the neighboring yard), hallucinatory hostile screaming at me ("He's driving you crazy!") and racing thoughts. At the end of the hour Celia cautiously and fearfully asked to shake my hand, and I assented. Her hand literally shook with what I sensed was her oscillation between caring and hating, between making contact and pulling away, but she said it made her feel better.

Celia remained more floridly psychotic, with strong wishes to run away, and she said she thought it had to do with her dilemma about mother—her overwhelming rage if she continued with her accustomed selfless caretaking activity and her terror of retaliatory annihilation should she refuse to do so. She said going crazy was a terrible price to pay for not being able to say no. I pointed out it was also a poor way to say no. Her hallucinations warned her against me; she said I was most dangerous because she liked me. Finally, the conflict became more specific; she had been regularly driving mother to the hospital for her treatments and wished to say no but could not. She recalled a childhood incident where she had hidden from mother but mother had found her, banged her about, and told her if she saw her again she would cook her in the oven and eat her for dinner. In response to things like this Celia said she learned to count patterns in the linoleum or to "be up on the ceiling," far away. In our 579th hour Celia told me she had managed to tell mother that she could not see her for the foreseeable future, and mother was surprisingly accepting. This too enraged Celia for she felt it came much too late; she had no forgiveness in her heart, only hatred. As she told me this, her hands alternately embraced the cushion on the couch where she sat or became menacing fists, eloquently expressing her simultaneous wishes to hug and to hit. She felt blind rage and recalled that after mother left and no longer terrorized her, father was so indifferent and isolating of himself in the house that their pet birds literally died for lack of food; she then learned to hoard food as though she were a castaway in the jungle.

Once again Celia abruptly and impulsively decided to stop smoking. Our 583rd hour, prior to a long holiday weekend, was a poignant one. She felt alone, terrified (particularly at night), and in need of protection. She quietly sobbed and gasped, in a way reminiscent of an inconsolable infant. Over the ensuing weekend she wrote me a letter which she gave me the following hour. In one part she said,

"I would like to kill a lot of people, and they don't know it, but really I don't want to kill you, I wish I could see you right now, I wish I could give you a big hug and tell you how I feel, that I am so lonely and so tired and I can't sleep and I am so scared."

The next hour she was in a tense, paranoid state, near to being overwhelmed. She reported difficulty falling asleep and then waking in a state of terror, without dream content. She couldn't decide whether or not she wanted to be with me—nothing I said seemed to make a difference—and she left the session early. She brought letters she had written in the intervals between the next two therapy hours. In the first she commented on how the separation cries of her nursery school children for their mothers made her feel astonishment and rage:

"My god, all that sadness for 3 hours [the length of the nursery school day]— how I must have felt, how I feel now, utterly lost, no one there, and so angry I could wrench trees right out of the ground, throw cars like Tonka toys, murder people and not blink an eye. Taking away cigarettes is too much. . . . Cigarettes are my mother, the big tit."

In the next hour she elaborated the idea of loss of her cigarette-mother, and described her massive rage and her need to protect others from it by getting away from everyone. She wanted to shoot herself in the head, which meant eliminating her thoughts and feelings. Again she wrote a letter, telling me she had resumed smoking:

"It really does piss me off that the one thing I enjoy could kill me, but that is probably an important part of it . . . I know it won't be you that kills me, it is the feelings that I think will kill me, feeling good, safe, loving you, wanting to hug you and never leave, I think of you sitting in your chair and I feel warm inside and safe and so sad I can hardly bear it, like I could cry forever."

After a diatribe about having to separate from the security of the hospital she added what she thought my response would be:

"You talk about all these people and places not being reliable, but I am here and you don't take advantage of that and feel good here."

and she concluded, as her rejoinder to my imagined comment, "Well, I know." In the ensuing hour she admitted to feeling like a frightened little girl in need of comfort who has to function like an adult and take care of others. The smoking, she realized, satisfied an urge to suck and made it easier for her to go to sleep. She confided that she had purchased some sheets with figures of lambs on them.

Celia returned to memories of her adolescence, and wondered if she might have begun hallucinating the summer her father was dying, when she was sent abroad. In the next hour she remembered that summer, particularly how she would visit an old baker, to whom she became very attached, each morning. He had an endearing pet name for her, and she recalled wishing that he would adopt her. She told me a number of instances of his warmth and caring for her. I had a familiar sensation of surprise and mild disorientation learning of this hitherto unmentioned oasis of caring in her life. But the very next hour Celia informed me that she had listened to her tape recording of the hour and realized that what she told me was what she had wanted to believe, whereas in fact she had only run errands for the baker.

Subsequent discussion led to her lifelong sense of helplessness to effect change, and the belief that the only thing one can do with painful reality is to negate it and to say it isn't true or doesn't matter. Subsequent to this hour Celia learned that a hospital staff member who had been very important to her and with whom she still had contact would be leaving, and she raged at me, wanted me to shut up, and wanted to avoid emotional contact with me because I represented the reality of her feelings and needs. I remarked that it appeared she was trying to relive with me her relationship with mother: I was supposed to be inconspicuous and not call attention to the need part of her, and if I violated this commandment the mother part of her would attack me. We talked of her feeling of being lost and of her wish for me to keep trying to find her, even when she continued in counterpoint to try to remain lost. Celia recalled her terrifying mother, tall and wiry, "wired up" all the time. I recalled some of her delusional preoccupations with electricity and some of the near serious mistakes she had made during a period when she did wiring; she laughed and related this to her wish and fear to hold on, adding,

"If the voltage is high and you hold on with both hands the current will go through your heart and kill you."

At this time Celia also described the empathy she felt for the nursery school children and their need for hugging when hurt. She sobbed and expressed anger about the loss of the staff member, her mother's departure for her new home, and about necessary goodbyes with her little charges. To her surprise Celia felt better about herself and our relationship, she told me that she had been able to study successfully for exams and that she had found a better housing situation in which to live.

Celia's paternal grandmother, the only person in the family she felt a strong kinship to, sustained a massive heart attack and died. Celia would not believe it, and commenced hallucinating. She was simultaneously enraged at my failure to "find" her and make her feel (and at her success in detaching and making me drowsy), and at my representation of feelings of love and caring, which reminded her of the loss of her grandmother. She wanted to beat me up no matter what position I took, and she added,

"The biggest mistake I ever made was to start seeing you."

As we approached her feelings she literally made fists at me, which meant

"Touch me [emotionally] and I'll clobber you!"

Eventually Celia was able to grieve appropriately and even to share feelings and memories of grandmother with other members of the family. In the process she split her feeling self and the self that refused to feel, and projected the latter onto her family, being convinced family members would show no emotional response and would ridicule her if she did. In fact, things did not go according to her scenario, and she began to suspect that some of her family's nonresponsiveness around her might relate to her own distant, off-putting attitudes.

Now Celia had to cope not only with the death of her grandmother but with helping her mother move and with moving into a new place of her own, as well as with the reasons for and consequences of a sudden decision to quit her job (which she told me about after the fact in hour 606). In response to my questions about quitting her job she said she had elected not to discuss it with me because of her conviction that I would oppose her, a conviction that was part of a more general image she had of me as unsympathetic to her sufferings and not wanting her to have enough time to eat, sleep, or think, an image that enraged her. She wanted to have nothing to do with me. Soon I became sleepy and she raged at me about that until we both realized that she was again repeating with me her relationship with mother, with roles reversed.

As mother's move impended, Celia's rage seemed to crowd out everything else. It became painfully apparent that our relationship or her paranoia were her only outlets for her rage. Celia feared the consequences of her rage, including imagined retaliation. Again she blamed me for making her feel, but she was surprised to discover at the beginning of an hour, a time when she usually cursed and expressed wishes not to be with me, that she was glad to see me. Celia rapidly alternated between wishes to hug me and wishes to hit me which were associated with reflexive fist clenching, stroking of her fist, and demonstrating her right-cross. At times her anger was so threatening to her that she literally sat on her hands without realizing what she was doing. Wherever she looked in the office she was reminded of her mother and her rage; she came so close to picking up a small statue and hurling it at me that I moved it away from her. This left her quite confused; for a time she couldn't "locate" her anger at all.

Nonetheless, around the time mother moved to another state, Celia began intermittently reporting how much better she was. She was more genuinely interested in people and ideas, and both the subjects she was taking and her classmates at graduate school were sources of interest and caring. As I had come to expect, such declarations were usually followed by anger; suspiciousness, wishes to run, to disrupt, and to detach; and eventually by attribution of the detachment to me, followed by rage when her treatment of me got the better of me and I would become sleepy during her hour.

At the school where she did her student teaching as part of her studies, Celia became very invested in the children and was quite upset when vacations and separations arose. She remembered mother's return from the hospital for a holiday visit: Her parents quarreled and father literally threw mother out of the house. Celia realized in retrospect that she had experienced incredible rage and also terror that she too would be thrown out; now she was particularly struck by the realization that neither parent had seemed at all aware that the children might have been upset by this scene. Celia felt terribly lonely at holiday time, claimed she just wanted to be with me, and imagined being part of my family, but in fact she spent the therapy hour staring out the window and soothing herself by elaborating visual patterns she perceived.

Celia's preoccupation with the death of her houseplants, and her related feeling that everything, including herself, was dead, made her realize she was sad about mother's move to another state. With mother gone she didn't have to hide anymore, but since hiding was a way of being alive, she began to imagine things to hide from and developed numerous "mindless" activities to avoid thinking. She became even more sad when she realized that, as bad as the terror she had experienced with mother had been, it was better than awareness of being left all alone. Though she had not loved mother, there was a sense of security and predictability about their relationship. She had learned how to anticipate mother's disturbances and to cope with them, and she had liked watching mother pursue some of her interests and activities. Though it was hardly love, in some way she had been attached and anchored.

In our 627th hour Celia spontaneously decided she needed to begin to talk with me about sex, since she had wishes to have children of her own. Through memories of her many remarkably similar experiences with men she elaborated a scenario of performing fellatio while transforming her feelings of passivity and helplessness, with urges to vomit, to hit, and to bite off the penis, into a sense of mastery and control through learning to feel disengaged and superior, while inwardly belittling the man for being so excited while she was indifferent, without thought and feeling. As she talked Celia experienced these feelings and wishes, and she covered her mouth, made a fist, and kept her eyes closed as part of a magical wish not to see her memories. She realized that she had perceived male sexual excitement as loss of control and as insanity, and had imagined her "job" to be one of keeping men sane.

Coincident with telling me she wanted more of what other people seemed to have in their lives, two men—a former hospital staff member and another old friend—asked Celia out. She enacted with me cutting off her thoughts and her sentences and detaching herself. I felt sleepy. We talked of her wish to deal with her anxiety by disabling the world and tranquilizing men or putting us to sleep. The date with the former staff member proved most distressing because he took her to a sadomasochistic movie. She felt betrayed, mostly by me; I had made her vulnerable. I, in turn, wondered why she had been unable to say no. But the following hour (633rd) Celia described a very positive, emotionally meaningful lunch date with her other old friend.

During a discussion at school Celia surprised herself by passionately espousing a caring point of view during a class argument. During her therapy hour she talked about feeling much calmer and about having a positive sense of the future and of choices. At the end of the hour she realized that she had been reporting facts and not dealing with their relevance to our relationship. She squirmed with discomfort as she tried to find some way to thank me for helping her. At graduate school Celia began to have a mind of her own, to show increasing excitement about learning and to realize that she was valued by both teachers and fellow students. She began to develop an impassioned orientation toward teaching, believing that a teacher must take into account the student's personality and needs, as well as his cultural and family background. (This was to prove both positive and negative in the years to come insofar as Celia tended to split the caring part of herself and to enact it against projected hostility in the setting of her work as educator, whereas with me she characteristically and equally passionately expressed its counterpart and left me to hold the bag of caring, so to speak.)

After a phone conversation with mother in which heightened awareness of Celia's hatred led her to conclude that she was losing control, we discussed her concept of control as being nonreactive; I reminded her that her expertise in ignoring her feelings had not kept her sane, and suggested that there might be another kind of control—one based on knowledge of one's emotions and selective action based on this knowledge. With obvious reluctance Celia began to tell me how important I was to her, and how held and secure it made her feel to be listened to and attended to for the first time in her life. She admitted that she slept better at night after a therapy hour when she talked about upsetting things; this was a significant acknowledgment since she ordinarily spent so much effort trying to convince me that I was driving her crazy by encouraging her to feel things (and not infrequently succeeding in making me wonder whether I was fostering a regression). The 644th hour concluded with a joking interaction, which was becoming more common, in which she told me that in spite of her lifelong conviction that no one would ever "get a rise" out of her, I had succeeded in doing so. This was followed by simultaneous wishes to hit and to hug me and then an impassioned "I was awfully lucky!"

Celia laughed sadistically at the commencement of our next hour. This prefaced enacting and talking about her wish not to look at or talk to me and to destroy all meaning. She was angry and brandished her fist, but by the end of the hour she acknowledged she was acting this way out of fear of being closer to me. In the next hour Celia was paranoid and believed that danger might lurk in the corners of the room; then she realized the danger was from her sad feelings, and went on to talk about the painful isolation of her adolescence. For several hours we were unable to make much contact. She perceived me as cold and critical, and I perceived her as angry and dissatisfied. She brought in a problem related to school but, try as I might, none of my comments seemed of any consequence; increasingly, I sensed in myself the coldness and dissatisfaction she was noting. Then she was late because she could not recall the time of our appointment and would not call to ask. Finally, when I suggested she was refusing to make sense, her rage and disappointment surfaced, as well as an underlying fantasy of being utterly dependent on me and not having to make any effort, a fantasy in which I would pick her up, hold her, and take care of her. The sadness and rage related to how little, by comparison with her fantasy she was actually offered.

Again Celia felt better. But this time we began to focus on her internal inconsistency about bearing feelings and on her relative comfort with such undependability. In our 655th hour I introduced her to the concept of having a unified and consistent orientation or set of goals. This concept both puzzled and annoyed her, and then she added ruefully that her inconstancy was her way of being elusive so that no one could ever find her. On the other hand, she realized that her increasing integration, particularly of her rage, was responsible for the virtual cessation of the hallucinations and for an increasing sense of calmness. For the first time she began to ask herself why she was in therapy, and what her interests and goals might be.

Celia became increasingly concerned about her mental flip-flopping and constant self-contradiction; she said she wished to be involved with me more consistently but had no idea what that might involve or how to go about it. In a fit of perhaps misguided zeal, in the 662nd hour I suggested she might be mentally lazy. Celia took great offense at this and proceeded to disrupt all coherent thinking and conversing. She related her rage to father's admonitions that she do better at school and his total lack of effort to understand what her problems were or to help her, recalling as an example that no one had ever tried to help her learn to tell time. Laboriously she strove to separate her feelings about father from those about me, and then went on to make clear that she wanted me to search for her and find her without any effort on her part, except what was necessary to continue to elude me, and that she felt it was my job to compensate her for what she had missed in life. This was symbolized by her wish to be upstairs with me and my family rather than in my basement office, which symbolized concretely the basement of her house to which she had been consigned by father for so much of her childhood, and represented her emotional deprivation. I responded that I wanted her to have an "upstairs" in her life too but that until she allowed herself to be reached in a consistent way it would not be possible. She sobbed and ignored the box of tissues I offered her until I pointed out the repudiation involved, at which time she accepted it and said she did wish to have contact. After the hour she felt better. In the following session she described the part of her "in the back of [her] head" that laughed, ridiculed, and reduced everything to nothing and to unreality, a kind of "flexible skin" that kept after her, and she vowed that she wanted to change it.

Year Five

With the 665th hour Celia began her fifth year of treatment. At the start of our 666th hour I commented about her habitual gaze aversion from me and her custom of staring out the window behind her at the start of each hour. She admitted this was her way of controlling feelings by making them nonexistent. She went on to recall her childhood terror when mother wandered around randomly, talking crazily, and her efforts to hide both literally and by turning off feelings so that she would not antagonize mother. During the course of the discussion Celia became increasingly terrified and paranoid. In the next hour she reported our discussion of the previous hour had left her feeling "shell-shocked" but it was clear that, far from slipping further into psychosis, she found the propensity to do so more ego alien, and that she was aware of more of a wish to sit with her upset feelings and not run away. Although she remained detached and somewhat fragmented in her thoughts, chopping up words and sentences, she was clearly distressed by her behavior and its outcome, which she now perceived more clearly as intolerable loneliness. She talked about what she had learned from her mother, which was not what things meant and what to want but, rather, that the world was so unpredictable and threatening that to feel or want anything at all, or even to think clearly, was intolerably frustrating. It was apparent that an enormous struggle was going on within her, and she fantasized about my coming over to her and removing a tiny baby from within her and nurturing it; a part of her, she said, wanted to sit next to me and sob and yell. But she also recognized another part of her—a part that wanted to hit, withdraw, and retaliate. After more memories with the common feature of a total absence of any relatedness between her parents and between her parents and herself, Celia's flatness began to make me sleepy and to feel like a spectator; she was paying as little attention to me as had been paid to her, and there was nothing I could do to reach her.

Celia's birthday approached. She recalled how mother, who was obsessed with fear that the children might die, was unable to remember any of their birthdays. Her father had once built as a gift a swing that went out over a steep hill in their yard, which neighborhood parents considered so dangerous that they forbade their children to use it, and he had given her a balance beam, which he placed on the concrete garage floor, and encouraged her to use it. Celia began to absentmindedly pound on her knee as she spoke. On her birthday I gave her a card with the following inscription: "We all deserve the opportunity to be special to someone. I hope you won't let the misfortunes of your past imprison you so that you won't have yours." Her immediate response was a fragmented combination of tense laughter, sadness, anger, and relatively flat words of thanks. I had upset her expectation that I would not remember and that she would have to remind me. She told me how, with family members, she always had to remind them. Then they would do the right thing, albeit not out of feeling for her. Although this made her angry it became clear that she was more at home with such treatment than she was with getting attention; even as we spoke, the good feeling she had about our interchange was insidiously subverted by feelings of fear, entrapment, and anger.

Around the 680th hour Celia was able to articulate a growing sense that she was entitled to be treated well and cared about and to report that she experienced a more consistent feeling of anger when she was not. She realized that she was no longer as helpless and hopeless as she had been in childhood, for she was now capable of making situations more productive and satisfying by speaking up. Together we wondered whether she was capable of further intimacy or whether the best she could do was to be like a squirrel that gets a nut and then runs. In hour 686 Celia reported a nightmare in which she was with a female former patient who in fact had sent her a birthday card. The woman was wheelchair-bound, her hands and feet amputated, although, at times they grew back slightly. Celia was hugging her and trying to estimate just how much she was capable of learning to do. She realized that the wheelchair-bound person was herself, and that some of her difficulty of late had been over the impotent wish to respond positively to my card.

The concept of future was now a meaningful one, and Celia talked about her own plans to become a full-fledged teacher the following year. Though she did not seem able to get sustenance from it, she reported much feedback that she was doing very well at school and in her work. Although she spoke of her anger at my leaving for a week's vacation, which presaged my longer summer vacation, her manner was affectless and disengaged and I felt and therefore uttered no response. Before our last hour Celia went to a bar and got drunk, and in the final session she said she had felt rejected.

When I forgot that Celia and the analytic patient who followed her had switched appointments, and in consequence had my couch, which looks ordinary enough when I am not using it for analysis, set up for my analysand, the sight of it evoked in Celia a flood of memories about sex and her body, but mostly awareness of how completely she tended to deny the existence of both. I reminded her of her need to act dead or be invisible to avoid provoking mother, and this triggered some terrifying childhood memories of bathing with mother while mother shaved and of imagining mother would kill them both. Celia seemed increasingly shut off, without affect, and she fought with me over anything and everything. Thoughts of running away and of committing suicide preoccupied her. In her rather predictable pattern, she would only allow a bit of emotional contact just before the end of the hour, when in a sense, it was too late. In response to her deadness I became sleepy; her associations revealed that she was trying to torture me as she had felt tortured as a child so that I would learn I could do nothing right and would struggle to be invisible in terms of body and mind, while pretending to be present; what solace I might get would have to be in fantasy. She did this by doing what she imagined mother had done, by withholding all love, all the positive things about her life, and all interest in me as a real person. She laughed with ridicule as we discussed these things, and she expressed her generalized hatred of people. We talked about her chronically hunched-over posture in the office, which turned out to involve efforts to deny the existence of body and sexuality. She was literally unable to sit back; when she tried she felt dizzy and nauseated, with powerful sensations of terror that she would be attacked, ripped apart, and annihilated. She told me this was why she had never felt safe enough to wear skirts. The experience was concretely real to her, and not available for reflection.

In the face of these difficulties things continued to go well at graduate school. Celia received superb evaluations, even from teachers she was convinced disliked her. She even reported having fun with others on occasion, and she was more aware of not wanting to continue to be alone. I kept pointing out the split between her wishes and goals in life and her behavior with me. Celia recognized that, in treating me as her mother had treated her, she was destroying what was most important to her, and she said, plaintively, that while she would like to put lots of people to sleep, I was not one of them.

School came to an end and Celia was saddened; she had had a wonderful experience; fellow students and teachers alike were fond of her and thought of her as gifted and creative. She experienced a sense of catastrophic depression, a feeling out of keeping with the end of what had probably been the best year of her life and with what might more accurately have been viewed as a new beginning. When I questioned her about this she told me, with her ridiculing laugh, that nothing good lasted or was real. She said it was like a carpet rolling up behind her (or, as she put it on another occasion, she felt she was "constantly erasing things"). When I pressed her further about the catastrophic feeling she said it had begun to dawn on her, with much anger and sadness, that perhaps she was not an awful person or an unlovable child, and that perhaps she had been the victim of a terrible rip-off. In our 715th hour Celia said that she wanted to kill herself, that I had "set her up" by making her aware of caring and loneliness but she knew she couldn't have what she now wanted in life because she hated everyone and everything. She blamed me for everything and felt sorry for herself and cheated. She said she deserved better than to be sent back to live with mother after father died and believed that had finished her. At the end of this 716th hour she felt a bit better; she was not so hostile to me and, in characteristic fashion, because she had to leave and knew she could not get what she wanted, she experienced wishes to stay and to hug me.

Celia was unexpectedly offered an unusual and interesting summer job opportunity related to her schoolwork, one that would require her to live at some distance. Although it would coincide with my summer vacation, it would necessitate, beginning almost immediately, interrupting all but a couple of appointments for an additional month as well. Celia expected me to fight with her over her excited wish to take advantage of the opportunity, but I responded that a consequence of her being able to care more about her life was that she was now beginning to have choices and conflict involving positive alternatives, conflicts I could not resolve for her but would try to help her to resolve. We talked about the sense of entrapment she had had in so many situations as a child, where there seemed to be no choices, and we discussed the positive aspects of the job as well as her very mixed feelings about remaining and trying to be involved with me. She was both grateful and dismayed that I did not intervene and save her from having to choose. With some inner struggle she decided to accept the job, but she became detached from her feelings and from me once more; again I became sleepy.

In our 721st and last regular hour for the summer Celia was more present and caring, and despite her usual feeling of rage and disruptive sadistic laughter she told me that for the first time in her entire life she felt optimistic and excited, and had even purchased a dress to wear to a job interview. She was certain she now had enough control so that she would not become psychotic during the summer. We both looked upon this interchange with a certain skepticism, and realized that part of the reason she could allow herself this degree of closeness was because she now had a legitimate, nonpsychotic reason to get away. At the conclusion of the hour she shook my hand, expressed her gratitude to me for having "put up with" her, and said she would miss me. I remarked that she had had to put up with me as well and that it hadn't been easy, and with a brief burst of the now-familiar sadistic laughter she departed.

Celia did very well at her summer job, and she found her experiences with deprived and disturbed children emotionally meaningful. When we resumed our work after 2 months, in hour 725, she had begun her new full-time job. Although she erupted with rageful wishes to trash our work and our relationship and leave me the way she had felt left, now the caring part of her realized that it was not I who did the leaving at all but that, in fact, I was the consistent and stable partner in our dyad.

In the 730th hour Celia and I began to talk about the stalemate between the constructive and destructive parts of her. The constructive part, largely consisting of nurturant longings, seemed passive and magical. Through a combination of my attention and activity and her fantasy, she might imagine I was taking care of her. Passive fantasy had been her form of self-nurturance as a child, and she looked upon it as normal. Her active emotional investment seemed to involve rage, hatred of and aversion to people, and the wish not to be psychotic again. I noted the absence of active loving feelings, although perhaps these were more covertly expressed in her work. Celia sadly contrasted herself with a warm, open child in her class, but she promptly put this subject out of mind. At the end of a subsequent hour, which she admitted she was filling with "chit-chat" about school, I reminded her about the absence of active self-motivation, and she angrily expressed her wish that I do it for her. Moreover, Celia continued to confuse thinking and feeling, and their products, her new awareness of pain and distress, with unnecessary suffering and even craziness, and she held me responsible for this. This led to what I now thought of as the therapeutic paradox: I was to actively and constructively represent caring and to gratify her fantasy of being mothered, whereas she would subtly but equally actively represent rage, destroy everything, and revert to a state of psychic nothingness, which was her form of parenting herself.

Celia seldom recalled her dreams, but in the 738th hour she reported a nightmare. Her wish not to think about such things was reflected in the fact that she had not written it down afterward—because in her dream she had already done so! In her dream Celia observed a person of indeterminate sex who was wearing a plastic raincoat and who had set herself or himself on fire in a suicide attempt. There were crazy and suicidal people all around her who paid no attention and did not care. Eventually someone put out the fire. The victim, who was amazed to find out that she or he hadn't died, tried to pretend everything was fine, but two grommet eyes had burned holes in her or his side and it was evident that the coat had melted into the person's body. Celia could not or would not reflect on the dream other than to describe it as "awful" and "weird," though she accepted my suggestion that it was about herself. Finally she recalled a childhood incident of nearly drowning when mother's sailboat tipped over, throwing her in the water with the sail on top of her; because she had followed mother's instructions and had worn a life preserver, she was trapped beneath the sail and couldn't get out. This incident made a lasting impression on her. We explored the dream over the next several therapy hours and elaborated from it Celia's three positions: a detached but lamenting observer of her own self-destruction; a part of her that hated being human, tried to extinguish thinking and feeling, and hated me for representing these things; and a part of her that longed for caring but would not care actively and wanted to believe that I was magically taking care of her.

Celia witnessed a serious auto accident and imagined that if she were the victim she would maintain to the rescuers that she was fine so they would not know that her legs were cut off; she added that she had to present such a "nothing is the matter" front in order to function normally at work. In subsequent hours Celia told me how totally she had formerly denied that anything was the matter, and how she had come to accept her problems in pieces (for example, that she hallucinated) but that she now saw the bigger picture of how crazy she was and that it horrified her. In her work she no longer strove to present a perfect facade but shared her problems more honestly with others, and when she had to speak before a group she focused for reassurance on someone who had a warm smile and showed clear interest in her, instead of joining her gaze with the most vacant and hostile members of the audience, as she once would have done.

Celia was furious at my penchant for pointing out what she already knew she did to avoid closeness, rather than being empathic with her loneliness and suffering. I noted that the angry affect, so long absent from her flat voice even when she expressed rage, was becoming perceptible. As I could see some truth in her observation, I attempted to be more empathic with the pain she told me about, but she attacked and found fault with my every effort. Finally, when she heard a caring tone in my voice, her head "exploded" and she realized that the empathic barrier was not in me but in herself. Over the subsequent 5 or so weeks Celia showed novel and notable signs of spontaneous movement and affect and, with them, associations clarifying just how much effort she ordinarily expended in playing dead. She sat a bit closer to me in the room, spontaneously clapped her hands when she said something, and wanted to examine an object of interest in the office. At times she even sat back and relaxed, and once, in an angry voice, she said, "Fuck you!" All these relatively unguarded gestures, as well as her increasing affect, terrified her; she feared she would be attacked. But she realized that it was she who had been systematically attacking everything both of us did or said as wrong, and that what really frightened her was the possibility that, if she moved closer in response to her wishes to hug me, *she* might attack *me*. I suggested that she required us both to be dead, with no movement, and that while she was relatively conscious of the dead role she had elected to play with mother in order to survive, she was less aware of how she terrorized herself into deadness and tried to do the same to me, as her mother had done to her. In response she elaborated wishes to drive me crazy, such as commanding me to "turn around in your chair, asshole!" and then making noises to frighten me.

At the end of the 750th hour Celia remarked how she was generally more aware now of bodily sensations of heat and cold, pain, and physical illness. She made the surprising revelation that there were now four men she liked. The school where she worked was coming to seem like a good home to her. When Celia experienced her longing for physical affection she felt like a child and wanted to cry, though she would not allow herself to do so. In the 769th hour I noted how restless her hands appeared, and she acknowledged wishes to touch me. She struggled to face me more directly as we talked, but this prompted feelings that she would be forced to talk about sex. After much discussion we concluded that this idea reflected her adolescent belief that in order to get any semblance of affection she was forced to perform sexually. I commented that it was affection and not sexual interest that we were talking about. The following hour she perceived me as a crazy man, out of control of my sexuality and sadism and not to be trusted, and she felt rage. Soon it became clear that this was a projection of her own wishes to abuse and hit me, and that she was chopping up her thoughts. She would not talk about the previous hour, and when she finally did, it turned out that she had forgotten all the parts related to affection, and had concluded that I had disrupted our relationship by prematurely forcing the subject of sex on her. This realization made her aware that it was easier for her to deal with abuse than affection; she recalled so little experience with the latter that, as a child, she hadn't known what to do with a stuffed animal or a doll.

Celia kept an appointment even though she was quite ill. With her sadistic laugh she repeated the familiar idea that she was being strong. I recast this idea as equating strength with being destructive to herself as a feeling human being. In subsequent hours, as her illness continued, Celia graphically portrayed her poor self-care in terms of her failure to sleep, eat, and when ill, take her temperature, and take medication. She was enraged that there was no one to care for her and equally enraged that she had needs, which reminded her of her hopeless feelings as a child and of the possibility of losing control, showing her needs, and inviting mother's wrath on herself. I was very concrete with her about the basic things she needed to do in each coming day to take care of herself. She feared she would have a coughing spell in the office and the issue of needing some water might arise; she felt she would die were this to happen, but also wished it would happen. She recalled hospital patients who pestered their doctor so insistently that the doctor rejected them. Quite uncharacteristically she sat back in her chair and relaxed, then, as she suddenly realized what she had done, her perception of reality changed, objects seemed to be floating, and she felt terrified, convinced that mother was lurking in the room.

In our 778th hour Celia told me the following dream which, again, she had tried first to forget and then to dismiss as "weird": A person was trying to construct a human being who would become the person's proxy or facade, by killing others, removing their vertebrae, and stringing all the vertebrae together. Through some form of X-ray or analysis the fraud was discovered. After much effort to deny that the dream had meaning, Celia realized that it represented her attempt to kill off her humanness and construct a facade.

At Thanksgiving Celia experienced rage after she acted as though she had no needs; made a feast for a large group, some of whom were strangers; and was not called by any of her family. She recalled worse Thanksgivings on skid row, particularly one when she had worked until 2 A.M. in a bar and had then become so paranoid that she could not even enter her apartment to sleep but had gone into a back alley, where she slept in the rain, under a shelter, with the garbage cans.

Again I had the feeling that nothing I did was helpful to Celia. She acted angry, destructive, and complaining no matter what position I took. In hour

783 she reported a dream in which she had carefully grown tomatoes in a rich soil; they flourished, but there were no blossoms. When she suddenly realized that they would blossom only in bad soil, she began to throw them away. Associations were to her devaluation of feelings, needs, and caring. We talked about how she would not allow even her basic needs to be met, much less the "flowers" or the "fruit." Presently I saw her absentmindedly and viciously pinching and squeezing her arm and called her attention to it. She was disquieted to learn that she had really hurt herself. She found this session disturbing and wondered how she could possibly deal with the massive contradictions she now perceived in herself. I commented that since she tended to attack whatever position I might take, I ended up feeling that she was trying to drive me crazy, as she had been; first I was expected to overlook gross contradictions as though they did not exist, I told her, but since even that would not spare me from her attack, my ultimate solution (beyond splitting, I thought to myself) would have to be to withdraw into myself. Celia commented, "You don't even have the luxury of showing that you are crazy," which, in turn, made me realize that to avoid further attack I would have to put on a facade, as she had done, and pretend everything was fine. Fortunately Celia had a wry sense of humor, and we had acquired a certain capacity to look with this perspective on her behavior.

Celia envisioned scenarios of "losing control" with me and crying or raging, but instead she continued to deaden herself. She remarked that she was frequently mistaken for a younger person because of her lack of affect, manifested by a kind of childlike voice and an unlined face (because she had never shown emotion). She longed to sit with me and cry for days on end, until she fell asleep, but she was terrified that if she cried she might never be able to leave the office and that if she raged she might assault me.

Celia had planned a holiday trip abroad with a friend. She gave me a small gift with a card before leaving and shook my hand, demonstrating the violent shaking I now associated with the tension of oscillating between holding on and breaking off. At the beginning of the separation Celia had the first dream she could recall that seemed to include me, which she told me on her return 10 days later (in our 794th hour). She was in my office, and there was a big window, against which lay a monstrous dead whale. It seemed normal to her that it be there, until my teenage daughter, a lively person, came along and Celia asked her what the whale looked like from outside. Then Celia saw me approach from another building and feared I would get angry at my daughter for talking to her. She readily related the dream to her deadness identity and to a childhood memory of seeing people pick apart a dead whale that had washed up on the beach. The dead whale became an important therapy metaphor for the state of being she continued to strive to achieve.

Once again Celia was flooded with memories from adolescence, with the theme of having been pawed, poked, raped, drugged, used in a variety of ways, with her own passive acquiescence, and treated like a nonfeeling, nonhuman object. Though our talk was punctuated by Celia's brief laugher and her idea that she was superior to everyone and everything because she had been "ca-pable" of not feeling the hurt, such a construction was less and less believable to her, and she experienced belated revulsion, fear, and rage. We concluded that she had a long "hit list" of people who had abused her. In the 811th hour she reported nightmares of trucks going in the wrong direction on freeways, and for the first time she herself made the connection—which for years I had been suggesting—between her utter lack of concern when being used and assaulted and her enormous paranoid fear of attack under safe circumstances. This was not the only integrative sign this hour: She said that she had the urge to punch me but at the same time was aware of liking me.

In subsequent hours Celia talked about her goals—her summer school plans, which focused both on education and on meeting more people; her wishes to first become a good teacher and eventually to expand her career in education beyond the classroom; and her hopes to have children of her own. This last she admitted with much reluctance, because she was aware of the problems involved, namely, finding a husband who would not abuse her, allowing herself to be close to him, and, even more fundamental, talking with me about the related issues which she rarely allowed herself even to think about. She had difficulty sleeping—but not for the familiar reason that she was haunted by hallucinations and delusions; rather, her insomnia was due to the fact that she worried about the real problems in her life. In the context of telling me this Celia revealed that her usual bedtime procedure had been to distract herself from her thoughts and feelings, usually with a book, and then gradually to become paranoid and preoccupied with efforts to construct some linkage between the sights and sounds out there.

With great difficulty Celia took the unprecedented step of telling her old-est, and perhaps only, male friend that she cared about him. She was initially crushed and subsequently enraged by his revelation that he did not reciprocate the feeling. She fled to a poker hangout where she proceeded to beat every man she could find (she had become a remarkable card player during her stays on skid rows). Celia's wishes to be a mature adult woman and her dealings with pubescent female students who were interested in boys and sex led her to make some experimental efforts to masturbate; she found the activity not only pleas-ureless but an unwelcome reminder that she had a body. When her best friend took a long trip Celia feared becoming crazy in response to her loneliness.

In hour 822 Celia reported a nightmare: She was having fun shopping in a store with her two dogs and talking to some school acquaintances, but P, a psychotic acquaintance from the hospital, told her that there was a dangerous plot against her and that she should leave. Then she was home, trying to call me, but the line was dead, having been cut. A man came to the door but the dogs did not bark. Despite her efforts to repel him he threw her on the floor and threw a powder on her that was going to kill her. The dream seemed so real to her that she had difficulty writing it down upon waking, and this heralded a period of continuing confusion on her part about whether she was in danger of being attacked or of becoming paranoid. In her interactions with mother, small acts of self-assertion resulted in alternating fears that mother would retaliate and paranoid convictions that mother was actually about to come and kill her. It was as though she were discovering painful feelings (sadness, anger, fear, bodily pain, aloneness) for the first time. She was more aware of menstrual cramps. She wanted to scream. By her former standards she was a "wimp." She wanted to run from the feelings but realized she would just be running to paranoia. In our 829th hour, at the end of the fifth year of our work, Celia was not only unaware of her feelings but was not sure if there was a wall behind her, could not sense the passage of time, and claimed that her voice sounded unreal. She realized she was fearful of the Scylla of feelings and the Charybdis of psychosis. Her customary angry response that I did not understand something she told me, something that she evidently thought was emotionally important but that she had presented without affect or urgency, was now tempered by awareness of her inadequate command of expressive language and affect.

Year Six

Celia's growing satisfaction in mothering her school children was associated with acutely painful thoughts about being motherless herself. She marveled at how she could have survived without ever being hugged. She realized that I served some of the mothering function but that she fought me off with what she referred to as her "mental diaphragm." Because she could not face a lonely Saturday night she went to a neighborhood bar and ended up going home with a neighbor and sleeping with him. Although the sex was pleasureless he was a kindly man, they talked, and Celia felt a degree of security and comfort from this contact. But the next day she felt rage at me because our bond seemed to be the only thing keeping her from running off and perhaps committing suicide. At a party at the home of one of her siblings she uncharacteristically shunned her mother out of anger, and was disturbed to realize that mother did not even seem to care enough to attack her in retaliation (father, at least, would have gotten angry at her). In realizing that was the only form of caring she knew, Celia had a new understanding of why mother's departure in her childhood had been followed by her quest after harmful people and situations. She imagined not coming to her therapy hour, killing herself, and sending a pretend self; we concluded that this, in a sense, was what she had actually done to survive as a child. When she told me she had not realized therapy would hurt so much, I responded that part of coming alive was experiencing the pain that had made her wish to be dead.

Memories of childhood longing to be held were followed by a recollection of putting her fingerprints on everything in her room with mascara, which she now concluded was a sad effort to find her boundaries and a sense of identity. She recalled two pleasurable memories: one of a maid showing her how to wash behind the ears at age 10 and the other of splashing pleasurably in the tub earlier in childhood. But in the latter instance she heard mother coming, realized there was water on the floor, and became terrified. She could recall nothing more. But her next associations, accompanied by obvious distress, were to having been given a doll of her own, hating it, and taking it to the tub and "drowning" it. In the subsequent 837th hour she continued to try to recall more about the bathtub incident; instead, her head became numb, she began to laugh and to have paranoid thoughts, and she told me of how terrified she had been of the movie *Jaws*. She recalled being so terrified as a child that she literally could not move from her bed and felt she did not know where the walls of the room were; she would count repeatedly to the number 8 in an effort to be secure.

When Celia's students and another teacher celebrated her birthday she tried to denigrate the experience. As she anticipated a birthday dinner with her family with feelings of envy related to their marriages and children and resentment that they did not seem aware of her feelings of deprivation, I commented that she never let anyone know who she was or what she wanted—and was not at all consistent about it herself. She felt it was too late for her, and wishes to kill herself alternated with fears of dying in an accident; however, she also experienced marked dissatisfaction with herself for not being more assertive of her needs. She feared her family would not only fail to comprehend but would get angry at her.

In the next hour (the 843rd) she was furious with me for what I had "forced her into." She had been superficial with the family at dinner but at the end had gotten uncharacteristically upset and had tried to leave abruptly. A brother had insisted on coming with her, and she had burst into tears, initiating a long conversation during which they shared a sense of mistrust of others and the belief that the ability to be detached and unfeeling represented control. Her brother had sympathized with her and hugged her. Even though Celia knew I hadn't done anything "bad" to her she angrily blamed me for all of this. Soon thereafter she reported a nightmare in which she entrusted the care of her students to someone else and went off and literally forgot their existence. When she remembered them and returned, two teachers opened the door and their expression made her realize that something terrible had happened to one of the students. Celia concluded her recitation of the dream by commenting that she just wanted to get drunk and let happen to her whatever might. I responded that I knew what had happened to the student: Since it had been unbearable for her to be left alone she had gone and gotten herself beaten into unconsciousness. Celia laughed and said that it was all right to be unconscious for a while, but she added that she was frightened that she might be going crazy.

In fact, Celia was psychotic at the start of hour 845. She had called me the previous night to inform me that an intruder was about to come get her, and that if she didn't show up for her appointment I should realize it wasn't because she didn't want to. With me she was paranoid but aware of it; she felt that someone was sneaking up on her, perhaps with a gun. As I encouraged her to share her feelings she began to own her rage and a remarkable transformation occurred: She felt saner. She reported rage and nausea over several incidents at school that had made her conscious of the distinction between good and bad mothering, particularly one in which her principal wanted to tone down a letter she was writing to the "bad" mother of one of her students. She was furious I had not given her a birthday card this year, as I had the last. I commented that she had used her mother's assault on her thoughts and feelings as a kind of mothering, a surcease from emotional pain, and that she now had to make a choice between the two mothers she ran back and forth between—the mother of attention to thoughts and feelings, even very painful ones, and the mother of nirvana, or destruction of her mind.

Celia's remaining (maternal) grandmother died suddenly. She was described as an antisocial recluse, liked by no one, who had lived alone with an accumulation of detritus. Celia felt sympathy for her mother, who was quite upset. Although she spoke in an emotionless, obfuscating manner, she told me she had been thinking that she didn't want to be crazy like those two. She said she could not stand to be alone and sad; I countered that she could not stand to be with someone else and sad. She imagined me with my arm around her, comforting her, but remarked that it would not make her feel better for she would not be able to stand it! Hatred of me, which readily resolved itself into hatred of my attentions and the feelings they elicited, predominated. Celia couldn't comprehend why I continued to pay attention to her when she showed so little sign of change, but at times she told me how important it was to her that I did.

An incident at school involving two delinquent older boys who were nearly out of control reminded her again of her years of being used and abused by men. When once again she talked about that activity as being sexual, I commented that perhaps it was sexual in the obvious physical sense but that its meaning had involved her relationship with her mother, an observation with which she agreed. She recalled her emptiness in childhood when mother left, and her redoubled efforts to preoccupy herself with numbers and patterns, and she surmised that, had she not become delinquent, she might have been even crazier than she ended up being, that, in other words, her delinquency was a somewhat successful effort to find mother again.

Over the course of the next 5 or so weeks, beginning with hour 857, Celia told me not only that she experienced pleasure in teaching but that her reputation with other faculty and with parents as a caring, creative, innovative teacher was growing. When the school year ended, those with whom she had been involved—students, their parents, and other teachers—were obviously grateful to her and very sad to part from her, and despite her tendency to minimize such occurrences, it was clear that Celia took much pleasure from her success. When she was a victim first of a man's negligence in an minor auto accident, and then of his efforts to evade responsibility and blame her, she defended herself actively and vigorously: however, she subsequently described this behavior as "losing it."

For the most part, the 3 months that included the conclusion of the school year and anticipation of my summer vacation were a long stalemate in which

Celia claimed she wanted it one way (home, caring, relationships) because she was so sad and lonely but acted the opposite (angry refusal to relate or to deal with feelings). We made some headway on her difficulty with expressive English, learning during a period of rage that she had long ago decided to speak pseudo-English, whereby nothing important was to be put into words and words themselves were to be used only for purposes of deception. At one point, in an effort to stimulate affect and thereby change the rigid ways she related to me, Celia decided to try to play checkers with me, despite merciless self-ridicule when she brought in the paraphrenalia. To her surprise she felt very good while playing, but when she was reminded, by contrast, of her childhood deprivations, she first "spaced out" and then went out and got drunk, and would not bring the checkers again.

Celia experienced some minor disappointments and rejections, and I had minor hand surgery, which left me with a cast for about 10 days. Celia was very upset, having been reminded of her parents' various illnesses and departures, and she wrote me a letter in which she tried to be genuine about her mental state (rather than to simulate precocious knowledge she did not feel or believe as she had done in other letters), even though the resulting self-contradictions were deeply disturbing to her for they showed her just how crazy she was. Among other things she said, in that letter:

"You shouldn't bother [with me] and should take a pain killer and sleep or at least not have to deal with me. . . . You know I do hear you and I feel I am being attacked because it is not too pleasant what you are saying. And you are right. But I just want to tell you to go to hell and take your damn caring with you because I want to blast everyone to hell especially someone who cares. . . . No one else notices when I attempt to blast them to hell because they don't care. . . . It is becoming clear what I want, what I don't want, what I didn't get, and what I need to do to clear up all the confusion. That clarity makes me more angry and resistant. I AM SO ANGRY it scares the hell out of me . . . that I might actually run into all those cars, throw something at you, kill myself . . . kill someone over a damn dryer at the laundromat [referring to an incident in which she had stood up for herself]."

With my encouragement Celia tried again to tape-record her sessions in order to help her reflect on her contradictions (she had not been able to sustain her earlier effort to do so), but she openly expressed wishes to be crazy, and to avoid thinking, feeling, remembering, and laughed derisively about these things. She kept "forgetting" either to bring the machine or to listen to the tapes. Finally, I pointed out (in the 876th hour) that she was making me feel as she must feel, that the only choices were unmitigated and endless suffering, anger, aloneness, and misery, or else some form of escape, physical or mental. This upset her and led her to try once again to clarify my importance to her, which she was amazed I did not seem to know. I remarked that I was important to her in a way that left me feeling entrapped in badness and hostility, as she had been. Our discussion made a considerable impression on her, and Celia became more aware that she seemed to want me to feel as she had felt as a child. She then dreamed that someone killed her brother, cooked his appendix, and gave it to her to eat as though this were normal; in the dream she was terribly upset, screamed, and then awoke. Although she attempted to maintain that the dream was meaningless, it turned out that the brother image represented things she liked and valued in her life, whereas her cannibalism represented the killing of caring; it was the part of her that was upset by my comments of the last hour that was shocked and screamed when she was given his appendix to eat. Nonetheless, there continued to be associations to her efforts to torture and reject me, since I was the only person who had ever cared enough to afford her the opportunity. Once again she feared that if things were different and she "really" depended on me, she might, as she put it, "fall apart," or "lose control," and punch me or throw things at me or else cry forever and never want me to leave.

In the 2 therapy hours before my weeklong vacation Celia was distant and disorganized, laughed inappropriately, caused her tape recorder to malfunction, projected extensively (would I speak to her, she asked, so she could know if I was here?), and was hallucinating again. Now she was much more aware that the hallucinating represented her rage; she heard cursing voices that told her to leave, and then turned on her when she confided their content to me. As we discussed the targets of her rage—her thinking, feeling, and caring, and the loneliness that would ensue when I left and she lost any touch with these elements of herself which she assigned to me—she pulled herself together a bit, and said, somewhat to my dismay, that she would hold herself together for my sake, so that she would not ruin my vacation; I said it was regrettable that she did not feel able to care on her own behalf.

While I was gone Celia used alcohol and marijuana in what I interpreted as self-medication, but she also struggled constructively, cleaning her apartment and preparing for a course. Although she picked up a man in a bar, she realized for the first time in her life that she had a choice of what to do next. Instead of sleeping with him, she simply dated him on two successive nights. In our 884th hour, after she had thought through my comments about her efforts at self-medication, she requested medication and I started her on 10 mg loxapine, as needed. There was a gradual transition over the next hours from a state of deadness—in the presence of which I had to struggle to remain wakeful, and in which she was confused and self-contradictory, unable to think or to finish a sentence—to a position of cessation of hallucinations and resumption of splitting. Celia began hour 888 by informing me with a worried, upset facial expression that she was really enjoying both her work and her courses. When I remarked on her discrepant expression, two parts emerged: the caring part, which did not want to be psychotic, wanted to relate to me, and was excited about her work, and the depressed and suicidal part, which was infuriated and felt "messed up" because she had stopped hallucinating and was once again experiencing caring feelings. Because she held me responsible for the "messing up," I clarified that, though I would be sad if she opted for psychosis and against using her human potential, I was not so much invested in taking sides in her internal struggle as I was in helping her to become more integrated and to be able to make a choice.

My summer vacation approached. Again we discussed what it was Celia wanted of me, and finally she concluded that she just wanted to have me around and to hear me talk—but did not necessarily want to have to listen to the content. I said it sounded as though she might like me to read her a bedtime story. In response she became very sad and said she wanted to cry, but of course she could not permit this. Next hour she forgot her tape recorder (again) but commented that she had been moved by our discussion of yesterday and that clarification of her wish to be read to made her aware of a plethora of painful feelings she had hardly been aware of in her childhood and did not want to face now. She broke off contact with me, and eventually I picked up the paper and read (to myself), an action that seemed satisfactory to her. After a long hiatus she told me that she had seen the Hitchcock movie *The Birds* the previous night and that it had reminded her of seeing it with her mother at age 6 or 7 and running from the room in terror. Mother did not bother to follow her.

As the long vacation separation approached, Celia reproached me for leaving, saying, "Look who you're leaving me with!"—a reference to the destructive, hateful part of herself, which she now more clearly recognized was intermittently represented in her hallucinations. And she added the following, as though speaking to someone else and in a manner she herself found "weird": "I'm going to make her suffer during the month!" She could now dramatize the struggle between the needy and the mocking angry parts of herself. This confused her; it had been simpler when she "knew" where the enemy was. I pointed out that she was holding tight to an internalized mother.

Our last hour was emotionally moving. Celia brought me a gift. She had come through a severe storm, and she talked of the strange sensation of making herself drive carefully because she cared about seeing me. She talked about her enthusiasm for a writing class she was taking, as well as about the esteem in which she was held by her teacher and classmates. But there were disquieting elements, particularly her mocking editorial laughter. I wondered if she was allowed to be more positive because the angry separating elements were now being enacted by our forthcoming separation. At the end of the hour she wanted to shake my hand and wondered if I objected; I responded that it was she who did.

Before our 896th reunion hour in the fall, Celia felt terrified and wanted to run away. She anticipated encountering anger and critical disapproval from me. Nonetheless, she told me how constructive her month had been: She had purchased a house of her own in a safe neighborhood, found a good job, and kept a positive sense of me within her, a caring presence that helped her make good decisions. The hostility she anticipated from me at the beginning of the hour turned out to be her own rage that she had allowed an alien internal presence to be more important than the rageful hallucinatory one. In the 900th and 901st hours it was clear that Celia was bringing a thoughtful, innovative, active and assertive self to her work and was experiencing excitement and pleasure there, as well as in contemplating the furnishing of her new house. By contrast she realized how unfocused she hitherto had been in her life. She kept forgetting to bring me her new address and phone number and neglected to furnish the new house. Her sarcastic editorial laugh pealed when I noted these things. We talked then about her repudiation of her human needs and her need instead to deprive herself and to suffer; once again she recalled how much her relationship with her mother and her self-control had been predicated on eradicating any signs of cognitive and emotional life within herself. She remembered early childhood efforts to "separate" from her terrifying mother in winter by building snow houses and barricading herself in them, shivering, but believing she was secure. As she proceeded, relatively unaware, to talk about her belief that "[her] children" required a pleasant learning environment and attention to their individual feelings and needs, I pointed out her need to live in environments that were not as good as the average prison, and how she seemed to continue to try to educate herself to survive with a terrifying, threatening, depriving mother. Celia managed to miss three of her hours the following week and to be late for the fourth, although she was aware that refusal to think and feel or have anything to do with others would lead to death or permanent insanity. She raged at me and talked about the curse of knowledge. When I commented about how she managed to deflect the rage from mother to me, she responded that she had talked to mother only yesterday, and added matter-of-factly that she could not feel or think in mother's presence. Celia commented that when she tried to recall mother's ashtray-throwing incident (when Celia was hospitalized during her second year of therapy with me) she ended up feeling angry at the hospital, not at mother.

Our 908th hour was more positive, and it was a mystery why until we recalled how many of her recent therapy hours Celia had made herself miss. She showed interest in my clothing and eye color, and she talked of wishes to touch my face to see if I was real, dismissing these as "crazy." Her wishes terrified her and she recalled submitting to mother's embraces, not knowing when they would end and fearing to object lest mother attack her. It struck her that a deeper component of this fear of expressing her objection to mother's embrace was that mother would not be upset at all if she did object, for she really didn't care about her.

Celia talked about her conflict between the wish to be messy and itinerant, without roots, and her wish to furnish and be at home in her new house. She had purchased a lovely dining table, but she feared using it lest she harm it. She dreamed that she had spilled coffee on the table and that, in order to avoid a contrast between the marred area and the rest of the tabletop, she rubbed coffee all over it and finally hacked it to pieces. She went on to talk of her belief that to care is crazy, and just exposes one to loss.

Celia talked about her struggle to communicate caring to a psychotic boy in one of her classes, a child who avoided emotional contact and was extra-ordinarily hostile. I remarked that she was talking of the two sides of herself, and her associations were to a belief that she would have to be on guard against wearing two mismatched shoes to a forthcoming parent's meeting, and to her despair about dealing with what seemed to be two equally mismatched parts of her self, parts totally unconnected by dialogue or compromise; so that she "was" either one or the other. In distress Celia remarked that she increasingly felt a sense of fear at being alone with a dangerous person—herself. I said I could readily understand. To help her objectify and differentiate, I suggested that she try to find names for the two parts of her self and that she try sitting in different chairs in the office when talking from each position; although her response to my suggestion, as to everything, was sporadic and temporary, this nonetheless seemed to help her to think about herself more. She called the two parts "black" and "red", and I prefaced them with *Ms.* when addressing her. Over the next 5 weeks or so we elaborated the characteristics of each persona. Ms. Black, the psychotic part, proved secretive. Celia still turned away from me from time, to time and she muttered or swore under her breath and let name-calling thoughts race in her head without reporting them. Ms. Black, who was thoughtless, ignorant, rigid, hateful, and destructive, possessed a noncommunicative vocabulary limited to name-calling. After participating for a while in this discussion Celia began to panic and said that I did not understand, that she would punish herself for this conversation once she got herself alone. Next hour she tried to tell me she had been destroyed by the conversation, but when I asked her to elaborate it turned out that, despite a familiar urge to get in her car and drive to a distant city, she had been more self-aware than usual and more frightened of herself rather than of delusional dangers. I pointed out that the wish to flee was a concrete manifestation and enactment of how she fragmented herself and alienated herself from people and from her mind. Celia felt like crying, and responded by remembering (and/or reconstructing) how much pain she was in as a child and how, in response, she had exercised the only power she had to attack the cause of the problem, namely, her self-awareness and connectedness to others.

In our 918th hour Celia professed that I was torturing and confusing her and that things were getting worse, but again, detailed examination of her life showed no evidence in support of her claim. In fact, during this time Celia continued to tell me stories about her teaching that clearly indicated both her caring and her considerable success in her work. Then she reported a nightmare: Her house was burning down; she walked down a dark, empty street with burns on her feet; but she did not seem to care about any of it and had no feeling. On waking, Celia was very distressed about the absence of feeling in the dream. With much hostility toward thinking further, and with derisive comments that I was "playing shrink" when I questioned her, she reported that she had made biscuits and tea as a treat for herself earlier in the evening. Somehow she had managed to oversalt the biscuits (she was, in fact, a talented cook), and then, not having pot holders, she had burned her hands slightly in removing them from the oven. She thought about Joan of Arc burning at the stake and hallucinating, and she realized that a friend had been reading to her from Shaw's play only several days before.

Celia was very upset about the stalemate between the parts of herself. She said she was falling apart and accused me of doing nothing. At the same time she remarked how she had avoided writing down her latest nightmare even though she had left pen and paper by her bedside. She was recurrently late to her appointments, and during therapy we would periodically become aware that she was twisting her fingers as though she was trying to break them. The caring part, which she referred to as "wimp," felt alone and in need of my help. She was frightened of herself, and did not seem to know how to fight back. I responded that if she were a child and I were present while she was being tormented by a madwoman I would certainly try to help, but now that the drama was so clearly within the confines of her adult self there was little I could do other than make her aware of it. Celia was very angry at me, full of pessimism and despair, and she talked of cutting the frequency of our appointments. But, surprisingly, in the subsequent hour she reported feeling a good deal better because she had allowed some contact between us and had assimilated some of my empathy and understanding. She added that my helping her to be clearer about the two parts of her gave her more of a sense of control. I pointed out that she usually conveyed the opposite message, that self-awareness and my role in promoting it were destroying her. She then told me of a dream in which we were traveling together in a car; I was driving and she was shifting the gears while I put in the clutch.

In her usual self-effacing style Celia reported pride in her accomplishments at school and praise from the principal who had observed her at work, and she then proceeded to begin attacking herself, claiming she had done terribly. She said that she was pleased with therapy of late, that she was shaken up by it but that it was helpful. Then Celia began to deaden herself, to devalue everything, and to attempt to convince me that she was going crazy. When I made some exclamation after she told me that she hated "shrinks" and that I was a fool, she said she didn't think that at all, and then proceeded absentmindedly to whip a broken rubber band violently against the back of her hand. When I called attention to what she was doing she recalled how, years ago, she would heat knives on the stove and methodically burn her hands with them! These oscillations continued, and when they centered on me Celia began to express increasing horror at Ms. Black, even criticizing herself for wanting to call me names; I had hitherto rarely heard this deployment of her critical faculties against her self-destructive part. She called this aspect of herself "mean" and "Neanderthal," but she felt frightened of opposing the hostile, destructive part of herself, just as she must have feared standing up to her mother. Then after this unusual reversal of name-calling she told me she felt that her mind was exploding and her thoughts were flying apart, and she was barely able to speak. I found myself increasingly confused about how to address Celia in terms of instrumentality; I felt as though I in fact needed to choose which of two people I was going to speak to, and I shared my perplexity aloud with her. Who was doing what to whom? Which was Celia? Should I, for example, say "You came late in order to propitiate the Neanderthal" or "You punished the needy part by being late"?

In the 927th hour, after some discussion of her teaching, Celia wanted to know if I taught too, and her wondering launched a somewhat surprising historical overview of our relationship; however, she always stopped just short of drawing conclusions, and once interrupted to ridicule what she had said. She recalled how disturbed she had been, how she would not let anyone get to know her, and how bent she had been on tricking people. She commented on my specialness to her, and on how persistent and reliable I had been, neither frightened of her (as she believed others had been) nor pretending I had all the answers (though sometimes she had wished me to), knowing just how hard to push her and when to wait. Not surprisingly, our next hour was much more chaotic. Celia had dreamed that she and I had a "normal" relationship and a relaxed, sane conversation in which she had a good time and there was no self-contradiction. She would not let herself write the dream down, however, and commented to me as follows:

"The mere thought of writing down something that I don't feel I have control of makes me so scared. I don't want to tell you anything. I don't want you to know anything about me. It is so crazy because you know me really well by now. . . . I pretend that you don't really know me at all, as though you are a stranger."

When Celia told me how she had cared for two children at school who had sustained playground injuries, I underscored both her capacity to care and her hostile refusal to take care of herself. She responded by observing that she had been walking around with a hole in her shoe, that she habitually fought with herself over driving without putting on her seat belt, that she allowed her house to remain a mess, and that she did not allow herself enough sleep and tried to believe that all she needed was cigarettes and that, underlying it all, she was not human. She commented on how she physically tortured her hands when expressing her caring part with me, and worried that she might actually break one of her fingers. She was appalled to acknowledge that the crude and destructive part was herself. In the next hour she had nothing to say to me. She did not know why she had bothered to come and began to contemplate reducing the frequency of our sessions. She said she was talking to herself, cursing at life, at everyone and everything, much the way her hallucinated voices had once sounded. She left after half the session so as spare us both the waste of our time. After 2 hours of this she began to achieve some perspective on her rage again, and to realize how terrified she was of this crazy, destructive part of her. She realized that the closer she allowed herself to feel to me the more destructive she would get. She felt better. I remarked that with her everything was external: The hostile, destructive part had been expressed in hallucinations and delusions, and the needy caring part was assigned to me or to the children she taught. This helped her to understand more about why she had such difficulty seeing either of us as real.

Celia wondered how she might better track and manage her rage, and in response I suggested looking at where it belonged, which led us to the image of and her relationship with her mother. Her response, in the next hour, was to tell me of redoubled self-destructiveness: almost letting her car run out of gas, unnecessarily getting herself lost, going home to a freezing house because she would neither get an automatic thermostat nor turn up the heat, and being obsessed with the urge to travel to a nearby city where the news media reported a mass murderer had been killing women. As she told me this she twisted her fingers and kept disrupting her sentences.

In our 939th hour Celia reported another nightmare: She had cancer, and was testing and diagnosing herself in the belief that she could do something about a condition about which she is in fact ignorant. She took a biopsy and put the specimen in a huge, drawerlike oven to incubate; it grew to be monstrous—long, thin slices of herself, black, gross, and disgusting. Again she pleaded total ignorance about the dream, but without much trouble we realized she was talking about fulmination of the cancerous killer part of herself and about her know-it-all attitude that allowed it to continue to grow unchecked.

Before the Christmas holiday Celia gave me a card. I understood it in the context of its presentation an hour later than she had consciously intended (because she "forgot" the pocketbook that contained it), which was followed by evasive and detached behavior. The wording of the card was as follows:

"Thank you for putting up with my endless stalling, confusing contradictions, and general nastiness. You have helped me come a long way. I have a real job that I do like very much and I live in a nice place without being crazy all of the time. I have a long way to go. It is clearer now what I want (that I even want anything is relatively new). I know that I need to quit stalling and get to work so I can find the people that I need and want to be with. Because of you I really believe that these people exist—you are one of them."

After the holiday Celia was diffusely and destructively angry; then she began to experience anger directed more specifically at the destructive part of herself, which had terrorized her during a long drive home from an evening with her family, and had made her fearful of driving off the road or hitting other cars. On reflection she decided that her anger was the only connecting link between the two parts of her, and I had the chilling thought that it must have been so with her mother as well. We talked of her need to fight with the mother part of herself since she had been unable to fight with her mother as a child, and she realized she hated crazy, destructive, selfish people. In our 954th hour, as we discussed her self-destructiveness yet again, she got angry at me for repetitively telling her the same simplistic things related to caring. I responded that it bored me too and that I knew this simpleminded level of discourse hardly began to tap the more sophisticated interactions we might both be capable of having. She said she felt ashamed and embarrassed over her "stupid" behavior, including her muttering, cursing, and inappropriate laughter, but she added, "If I lock up this Neanderthal part, then I will have lost the only part that has ever taken care of me, and I will feel intolerably alone." In hour 957 Celia told me that she was having more success "tying up" the destructive mother part of herself. When traveling in her car recently she had felt needy and close to tears, and she had allowed herself to pull over to the side of the road and cry. We were now able to joke some about the "awful thing" I had "done to" her by "trapping" her into having caring feelings and an investment in our relationship. She wondered how a brokenhearted person could learn to care again, and I encouraged her to talk more about her broken heart. She felt that the last straw had occurred when she was in fourth grade, after mother was hospitalized. Celia felt different from everyone else, and was convinced no one liked her. Because of a quarrel involving her father and the neighbor who was mother of Celia's best (and probably only) friend, Celia and her friend were no longer allowed to play together. Reluctantly and self-mockingly she acknowledged to me that she now had a favorite TV serial, a program about a caring veterinarian.

Celia went to a party and became involved with others in a constructive and satisfying way; she danced and actually allowed herself to enjoy the experience. This led to a variety of fantasies about spending time with me. We would walk together, see sights, sit in cafés, drink coffee, and get to know one another. But she began the next hour with her usual *sotto voce* cursing. Now she acknowledged that cursing was her effort to drive out of her mind all the thoughts and feelings she wished to share with me, all her crazy, silly daydreams. But she found the insecure state that resulted from such self-attack disquieting. After another hour that began with the usual cursing she spontaneously apologized, and admitted she was attacking the warm, positive impulses she experienced when she first saw me. She realized that the really stupid part of her was the the the destructive know-nothing, feel-nothing part; now there was an inner war over what constituted dumbness and stupidity.

Celia began to anticipate my next midwinter vacation. Realizing she needed my help to keep track of her feelings and to counter the only parenting she knew, her own internalized hostility, she felt very sad, and said this would be our most difficult separation. As she expressed her fear that without my help she would be unable to continue to feel, her concern began to sound like a heartbroken lament, I can't live without you. I brought this to her attention, and she remembered sitting on her bed after mother left, so overwhelmed by her feelings that she was literally immobilized; she eventually tried to cope by imagining boxes surrounding her, which we realized represented her efforts to construct holding parents. In hour 976, our last, she did not want to have anything to do with me or to feel, which she believed would lead to crying. In order to achieve these objectives we were not supposed to move (I was not supposed to leave). She almost literally felt that if anything "happened," she would be heartbroken. At the end of the hour she admonished me to take care of myself so that nothing would happen to me, and I responded that she needed to take care of herself, which meant bearing her feelings. More concretely, in the light of comments she had made about how she did not care for herself, I suggested that she make her bed, get a bedside reading light, and turn up the thermostat in her house. When we resumed, Celia told me that she had begun to torture and torment herself with sadistic thinking after I left, but that she had taken my concrete suggestions and they had helped.

Celia was amazed at how horrified and disbelieving her students were when they read a story of a little girl who was abused by her parents; her response, in contrast, was envy because the girl had two other caring people in her life. Once again we returned to her overwhelming heartbroken sadness. She remembered as a child sneaking into the kitchen when she felt it was safe, cooking herself little snacks, and eating them when no one was looking. As we discussed this, the fact emerged that no one had ever made lunch for her; then, in the subsequent hour, we discussed how poor her current nutrition was. Although Celia was an excellent cook, she rarely made meals for herself. Once again she struggled with her conflict over crying and allowing herself to be comforted. Around this time I began to realize that Celia's protestations about caring and her hostility to being with me had lost much of their sting; when she commenced a new litany, and I responded that I no longer found her negativism so believable, she responded that she did not either and that she was protecting herself from "falling apart" and crying. She talked of the difficulty she was having at work, where she was now so valued and praised that it forced her to consider seriously the possibility that she might be of value, a thought that in turn threatened to precipitate serious lamentation over her childhood deprivation. She imagined having me sit next to her and put my arm around her so that she would feel secure and be able to fall asleep. But following this fantasy Celia panicked and became paranoid, until she realized that her image of me had changed into that of her mother, with long fingernails, ready to strangle her.

Year Seven

We began the seventh year of work with the 987th hour. Celia realized while viewing a movie that she was not really interested in sex, but that one had to do it in order to have an intimate relationship. When she bumped into a chair in the waiting room on entering the office (hour 993), she attributed it to letting herself think about talking about sex. She feared if she did so I would change and the sense of security and home that she experienced with me would vanish. But as she continued to pursue the subject it soon became apparent that, once again, the issue was not about sex at all but about how she ran away after mother left and got men to abuse her and force her to have oral intercourse, which she did to calm the "crazed" man though it made her choke and want to vomit. As she talked we realized that in these behaviors she had been seeking her mother and trying to placate her in order to get nurturance. Celia began to cry and to talk about wanting a mother. She knew she had been breast-fed and began to wonder what it had been like. She felt relieved though shaky; the subject of sex, which had not made any sense to her, was beginning to. She felt better next hour although it became clear as we talked that part of her agenda was to please me and defy the prediction that she would inevitably act crazy in the therapy hour after a session in which something positive happened. She began to be frightened of me. The next hour she came in muttering and admitted she was very angry at me, though she was not certain why. Then she realized that her birthday was again approaching and she had wishes to be with me and have me tell her about myself. She wondered what I did on vacations and hesitantly asked some seemingly innocuous questions, such as whether I read all the time. When I told her a few things I like to do, she got very upset and admonished me not to tell her more because it made me "more human" to her. She longed for a mother who would make the effort to find her and mother her in spite of herself, hold her and never let her go no matter how badly she acted. With reluctance she called family and friends and let them know she would like to be taken out to dinner for her birthday.

On Celia's birthday (our 998th hour) I gave her a card with the following notation: "I am sorry I can't be the loving mother you never had. And I can't take away your memories and feelings about never having had one. But I would like to help you put these things where they belong so you can get some love in the future." Celia was very touched and literally clung to the card for the entire hour, which was at times interrupted by the feeling that mother was about to take it from her, and at other times by her own wish to get away (she told me that she kept the previous card I had given her on her person for half a year). Celia received many sincere birthday greetings from people at school as well. She wondered what it had been like as a child to have no one to pick her up, to put her to bed, to respond to her emotions; there were no "edges" or "boundaries," and she did not know who she was. She described her determination to take care of herself the previous night: "I was going to do it even if it killed me!"

After being late for her hour and making various excuses for not having brought a pad, as she had intended, so she could draw a picture, she asked to borrow one. I declined, commenting that she needed to learn to take more responsibility for caring in her life. She became furious and hurt, but with my help she sorted out her hyperresponsible attitude with others from her wish to act irresponsible, assign caring to me, and get revenge by driving me crazy in an effort to care for her. I expressed my perplexity about how best to deal with her and said, somewhat facetiously, that I needed a consultation from her. In response she spent the following weekend in serious thought, and brought me the first in a series of wonderfully artistic and articulate documents, illustrated as though they were children's stories, accompanied by the comment that her holding on to mother was the barrier between us, and that she needed to face her rage and tears at having had no mother. The following are excerpts from this document, written in part in the style of a consultation:

"Celia is wasting, on average, 180 minutes of her 200 minutes a week of therapy time. Time is a major issue—biological clocks are ticking . . . other clocks are ticking as well (how long can a person stay in therapy?). I don't want to spend my life doing a Woody Allen impersonation. Then there is the . . . 'how old was she when she died' clock that I haven't really noticed until now. The pendulum has been swinging for 35 years despite efforts to the contrary . . . swinging without any joy, love, sadness, company. . . . Already I have lost out on a lot of 'tick tocks'—I want the other 180 minutes with you. I want the rest of my life also [then, after what was an actual time pause, she returns to the writing task]. Writing this is doing me in. I just spent four hours trying to escape. I started feeling more and more helpless . . . hopeless. I want to die. . . . Back to the consultation. Problems: Wasted time. Being late, talking nonsense, refusing to relate things to me, getting angry at you rather than my mother et al., never allowing closeness. . . . When you aren't there I want lots of things. The minute you show up I don't want anything but to drive you nuts and run . . . [The following is written in black to indicate the thoughts of Ms. Black:] I hate people. I hate you for spending all this time chasing me . . . I'm sick of you making trouble. [then, in red] I miss people. I like people a lot. They are essential in my life. You are the most important person in my life . . . I am aware that this puts you in a very difficult position. If you stop chasing after me I get angry and if you chase me I keep running. I do get a sadistic, nasty pleasure out of bugging you (by not doing anything or coming close up one minute and backing off the next. The revenge factor. I finally found someone who will keep chasing me . . . like I had to with my mother. So I waste my time getting revenge on you (who has never hurt me in any way) and in reality getting revenge on myself, carrying out my mother's misdirected revenge on me. [Again she writes in black]. This is a bunch of bullshit. I am getting further and further away from my feelings and from you. It makes me want to die when I think how badly I want to see you and cry, and to understand that I only feel that because I can't see you."

In hour 1,004 we talked about clinging to mother and Celia's illusion that if she was compliant and treated herself badly, mother might yet care. Reciprocally, she realized that her destructive rage was a barrier against having to deal with the powerful positive feelings she had toward me. She remarked, half facetiously, that the "courses" she was taking with me were "feelings 101" and "elementary language."

Year Eight

As our seventh year ended and the eighth commenced Celia told me that she was taking better care of herself. When toast got stuck in her toaster she unplugged it before fishing for it with a knife, whereas in the past she would not have bothered, thinking to herself, "If it won't kill me what does it matter, it's only a shock!" A gang rape was in the news and Celia reported mother's comment: "She deserved it." But a mugger was operating in her neighborhood, and despite warnings, Celia had trouble taking precautions. As we talked she remembered some of the times she had been beaten, robbed, and raped, and although, at the time she had reacted without feeling, now she felt overwhelming terror and aloneness.

Celia was distressed when I got up to adjust the thermostat during a session, and again when I asked her permission to write about her in this book. These things signified we were human; if she was in my book then I thought about her, her life was real and she had needs. Over the course of several hours Celia kept returning to the issue of the book, gradually elaborating how it flew in the face of her reflexive commitment to mindlessness, thoughtlessness, and not facing reality. I responded that she must be very angry at her family for not thinking about her, and that her responses to my actions suggested that she was fragile and that I needed to be constricted so as not to upset her. This idea was particularly upsetting to her, for it called into question her cherished belief that she was tough. In an act of bravado Celia decided she would get up and walk around the room, but she could not so much as stand without becoming terrified, not because she felt threatened from without, as she had imagined she might, but because it made her feel powerful. She castigated me for slight variations in the way I came into the waiting room to fetch her. I suggested that this was the mother part of her trying to terrorize me into immobility. She felt "hit" by her emotions when she came in the door, and as she told me this she reflexively banged her hand very hard on the back of the the wooden chair. Characteristically, Celia's paralytic immobility would abruptly shift, usually near the end of the hour, and she would articulate her loneliness; her wish not to leave but to be taken care of, read to, and put to bed; and her wish to be able to cry. Her old escapes from loneliness were not working anymore and she realized once again that she needed to face her brokenhearted feeling. I interpreted the warfare within her between the needy little girl and the threatening punitive mother, and in response—much to both our surprise—she burst out chastisingly, to herself, "You are not to have anything to do with him!" During another similar discussion she suddenly erupted with "Don't let the asshole get near you!"

Celia began to articulate fears that she might not be able to change. She missed a therapy hour because she sat paralyzed at her desk. Many of her hours were deadly boring, and I had to struggle with sleepiness. On the other hand, she reported that on a school outing a little girl had gotten dirt in her eye. The girl's mother, who was present, would not let her daughter touch her eye lest she be contaminated and harmed, but Celia had said, "Just cry, and it will all come out!"

As the boring immobility and stalemate between the two parts of Celia continued, along with her diffuse anger at me no matter what I did, I observed aloud that I was of little use to her and that she did not seem to want anything I had to offer. Celia supposed that what she wanted was for me to experience what she had been made to bear—inability to move, boredom, fear of going to sleep, and futile hopelessness to alter the situation. Then she spontaneously decided to create and tell me a story. It was a bleak tale of a little donkey and his caring mother. The mother was shot by a bad boy, leaving the little donkey all alone, staring into the mud and rain. I commented that this was a story about heartbreak and the end of the world.

Celia enrolled for a fascinating educational trip during our summer separation, but she was uncharacteristically fearful that she would die in an airplane crash. She realized for the first time that she valued her life and did not want to die; moreover, she would not want me to think we had failed. She proceeded to try to face just how ill she had been, and to tell me how proud of herself she was for the last 2 constructive years. She reported a nightmare about wandering disoriented in a desert, opening one door after another only to be yelled at by frightening figures. Once she locked herself out of her house and then became aware of an urge to do it again, as well as of long-standing compulsions to crash her car, jump down stairs, and the like. After she managed to drop a heavy bookshelf on herself, we realized that her fear of the plane crash also represented a wish, and I commented on her continued tendency to disown, externalize, and enact this destructive part of herself. We realized that the "crazy" part of her not only did not think, but had no words and that she would have to struggle to speak for it. In the effort to curtail mindless action and to articulate the "crazy" part instead, she said she wanted to make me crazy, confused, sleepy, and alienated. A result of such verbalization was that Celia experienced her craziness more directly. I, in turn, felt relief, and told her that when she spoke for that part I felt less crazy, for her words were more synchronous with her actions and with my experience of her and thus she made sense to me. I said it was clear that the crazy part of her and I were enemies, and it was a relief to have it be so obvious. In our final hour (the 1,050th) before the summer separation Celia reported a TV program she had seen about primitive countries that simultaneously harbor two incompatible wishes of their government, and so are unable to have a single government with a "loyal opposition" but instead suffer repeated coups; she realized this was a description of herself.

When we resumed in the fall Celia had just returned from her trip, and she looked as good as I had ever seen her. She was tanned and had lost weight. She was enthusiastic and excited and talked about her adventures, fun, and new relationships, at least one of which was destined to endure. Most of all, she had felt good about herself in relation to the others in her group, for she had discovered that without having to conceal or deny feelings and problems she was nonetheless the most stable and reliable member. She reported a dream in which she was trying to communicate her activities and excitement to Dr. A, the superintendent of her school system, a man who in reality she experienced as unsupportive of her work. She was upset to discover that he was dead, that he was just a facade. Then she had to drive a truck with an old friend in the back seat, even though she could not see through the windshield and the brakes did not work. Finally, she decided to stop and try to fix things. She thought that the dream symbolized her crazy life until now and that the first part represented the war between the two parts of herself.

But the ambience of Celia's therapy hours soon reverted to deadness and immobilization. When she talked about her alive, active, exciting class in comparison to the class of another teacher who was dull and repressive, I pointed out how she seemed to require an external destructive or deadening force in her life to represent the psychotic part of herself in order to function well, and how she had to express that part directly when such an external force was not present. This distressed her a good deal, and was followed by a dream in which I appeared, a fact that bothered her because it indicated my importance. We were sleeping in separate sleeping bags, entirely zipped up, on a beach on the northern coast. We had been there a long time, there was water and a line of seaweed over much of us, and she was half awake. This clear illustration of our relationship was most troubling to Celia. She commented on our disconnection and dormancy, the chronicity, and the fact that she could observe what was happening.

Two hours later, when we were discussing the seeming paradox that though she loved children very much she seemed determined to destroy the child part of herself, she recalled how her grandfather would bribe her and her brothers, when they were small, to dive in deep water to fetch him mussels, along with imagery suggesting that she perceived this as an expression of some unconscious lethal wishes he had toward them. She cursed at the beginning of her hour about having to be there, and again at the end when she realized she had to leave. We were both painfully aware of the immobilizing contradictions, and Celia lamented with seeming sincerity that she did not think she could change but could not tolerate remaining like this indefinitely, that she would probably end up killing herself, and that the changes she had made, while real, were not enough. She wondered if she should stop therapy. Over a weekend separation she missed me and pretended the teddy bear she now used for comfort represented me, but in the course of telling me about it she called herself a "stupid jerk." She realized both sides of her agreed that she was a "stupid jerk" but for diametrically opposite reasons; there was no inner dialogue.

With difficulty Celia acknowledged some curiosity about me, and then it dawned on her, quite by surprise, that I was curious about her as well. I pointed out that mutual curiosity was one of the foundations of a relationship, but that in order to satisfy it one had to take risks in the relationship, which was especially difficult for her because her personality was organized around her fear of getting to know mother better. Celia began to talk about her future and faced for the first time the likelihood that despite her love of children she would probably never be able to have any of her own. I talked about her need to externalize the hostile crazy part of herself and wondered aloud if, just as the deprivation inherent in the end of the therapy hour seemed to liberate her briefly to acknowledge and express her needs, so menopause (or perhaps lung cancer and impending death as a result of her heavy smoking) might liberate her to experience, without so much hostility toward herself, her sense of heartbreak, and the wishes for things to be different.

After some discussion Celia agreed to try for the third time to tape her sessions so that she could study and remember them better (the second effort, like the first, having been rather quickly aborted). But subsequent hours involved a comedy (perhaps tragedy would be a more apt term) of errors in which she did everything imaginable to forget the machine, make it malfunction, or not listen to the tapes. She was aware of wanting to smash the tape recorder and was certain that listening to our discussions would be acutely unpleasant. Yet after hearing the first tape she admitted not only that she had enjoyed listening but that she had derived comfort and a sense of security and safety at night from listening to my voice, as though I were there. She suspected that she was being destructive to the recording process in response to her enjoyment of listening to the tapes. She described herself and mother as homewreckers, committed to destroying anything that felt good or was enjoyable; while telling me this she unconsciously twisted her hand in a most painful manner, made menacing gestures toward the tape recorder, and talked about wishes both to hug me and to hit me and break my things. Then she went on to talk about how much work is involved in chasing after children and getting them to do what is good for them. I commented that this was what she had needed and lacked in the past, but that now there was no way I or anyone else could make her do anything she did not wish to do. She shared painful memories of her childhood and expressed anger that I could not be the parent she never had.

Celia had talked of wishes to fall asleep in the office if only she had a blanket, and she hinted, without outright asking, that she would like some of the old science magazines from my waiting room for her class when I was done with them. I had intermittently considered having a blanket available on my couch, and her comments galvanized me into action. I also left some magazines for her in a box in the waiting room. She was touched and thanked me but forgot to take the magazines with her. The next hour Celia was very threatened by the presence of the blanket, even a bit paranoid, with some perceptual alteration and a vague sense of threat in the office, but it was clear that what frightened her was the intensity of her heartbroken childlike longing to cry, be comforted, and fall asleep, to have a home despite her vigilant suppressive mothering part. She actually struggled to put the blanket over herself, but when I observed her striking motoric inability to clutch and hold it and contrasted her difficulty holding onto caring feelings with her adeptness at clutching and monopolizing destructiveness, she felt even more tearful. Again she forgot to take the magazines, and again I left them in the waiting room.

Early in the 1,076th hour Celia said she felt cold, and since I agreed with her that the room seemed cool, I got up to adjust the heat. This upset her, and she angrily began to talk about how she didn't want anything from me. She continued repudiating any need for me at the start of the next hour, swearing and admonishing me to get rid of the blanket. But her protestations seemed transparent and I suggested that she was not really behind them. She responded that the power of her repudiation had made her unable to sleep the night before, and fearful that someone was outside her bedroom with a knife. She decided that she was exhausted and wanted to sleep, and told me to occupy myself with some other work, but when she unfolded the blanket and put it over her she became terrified that someone was behind her. I commented that it was the killer part of herself and that it began by repudiating her feelings and ended up wanting to kill her so she could prove nothing could make her feel.

After missing most of another session because she made herself sit soundlessly in the waiting room after erroneously believing she had pushed the buzzer to let me know of her arrival for her hour, Celia got angry that she was allowing herself so little. After reluctant acknowledgment (in the 1,098th hour) of wishes to get married and have a family, she did not want to pursue a question that involved thinking, was full of contradictions about what she wanted, used vague terminology, destroyed the order of my words in her head, and experienced me as critical. Finally, she covered herself with the blanket but told me it made her feel worse, by which she seemed to mean that it made her more aware of the magnitude of her needs. At the end of this mutually frustrating hour Celia summarized that she tended to use the first 10 minutes of each hour being late and the next 30 avoiding contact, and that the feelings she showed during the last 10 minutes were meaningless since they were predicated on knowing she could soon leave. She concluded that she hated everyone and "nothing in a million years will make a difference." The next hour she apologized; talked about her efforts to frustrate me, split me into pieces with her contradictions, and drive me crazy; and said it distressed her. But as the Christmas holiday approached, Celia's delusional and hallucinatory thinking became more apparent, along with anger at me because I did not appreciate how hard she was trying in the face of "them," the multiple male and female voices that ridiculed her and told her to pack all her things and prepare to leave.

Over subsequent hours Celia was intermittently able to discuss her rage and recall the narcissistic preoccupation about holidays that characterized her parents. Father bought lavish but personally meaningless gifts, for which he expected profuse gratitude, and mother, despite or perhaps because of her obvious anger at the burdens placed upon her, was menacingly insistent that the children enjoy the holiday. Celia brought me a holiday bouquet; her fantasy had been to bring two plants (one a cactus) growing side by side in representation of herself. When she shook my hand at the end of the hour her hand trembled in reflection of her ambivalence.

After a long holiday weekend separation Celia told me she had gotten drunk and had slept with a "loser" who lived in her neighborhood and had been pursuing her for a year. I remarked that she had once again forced herself to be physically intimate with someone she did not like. She began to hallucinate, cursing critical commentary on her relationship with me. She made it clear over the holiday she had felt rejected by me and excluded from my family. In reviewing our prolonged stalemate, I again suggested medication; after a discussion of her wish to reject it and her acknowledged fear that it might make her feel better, Celia reluctantly agreed. We began a 6-mg dose of trifluoperazine, over the next 36 treatment hours or (2½ months) the dose was gradually increased to 20 mg.

Almost immediately Celia's hallucinations diminished; she became calmer and began to sleep better, and gradually she became better able to focus attention, to concentrate and to organize her life. But these changes and the idea that she was allowing someone or something to influence her were terrifying. Though she had looked forward to seeing me, in hour 1,110 she hallucinated, lost her thoughts, spoke vaguely, and could not focus. She recalled struggles in the hospital to fight off the effects of a dose of trifluoperazine designed to calm her during an out-of-control paranoid episode. I wondered aloud about my own craziness and masochism in continuing to try to help her in light of what she was telling me, and we returned again to her enactment of revenge; her turning the tables of her childhood. She wanted to shake my hand at the end of the hour, but the shake was punctuated by the usual rhythmic disruptive tugs. In our next hour she told me it had frightened her to do so, and had reminded her of feeling captured by mother, but, at the same time, she had enjoyed it.

As she became more aware again of her thoughts and feelings Celia was disturbed that the medication was making her "too calm. She acted mellower, and wanted to end each hour by shaking my hand. As she told me how effectively she had calmed a paranoid man in a store, while other customers had stood around, paralyzed, I commented on the absence of effective inner dialogue between the parts of herself and her inability to calm her destructive aspect. She tried sitting closer to me and had a fantasy of being dragged back into the corner by her hair, which seemed so vivid she was more or less convinced it was a memory. She realized she was angry but began to forget and to fragment her thoughts. She admitted she had to "kick [herself] in the head" before anyone else could. Another time she wanted to lie down on the couch and nap, but when she tried to do so she lost sight of me, sensed danger, and had to sit up. She realized she was the attacker, and with my encouragement was able to articulate her hatred and ridicule, and particularly her hatred of the trifluoperazine, which was making her feel "strange."

Again I encouraged Celia to identify and separate the parts of her by moving from one chair to another when speaking for different parts of herself. She began by swearing upon seeing me, and by first enacting (but soon describing) the wish not to think and feel. In the destructive chair she talked with a sense of omnipotence about her contempt for human beings, relationships, and her own well-being, and about her capacity to destroy caring. She also told me she had made a new female friend, had joined a health club (exercising had hitherto been unheard of since it made her more aware of her body and feelings), had cleaned her house, and was expressing anger more appropriately at people who mistreated her. She related some of this improvement to the medication, but at the end of the hour she reported a "splitting headache."

About 3 weeks after commencing trifluoperazine (in hour 1,120) Celia began to recall disturbing memories of performing fellatio, and to speculate that this had been a repetition of her breast-feeding experiences. After stating this impression she felt I had changed and become a different person. After the hour she most uncharacteristically remained in the waiting room, crying and debating whether to knock on my door. In the next session (hour 1,121) she had many associations to the idea of being force-fed with the injunction that she had to pretend to enjoy the experience, including feelings of suffocation, gagging, and wishes to bite the feeding instrument off. She recalled her thin, breastless mother, with nothing to give, but with a powerful investment in believing she was a good mother nonetheless. I reminded Celia of her rage at Christmas over her parents' narcissistic investment and her need to pretend everything was wonderful in order to make them feel good. We discussed her confusion between closeness initiated by love and by forced compliance. In the middle of the discussion Celia had a sudden urge to suck her thumb, which shocked her, and she recalled having done so until the fifth or sixth grade. She also recalled a childhood fantasy that mother was hospitalized because she had lost her thumb.

In hour 1,122 Celia told me that when she lay in her bed, clutching her teddybear and with the covers pulled over her, she now felt relatively and unambivalently at home—but she had to editorialize that she considered this abnormal. She reported two dreams: She and her brother were attempting to escape from her home of origin through an underground garage, but mother came along in a car and flattened them. Celia had no thoughts about this dream, and when I inquired it turned out she had forgotten our recent discussions about feeding. In the second dream she came to my house for an appointment, but there was a party and she could find no place to park. When she finally came in she could not find me. The house was very neat. She began to smoke but became uneasy about doing so and ran out.

After attempting to portray the trifluoperazine as bad for her (at the start of hour 1,123), Celia admitted that the problem was that it was "making" her feel and think. She returned to the issue of feeding and of running away from home after mother left and engaging in a series of enslavements characterized by sucking a penis to ejaculation. Celia was angry at me for not being there to rescue her, and added that it was too late now for she was dead. The following hour she reported a dream of being buried in the sand. She was intentionally late for her next hour (the 1,126th), and in the face of intense angry wishes to withhold she reported dreaming of a trip up a jungle river with two guides. On the last part of the journey they went over rapids, and she fell into the water and was rescued, near death. No one was present who could pump the water out and resuscitate her, and she died! Celia had actually been contemplating a jungle vacation, and the woman who was her tentative companion had just backed out. She told me she wanted to take the trip so that she could bring me back a native statue, as she knew I liked such things. I remarked that she was willing to go around the world and take grave risks to bring me a statue but that she did not want to come to her hour on time and bring a dream! Celia recalled two instances with her mother where she had nearly drowned, but she felt certain the dream represented her breast-feeding experience. She also feared that I was the guide of her dream and that I could not save her. I commented that, on our trip, she was not just a passive passenger, that she had to work and to think. Suddenly, she recalled imagery of mother's insane behavior in the kitchen, cursing, threatening, throwing things, making bizarre decorations; Mother would bake and then make the children sit in a circle on the floor and, one by one, lick the remains of the batter from her finger. Further associations led to the idea that she was resisting what I "forced on" her in our relationship, though she knew I was not really forcing her. Celia recalled bathing in the tub with mother at around 3 or 4 years of age and feeling terrified; perhaps mother had been shaving. Her sister had recently been born, and Celia had watched her lose a piece of umbilical cord shortly after coming home from the hospital, and had imagined that mother had done something to her. These discussions were punctuated by feelings of terror, episodic deadness, and mental blank-ness.

Celia had the urge to sleep with her longstanding male friend, and we began to see that getting herself assaulted, performing oral sex, and proving that it did not bother her was a way to avoid thought and memory—and perhaps served, I suggested, to assuage her doubts about her gender. To my surprise Celia assented to this interpretation almost eagerly, and began to talk about the feeling that she had been "ripped off" and forced to be a girl. She recalled childhood activities with a blowtorch in her basement, which she now believed were efforts to construct a penis. She recalled believing that her parents wanted to get rid of females. She felt the need to service men. She was apprehensive that I might want a "blow job," and her perceptions of the room began to change; things began to move around. She acknowledged that she had been studying penises all her life, and that she believed she once had one but lost it. She felt rage at father who favored her brothers, and she believed that boys got everything.

Celia was confused, self-contradictory, and filled with rage. There were suicidal thoughts. She got drunk, stayed in bed, wandered about, and was vague and out of touch. And then she wrote me a letter:

"It terrifies me that I might push you to the point where you tell me that you have had enough. . . . I don't trust myself and I know that you don't trust me at all. . . . I dreamed that I was searching for something but there was this demon following me around in the shadows killing people. It was like some robot that ripped the tops of people's heads off and ate their brains. Really gruesome. It ate people's hands, too. It crept around and I could never quite make it out but I saw it doing the killing. It was terrifying because I couldn't find anyone to help kill it because it kept killing everyone that I saw or talked to. What a vivid picture of what I am doing! I can barely think about it. . . . The monster is obviously me and I can't kill it and you can't kill it because all it does is constantly try to kill you. . . . I don't think you really understand what a monster I am. You are the recipient of all its wrath. . . . I get you where it hurts. I get you to care about me and try to help and then kick you in the head over and over. . . . There is a part of me that is getting kicked in the head as well. . . . I expect you to sit there and take all this abuse for so long. Obviously you won't because you are a sane person. . . . Maybe if I am not working through the summer we should stop."

As we discussed this letter we agreed that Celia had learned about caring, and also about how crazy she was, and that part of the reason she wanted to quit was that she could not stand being aware of and responsible for how destructive she was. When Celia expressed her concern that she might drive me crazy, I commented that there were differences between my investment in her and hers in her mother, differences that made this impossible. This simultaneously reassured and enraged her.

Celia calmed somewhat, and returned in hour 1,136 to the subject of castration. Gradually we learned that unconsciously she believed that all children are initially the same sex (male), that males ("pricks, brains in their crotch") have power and control, and that some get "ripped off" and become eunuchs. (I wrote in my notes, unconsciously, I believe: "It is like pulling teeth to get her to continue to think about all this.") Amidst much anger and negativity Celia began to realize that she had continued unconsciously to believe she was a man, and that getting a penis inside her was her way of affirming her belief. Her promiscuity—getting beaten and "ripped off" and trying to control the penis and thereby make it her own—was a reenactment of the struggle with her mother. Awareness of the belief that she had once had a penis and that it had been "ripped off" because she was bad made her feel sad for herself. It also emerged that she felt she controlled me by withholding her thoughts and feelings; by offering, then withdrawing; by "ripping me off" and by reversing roles and making me the impotent female or eunuch, which she did partly in the hope that someday I would tell her that it was all a delusion that she was female, that she really had a penis. Despite this confusion it depressed Celia to realize that she unconsciously assumed she had a penis; it became clear that she had an investment in sexual differentiation, and preferred that men look like men and women like women. Her wish was not so much to be a sexually differentiated man but to be a creature with a penis, but with no muscles or breasts. When I suggested that she wanted to be a little boy, she agreed and elaborated on how much little boys received in her family in contrast to little girls.

In hour 1,144 Celia reported a dream in which she was custodian of some things at school that were being sold to a rich man who valued them. These included lovely scarves, soft and feminine, an antique silver iron, and a hammer. Another man wanted to rip them off. Celia was entrusted with the dangerous task of getting the things out, one by one, by reciting a special number. After we struggled through her customary litany about the meaninglessness of the dream she guessed that I was the wealthy man and that the things represented her disowned insides. She reluctantly acknowledged that what she was now learning about herself was making her feel better, but then she shut down emotionally and wanted to withhold her "secrets" from me and leave. She said her head ached as though she had been hit (she reflexively gouged at her temples) and suddenly she recalled several instances when mother had hit her.

Year Nine

We began the ninth year of Celia's therapy. She reported a "splitting headache" as she contemplated both the part of her that wanted to be close and the part of her enraged at humanity. She missed hours and made the tape recorder malfunction. She picked fights with me over everything and wanted to "kick [my] balls." She reported a dream in which she had to have a finger chopped off because of skin cancer, but it didn't matter because the cancer had spread and she was going to die anyway. She insisted on stopping trifluoperazine since it made her feel drunk and sleepy. I pointed out all the ways the trifluoperazine seemed to have helped, but because Celia was so adamant, and because I felt that at this point she needed to bear the consequences of her decisions, I reluctantly assented. Over the course of the next several therapy hours she reported feeling more alert but sleeping less well and feeling more disorganized; but, perhaps most importantly, the meaningful thinking and content that had characterized our recent sessions more or less ceased, and the familiar deadened, stalemated quality returned.

In hour 1,149 Celia would not think, and expressed a sense of hopelessness and helplessness to alter her situation. I challenged her posture as passive victim, and wondered aloud what else she could expect considering that she had stopped tape-recording, stopped trifluoperazine, and stopped thinking. She responded that she was very upset about my next vacation, which she associated with mother's departure when she was 9, and that rather than have thoughts and feelings about it she might be better off if she stopped seeing me entirely. At the end of the hour she decided to resume the trifluoperazine, and we agreed on a 10-mg dose. But her destructiveness escalated, and after a weekend separation Celia reluctantly revealed that she had slept with her old boy-friend, had been talking to herself, and had had the urge to run away and go crazy, but that now the prospect of doing so frightened her much more than it had in the past for she thought it might be permanent. She realized that she was trying to destroy herself and to say "Fuck you" to me. She said she had not taken the trifluoperazine we had agreed upon; she thought that 10 mg was too much, but she agreed to take 5 mg. Celia talked about the conflict she was involved in at school over whether a psychotic child should have therapy, and about the opposition she encountered from the school administration, as well as from the parents, when she recommended such a course. She was convinced they hated her and were going to kill her. I pointed out the reversal of roles in our relationship, and this made her aware of her wish to kill, which was literally making the muscles of her arms ache with tension and which terrified her.

Celia reported a fantasy that mother was hiding in the corner, and Celia was playing dead; she also verbalized more active wishes to throw me around, choke me, and make me feel as mother had made her feel. She decided she would increase the dose of trifluoperazine, but near the end of our next hour, after she told me she would miss me and felt safe with me, she said that she was hallucinating again and that "they" were telling her she should keep away from me for I intended to kill her. In the final hour before our 2½-week separation Celia sat in her corner hallucinating her Greek chorus of voices reviling both of us. when I urged her to face the anger more directly she began to articulate her rage at me for leaving, and her wish to beat, terrorize, and immobilize me as her mother had done to her; but, characteristically, she could not focus the rage on mother herself. In fact, it was near mother's birthday, and Celia was preoccupied with efforts to commemorate the occasion in some positive way. As was characteristic, she felt a bit better and closer to me at the very end of the hour; she talked of how frightened she was of her psychotic part, and she wished me a good vacation and assured me she would not act self-destructively while I was gone.

Our reunion was discouraging to both of us. Celia was distant and pessimistic. She informed me that she had stopped taking the small dose of trifluoperazine she had agreed upon as soon as we separated, for reasons she could not or would not clarify, and that she had continued to hallucinate intermittently. Though she had not gotten into any overt trouble, she reported having walked in front of her car after parking it on a hill without setting the hand brake and nearly running herself over. On another occasion, while playing with friends, she had accidentally gotten hit in the head with a basketball so hard that her ears rang; her companions were shocked not so much at the injury but at her utter absence of reaction to it. When she said I looked like I felt there was nothing I could do, I readily assented. She felt sad, as though we were saying goodbye and she were attending her own funeral. She began the next hour with some vague comments about falling apart, getting crazy, and having difficulty functioning. She had not brought the tape recorder. When I was silent she got furious, and then commented about the endless chasing game we had been playing. Again I was silent. Finally she said that it was pointless, that she was not going to change, and that although she was sad and would miss me, tomorrow would be our last hour! She spontaneously added that she did not believe this was her reaction to my vacation, and that she did not want me to worry, for she was not going to kill herself. I shared my sadness at her decision to stop, and acknowledged that I had been concerned about her suicide potential.

Celia reconsidered her decision. She told me her fantasy had been to quit therapy, stop caring, quit her job, and drive off in a van. We agreed that such a trip was from the "city" of caring and living to one of hatred, insanity, and perhaps suicide. When she talked about how little it would probably disturb her family if this were to happen, I said I cared and did not want that to happen to her. She was clearly and deeply touched, said she knew, and cried a bit. She said she wanted to continue to see me but she could make no guarantees. When she left her session she discovered she had locked herself out of her car, and had to return to the office where I helped her call a locksmith. The next hour, after her preliminary curses, she said she had been relieved to find herself locked out of her car; she was certain it had been her unconscious effort to keep herself from quitting. What relieved her most was that this was the first instance she could recall in which her unconscious motivation had been constructive!

Nonetheless our impasse continued. The apparent significant change, however, was that Celia was no longer psychotic; she told me, to her surprise, that she had never been this depressed before without accompanying delusions and hallucinations. We discussed the destructive lost-and-found chase we had been involved in, and its relationship to her endless chase after her mother. Celia felt she had been misusing therapy to discharge her anger at mother. Nonetheless she thought she wanted to cut the frequency of our meetings to once a week; I did not oppose her wish but expressed my puzzlement about what would be accomplished.

Celia began some constructive planning, including contemplation of ways in which she might communicate more honestly with her mother. She informed mother that she had not been talking with her because she was so angry at her, and, even more uncharacteristically, told mother she had seriously been considering killing herself. To her surprise and even dismay mother seemed concerned, and wondered what she could do. Then mother reverted to form and, to Celia's combined dismay and relief, quickly forgot what Celia had told her, leaving Celia to conclude that she was virtually incapable of feeling angry at mother.

Celia worried about whether she could manage seeing me less frequently. She reported a dream of living on another planet where things were wonderful and she felt happy, and I wondered if she thought she would leave the angry, destructive part of her in the office when she saw me less often. In our final hour (the 1,168th) before the change in frequency Celia volunteered that she had changed in many ways as a result of our relationship, and that her goal was to sustain and expand some of these changes while seeing me less often. She listed being much less self-destructive, caring about and needing others, no longer wanting to be psychotic, and knowing what steps to take to prevent it; in short, she had greater self-awareness and real control over her life.

Celia and I then met weekly until we both came to realize that her stalemated, nonallied, distant, and at times even mildly hostile relationship with me was her way of conveying that she felt unable to work further to achieve the intimacy she claimed she wanted, and that continuing a relationship of lesser frequency so she would have a "home" where she might report the progress in her life would be so frustrating to her that it would evoke gratuitous hostility. The remaining year and a half of our relationship will be summarized briefly.

Celia and I were able to clarify her motives for decreasing the frequency of therapy. First and most obvious was her genuine doubt that she was capable of more intimacy, along with her terror of what might transpire were she to try, which at various times she conceptualized either as more craziness and hospitalization or else as unbearable feelings, including destructive rage. Her second motive was to prove to herself that she could manage a constructive and reasonably satisfying existence on her own, without me. Not surprisingly there seemed to be two components to this wish. The first was adolescent-like—a need to test her capacity for constructive independent living. As she had never been on her own in a nonpsychotic state, Celia needed to know that she could do it, and that dependency and independency alike could be matters of mature choice and not something forced on a person. Over the remaining year and a half that we met at weekly intervals and the almost two years since we terminated, Celia succeeded in proving this to our satisfaction, and experienced appropriate pride and self-esteem in her accomplishment. The second component of this motive to decrease the frequency of her therapy hours was the familiar psychotic wish to triumph over her dependency and need for anyone. However, we both noted the paradox that she seemed to need to prove this to another person, that she had to keep me around to witness her independence. Gradually we both became convinced that she had fully internalized a self-caring attitude, which would persist whether or not she continued therapy—though it seemed that much of this attitude came from a now internalized sense that she was doing it for me, and that I would be angry at her if she did not take good care of herself.

Some 7 months after we decreased the frequency of appointments, Celia gave me one of her illustrated letters, her first year-end assessment, as a kind of Christmas gift. After summarizing considerable success in her work, some good friendships, and more pleasure in socializing, she concluded as follows:

"From the quiet room to this. That is saying a lot. For a huge chunk of each day I am happy, enjoying myself, challenged. You stuck by me. Thank you for your amazing patience and caring. . . . I did everything I could to drive you away, and I continue to keep you at a distance with all the ways I have worked out over the years. But at the same time I take little pieces of our friendship and use them to patch my heart. . . . You have given me a good life with friends and a satisfying job. You have also, like you said a long time ago, given me choices. I have tried out for a while now what my life is like where I have slammed the brakes on. It is a hell of a lot more than I had before. It is better than being dead or psychotic, and better than many people have. Part of me wants to rip it all up; destroy you and my feelings, destroy myself. My happiness with what I have now fuels the great rage that wants to undo. . . . Part of me wants much more and is so desperately sad, and thinks that I can go further than this. Thank you . . ."

Somewhat to my surprise, there was no recurrence of psychosis, that is, hallucinations or delusions, from the time we reduced the frequency of sessions to weekly, to the time of termination, and none in the 2 years since. Celia has reported an increasing sense of control over her sanity, as well as further progressive expansion in the areas of close friendships and work. The notable paradox or split between her professional life and her relationship with me continued. Her work adjustment seemed based both on genuine caring for the children she taught, and on an identity as an educational crusader; she adopted a kind of adversarial stance against the stereotypic passive, uncaring attitudes of other educators and parents. That this could not simply be dismissed as paranoia was evidenced by her meteoric career advancement and by the high esteem in which she was held by everyone in the community—other educators, parents, and the children she taught. It became increasingly clear that the extent of her professional ambition and effort would be the only limiting factor in the success of her career.

Meanwhile, Celia continued intermittently to experience a sense of suffering (loneliness, rage, and despair), which impressed me as more appropriate to her childhood than to the rather full life she now led, and to have periods of despair so intense she contemplated suicide. Her capacity to acknowledge and talk about the role of her anger and the resulting distance she maintained from others in the perpetuation of these feelings was limited; instead, she periodically tended to hold me responsible for the suffering and to get angry at me for not being sufficiently empathic with her, as though the distance in our relationship was the result of my lack of caring.

In the course of the year Celia concluded that because of her age and the genetic possibility of having a schizophrenic offspring she would probably never have children of her own, but that she was heterosexual. Female friends were not enough for her, and life would not be really satisfying without intimacy with a man. Although she wondered, mostly privately, about the wisdom of her decision to diminish the intensity of our work, and claimed she knew she was unlikely to be able to attain her goal of intimacy with a man without further intensive treatment, each gesture in that direction or toward me was regularly followed by some form of destructiveness. She was often late for appointments and missed hours without informing me. During our sessions her gaze was usually averted, her affect flat, and she volunteered little beyond accounts of her struggles at work. She seemed to be saying "I won't" or "I don't want to" to any kind of intensive emotional involvement. Finally, I pointed out that her angry negative behavior seemed to convey what she was unable to say in so many words, namely, that she did not wish further treatment of any kind.

Now it turned out that Celia did not want to experience the intense sadness of termination either. The "I won't" and "I don't want to" seemed directed against *any* change in our relationship, any interaction between us that would arouse intense emotion. She seemed to want to continue our contact endlessly without movement or emotion. Because this did not seem therapeutic to either of us, it was with a mixed sense of accomplishment and regret that we agreed not to termination, for Celia seemed no more capable of saying goodbye than she was of continuing our work, but to a kind of suspended animation in which she might visit and report to me every half-year or so, in the hope that, eventually, she might be able to reach a more definitive decision of one kind or another.

Celia and I both harbored doubts about her capacity to make a successful

and lasting termination of therapy out of this seemingly chronic state of in-
decision, both because of the limitation of our work on intimacy and because
of the evident continued existence of a destructive psychotic part of her personality, albeit one that was much more under the control of a more mature and
constructive sense of self.

After cessation of our work Celia wrote me a letter in which she described
some of the changes in herself:

"I have my job and more and more I am realizing that I am really good at
this. . . . I do have friends now . . . and I am getting closer to [them] than I ever
did before . . . the feelings are not overwhelming. . . . There are nights where I
get so depressed and feel hopeless and angry and want to die, but I can survive
these times, I have control and know more clearly that the feelings will not kill
me. I do not take drastic action anymore, I ride out the night and somehow pull
myself together. Often I don't pay attention to my feelings and it is only when
I get very close to being psychotic when I force myself to figure out what is
going on. You helped me to do this many, many times. I can do it myself now.
Thank you for your patience and caring. Thank you for giving me choices. You
sat there for years waiting for me to show up, to be there. You ran the risk of
holding out your caring and being rejected over and over and over. I know that
I didn't entirely arrive, but I am happy, and the day to day is often very
satisfying and rewarding. . . . I know that it is not ideal that I carry you around
in my head as a watchdog..I have you there to look out for me. Ideally it should
be me that does this but the part of me that wants to destroy all caring and all
life is very powerful and I need you there in my mind as a third party . . ."

Celia initiated several meetings about a year after therapy was suspended.
It was apparent that her personal growth had continued, and although she still
suffered from bouts of despair and suicidal thinking, which she related to the
absence of a meaningful relationship with a man, she had achieved some
rather remarkable success both in her work and in personal friendships. According to her subjective report, she no longer experienced delusions, hallucinations, or periods of psychotic disorganization. Despite her expressed desire for intimacy she recognized from the familiar signs of negativity in herself
when we approached the subject that she remained unready to resume a
therapy whose goal was to work toward that end—and yet she remained
unwilling to terminate with me.

Nine more months elapsed and Celia made another appointment. She was
very pleased to tell me that she had made a very satisfying relationship with a
man she had been introduced to by a friend; a man whom she described as kind
and intelligent. He lived in another part of the country, and they had spent
several periods of time together. They shared much in common and had
reached a mutual decision that in order to decide whether they wanted to make
a commitment to one another they would first need to live together. This
awareness coincided fortuitously with Celia's conclusion that in order to advance her career she needed to change jobs and further educate herself; she felt
that this might just as well be done in the city where this man lived. She had

come to tell me this, knowing I would be pleased, and, since she had already made preparations to move, to say goodbye. What was most surprising to both of us was her statement that she had a sexual relationship that satisfied her and that it was predicated on her realization that she could not allow herself to lose her mind during sex; in order to retain her sanity she felt she had to reserve the right to ask her partner to stop lovemaking at any time, a condition he was willing to honor.

In the course of leaving her job Celia had been amazed to learn how professionally valued and personally cared about she had become to many people. While she still felt that I was not someone she could ever say goodbye to, and that she would want to keep me posted as her life continued to evolve, she stated that this was a genuine termination of therapy, and expressed herself with moving tears of farewell and gratitude.

After another half year I received a brief letter posted from the distant city in which Celia and her friend now lived. In it she said that their relationship and her work were both fulfilling, and she hoped all was well with me.

Part VI

Conclusion

Chapter 22

Systems and Interventions in Schizophrenia: A Reprise

I have argued that the illness we call schizophrenia is a simultaneous expression of a number of independent but interlocking hierarchical systems: the psychological system we call the human mind and personality, which itself may be conceptualized as an epigenetic transformational hierarchy; the interpersonal system; the family system; the social and cultural systems; and the organization of the brain or central nervous system. While it is *necessary* to view schizophrenia as an organic process, this perspective is not *sufficient*, and the common belief that this illness is nothing more than an organic toxic affliction visited on an otherwise "normal" person, his family and society, is both incorrect and misleading.

Our journey began with a demonstration that it is not only possible to study and in some instances effectively treat schizophrenia by focusing primarily at the psychological level of the person, with suitable assistance from disciplines organized around the organic, familial, and sociocultural levels, but that there are special advantages to doing so. The degree of integration of knowledge, and depth of analysis provided by a systems-theory-informed psychologically oriented case study can be acquired in no other way. Analogously, successful treatment by methods that are primarily though not exclusively psychological maximizes the maturational and compensatory capabilities of our patients and most closely approaches what we like to think of as "cure."

I draw no extreme conclusions from these observations, for methodology derived primarily from knowledge of the psychological system is not applicable in all cases, and I remain skeptical of monistic modes of thinking about human conditions such as schizophrenia, whatever form they take. We have traversed two centuries of disintegration and oscillation between exclusively organic and exclusively psychological conceptions of schizophrenia and, most recently, a half century during which there has been a breathtaking shift from a more or less exclusively psychological or psychoanalytic viewpoint to the currently popular trend toward neuroscientific reductionism with its associated belief that schizophrenic mentation and affect are epiphenomena. The real challenge to those of us who come from separate scientific cultures and speak in different scientific tongues is to find a separate and equal place for each of our viewpoints, so that each retains respect and integrity, and each has the opportunity to enrich the others and to contribute to a broader view of schizophrenia.

The humanistic emphasis of this book is both the focal point from which one commences to think about and interact with a schizophrenic person and the representative of one level of the systems hierarchy that comprises schizophrenia; one component of a broader perspective. When Bleuler in 1911 characterized schizophrenia as a group of conditions not all of which were necessarily characterized by progressive dementia, he was implying the likelihood that the characteristic combination of behavior and symptomatology might be reached by a multiplicity of routes or pathways with very different etiologic starting points. In these pages I have also proposed a multiple perspective view of schizophrenia, albeit one with implications quite different from his. Hierarchical systems theory retains the humanistic perspective of the psychological and social disciplines as a central focus and entry point into an understanding of schizophrenia while valuing and finding a separate but equal place in theory making and treatment for the contributions of the other human sciences. These are part of a hierarchy of creatively re-organized systems, each of which is dependent on the ingredients of a more microscopic or concrete or temporally antecedent, lower-level system, but is neither reducible to nor predictable from it. The enrichment of understanding afforded by this interactive, broadly evolutionary multiplicity of perspectives stems from more than a simple summation of its individual scientific parts. While we are traditionally accustomed to wondering what schizophrenia *is*, hierarchical systems theory exposes the monistic fallacy that it is any single thing, and directs us instead to the more ambiguous conclusion, consistent with the viewpoints of relativism and uncertainty of modern physics, that schizophrenia is a very different condition when viewed at different hierarchical levels of organization. Perhaps it would be more accurate to refer to it as a complementary set of conditions, or as a multidimensional phenomenon. As in the fable of the blind men and the elephant, our picture of schizophrenia will approach completeness when we examine as many of these separate but interrelated facets as possible. The viewpoint or definition appropriate to one level is not necessarily more valid than that of another, unsettling as the idea may be to those who still retain concrete and prerelativistic viewpoints about "truth," and particularly to those who concretely rely upon the medical definition of disease as synonymous with somatic lesion.

At the organic level of brain structure and function schizophrenia seems to be a configuration of abnormal structures and circuits in the brain, perhaps subtle alterations in the limbic system and related frontal-cortical pathways, which are apparently (at least in part) inherited, and partly the product of environmental forces in the course of early development, conceptualized as physical processes. One striking conclusion to be tentatively drawn from current organic research is that these changes are so subtle that in many respects they are closer to so-called normal variations in character and personality than they are to the gross lesions we are accustomed to visualizing when we think of pathology. Perhaps it is time to discard our traditional dichotomy between organic and nonorganic forms of psychopathology.

At the level of individual psychology, schizophrenia is the structure and dynamics of a human being who is unable to care for himself or to function adaptively in the world; who is unable to organize his mind and differentiate it from that of others sufficiently to form a stable sense of self; who is both passive about and deeply averse to making the dependent human attachment and doing the mental work necessary for remediation; and who expresses his mental primitivism in characteristic ways.

At the levels of dyadic human relations and the family, schizophrenia represents the pathological protosymbiotic bonding of this passive, self-destructive, functionally incompetent person with one or more others whose sense of self and capacity to function adaptively depends on the active maintenance of a relationship with him. Ironic as it may seem in this context, there appears to be a place for all of us in the world.

Finally, at the sociocultural level, schizophrenia is a defect in the family subsystem of the larger sociocultural system that is at once reflected, enacted, denied, and compensated for so as to maintain the integrity and equilibrium of the larger social order.

If we examine the characteristic features of schizophrenia at each level of the human systems hierarchy we find both constant or enduring elements and novel or emergent ones. The constant elements are those that first manifest themselves as constitutional vulnerabilities at the organic-psychological interface at the dawn of mental life. These include severe impairment of integration and differentiation, with a related absence of coherent self sense, object sense, and reality sense; difficulty with stimulus intensity and regulation, both external and internal; aversion to mental work and mental contents; and aversion to other people. In Chapter 7 I hypothesized that these elements can be grouped into two basic vulnerabilities: one in the area of mental organization and affinity, the other in the area of stimulus intensity and regulation.

At the dyadic and family systems levels, new elements emerge which simultaneously reverberate with, express or enact, and compensate for the deficits of the organic and self-psychological levels, thereby enabling a pathological adaptation or relationship between the schizophrenic and others. The family level supplies the activity, organization, and adaptation which are missing at the individual level. Its provision of sensorimotor–affective thinking and archaic projective-introjective modes of relating compensates for the schizophrenic's basic maladaptive disorganization and inactivity. The family supplies the missing reality sense (denial and inversion) and, for the incoherent schizophrenic, a fragmented, archaic narcissistic sense of personal identity (devalued and grandiose) as well. It compensates for the schizophrenic's missing stimulus-regulating capacity, both external (sensation and perception) and internal (drive and affect), in the case of the former by encouraging his avoidance modes and overprotecting him, and in the latter by initiating and encouraging a process of inner totalitarian invalidation and suppression. Finally, the family supplies the schizophrenic with the caretaking he is unable to provide for himself, in the form of infantilization that enables him to enact his aversion to human contact and to avoid potentially growth-promoting confrontations with his problems.

At the sociocultural level, elements are supplied that maintain the pathological adaptation of the schizophrenic and his family. While on the surface of things it would appear that a concerned society and culture attend to the problem of schizophrenia and struggle to find a solution to it, in fact, society denies the existence of the schizophrenic as an individual as well as of the familial problems that constitute the illness, defines pathological modes of thinking and relating as normal, abets the repressive way the family deals with its schizophrenic member, and compensates for the problems of each. Society even goes so far as to define a reflected and enacted version of the illness itself and the family response to it as "treatment." In other words, from a hierarchical systems standpoint the concept of pathology is relativistic; what we might deem pathological from the standpoint of individual development and actualization of potential may be normal or at least unremarkable at the level of society and culture, thus reflecting an intersystemic conflict of definition and expression which has major implications for our efforts to distinguish between good and bad treatment, or to say it differently, between treatment designed to foster individual autonomy and treatment designed to stabilize a defective family unit and maintain social homeostasis, and to decide which is our goal.

In Chapter 9 I described how the concept of pathological symbiosis is central to an understanding of schizophrenia (and the primitive personality disorders as well). Now we might use the information gained from our review of the more macroscopic levels of family and social functioning to broadly redefine the symbiosis concept. The symbiotic bond formed with the schizophrenic at the interpersonal-familial hierarchical level of function and structure compensates for deficits at the lower, more molecular individual psychic level by providing organization-affinity and stimulus regulation and control. Symbiosis is a particular instance of a larger phenomenon of mutual adaptation characteristic of hierarchical systems, namely, the provision of homeostatic processes and structures at a higher level to compensate for incomplete organization (differentiation and integration), both structural and functional, at a lower one.

Hierarchical systems theory also enables a larger view of some other familiar psychoanalytic concepts, for example, transference and countertransference. In schizophrenia and, I suspect, in many if not most other forms of psychopathology as well, the transference repeats a particular configuration which was actualized in the infant's earliest relationships based on interaction of constitutional factors as well as caregiver idiosyncracies. The countertransference responses of the analyst or therapist, in turn, will reflect, along with idiosyncratic elements, his natural tendency to enact normative socio-cultural responses both to schizophrenia as an illness and to schizophrenic families as a generic social entity.

By using hierarchical systems theory, we come to realize how the theories and associated treatment modalities characteristic of the various human sciences that impinge on schizophrenia may either complement each other and enrich the treatment of schizophrenia or may be destructively antagonistic to one another and unwittingly enact and perpetuate the illness process.

Organic treatment of schizophrenia, unleavened with the viewpoints of other system levels, tends to reify the underlying disease process. Even the possibility of early intervention based on identification of at-risk individuals by such things as biological markers should not stir undue optimism, for the families of the adult schizophrenics we treat, who are the potential intermediaries in any childhood intervention effort, seem deeply committed, at a survival level, to a pathological mode of functioning based on denial and inversion of reality. Unless the form of such intervention is shaped by knowledge of the psychological, familial, and sociocultural levels of schizophrenia, families "at risk" cannot be expected to participate enthusiastically in early remediation efforts that involve the whole personality, and are more likely to manifest an unintegrated response characterized by interpreting the problem as some sort of wart on what they believe to be an otherwise normal personality and family. The case studies in this book eloquently attest to the fact that, even under optimal treatment conditions and when problems have become impossible to avoid, families tend to be refractory to outside intervention. The Swados family, for example (Swados, 1991), was the recipient of considerable outside intervention in the form of schools, doctors, hospitals, and social agencies, and yet its pattern of denial and blaming remained impenetrable and (at least in the case of Elizabeth Swados and her schizophrenic brother) no new learning appears to have occurred.

Just as family attitudes pose a considerable obstacle to effective implementation of treatment of individual instances of schizophrenia, so specific efforts to modify existing social attitudes and practices regarding treatment—including revitalization of the psychological level of treatment in some mental hospitals, provision of increased funding for it, and efforts to enhance communication among members of the various human science professions, are likely to be of little avail unless they are accompanied not only by an awareness of the way society, in the guise of treatment, actually amplifies and reverberates the individual and familial pathology of schizophrenia, but also by an understanding of the reasons why this is so. To comprehend this we must view schizophrenia from a sociocultural perspective, that is, in terms of the threat it poses to the integrity of the nuclear family, which in turn is an essential element of social organization and order. Family integrity is constantly under potential or actual siege from the competing agendas, conflicts, and hostilities of its individual members. I am suggesting that there is an inherent intersystemic conflict between the value of self-actualization, which characterizes the level of personal psychology, especially in Western civilization, and is reflected in disciplines such as psychoanalysis, and the value of family stability, which characterizes the sociocultural level. Thus far, society and culture have lacked effective means to deal with these potentially fragmenting, divisive forces in a way that simultaneously preserves the social fabric and guarantees individual rights; it is possible that the question has never seriously been addressed. How society has chosen to respond may be seen in the myth of the happy family and the myth of treatment (which I describe in Chapters 10 and 11). Perpetuation of these ideas relies heavily on a combination of denial, rejection, and autocratic suppression. The difficulty and relative recency with which society has come to recognize the legitimacy and necessity of divorce and the widespread existence of gross physical child abuse in its various forms (to say nothing of the more subtle forms of abuse described in this book) attests to the truth of this idea. How can we expect a society to confront the subtle but individually devastating psychological maltreatment of children by parents, and the related and even less obvious limitations schizophrenic family organization imposes on autonomy and growth of its non-schizophrenic members, when it has the greatest difficulty acknowledging and intervening in the most gross and horrifying instances of physical abuse committed with direct intent to do harm?

If society can reorient itself to be more truly respectful of the individual autonomy of its members—and our knowledge of what is at stake in preservating the social fabric and the lessons of history with regard to the ubiquitous conflict between individual freedoms and the continuity of empires, nations, and institutions suggest that this is not a broadly held agenda and that we ought not to be overly optimistic in this regard—a better understanding of and support for effective treatment of schizophrenia may be possible. Such treatment comprises the effort of a primitive social system (the mental hospital), sometimes in concert with a (hopefully) better integrated and differentiated individual psychological system (a therapist), to objectify and to work with, on the one hand, the constitutional vulnerability of the schizophrenic and its elaboration in the course of his interpersonal and social development and, on the other hand, the pressures exerted by his family in particular and by our society in general to maintain rather than ameliorate the pathological status quo. In responding to this squeeze play between individual development of the schizophrenic on the one hand, and stabilization of the family and society on the other, the therapeutic "systems" (that is, the therapist and the hospital) must also treat themselves. Without such treatment they have the potential to regress and to become more structurally and functionally primitive as they resonate to, enact, and pathologically attempt to compensate for the difficulties of patient, on the one hand, and family and society, on the other.

The reader who has followed the hierarchical systems model of schizophrenia that I have presented will appreciate that I am not recommending that all schizophrenics and their families, or even most of them, be treated with a combination of long-term hospitalization and individual and family therapy but, rather that the decision about how to treat (the triage pathway involving critical choices that I outline in Chapter 12) be made with as enlightened an appreciation of the balance of forces involved as possible, and not as a blind enactment of the illness process rationalized in the guise of treatment. Often— and hopefully in as individually humane and culturally constructive manner as possible—it will be most judicious to knowingly join with existing personal, familial, and social forces in efforts to stabilize the illness as it is individually expressed and interpersonally and socially enacted and compensated for. To say it differently, treatment of schizophrenia occurs in the potentially creative area of tension generated by the capacity of the treating system—be it individual therapist, hospital, psychopharmacologist, family therapist, or some combination—to objectify and question what would otherwise be an unexamined but pathological enmeshment of schizophrenic pathology and familial and social norms. A creative response to such enmeshment might be to heighten awareness and to promote learning of more autonomous ways of being and relating, or it might involve the conscious choice of perpetuating, in the most benign ways possible, the fit between schizophrenic and society that the family and the culture have already created.

The gravity of the problem presented by the constitutional core of schizophrenia, and the problems and conflicts it presents at each level of the human systems hierarchy as well as between systems themselves, cannot be overestimated. I have tried to demonstrate the value of a hierarchical systems approach in enabling us to both observe and objectify the illness process at each system level and to comprehend what might be transformational forces as contrasted with enactments of the illness rationalized as interventions. While we may be optimistic that we possess the means to intervene in at least some cases of schizophrenia in a way that may make a substantial difference, enabling a person whose development has been vitally aborted to flower in a way that is not only fulfilling to him but productive to society, it is sobering to contemplate the possibility of mitigating the powerful array of forces in the schizophrenic himself, his family, and our society and culture, which are suppressive of the individual schizophrenic person, in order to preserve a larger homeostatsis.

References

Adler, L., Pachtman, E., Franks, R., Pacevich, M., Waldo, M., & Freedman, R. (1982). Neurophysiological evidence for a defect in neuronal mechanisms involved in sensory gating in schizophrenia. *Biol. Psychiatry, 17*:639–654.

Aggleton, J., & Mishkin, M. (1986). The amygdala: sensory gateway to the emotions. In R. Plutchik & H. Kellerman (Eds.), *Emotion: Theory, Research, and Experience: Vol. 3. Biological Foundations of Emotion*. Orlando: Academic Press, pp. 281–299.

Alanen, Y. (1966). The family in the pathogenesis of schizophrenia and neurotic disorders. *Acta Psychiatr. Scand., 42* (Suppl. 189).

Alzheimer, A. (1897). Beitrage zur pathologischen anatomie der hirnrinde und zur anatomischen grundlage einiger psychosen. *Monatsschrift für Psychiatrie und Neurologie, 2*:82–119.

Andreasen, N. (1988). Brain imaging: Applications in psychiatry. *Science, 239*:1381–1388.

——— (1991). Assessment issues and the cost of schizophrenia. *Schizophr. Bull., 17*:475–481.

Andreasen, N., Nasrallah, H., Dunn, V., Olson, S., Grove, W., Ehrhardt, J., Coffman, J., & Crossett, J. (1986). Structural abnormalities in a magnetic resonance imaging study. *Arch. Gen. Psychiatry, 43*:136–144.

Angermeyer, M., Kuhn, L., & Goldstein, J. (1990). Gender and the course of schizophrenia: Differences in treatment outcomes. *Schizophr. Bull., 16*:293–307.

Arieti, S. (1967). New views on the psychodynamics of schizophrenia. *Am. J. Psychiatry, 123*:453–458.

Arlow, J., & Brenner, C. (1964). *Psychoanalytic Concepts and the Structural Theory*. New York: International Universities Press.

——— (1969). The psychotherapy of the psychoses: A proposed revision. *Int. J. Psychoanal., 50*:5–14.

Balint, M. (1965). *Primary Love and Psycho-Analytic Technique*. New York: Liveright.

Basser, L. (1962). Hemiplegia of early onset and the faculty of speech with special reference to the effects of hemispherectomy. *Brain, 85*:427–460.

Bassuk, E., & Gerson, S. (1978). Deinstitutionalization and mental health services. *Scientific American, 238*:46–53.

473

Bateson, G., Jackson, D., Haley, J., & Weakland, J. (1956). Towards a theory of schizo-phrenia. *Behav. Sci., 1*:251–264.

Beiser, M. (1992, March). Paper presented at the Massachusetts Mental Health Center, Boston, MA.

Benes, F., Davidson, J., & Bird, E. (1986). Quantitative cytoarchitectural studies of the cerebral cortex of schizophrenics. *Arch. Gen. Psychiatry, 43*:31–35.

Berenbaum, H., Oltmanns, T., & Gottesman, I. (1987). A twin study perspective on positive and negative symptoms of schizophrenia. In P. Harvey & E. Walker (Eds.), *Positive and Negative Symptoms in Psychoses: Description, Research and Future Directions*. New York: Erlbaum, pp. 50–67.

Bergman, P., & Escalona, S. (1949). Unusual sensitivities in very young children. *Psychoanal. Study Child, 3/4*:333–352.

Bertalanffy, Ludwig von (1952). *Problems of Life*. New York: John Wiley.

—— (1967a). *Robots, Men and Minds*. New York: Braziller.

—— (1967b). The role of systems theory in present-day science, technology and philosophy. In K. Schaefer, H. Hensel, & R. Brady, (Eds.), *Toward a Man-Centered Medical Science*. Mt. Kisco, NY: Futura, pp. 11–16.

—— (1968). *General Systems Theory*. New York: Braziller.

Binswanger, L. (1956). Freud's psychosentherapie. *Psyche, 10*:357–366.

Bion, W. (1957). Differentiation of the psychotic from the non-psychotic personalities. *Int. J. Psychoanal., 38*:266–275.

—— (1959a). Attacks on linking. *Int. J. Psychoanal., 40*:308–315.

—— (1959b). *Experiences in Groups*. London: Tavistock.

—— (1962a). The psychoanalytic theory of thinking: II. A theory of thinking. *Int. J. Psychoanal., 43*:306–310.

—— (1962b). *Learning From Experience*. New York: Basic Books.

—— (1965). *Transformations*. New York: Basic Books.

Bleuler, E. (1911). *Dementia Praecox or the Group of the Schizophrenias*. New York: International Universities Press, 1950.

Bleuler, M. (1968). A 23-year longitudinal study of 208 schizophrenics and impressions in regard to the nature of schizophrenia. In D. Rosenthal & S. Kety (Eds.), *The Transmission of Schizophrenia*. Oxford, UK: Pergamon Press, pp. 3–12.

—— (1978). *The Schizophrenic Disorders: Long Term Patient and Family Studies*. New Haven, CT: Yale University Press.

Bogerts, B., Meertz, E., & Schonfeldt-Bausch, R. (1985). Basal ganglia and limbic system pathology in schizophrenia: A morphometric study of brain volume and shrinkage. *Arch. Gen. Psychiatry, 42*:784–791.

Bookhammer, R., Meyers, R., Shober, C., & Piotrowsky, Z. (1966). A five-year follow-up study of schizophrenics treated by Rosen's "direct analysis:" Compared with controls. *Am. J. Psychiatry, 123*:602–604.

Bowen, M. (1960). A family concept of schizophrenia. In D. Jackson (Ed.), *The Etiology of Schizophrenia*. New York: Basic Books, pp. 346–372.

—— (1965). Family psychotherapy with schizophrenia in the hospital and in private practice. In I. Boszormenyi-Nagy & J. Framo (Eds.), *Intensive Family Therapy*. New York: Harper and Row, pp. 213–243.

Boyer, L. B. (1983). *The Regressed Patient*. New York: Aronson.

Boyer, L., & Giovachinni, P. (1967), *Psychoanalytic Treatment of Schizophrenic and Characterological Disorders*. New York: Science House.

Bracha, H., Torrey, E. F., Bigelow, L., Lohr, J., & Linington, B. (1991). Subtle signs of prenatal maldevelopment of the hand ectoderm in schizophrenia: A preliminary monozygotic twin study. *Biol. Psychiatry, 30*:719–725.

Breier, A., Schreiber, J., Dyer, J., & Pickar, D. (1991). National Institute of Mental Health longitudinal study of chronic schizophrenia. *Arch. Gen. Psychiatry, 48*:239–246.

Broff, D., & Geyer, M. (1978). Sensorimotor gating and schizophrenia: Human and animal model studies. *Arch. Gen. Psychiatry, 47*:181–188.

Bronson, E., & Desjardins, C. (1968). Aggression in adult mice: Modification by neonatal injections of gonadal hormones. *Science, 161*:705–706.

Brown, R., Colter, N., Corsellis, J., Crow, T., Frith, C., Jagoe, R., Johnstone, E., & Marsh, L. (1986). Postmortem evidence of structural brain changes in schizophrenia: Differences in brain weight, temporal horn area and parahippocampal gyrus compared with affective disorder. *Arch. Gen. Psychiatry, 43*:36–42.

Bruton, C., Crow, T., Frith, C., Johnstone, E., Owens, D., & Roberts, G. (1990). Schizophrenia and the brain: a prospective clinico-neuropathology study. *Psychol. Med., 20*:285–304.

Buchsbaum, M. (1990). The frontal lobes, basal ganglia, and temporal lobes as sites for schizophrenia. *Schizophr. Bull., 16*:379–389.

Burnham, D., Gibson, R., & Gladstone, A. (1969). *Schizophrenia and the Need-Fear Dilemma.* New York: International Universities Press.

Bygott, J. (1974). *Agonistic Behavior and Social Relationships among Adult Male Chimpanzees.* Unpublished doctoral dissertation, Cambridge University.

Caldwell, C., & Gottesman, I. (1990). Schizophrenics kill themselves too: A review of risk factors for suicide. *Schizophr. Bull., 16*:571–589.

Campbell, D. (1974). "Downward causation" in hierarchically organized biological systems. In F. Ayala & T. Dobshansky (Eds.), *Studies in the Philosophy of Biology.* London: Macmillan, pp. 179–186.

Cannon, W. (1935). Stresses and strains of homeostasis. *Am. J. Med. Sci., 189*:1–14.

Carew, T., Walters, E., & Kandel, E. (1981). Associative learning in *Aplysia*: Cellular correlates supporting a conditioned fear hypothesis. *Science, 211*:501–504.

Carone, B., Harrow, M., & Westermeyer, J. (1991). Posthospital course and outcome in schizophrenia. *Arch. Gen. Psychiatry, 48*:247–253.

Cleghorn, J. M., Garnett, E., Nahmas, C., Firnau, G., Brown, G., Kaplan, R., Szechtman, H., & Szechtman, B. (1989). Increased frontal and reduced parietal glucose metabolism in acute untreated schizophrenics. *Psychiatry Res., 28*, 119–133.

Clerk, G. (1972). An ego psychological approach to the problem of oral aggression. *Int. J. Psychoanal., 53*:77–82.

Coffman, J., & Nasrallah, H. (1986). Magnetic resonance brain imaging in schizophrenia. In H. Nasrallah & D. Weinberg (Eds.), *Handbook of Schizophrenia: Vol. I. The Neurology of Schizophrenia.* New York: Elsevier Science, pp. 251–256.

Craig, T. (1982). An epidemiologic study of problems associated with violence among psychiatric inpatients. *Am. J. Psychiatry, 139*:1262–1266.

Creese, I., Burt, D., & Snyder, S. (1976). Dopamine receptors and average clinical doses. *Science, 194*:545–546.

Crichton-Browne, J. (1879). On the weight of the brain and its component parts in the insane. *Brain, 2*:42–67.

Crow, T. (1980). Molecular pathology of schizophrenia: More than one disease process? *Br. Med. J., 280*:166–168.

Crow, T., & Johnstone, E. (1987). Schizophrenia: Nature of the disease process and its biological correlates. In F. Plum (Ed.), *Handbook of Physiology: The Nervous System, Vol 6*. Baltimore: American Physiological Society, pp. 843–869.

Davis, M., & Fernald, R. (1990). Social control of neuronal soma size. *J. Neurobiol., 21*:1180–1188.

Dawson, M., & Nuechterlein, K. (1984). Psychophysiological dysfunctions in the developmental course of schizophrenic disorders. *Schizophr. Bull., 10*:204–232.

Delay, J., & Deniker, P. (1952). Trente-huit cas de psychoses traitées par la cure prolongée et continue de 4560 RP. In *Comptes rendus du 50eme congres des medicins alienistes et neurologistes de France et des pays de langue Francaise*. Paris: Masson et Cie.

Delay, J., Deniker, P., & Harl, J. (1952). Utilization thérapeutique psychiatrique d'une phénothiazine d'action centrale elective (4560 RP). *Ann. Med. Psychol., 110*:112–117.

Delbruck, M. (1970). A physicist's renewed look at biology: Twenty years later. *Science, 168*:1312–1315.

DeLisi, L., Dauphinius, I., & Hauser, P. (1989). Gender differences in the brain: Are they relevant to the pathogenesis of schizophrenia? *Compr. Psychiatry, 30*:197–208.

Devereaux, G. (1978). *Ethnopsychoanalysis*. Berkeley, CA: University of California Press.

Diamond, M. C. (1988). *Enriching Heredity: The Impact of the Environment on the Anatomy of the Brain*. New York: Free Press.

Diefendorff, A., & Dodge, R. (1908). An experimental study of the ocular reactions of the insane from photographic records. *Brain, 31*:451–489.

Donnelly, E., Weinberger, D., Waldman, I., & Wyatt, R. J. (1980). Cognitive impairment associated with morphological brain abnormalities on computed tomography in chronic schizophrenic patients. *J. Nerv. Ment. Dis., 168*:305–308.

Drake, R., & Sederer, L. (1986). The adverse effects of intensive treatment of chronic schizophrenia. *Compr. Psychiatry, 27*:313–326.

Edelson, M. (1984). *Hypothesis and Evidence in Psychoanalysis*. Chicago: University of Chicago Press.

——— (1988). *Psychoanalysis: A Theory in Crisis*. Chicago: University of Chicago Press.

Eigen, M. (1986). *The Psychotic Core*. New York: Aronson.

Eisenberg, L. (1986). Mindlessness and brainlessness in psychiatry. *Br. J. Psychiatry, 148*:497–508.

Eissler, K. (1951). Remarks on the psycho-analysis of schizophrenia. *Int. J. Psychoanal., 32*:139–156.

——— (1953). The effect of the structure of the ego on psychoanalytic technique. *J. Am. Psychoanal. Assoc., 1*:104–143.

Ellenberger, H. (1967). The evolution of depth psychology. In I. Galdston (Ed.), *Historic Derivations of Modern Psychiatry*. New York: McGraw-Hill, pp. 159–184.

Engel, G. L. (1977). The need for a new medical model: A challenge for biomedicine. *Science, 196*:129–136.

——— (1980). The clinical application of the biopsychosocial model. *Am. J. Psychiatry, 137*:535–544.

Eysenck, H. (1965). The effects of psychotherapy. *Int. J. Psychiatry, 1*:99–178.

Fairbairn, W. R. D. (1952). *Psychoanalytic Studies of the Personality*. London: Tavistock.

Faraone, S., & Tsuang, M. (1985). Quantitative models of the genetic transmission of schizophrenia. *Psychol. Bull., 98*:41–66.

Farmer, A., McGuffin, P., & Gottesman, I. (1984). Searching for the split in schizophrenia: A twin study. *Psychiatry Res., 13*:109–118.

Federn, P. (1934). The analysis of psychotics. *Int. J. Psychoanal., 15*:209–214.

——— (1952). *Ego Psychology and the Psychoses.* New York: Basic Books.

Feighner, J., Robins, E., & Guze, S. (1972). Diagnostic criteria for use in psychiatric research. *Arch. Gen. Psychiatry, 26*:57–63.

Flavell, J. (1963). *The Developmental Psychology of Jean Piaget.* Princeton, NJ: Van Nostrand.

Flor-Henry, P. (1978). Gender, hemispheric specialization, and psychopathology. *Soc. Sci. Med., 12*:155–162.

——— (1990). Influence of gender in schizophrenia as related to other psychopathological syndromes. *Schizophr. Bull., 16*:211–227.

Fonberg, E. (1986). Amygdala, emotions, motivation, and depressive states. In R. Plutchik & H. Kellerman (Eds.), *Emotion: Theory, Research, and Experience: Vol. 3. Biological Foundations of Emotion.* Orlando: Academic Press, pp. 301–331.

Fotrell, E. (1980). A study of violent behavior among patients in psychiatric hospitals. *Br. J. Psychiatry, 136*:216–221.

Freedman, R., Adler, L., Gerhardt, G., Waldo, M., Baker, N., Rose, G., Drebing, C., Nagamoto, H., Bickford-Wimer, P., & Franks, R. (1987). Neurobiological studies of sensory gating in schizophrenia. *Schizophr. Bull., 13*:669–678.

Freeman, T. (1970). The psychopathology of the psychoses: A reply to Arlow and Brenner. *Int. J. Psychoanal., 51*:407–415.

Freud, S. (1891). *On Aphasia.* New York: International Universities Press.

——— (1894). The neuro-psychoses of defence. In J. Strachey (Ed. & Trans.), *The Standard Edition of the Complete Psychological Works of Sigmund Freud* (Vol. 3, pp. 45–61). London: Hogarth Press, 1962.

——— (1895). Project for a scientific psychology. In J. Strachey (Ed. & Trans.), *The Standard Edition of the Complete Psychological Works of Sigmund Freud* (Vol. 1, pp. 283–397). London: Hogarth Press, 1966.

——— (1896). Further remarks on the neuro-psychoses of defence. In J. Strachey (Ed. & Trans.), *The Standard Edition of the Complete Psychological Works of Sigmund Freud* (Vol. 3, pp. 159–185). London: Hogarth Press, 1962.

——— (1905). On psychotherapy. In J. Strachey (Ed. & Trans.), *The Standard Edition of the Complete Psychological Works of Sigmund Freud* (Vol. 7, pp. 257–268). London: Hogarth Press, 1953.

——— (1911). Psycho-analytic notes on an a case of paranoia (dementia paranoides). In J. Strachey (Ed. & Trans.), *The Standard Edition of the Complete Psychological Works of Sigmund Freud* (Vol. 12, pp. 3–88). London: Hogarth Press, 1958.

——— (1913). On beginning the treatment. In J. Strachey (Ed. & Trans.), *The Standard Edition of the Complete Psychological Works of Sigmund Freud* (Vol. 12, pp. 121–144). London: Hogarth Press, 1958.

——— (1914). On narcissism. In J. Strachey (Ed. & Trans.), *The Standard Edition of the Complete Psychological Works of Sigmund Freud* (Vol. 14, pp. 67–102). London: Hogarth Press, 1957.

——— (1915a). The unconscious. In J. Strachey (Ed. & Trans.), *The Standard Edition of the Complete Psychological Works of Sigmund Freud* (Vol. 14, pp. 159–215). London: Hogarth Press, 1957.

——— (1915b). Instincts and their vicissitudes. In J. Strachey (Ed. & Trans.), *The*

Standard Edition of the Complete Psychological Works of Sigmund Freud (Vol. 14, pp. 109–140). London: Hogarth Press, 1957.

—— (1916–1917). Introductory lectures on psycho-analysis. In J. Strachey (Ed. & Trans.), *The Standard Edition of the Complete Psychological Works of Sigmund Freud* (Vols. 15 & 16). London: Hogarth Press, 1963.

—— (1920). Beyond the pleasure principle. In J. Strachey (Ed. & Trans.), *The Standard Edition of the Complete Psychological Works of Sigmund Freud* (Vol. 18, pp. 3–64). London: Hogarth Press, 1961.

—— (1923). The ego and the id. In J. Strachey (Ed. & Trans.), *The Standard Edition of the Complete Psychological Works of Sigmund Freud* (Vol. 19, pp. 3–66). London: Hogarth Press, 1961.

—— (1924a). Neurosis and psychosis. In J. Strachey (Ed. & Trans.), *The Standard Edition of the Complete Psychological Works of Sigmund Freud* (Vol. 19, pp. 149–153). London: Hogarth Press, 1961.

—— (1924b). The loss of reality in neurosis and psychosis. In J. Strachey (Ed. & Trans.), *The Standard Edition of the Complete Psychological Works of Sigmund Freud* (Vol. 19, pp. 183–187). London: Hogarth Press, 1961.

—— (1926). Inhibitions, symptoms and anxiety. In J. Strachey (Ed. & Trans.), *The Standard Edition of the Complete Psychological Works of Sigmund Freud* (Vol. 20, pp. 77–174). London: Hogarth Press, 1959.

—— (1937). Analysis terminable and interminable. In J. Strachey (Ed. & Trans.), *The Standard Edition of the Complete Psychological Works of Sigmund Freud* (Vol. 23, pp. 209–253). London: Hogarth Press, 1964.

—— (1940). An outline of psychoanalysis. In J. Strachey (Ed. & Trans.), *The Standard Edition of the Complete Psychological Works of Sigmund Freud* (Vol. 23, pp. 144–207). London: Hogarth Press, 1964.

Fromm-Reichmann, F. (1939). Transference problems in schizophrenics. *Psychoanal. Q.*, 8:412–426.

—— (1948). Notes on the development of treatment of schizophrenics by psycho-analytic psychotherapy. *Psychiatry*, *11*:263–273.

—— (1952). Some aspects of psychoanalytic psychotherapy with schizophrenics. In E. Brody & F. Redlich (Eds.), *Psychotherapy with Schizophrenics*. New York: International Universities Press, pp. 89–111.

Fuxe, K., Agnati, L., Harfstrand, A., Cintra, A., Aronsson, M., Zoli, M., & Gustafsson, J.-A. (1988). Principles for the hormone regulation of wiring transmission and volume transmission in the central nervous system. In D. Ganten & D. Pfaff (Eds.), *Neuroendocrinology of Mood*. Berlin: Springer-Verlag, pp. 1–53.

Gardner, E. (1992). Neuroanatomical specificity of action of the atypical antipsychotics. In J-P. Lindenmayer & S. Kay (Eds.), *New Biological Vistas in Schizophrenia: Clinical and Experimental Psychiatry Monograph 6*. New York: Brunner/Mazel, pp. 158–181.

Gedo, J. (1979a). *Beyond Interpretation*. New York: International Universities Press.

—— (1979b). A psychoanalyst reports at mid-career. *Am. J. Psychiatry*, *136*:646–649.

—— (1984). *Psychoanalysis and Its Discontents*. New York: Guilford Press.

—— (1986). *Conceptual Issues in Psychoanalysis*. Hillsdale, NJ: Analytic Press.

—— (1988). *The Mind in Disorder*. Hillsdale, NJ: Analytic Press.

Gedo, J., & Goldberg, A. (1973). *Models of the Mind*. Chicago: University of Chicago Press.

Gibson, R. (1966). The ego defect in schizophrenia. In G. Usdin (Ed.), *Psychoneurosis and Schizophrenia*. Philadelphia: Lippincott, pp. 88–97.

—— (1989). The application of psychoanalytic principles to the hospitalized patient. In A-L. Silver (Ed.), *Psychoanalysis and Psychosis*. Madison, CT: International Universities Press, pp. 183–206.

Gill, M. (1976). Metapsychology is not psychology. *Psychol. Issues*, 36:71–105.

—— (1984). Psychoanalysis and psychotherapy: A revision. *Int. Rev. Psychoanal.*, 11:161–179.

Giovacchini, P. (1983). The persistent psychosis—schizophrenia: With special attention to schizophrenic disorders. *Psychoanal. Inq.*, 3:9–36.

Gittelman-Klein, R., & Klein, D. (1969). Premorbid asocial adjustment and prognosis in schizophrenia. *J. Psychiatr. Res.*, 7:35–53.

Gleick, J. (1987). *Chaos: Making a New Science*. New York: Viking-Penguin.

Golden, C., Graber, B., Moses, J., & Zatz, L. (1980). Differentiation of chronic schizophrenia with and without ventricular enlargement by the Luria- Nebraska neuropsychological battery. *Int. J. Neurosci.*, 11:131–138.

Goldstein, G. (1978). Cognitive and perceptual differences between schizophrenics and organics. *Schizophr. Bull.*, 4:160–185.

Goldstein, J., & Link, B. (1988). Gender differences in the clinical expression of schizophrenia. *J. Psychiatr. Res.*, 22:141–155.

Goldstein, J., & Tsuang, M. (1990). Gender and schizophrenia: An introduction and synthesis of findings. *Schizophr. Bull.*, 16:179–183.

Gottesman, I., McGuffin, P., & Farmer, E. (1987). Clinical genetics as clues to the "real" genetics of schizophrenia. *Schizophr. Bull.*, 13:23–47.

Gottesman, I., & Shields, J. (1982). *Schizophrenia: The Epigenetic Puzzle*. London: Cambridge University Press.

Gould, L. (1948). Verbal hallucinations and activity of vocal musculature: An electromyographic study. *Am. J. Psychiatry*, 105:367–373.

—— (1949). Auditory hallucinations and subvocal speech: Objective study in a case of schizophrenia. *J. Nerv. Ment. Dis.*, 109:418–427.

Green, H. (1964). *I Never Promised You a Rose Garden*. New York: Holt, Rinehart & Winston.

Greenspan, S. (1988). The development of the ego: Insights from clinical work with infants and young children. *J. Am. Psychoanal. Assoc.*, 36(Suppl.): 3–56.

—— (1989a). The development of the ego: Biological and environmental specificity in the psychopathological developmental process and the selection and construction of ego defenses. *J. Am. Psychoanal. Assoc.*, 37:608–638.

—— (1989b). *The Development of the Ego: Implications for Personality Theory, Psychopathology, and the Psychotherapeutic Process*. Madison, CT: International Universities Press.

Grinker, R. (1973). Changing styles in psychoses and borderline states. *Psychiatry*, 130:151–152.

Grinspoon, L., Ewalt, J., & Shader, R. (1972). *Schizophrenia: Pharmacotherapy and Psychotherapy*. Baltimore: Williams & Wilkins.

Grossman, W. (1993). Hierarchies, boundaries and representations in a Freudian model of mental organization. In J. Gedo & A. Wilson (Eds.), *Hierarchical Conceptions in Psychoanalysis: Theory, Research, and Clinical Practice*. New York: Guilford Press, pp. 170–202.

Grotstein, J. (1977). The psychoanalytic concept of schizophrenia: II. Reconciliation. *Int. J. Psychoanal., 58*:427–452.

—— (1989). A revised psychoanalytic conception of schizophrenia: An interdisciplinary update. *Psychoanal. Psychol., 6*:253–275.

—— (1990). The "black hole" as the basic psychotic experience: Some newer psychoanalytic and neuroscience perspective on psychosis. *J. Am. Acad. Psychoanal., 18*:29–46.

Grunbaum, A. (1984). *The Foundations of Psychoanalysis.* Berkeley, CA: University of California Press.

Gunderson, J. (Reporter). (1974). The influence of theoretical models of schizophrenia on treatment practice. *J. Am. Psychoanal. Assoc., 22*:182–199.

Gunderson, J., Frank, A., Katz, H., Vannicelli, M., Frosch, J., & Knapp, P. (1984). Effects of psychotherapy in schizophrenia: II. Comparative outcome of two forms of treatment. *Schizophr. Bull., 10*:564–598.

Gunderson, J., & Mosher, L. (1975). The cost of schizophrenia. *Am. J. Psychiatry, 132*:901–906.

Gur, R. E., Gur, R. C., Skolnick, B., Caroff, S., Obrist, W., Rersnick, S., & Reivich, M. (1985). Brain function in psychiatric disorders: III. Regional cerebral blood flow in unmedicated schizophrenics. *Arch. Gen. Psychiatry, 42*:329–334.

Haas, G., Glick, I., Clarkin, J., Spencer, H., & Lewis, A. (1990). Gender and schizophrenia outcome: A clinical trial of an inpatient family intervention. *Schizophr. Bull., 16*:277–292.

Haas, G., Hien, D., Waked, W., Sweeney, J., Werden, P., & Frances, A. (1989). Sex differences in schizophrenia. *Schizophr. Res., 2*:11.

Haber, S. (1981). Social factors in evaluating the effects of biological manipulations on aggressive behavior in nonhuman primates. In D. Hamburg & M. Trudeau (Eds.), *Biobehavioral Aspects of Aggression.* New York: Alan R. Liss.

Hanfmann, E., & Kasanin, J. (1942). *Conceptual Thinking in Schizophrenia, Monograph 67.* New York: Nervous and Mental Disease Publishing Co.

Harding, C., Brooks, G., Ashikaga, T., Strauss, J., & Brier, A. (1987). The Vermont longitudinal study of persons with severe mental illness: II. Long-term outcome of subjects who retrospectively met DSM-III criteria for schizophrenia. *Am. J. Psychiatry, 144*:727–735.

Harlow, H. (1958). The nature of love. *Am. Psychol., 13*:673–685.

Harlow, H., & Harlow, M. (1962). Social deprivation in monkeys. *Sci. Am., 207*:136–146.

Harlow, H., Rowland, G., & Griffin, G. (1964). The effect of total social deprivation on the development of monkey behavior. In P. Solomon & B. Glueck (Eds.), *Recent Research on Schizophrenia: Psychiatric Research Report 19.* Washington, DC: American Psychiatric Association, pp. 116–135.

Hartmann, H. (1950). Comments on the psychoanalytic theory of the ego. *Psychoanal. Study Child, 5*:74–96.

—— (1953). Contribution to the metapsychology of schizophrenia. *Psychoanal. Study Child, 8*:177–198.

Haug, J. (1962). Pneumoencephalographic studies in mental disease. *Acta Psychiatr. Scand., 38*:1–114.

Havens, L. (1962). The placement and movement of hallucinations in space: Phenomenology and theory. *Int. J. Psychoanal., 43*:426–435.

Heaton, R., Baade, L., & Johnson, K. (1978). Neuropsychological test results associated with psychiatric disorders in adults. *Psychol. Bull., 85*:141–162.

Heisenberg, W. (1958). *Physics and Philosophy: The Revolution in Modern Science.* New York: Harper & Row.

Hendrick, I. (1951). Early development of the ego: Identification in infancy. *Psychoanal. Q., 20*:44–61.

Heston, L. (1966). Psychiatric disorders in foster home reared children of schizophrenic mothers. *Br. J. Psychiatry, 112*:819–825.

―――― (1970). The genetics of schizophrenia and schizoid disease. *Science, 167*:249–256.

Hill, L. (1955). *Psychotherapeutic Intervention in Schizophrenia.* Chicago: University of Chicago Press.

Hirsch, S. (1979). Do parents cause schizophrenia? *Trends in Neurosci., 2*:49–52.

Hofer, M. (1981). *The Roots of Human Behavior.* San Francisco: Freeman.

Holzman, P. (1975). Problems of psychoanalytic theories. In J. Gunderson & L. Mosher (Eds.), *Psychotherapy of Schizophrenia.* New York: Aronson, pp. 209–222.

―――― (1987). Recent studies of psychophysiology in schizophrenia. *Schizophr. Bull., 13*:49–75.

Holzman, P., Proctor, L., & Hughes, D. (1973). Eye tracking patterns in schizophrenia. *Science, 181*:179–181.

Horwitz, W., Polatin, P., Kolb, L., & Hoch, P. (1958). A study of cases of schizophrenia treated by direct analysis. *Am. J. Psychiatry, 114*:780–783.

Hubel, D., & Wiesel, T. (1977). Functional architecture of Macaque monkey visual cortex. *Proc. R. Soc. Lond., 198*:1–59.

Huber, G., Gross, G., & Schuttler, R. (1975). A long-term follow-up study of schizophrenia: Psychiatric course of illness and prognosis. *Acta Psychiatr. Scand., 52*:49–57.

Huber, G., Gross, G., Schuttler, R., & Linz, M. (1980). Longitudinal studies of schizophrenic patients. *Schizophr. Bull., 6*:592–605.

Huxley, T. (1898). *Method and Results: Collected Essays, Vol. I.* London: Macmillan.

Ingvar, D., & Franzen, G. (1974). Abnormalities of cerebral blood flow in patients with chronic schizophrenia. *Acta Psychiatr. Scand., 50*:425–462.

Jackson, D. (1960). *Etiology of Schizophrenia.* New York: Basic Books.

Jackson, J. H. (1931–1932). *Selected Writings of John Hughlings Jackson* (J. Taylor, G. Holmes, & F. Walshe, Eds.) New York: Basic Books, 1958.

Jacobi, W., & Winkler, H. (1927). Encaphalographische studies au chronisch schizophrenen. *Archiv für Psychiatrie und Nevenkrankheiten, 81*:299–332.

Jacobson, E. (1953). Metapsychology of psychotic depression. In P. Greenacre (Ed.), *Affective Disorders.* New York: International Universities Press, pp. 49–83.

―――― (1971). *Depression.* New York: International Universities Press.

Johnson, A., Giffin, M., Watson, E. J., & Beckett, P. (1956). Studies in schizophrenia at the Mayo Clinic. II. Observations on ego functions in schizophrenia. *Psychiatry, 19*:143–148.

Johnstone, E., Crow, T., Frith, C., Husband, J., & Kreel, L. (1976). Cerebral ventricular size and cognitive impairment in chronic schizophrenia. *Lancet, 2*:924–926.

Jones, E. (1953). *The Life and Work of Sigmund Freud.* New York: Basic Books.

Joselyn, W. (1973). Androgen-induced social dominance in infant female rhesus monkeys. *J. Child Psychol. Psychiatry, 14*:137–145.

Josiassen, R., Roemer, R., Johnson, M., & Shagass, C. (1990). Are gender differences in schizophrenia related to brain-event related potentials? *Schizophr. Bull., 16*:229–246.

Kandel, E. (1978). *A Cell Biological Approach to Learning.* Baltimore, MD: Society for Neuroscience.

―――― (1979). Psychotherapy and the single synapse. *N. Engl. J. Med., 301*:1029–1037.

Kantrowitz, J., Katz, A., & Paolitto, F. (1990). Follow-up of psychoanalysis five to ten years after termination: I. Stability of change. *J. Am. Psychoanal. Assoc., 38*:471–496.

Karon, B., & VandenBos, G. (1981). *Psychotherapy of Schizophrenia: The Treatment of Choice.* New York: Aronson.

Karson, C., & Bigelow, L. (1987). Violent behavior in schizophrenic inpatients. *J. Nerv. Ment. Dis., 175*:161–164.

Kasanin, J. (1944). *Language and Thought in Schizophrenia.* New York: Norton.

Katan, M. (1954). The importance of the non-psychotic part of the personality in schizophrenia. *Int. J. Psychoanal., 35*:119–128.

Kendler, K. (1992). The genetics of schizophrenia: An overview. In S. Steinhauer, J. Gruzelier, & J. Zubin (Eds.), *Neuropsychology, Psychophysiology and Information Processing: Handbook of Schizophrenia, Vol. 5.* New York: Elsevier Science, pp. 437–462.

Kernberg, O. (1972). Early ego integration and object relations. *Ann. NY Acad. Sci., 193*:233–247.

―――― (1975). *Borderline Conditions and Pathological Narcissism.* New York: Aronson.

Kessler, S. (1980). The genetics of schizophrenia: A review. *Schizophr. Bull., 6*:404–416.

Kestenbaum, C. (1986). Thoughts on the precursors of affective and cognitive disturbance in schizophrenia. In D. Feinsilver (Ed.), *Towards a Comprehensive Model for Schizophrenic Disorders: Psychoanalytic Essays in Memory of Ping-Nie-Pao.* Hillsdale, NJ: Analytic Press, pp. 211–236.

Kety, S. (1978). The biological and adoptive families of adopted individuals who become schizophrenic: Prevalence of mental illness and other characteristics. In L. Wynne (Ed.), *The Nature of Schizophrenia: New Approaches to Research and Treatment.* New York: Wiley, pp. 25–37.

―――― (1983). Observations on genetic and environmental influences in the etiology of mental disorders from studies on adoptees and their relatives. In S. Kety, L. Rowland, R. Sedman, & S. Matthysse (Eds.), *Genetics of Neurological and Psychiatric Disorders.* New York: Raven Press, pp. 105–114.

Kety, S., Rosenthal, D., Wender, P., & Schulsinger, F. (1972). Mental illness in the biological and adoptive families of adopted schizophrenics. *Am. J. Psychiatry, 128*:302–306.

Kety, S., Rosenthal, D., Wender, P., Schulsinger, F., & Jacobsen, B. (1975). Mental illness in the biologic and adoptive families of adopted individuals who became schizophrenic: A preliminary report based on psychiatric interviews. In R. Fieve, D. Rosenthal, & H. Brill (Eds.), *Genetic Research in Psychiatry.* Baltimore: Johns Hopkins University Press, pp. 147–165.

Kinney, D., & Matthysse, S. (1978). Genetic transmission of schizophrenia. *Annu. Rev. Med., 29*:459–473.

Kirch, D., & Weinberger, D. (1986). Anatomical neuropathology in schizophrenia: Postmortem findings. In H. Nasrallah & D. Weinberger (Eds.), *Handbook of*

Schizophrenia: Vol. I. The Neurology of Schizophrenia. New York: Elsevier Science, pp. 325–348.

Kirk, S., & Thierren, M. (1975). Community mental health myths and the fate of formerly hospitalized mental patients. *Psychiatry, 38*:209–217.

Klein, M. (1948). *Contributions to Psycho-Analysis, 1921–1945*. London: Hogarth Press.

Kling, A. (1986). The anatomy of aggression and affiliation. In R. Plutchik & H. Kellerman (Eds.), *Emotion: Theory, Research, and Experience: Vol. 3. Biological Foundations of Emotion*. Orlando: Academic Press, pp. 237–264.

Knight, R. (1946). Psychotherapy of an adolescent catatonic schizophrenia with mutism. *Psychiatry, 9*:323–339.

——— (1953). Management and psychotherapy of the borderline schizophrenic patient. *Bull. Menninger Clin., 17*:139–150.

Knox, R. (1989). Liver transplant from live donor prompts optimism and caution. *Boston Globe*, November 29.

Koestler, A., & Smythies, J. (1969). *Beyond Reductionism: New Perspectives in the Life Sciences*. New York: Macmillan.

Kohut, H. (1971). *The Analysis of the Self*. New York: International Universities Press.

——— (1973). *The Restoration of the Self*. New York: International Universities Press.

Kolb, L. (1987). A neuropsychological hypothesis explaining posttraumatic stress disorders. *Am. J. Psychiatry, 144*:989–995.

Kopala, L., & Clark, C. (1990). Implications of olfactory agnosia for understanding sex differences in schizophrenia. *Schizophr. Bull., 16*:255–261.

Kraepelin, E. (1896). *Dementia Praecox and Paraphrenia* (R. M. Barclay, Trans.). Edinburgh: E. & S. Livingstone; New York: R. E. Krieger, 1919.

Kringlen, E. (1987). Contributions of genetic studies on schizophrenia. In H. Hafner, W. Gattaz, & W. Janzarik (Eds.), *Search for the Causes of Schizophrenia*. Berlin: Springer-Verlag, pp. 123–142.

Laborit, H., Huguenard, P., & Alluaume, R. (1952). Un nouveau stabilisateur vegetatif, le 4560 RP. *Presse Medicale, 60*:206–208.

Langfeldt, G. (1939). *The Schizophreniform States*. Copenhagen: Munksgaard.

Lazarus, R. (1966). *Psychological Stress and the Coping Process*. New York: McGraw-Hill.

Levenson, E. (1989). Whatever happened to the cat? Interpersonal perspectives on the self. *Contemp. Psychoanal., 25*:537–553.

Leventhal, B., & Brodie, K. (1981). The pharmacology of violence. In D. Hamburg & M. Trudeau (Eds.), *Biobehavioral Aspects of Aggression*. New York: Alan R. Liss, pp. 85–106.

Levin, F., & Vuckovich, D. (1987). Brain plasticity, learning, and psychoanalysis: Some mechanisms of integration and coordination within the central nervous system. *Annu. Psychoanal., 15*:49–96.

Lewine, R. (1980). Sex differences in the age of symptom onset and first hospitalization in schizophrenia. *Am. J. Orthopsychiatry, 50*:316–322.

——— (1988). Gender and schizophrenia. In M. Tsuang & J. Simpson (Eds.), *Handbook of Schizophrenia: Vol. 3. Nosology, Epidemiology, and Genetics*. Amsterdam: Elsevier Press, pp. 379–397.

Liberman, R., Barringer, D. M., Marder, S., Dawson, M., Nuechterlein, K., & Doane, J. (1984). The nature and problem of schizophrenia. In A. Bellack (Ed.) *Schizophrenia: Treatment, Management, and Rehabilitation*. Orlando: Grune & Stratton, pp. 1–34.

Lidz, T. (1973). *The Origin and Treatment of Schizophrenic Disorders*. New York: Basic Books.

———— (1990). Optimism in treatment of schizophrenia still premature, says expert. *Psychiatric News 25*(6):26,33.

Lidz, T., Cornelison, A., Fleck, S., & Terry, D.(1957). The intrafamilial environment of schizophrenic patients: II. Marital schism and marital skew. *Am. J. Psychiatry, 114*:241–248.

Lidz, T., & Fleck, S. (1965). *Schizophrenia and the Family*. New York: International Universities Press.

Lindner, R. (1955). *The Fifty Minute Hour*. New York: Holt, Rinehart & Winston.

Loewald, H. (1971). On motivation and instinct theory. *Psychoanal. Study Child, 26*:91–128.

London, N. (1973). An essay on psychoanalytic theory: Two theories of schizophrenia: Part II. Discussion and restatement of the specific theory of schizophrenia. *Int. J. Psychoanal., 54*:179–193.

———— (1983). Psychoanalytic psychotherapy of schizophrenia: A psychoanalytic view from without. *Psychoanal. Inq., 3*:91–104.

MacLean, P. (1985). Brain evolution relating to family, play, and the separation call. *Arch. Gen. Psychiatry, 42*:405–417.

———— (1990). *The Triune Brain in Evolution*. New York: Plenum Press.

Mahler, M. (1968). *On Human Symbiosis and the Vicissitudes of Individuation: Vol. I. Infantile Psychosis*. New York: International Universities Press.

Main, T. F. (1957). The ailment. *Br. J. Med. Psychol., 30*:129–145.

Malec, J. (1978). Neuropsychological assessment of schizophrenia versus brain damage: A review. *J. Nerv. Ment. Dis., 166*:507–516.

Mandelbrot, B. (1977). *The Fractal Geometry of Nature*. New York: Freeman.

Marlowe, W., Mancall, E., & Thomas, J. (1975). Complete Kluver-Bucy syndrome in man. *Cortex, 11*:53–59.

Marsella, A., & Snyder, K. (1981). Stress, social supports, and schizophrenic disorders: Toward an interactional model. *Schizophr. Bull., 7*:152–163.

Mason, W., & Sponholz, R. (1963). Monkeys raised in isolation. *J. Psychiatr. Res., 1*:98–306.

May, P. (1968). *Treatment of Schizophrenia: A Comparative Study of Five Treatment Methods*. New York: Science House.

Mazur, A. (1976). Effects of testosterone on status in primate groups. *Folia Primatol., 26*:214–226.

McCarley, R., Faux, S., Shenton, M., Nestor, P., & Adams, J. (1991). Event-related potentials in schizophrenia: Their biological and clinical correlates and a new model of schizophrenic pathophysiology. *Schizophr. Res., 4*:209–231.

McCarley, R. Lecture at Cambridge City Hospital, Cambridge, MA, January 15, 1992.

McGlashan, T. (1984). The Chestnut Lodge follow-up study: II. Long-term outcome of schizophrenia and the affective disorders. *Arch. Gen. Psychiatry, 41*:586–601.

———— (1988). Selective review of recent North American long-term follow-up studies of schizophrenia. *Schizophr. Bull., 14*:515–542.

McGlashan, T., & Bardenstein, K. (1990). Gender differences in affective, schizoaffective, and schizophrenic disorders. *Schizophr. Bull., 16*: 319–330.

McGlashan, T., & Keats, C. (1989). *Schizophrenia: Treatment Process and Outcome*. Washington, DC: American Psychiatric Press.

McGue, M., & Gottesman, I. (1989). Genetic linkage in schizophrenia: Perspectives from genetic epidemiology. *Schizophr. Bull., 15*:453–464.

Meehl, P. (1962). Schizotaxia, schizotypy, and schizophrenia. *Am. Psychol., 17*:827–837.

Meissner, W. W. (1985). Review of *The Regressed Patient* by L. B. Boyer. *Psychoanal. Q., 54*:89–91.

Mesulam, M. M. (1990). Schizophrenia and the brain. *N. Engl. J. Med., 322*:842–845.

Moore, B., & Fine, B. (Eds.). (1990). *Psychoanalytic Terms and Concepts*. New Haven, CT: Yale University Press.

Moran, M. (1991). Chaos and psychoanalysis: The fluidic nature of mind. *Int. Rev. Psychoanal., 18*:211–221.

Morrison, J., Winokur, G., Crowe, R., & Clancy, J. (1973). The Iowa 500: The first follow-up. *Arch. Gen. Psychiatry, 29*:678–682.

Nasrallah, H., Andreasen, N., Coffman, J., Olson, S., Dunn, V., Erhardt, J., & Chapman, S. (1986). A controlled magnetic resonance imaging study of corpus callosum thickness in schizophrenia. *Biol. Psychiatry, 21*:274–282.

Nozick, R. (1981). *Philosophical Explanations*. Cambridge, MA: Harvard University Press.

Nuechterlein, K., & Dawson, M. (1984). Information processing and attentional functioning in the developmental course of schizophrenic disorders. *Schizophr. Bull., 10*:160–203.

Nuechterlein, K., Dawson, M., Gitlin, M., Ventura, J., Goldstein, M., Snyder, K., Yee, C., & Mintz, J. (1992). Developmental processes in schizophrenic disorders: Longitudinal studies of vulnerability and stress. *Schizophr. Bull., 18*:387–425.

Nunberg, H. (1921). The course of the libidinal conflict in a case of schizophrenia. In H. Nunberg (Ed.), *Practice and Theory of Psychoanalysis*. New York: Nervous and Mental Disease Monographs, 1948, pp. 24–49.

Ogden, T. (1980). On the nature of schizophrenic conflict. *Int. J. Psychoanal., 61*:513–533.

Ornitz, E., & Pynoos, R. (1989). Startle modulation in children with posttraumatic stress disorder. *Am. J. Psychiatry, 146*:866–870.

Pao, P. N. (1979). *Schizophrenic Disorders*. New York: International Universities Press.

Pardes, H., Kaufman, C., Pincus, H., & West, A. (1989) Genetics and psychiatry: Past discoveries, current dilemmas, and future directions. *Am. J. Psychiatry, 146*:435–443

Parish, E. (1897). *Hallucinations and Illusions*. London: Walter Scott.

Parke, R., & Slaby, R. (1983). The development of aggression. In P. Mussen (Ed.), *Handbook of Child Psychology, Vol. 4*. New York: Wiley, pp. 547–642.

Parkenberg, B. (1987). Post-mortem study of chronic schizophrenic brains. *Br. J. Psychiatry, 151*: 744–752.

Parnas, J., Schulsinger, F., Teasdale, T., Schulsinger, H., Feldman, P., Mednick, S. (1982). Perinatal complications and clinical outcome within the schizophrenia spectrum. *Br. J. Psychiatry, 140*:416–420.

Pearlson, G., Garbacz, D., Moberg, P., Ahn, H., & DePaulo, J. R. (1985). Symptomatic, familial, perinatal, and social correlates of computerized axial tomography (CAT) changes in schizophrenics and bipolars. *J. Nerv. Ment. Dis., 173*:42–55.

Perls, F., Hefferline, R., & Goodman, P. (1951). *Gestalt Therapy: Excitement and Growth in the Human Personality*. New York: Dell.

Peterfreund, E. (1978). Some critical comments on psychoanalytic conceptualizations of infancy. *Int. J. Psychoanal., 61*:477–491.

Plomin, R. (1989). Environment and genes: determinants of behavior. *Am. Psychol., 44*: 105–111.

Popper, K. (1963). *Conjectures and Refutations.* New York: Basic Books.

Popper, K., & Eccles, J. (1981). *The Self and Its Brain.* New York: Springer International.

Rado, S. (1962). Theory and therapy: The theory of schizotypal organization and its application to the treatment of decompensated schizotypal behavior. In S. Rado (Ed.), *Psychoanalysis of Behavior, Vol. 2.* New York: Grune & Stratton, pp. 127–140.

Ram, R., Bromet, E., Eaton, W., Pato, C., & Schwartz, J. (1992). The natural course of schizophrenia: A review of first admission studies. *Schizophr. Bull., 18*:185–207.

Rao, D., Morton, N., Gottesman, I., & Lew, R. (1981). Pathological analysis of qualitative data on pairs of relatives: Applicability to schizophrenia. *Hum. Hered., 31*: 325–333.

Rapaport, D. (1958). The theory of ego autonomy: A generalization. *Bull. Menninger Clin., 22*:13–35.

——— (1960). *The Structure of Psychoanalytic Theory: A Systematizing Attempt.* New York: International Universities Press.

Reichard, S. (1956). A re-examination of "Studies in Hysteria." *Psychoanal. Q., 25*:155–177.

Reveley, A., Reveley, M., Clifford, C., & Murray, R. (1982). Cerebral ventricular size in twins discordant for schizophrenia. *Lancet, 1*: 540–541.

Reveley, A. M., Reveley, M., & Murray, R. (1983). Enlargement of cerebral ventricles in schizophrenia is confined to those without known genetic predisposition. *Lancet, 2*:525.

Rieder, R., Donnelly, E., Herdt, J., & Waldman, N. (1979). Sulcal prominence in young chronic schizophrenic patients: CT scan findings associated with impairment on neuropsychological tests. *Psychiatr. Res., 1*:1–8.

Ritvo, E. (1983). The syndrome of autism: A medical model. *Integrative Psychiatry, 1*:103–122.

——— (1985). Evidence for autosomal recessive inheritance in 46 families with multiple incidences of autism. *Am. J. Psychiatry, 142*:187–192.

Robbins, M. (1969). On the psychology of artistic creativity. *Psychoanal. Study Child, 24*:227–251.

——— (1981a). The symbiosis concept and the commencement of normal and pathological ego functioning and object relations: I. Infancy. *Int. Rev. Psychoanal., 8*:365–377.

——— (1981b). The symbiosis concept and the commencement of normal and pathological ego functioning and object relations: II. Developments subsequent to infancy and pathological processes. *Int. Rev. Psychoanal., 8*:379–391.

——— (1983). Toward a new mind model for the primitive personalities. *Int. J. Psychoanal., 64*:127–148.

——— (1988). The adaptive significance of destructiveness in primitive personalities. *J. Am. Psychoanal. Assoc., 36*:627–652.

——— (1989). Primitive personality organization as an interpersonally adaptive modification of cognition and affect. *Int. J. Psychoanal., 70*:443–457.

—— (1992). Psychoanalytic and biological approaches to mental illness: Schizophrenia. *J. Am. Psychoanal. Assoc., 40*:425–454.

—— (1993). Disturbances of affect representation in primitive personalities. In J. Gedo & A. Wilson (Eds.), *Hierarchical Conceptions in Psychoanalysis*. New York: Guilford Press, pp. 235–262.

Roberts, G., Colter, N., Lofthouse, R., Johnstone, E., & Crow, T. (1987). Is there gliosis in schizophrenia? Investigation of the temporal lobe. *Biol. Psychiatry, 22*:1459–1486.

Robins, E., & Guze, S. (1970). Establishment of diagnostic validity in psychiatric illness: Its application to schizophrenia. *Am. J. Psychiatry, 126*:983–987.

Rolls, E. (1986). Neural systems involved in emotion in primates. In R. Plutchik & H. Kellerman (Eds.), *Emotion: Theory, Research, and Experience: Vol. 3. Biological Foundations of Emotion*. Orlando: Academic Press, pp. 125–143.

Rose, R., Haladay, J., & Bernstein, J. (1971). Plasma testosterone, dominance rank, and aggressive behavior in rhesus monkeys. *Nature, 231*:366.

Rosen, J. (1947). The treatment of schizophrenic psychosis by direct analytic therapy. *Psychoanal. Q., 21*:3–25.

—— (1953). *Direct Analysis: Selected Papers*. New York: Grune & Stratton.

Rosenfeld, H. (1965). *Psychotic States*. London: Hogarth Press.

Rosenthal, D. (1963). *The Genain Quadruplets*. New York: Basic Books.

Rosenthal, D., Wender, P., Kety, S., & Schulsinger, F. (1971). The adopted away offspring of schizophrenics. *Am. J. Psychiatry, 128*:397–411.

Rossi, M., Jacobs, M., Monteleone, M., Olsen, R., Surber, R., Winkler, E., & Wommack, A. (1986). Characteristics of psychiatric patients who engage in assaultive or other fear-inducing behaviors. *J. Nerv. Ment. Dis., 174*:154–160.

Rousseau, J. (1762). *The Social Contract*. New York: Dutton, 1950.

Sandler, J., with Freud, A. (1983). Discussions in the Hampstead Index of *The Ego and The Mechanisms of Defense*. *J. Am. Psychoanal. Assoc., 31*(Suppl.):19–146.

Sartorius, N., Jablensky, A., Korten, A., Ernberg, G., Anker, M., Cooper, J., & Day, R. (1986). Early manifestations and first-contact incidence of schizophrenia in different cultures. *Psychol. Med., 16*:909–928.

Scheflen, A. (1960). *A Psychotherapy of Schizophrenia: Direct Analysis*. Springfield, IL: Thomas.

Schneider, K. (1959). *Clinical Psychopathology*. New York: Grune & Stratton.

Schwing, G. (1954). *A Way to the Soul of the Mentally Ill*. New York: International Universities Press.

Scull, A. (1989). *Social Order/Mental Disorder*. Berkeley: University of California Press.

Searles, H. (1965). *Collected Papers on Schizophrenia and Related Subjects*. London: Hogarth Press.

Sechehaye, M. (1951). *Symbolic Realization*. New York: International Universities Press.

Seeman, M. (1982). Gender differences in schizophrenia. *Can. J. Psychiatry, 27*:107–111.

—— (1985). Interaction of sex, age, and neuroleptic dose. *Compr. Psychiatry, 24*:124–128.

—— (1986). Current outcome in schizophrenia: Women vs. men. *Acta Psychiatr. Scand., 73*:609–617.

Seeman, M., & Lang, M. (1990). The role of estrogens in schizophrenia gender differences. *Schizophr. Bull., 16*:185–194.

Seidman, L. (1983). Schizophrenia and brain dysfunction: An integration of recent neurodiagnostic findings. *Psychol. Bull.*, *94*:195–238.

Selye, H. (1950). *The Physiology and Pathology of Exposure to Systemic Stress.* Montreal: Acta.

—— (1956). *The Stress of Life.* New York: McGraw-Hill.

Shader, R., Jackson, A., Harmatz, J., & Applebaum, P. (1977). Patterns of violent behavior among schizophrenic inpatients. *Dis. Nerv. Syst.*, *38*:13–16.

Shapiro, T. (1989). Paper presented at McLean Hospital, Belmont, MA, December 8.

Sharfstein, S. (1991). Prospective cost allocation for the chronic schizophrenic patient. *Schizophr. Bull.*, *17*:395–400.

Shelton, R., Karson, C., Doran, A., Pickar, D., Bigelow, L., & Weinberger, D. (1988). Cerebral structural pathology in schizophrenia: Evidence for a selective prefrontal cortical defect. *Am. J. Psychiatry*, *145*:154–163.

Shelton, R., & Weinberger, D. (1986). X-ray computerized tomography studies of schizophrenia: A review and synthesis. In H. Nasrallah & D. Weinberger (Eds.), *Handbook of Schizophrenia: Vol. I. The Neurology of Schizophrenia.* New York: Elsevier Science, pp. 207–250.

Sherwin, B. (1988). Affective changes with estrogen and androgen replacement therapy in surgically menopausal women. *J. Affective Disord.*, *14*:177–187.

Siever, L., & Coursey, R. (1985). Biological markers for schizophrenia and the biological high-risk approach. *J. Nerv. Ment. Dis.*, *173*:4–16.

Snyder, S., Banerjee, S., Yamamura, H., & Greenberg, D. (1974). Drugs, neurotransmitters and schizophrenia. *Science, 184*:1243–1253.

Southard, E. (1910). A study of the dementia praecox group in the light of certain cases showing anomalies or sclerosis in particular brain regions. *Am. J. Insanity, 67*:119–176.

—— (1912). Psychopathology and neuropathology: the problems of teaching and research contrasted. *Am. J. Psychol., 23*:230–235.

—— (1914). On the topographical distribution of cortex lesions and anomalies in dementia praecox, with some account of their functional significance. *Am. J. Insanity, 71*:603–671.

Spence, D. P. (1982). *Narrative Truth and Historical Truth: Meaning and Interpretation in Psychoanalysis.* New York: Norton.

Sperry, R. W. (1969). A modified concept of consciousness. *Psychol. Rev.*, *76*:532–536.

Spotnitz, H. (1976). *Psychotherapy of the Pre-Oedipal Conditions: Schizophrenia and Severe Character Disorders.* New York: Aronson.

Spring, B., Weinstein, L., Freeman, F., & Thompson, S. (1992). Selective attention in schizophrenia. In S. Steinhauer, J. Gruzelier, & J. Zubin (Eds.), *Neuropsychology, Psychophysiology and Information Processing: Vol. 5. Handbook of Schizophrenia.* New York: Elsevier Science, pp. 371–396.

Spruiell, V. (1993). Deterministic chaos and the sciences of complexity: Psychoanalysis in the midst of a general scientific revolution. *J. Am. Psychoanal. Assoc., 41*:1–44.

Stanton, A., Gunderson, J., Knapp, P., Frank, A., Vanicelli, M., Schnitzer, R., & Rosenthal, R. (1984). Effects of psychotherapy in schizophrenia: I. Design and implementation of a controlled study. *Schizophr. Bull., 10*:520–562.

Stanton, A., & Schwartz, M. (1954). *The Mental Hospital.* New York: Basic Books.

Stern, D. (1985). *The Interpersonal World of the Infant.* New York: Basic Books.

Stevens, J. (1982). Neuropathology of schizophrenia. *Arch. Gen. Psychiatry, 39*:1131–1139.

Stierlin, H. (1975). Schizophrenic core disturbances. In J. Gunderson & L. Mosher (Eds.), *Psychotherapy of Schizophrenia*. New York: Aronson, pp. 317–322.

Stone, M. (1986). Exploratory psychotherapy in schizophrenia-spectrum patients: A reevaluation in the light of long-term follow-up of schizophrenic and borderline patients. *Bull. Menninger Clin., 50*:287– 346.

Strauss, J., & Carpenter, W. (1972). The prediction of outcome in schizophrenia. *Arch. Gen. Psychiatry, 27*:739–746.

——— (1977). Prediction of outcome in schizophrenia, III: Five-year outcome and its predictors. *Arch. Gen. Psychiatry, 34*:159–163.

——— (1981). *Schizophrenia*. New York: Plenum.

Strauss, J., Carpenter, W., & Bartko, J. (1974). The diagnosis and understanding of schizophrenia: Part II. Speculations on the processes that underlie schizophrenic symptoms and signs. *Schizophr. Bull., 11*:61–76

Suddath, R., Casanova, M., Goldberg, T., Daniel, D., Kelsoe, J., & Weinberger, D. (1989). Temporal lobe pathology in schizophrenia: A quantitative magnetic resonance imagery study. *Am. J. Psychiatry, 146*:454–472.

Suddath, R., Christison, G., Torrey, E., Casanova, M., & Weinberger, D. (1990). Cerebral anatomical abnormalities in monozygotic twins discordant for schizophrenia. *N. Engl. J. Med., 322*:789–794.

Sullivan, H. S. (1929) *The Interpersonal Theory of Psychiatry*. Washington, DC: William Alanson White, 1953.

——— (1956). *Clinical Studies in Psychiatry*. New York: Norton.

——— (1962). *Schizophrenia as a Human Process*. New York: Norton.

Suttie, I. D. (1935). *The Origins of Love and Hate*. London: Kegan Paul, Trench, Trubner.

Swaab, D., & Fliers, E. (1985). A sexually dimorphic nucleus in the human brain. *Science, 228*:1112–1115.

Swados, E. (1991). *The Four of Us*. New York: Farrar, Straus & Giroux.

Tamminga, A., Thaku, G., Buchanan, R., Kirkpatrick, B., Alphs, L., Chase, N., & Carpenter, W. (1992). Limbic system abnormalities identified in schizophrenia using positron emission tomography with fluorodeoxyglucose and neocortical alterations with deficit syndrome. *Arch. Gen. Psychiatry, 49*:522–530.

Tardiff, K., & Sweillam, A. (1980). Assault, suicide, and mental illness. *Arch. Gen. Psychiatry, 37*:164–169.

——— (1982). Assaultive behavior among chronic inpatients. *Am. J. Psychiatry, 139*:212–215.

Tausk, O. (1919). On the origin of the "influencing machine" in schizophrenia. *Psychoanal. Q., 2*:519–556.

Tienari, P., Sorri, A., Lahti, I., Naarla, M., Wahlberg, E., Moring, J., Pohjola, J., & Wynne, L. (1987). Genetic and psychosocial factors in schizophrenia: The Finnish adoptive family study. *Schizophr. Bull., 13*:477–484.

Tienari, P., Sorri, A., Lahti, I., Naarla, M., Wahlberg, E., Ronkko, T., Pohjola, J., & Moring, J. (1985). The Finnish adoptive family study of schizophrenia. *Yale J. Biol. Med., 58*:227–237.

Torrey, E. F. (1988). *Surviving Schizophrenia: A Family Manual*. New York: Harper & Row.

——— (1992). Are we overestimating the genetic contribution to schizophrenia? *Schizophr. Bull., 18*:159–170.

Torrey, E. F., & Peterson, M. (1974). Schizophrenia and the limbic system. *Lancet, 2*:942–946.

Tsuang, M., Gilbertson, M., & Faraone, S. (1991). The genetics of schizophrenia: Current knowledge and future directions. *Schizophr. Res., 4*:157–171.

Tsuang, M., Woolson, R., & Fleming, J. (1979). Long-term outcome of major psychoses: I. Schizophrenia and affective disorders compared with psychiatrically symptom-free surgical conditions. *Arch. Gen. Psychiatry, 36*:1295–1301.

Van Praag, H. (1992). Introduction. In J-P. Lindenmayer & S. Kay (Eds.), *New Biological Vistas in Schizophrenia: Clinical and Experimental Psychiatry Monograph 6.* New York: Brunner/Mazel, pp. xi–xiii.

Vital-Durand, F. (1975). Toward a definition of neural plasticity: theoretical and practical limitations. In F. Vital-Durand & M. Jeannerod (Eds.), *Aspects of Neural Plasticity.* Paris: Editions INSERM, pp. 251–260.

Venables, P. (1987). Cognitive and attentional disorders in the development of schizophrenia. In H. Hafner, W. Gattaz, & W. Janzarik (Eds.). *Search for the Causes of Schizophrenia.* Berlin: Springer-Verlag, pp. 203–213.

Walker, E., & Lewine, R. (1990). Prediction of adult-onset schizophrenia from childhood home movies of the patient. *Am. J. Psychiatry, 147*:1052–1056.

Wallerstein, R. (1986). *42 Lives in Treatment: A Study of Psychoanalysis and Psychotherapy.* New York: Guilford Press.

Weiger, W., & Bear, D. (1988). An approach to the neurology of aggression. *J. Psychiatr. Res., 22*:86–98.

Weinberger, D. (1988). Schizophrenia and the frontal lobes. *Trends Neurosci., 11*:367–370.

Weinberger, D., & Berman, K. (1988). Speculation on the meaning of metabolic "hypofrontality" in schizophrenia. *Schizophr. Bull., 14*:157–168.

Weinberger, D., Berman, K., Suddath, R., & Torrey, E. (1992). Evidence of dysfunction of a prefrontal-limbic network in schizophrenia: A magnetic resonance imagery and regional cerebral blood flow study of discordant monozygotic twins. *Am. J. Psychiatry, 149*:890–897.

Weiner, H. (1970). The mind–body unity in the light of recent physiological evidence. *Psychother. Psychosom., 18*:117–122.

—— (1972). Some comments on the transduction of experience by the brain: Implications for our understanding of the relationship of mind to body. *Psychosom. Med.,* 34:355–375.

Weiss, P. (1959). Animal behavior as system reaction: Orientation toward light and gravity in the resting postures of butterflies (*Vanessa*). *General Systems: Yearbook of the Society for General Systems Research, 4*:1–44.

—— (1969). The living system: Determinism stratified. In A. Koestler & J. Smythies (Eds.), *Beyond Reductionism.* New York: Macmillan, pp. 3–55.

—— (1977). The system of nature and the nature of systems: Empirical wholism and practical reductionism harmonized. In K. Schaefer, H. Hensel, & R. Brady (Eds.), *Toward a Man-Centered Medical Science.* Mt. Kisco, NY: Futura, pp. 17–64.

Wender, P., Rosenthal, D., Rainer, J., Greenhill, L., Sarlin, M. B. (1977). Schizophrenic's adopting parents: Psychiatric status. *Arch. Gen. Psychiatry, 34*:777–784.

Werner, H. (1940). *Comparative Psychology of Mental Development.* New York: International Universities Press.

Wexler, M. (1971). Schizophrenia: Conflict and deficiency. *Psychoanal. Q., 40*:83–99.

—— (1975). The evolution of a deficiency view of schizophrenia. In J. Gunderson & L. Mosher (Eds.), *Psychotherapy of Schizophrenia.* New York: Aronson, pp. 161–174.

Whitaker, C., & Malone, T. (1953). *The Roots of Psychotherapy.* New York: Blakiston.

Will, O. (1973). Changing styles in the treatment of schizophrenia. *Am. J. Psychiatry,* *130*:153–155.

Willick, M. (1990). Psychoanalytic concepts of the etiology of severe mental illness. *J. Am. Psychoanal. Assoc., 38*:1049–1081.

Winnicott, D. W. (1947). Hate in the countertransference. In *Collected Papers: Through Paediatrics to Psychoanalysis*. London: Tavistock, 1958, pp. 194–203.

—— (1951). Transitional objects and transitional phenomena. In *Collected Papers: Through Paediatrics to Psychoanalysis*. London: Tavistock, 1958, pp. 229–252.

—— (1960a). Ego distortion in terms of true and false self. In *The Maturational Processes and the Facilitating Environment*. New York: International Universities Press, 1965, pp. 140–152.

—— (1960b). Counter-transference. In *The Maturational Processes and the Facilitating Environment*. New York: International Universities Press, 1965, pp. 158–165.

—— (1960c). The theory of the parent–infant relationship. *Int. J. Psychoanal., 41*:585–595.

—— (1971). *Therapeutic Consultations in Child Psychiatry*. London: Hogarth Press.

Wynne, L., Ryckoff, I., Day, J., & Hirsch, S. (1958). Pseudo-mutuality in the family relations of schizophrenics. *Psychiatry, 21*:205–220.

Wynne, L., & Singer, M. (1963). Thought disorder and family relations of schizophrenics: I. A research strategy. II. A classification of forms of thinking. *Arch. Gen. Psychiatry, 9*:191–206.

Zipursky, R., Lim, K., Sullivan, E., Brown, R., & Pfefferbaum, A. (1992). Widespread cerebral gray matter volume deficits in schizophrenia. *Arch. Gen. Psychiatry, 49*:195–205.

Zubin, J., & Spring, B. (1977). Vulnerability: A new view of schizophrenia. *J. Abnorm. Psychol., 86*:103–126.

Name Index

Subject Index

499